PROGRESS IN BRAIN RESEARCH

VOLUME 37

BASIC ASPECTS OF CENTRAL VESTIBULAR MECHANISMS

PROGRESS IN BRAIN RESEARCH

PROGRESS IN BRAIN RESEARCH

VOLUME 37

BASIC ASPECTS OF
CENTRAL VESTIBULAR MECHANISMS

PROCEEDINGS OF A SYMPOSIUM HELD IN PISA
ON 15th—17th OF JULY 1971 AS PART OF THE
XXV INTERNATIONAL CONGRESS OF
PHYSIOLOGICAL SCIENCES

EDITED BY

A. BRODAL

Anatomical Institute, University of Oslo, Oslo, Norway

AND

O. POMPEIANO

Institute of Physiology II, University of Pisa, Pisa, Italy

ELSEVIER PUBLISHING COMPANY

AMSTERDAM / LONDON / NEW YORK

1972

ELSEVIER PUBLISHING COMPANY
335 JAN VAN GALENSTRAAT,
P.O. BOX 211, AMSTERDAM, THE NETHERLANDS

AMERICAN ELSEVIER PUBLISHING COMPANY, INC.
52 VANDERBILT AVENUE, NEW YORK, N.Y. 10017

Science

LIBRARY OF CONGRESS CARD NUMBER 77-190680

ISBN 0-444-41048-1

WITH 229 ILLUSTRATIONS AND 8 TABLES

PRINTED IN THE NETHERLANDS

List of Contributors

P. BACH-Y-RITA, Smith-Kettlewell Institute of Visual Sciences, University of the Pacific, Graduate School of Medical Sciences, San Francisco, Calif. (U.S.A.).

A. BRODAL, Anatomical Institute, University of Oslo, Oslo (Norway).

B. COHEN, Department of Neurology, Mount Sinai School of Medicine, New York, N.Y. (U.S.A.).

N. CORVAJA, Institute of Physiology II, University of Pisa, Pisa (Italy).

I. S. CURTHOYS, Department of Neurology, School of Medicine, University of California, Los Angeles, Calif. (U.S.A.).

J. DICHGANS, Department of Neurology and Section of Neurophysiology, University of Freiburg, Freiburg i.Br. (G.F.R.).

L. P. FELPEL, The Rockefeller University, New York, N.Y. (U.S.A.).

S. GRILLNER, Department of Physiology, University of Göteborg, Göteborg (Sweden).

I. GROFOVÁ, Anatomical Institute, University of Oslo, Oslo (Norway).

O.-J. GRÜSSER, Institute of Physiology, Free University of Berlin, Berlin (G.F.R.).

U. GRÜSSER-CORNHELS, Institute of Physiology, Free University of Berlin, Berlin (G.F.R.).

S. M. HIGHSTEIN, Department of Physiology, Faculty of Medicine, University of Tokyo, Hongo, Bunkyo-ku, Tokyo (Japan).

D. E. HILLMAN, Division of Neurobiology, Department of Physiology and Biophysics, University of Iowa, Iowa City, Iowa (U.S.A.).

T. HONGO, Department of Physiology, Tokyo Medical and Dental University, Yushima, Bunkyo-ku, Tokyo (Japan).

M. ITO, Department of Physiology, Faculty of Medicine, University of Tokyo, Hongo, Bunkyo-ku, Tokyo (Japan).

S. IURATO, Departments of Bioacoustics and of Histology and Embryology, University of Bari, Bari (Italy).

H. H. KORNHUBER, Department of Neurology and Section of Neurophysiology, University of Ulm, Ulm/Donau (G.F.R.).

R. LLINÁS, Division of Neurobiology, Department of Physiology and Biophysics, University of Iowa, Iowa City, Iowa (U.S.A.).

O. LOWENSTEIN, Department of Zoology and Comparative Physiology, University of Birmingham, Birmingham (Great Britain).

L. LUCIANO, Laboratory of Electron Microscopy, Department of Anatomy, University of Hannover, Hannover (G.F.R.).

C. H. MARKHAM, Department of Neurology, School of Medicine, University of California, Los Angeles, Calif. (U.S.A.).

W. R. MEHLER, Experimental Pathology Branch, NASA, Ames Research Center, Moffett Field, Calif. (U.S.A.).

G. MELVILL JONES, Canadian Defence Research Board, Aviation Medical Research Unit, Department of Physiology, McGill University, Montreal, Quebec (Canada).

C. M. OMAN, Man-Vehicle Laboratory, Department of Aeronautics and Astronautics, Massachusetts Institute of Technology, Cambridge, Mass. (U.S.A.).

E. PANNESE, Institute of Human Anatomy II, University of Milan, Milan (Italy).

B. W. PETERSON, The Rockefeller University, New York, N.Y. (U.S.A.).

O. POMPEIANO, Institute of Physiology II, University of Pisa, Pisa (Italy).

W. PRECHT, Max-Planck-Institute for Brain Research, Frankfurt a.M. (G.F.R.).

E. REALE, Laboratory of Electron Microscopy, Department of Anatomy, University of Hannover, Hannover (G.F.R.).

C. L. SCHMIDT, Department of Neurology and Section of Neurophysiology, University of Freiburg, Freiburg i.Br. (G.F.R.).

H. SHIMAZU, Department of Neurophysiology, Institute of Brain Research, School of Medicine, University of Tokyo, Hongo, Bunkyo-ku, Tokyo (Japan).

J.-I. SUZUKI, Department of Otolaryngology, Teikyo University School of Medicine, Tokyo (Japan).

E. TARLOV, Neurosurgical Service, Massachusetts General Hospital, Boston, Mass. (U.S.A.).

T. UEMURA, Department of Neurology, Mount Sinai School of Medicine, New York, N.Y. (U.S.A.).

I. H. WAGMAN, Department of Animal Physiology, University of California, Davis, California (U.S.A.).

F. WALBERG, Anatomical Institute, University of Oslo, Oslo (Norway).

J. WERSÄLL, Department of Otolaryngology and King Gustaf Vth Research Institute, Karolinska Sjukhuset, Stockholm (Sweden).

V. J. WILSON, The Rockefeller University, New York, N.Y. (U.S.A.).

E. R. WIST, Department of Neurology and Section of Neurophysiology, University of Freiburg, Freiburg i.Br. (G.F.R.).

L. R. YOUNG, Man-Vehicle Laboratory, Department of Aeronautics and Astronautics, Massachusetts Institute of Technology, Cambridge, Mass. (U.S.A.).

Preface

In the last 10 years vestibular mechanisms have been dealt with in several symposia. In view of the marked expansion in the field of vestibular research in recent years we felt that it might be timely to arrange another symposium, in conjunction with the XXV International Congress of Physiological Sciences. It was clear that even restricting our scope to the area of "Basic Aspects of Central Vestibular Mechanisms" this subject could not be treated exhaustively. Nevertheless, we believe that the most important points have been covered, and that the material presented during the symposium gives a true and fairly complete picture of present knowledge of the basic aspects of central vestibular mechanisms. This volume contains the papers delivered at the symposium. It was decided not to publish the often lively discussions which followed the presentation of the papers. However, participants desiring to do so could submit written accounts of essential points which they contributed during the discussions. These are included as comments in the volume.

In retrospect, it is of some interest to note that the proceedings of the Pisa Symposium will appear almost exactly 10 years after the publication of the monograph by Brodal, Pompeiano and Walberg: "The Vestibular Nuclei and their Connections, Anatomy and Functional Correlations". It has been a great satisfaction to us that this volume has apparently been useful for many workers in the field, especially perhaps for neurophysiologists looking for a condensed account of the anatomy of the vestibular nuclei. We hope that the present monograph will for some years to come serve at a complement to our book, and that it will also prove to be a valuable source of reference for people working in the field.

A comparison of the contents of our monograph from 1962 with those of the present book is a good illustration of the amazing wealth of new data which has accumulated since 1962 in the field of vestibular research. For example, at that time electron-microscopic studies had been performed only on the normal structure of the sensory apparatus, only a few studies using microelectrode recordings had appeared, and data of the pharmacology of vestibular mechanisms were very scanty. Today the situation is totally different.

In general it may be said that on all points where progress has been made, the situation has turned out to be far more complex than one imagined 10 years ago. The organization of the vestibular nuclei seems to be infinitely complex both structurally and functionally. An increasing body of data, morphological and functional, demonstrates that the vestibular nuclei are indeed composed of a number of minor units, which differ morphologically as well as functionally. It is interesting to note that even some of the small cell groups which we distinguished morphologically in 1957 are now being studied physiologically. In view of this complexity it is encouraging to see that, where carefully performed, anatomical and functional studies are generally in

VIII PREFACE

agreement. Furthermore, there appears to be a satisfactory agreement with the chemical data so far available.

In spite of the great progress made, there are still many unsolved problems. Indeed, the problems are perhaps greater than ever, because we now have to deal with ever more basic features in the organization. For example, in the field of morphology more precise information is needed especially as concerns synaptic relations, and we must know more about possible interconnections between the vestibular nuclear units. In the functional field, there is a great demand for studies of the cooperation between units on the cellular and nuclear level, of correlations of the multiple effects of stimulation, preferably natural, and of the concerted actions of impulses from different sources which impinge upon a cell or nucleus. The manyfold relations, morphological and functional, between the vestibular nuclei and other parts of the nervous system, in addition to the spinal cord and the oculomotor nuclei, for example their influence on sensory mechanisms, deserve increased attention. It is too optimistic to expect that research in the next 10 years should increase our understanding of the role of the vestibular mechanisms in the activity of the entire nervous system?

The meetings of the Symposium were held in the Scuola Normale Superiore in Pisa. We are most grateful to Professor G. Bernardini and Professor L. A. Radicati, Rector and Dean, of this center of European culture, for having permitted us to enjoy the lovely atmosphere of their historical building at the Piazza dei Cavelieri. We also thank Professor A. Faedo, Rector of the University of Pisa, for his valuable assistance in the organization of the Symposium.

The Italian National Research Council and the International Brain Research Organization kindly agreed to sponsor the Symposium. This, as well as the financial support of the Italian National Research Council and of the firms Carlo Erba, Farmitalia, Montedison and Roche, are gratefully acknowledged. Last but not least, let us thank the assistants, secretaries and technicians of the Institute of Physiology in Pisa for their efficient cooperation in preparing the Symposium.

Pisa, July 1971   A. Brodal and O. Pompeiano

Contents

CONTENTS   XI

I. INTRODUCTORY REVIEWS OF SOME ASPECTS OF VESTIBULAR MECHANISMS

Morphology of the Vestibular Receptors in Mammals

J. WERSÄLL

Department of Otolaryngology and King Gustaf Vth Research Institute, Karolinska Sjukhuset, Stockholm, Sweden

The mammalian vestibular sensory epithelia have been thoroughly studied by means of light and electron microscopy since the first electron microscopic publications appeared (Wersäll, 1954, 1956; Wersäll *et al.*, 1954; Smith, 1956). The aim of the present paper is to summarize some morphological findings which seem to be of special importance for the understanding of the physiology of the vestibular sensory cells.

Sensory areas of the vestibular sense organ

The otocyst in mammals changes during the early embryonic stage from a vesicle to a system of canals and sacs. The 3 semicircular canals, the utricle and saccule each contain sensory areas; the 3 cristae ampullares of the semicircular canal, the macula utriculi and the macula sacculi are innervated by branches from the vestibular nerve.

Each *semicircular canal* widens in one end to an *ampulla*. The floor of the ampulla is crossed by a saddle-shaped crest formed by connective tissue, vessels and nerve fibres (Figs. 1, 2). The major part of the crest is covered by a highly specialized sensory epithelium containing two types of hair-bearing sensory cells, type I and type II (Wersäll, 1956) and supporting cells. Between the surface of the crista and the wall of the ampulla lies a gelatinous substance, the cupula (Fig. 2). The periphery of the sensory epithelium is surrounded by epithelial cells, the structure of which indicate secretory and reabsorbtive function (Dohlman, 1965, Kimura *et al.*, 1963). Large areas around the cristae ampullaris and in the wall of the sacs are pigmented.

The *utricle* is an elongated sac traversing the superior part of the vestibule. The anterior part of the utricle widens to a recess in which the sensory area, the *macula utriculi* is located.

The *macula utriculi* (Fig. 3) is shaped like a spade, its anterior wider part forms a sharp angle with the main part. The plane of the major part of the utricle is almost horizontal when the head is in the erect position.

The macula utriculi is composed of connective tissue, penetrated by vessels and nerves and in its anterior part resting on bone. The epithelial cover is composed of a sensory epithelium similar in structure to that of the crista ampullaris, surrounded by supporting cells and cells with a pronounced secretory or reabsorbtive function. The epithelium is covered by a gelatinous structure in which are embedded a densely

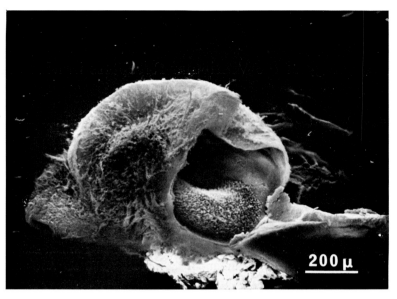

Fig. 1. Ampulla of the lateral semicircular canal from the labyrinth in guinea pig. The wall of the ampulla is opened to expose the saddle shaped crista ampullaris. Scanning electron microscopy.

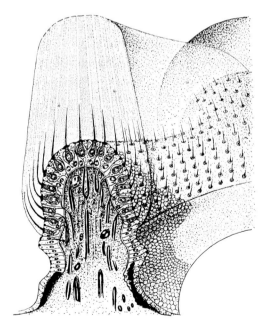

Fig. 2. Crista ampullaris covered by hair bearing sensory cells. The hairs protrude into the gelatinous cupula filling out the space between the epithelial surface and the ampullar wall. Schematic drawing.
From Wersäll (1956).

MORPHOLOGY OF THE VESTIBULAR RECEPTORS 5

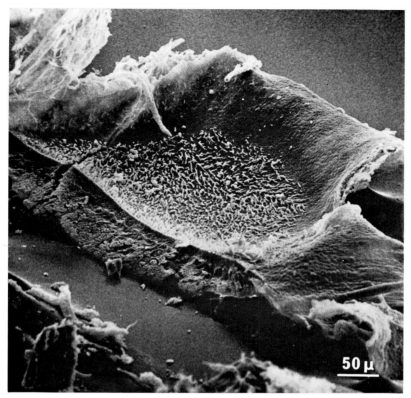

Fig. 3. Scanning electron microscopic survey showing the main horizontal part of the macula utriculi in guinea pig. A fracture goes through the macula. The statoconium membrane was taken away during preparation to show the hair bundle on the surface. From Wersäll *et al.* (1970).

packed mass of calcite crystals (Figs. 4, 5), the statoconia (Carlström and Engström, 1955). The whole structure is called the statoconium membrane.

The *saccule* is a flattened sac located in a shallow groove on the medial side of the vestibule. The sensory area of the saccule, the *macula sacculi*, is hook-shaped with one longer oval surface with its main axis directed posteriorly inferiorly and a shorter limb bent in a superior direction. The sensory epithelium of the macula sacculi is coated with a statoconium membrane.

The vestibular ganglion and nerve

The *vestibular ganglion* cells are partly separated into a superior and inferior division of the vestibular ganglion. The ganglion cells are bipolar. The cells as well as their central and peripheral axons are myelinated. The central axons form the vestibular nerve. The peripheral axons form a number of branches supplying the sensory area of the vestibular sense organ. A certain variation is found in the route of the peripheral axons in the temporal bone which reflects anatomically a variation in the size and

References pp. 16–17

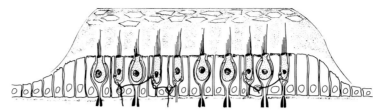

Fig. 4. Macula with type I and type II sensory cells. The sensory hairs protrude into the gelatinous substance covering the epithelial surface in which statoconia are embedded. Schematic drawing.

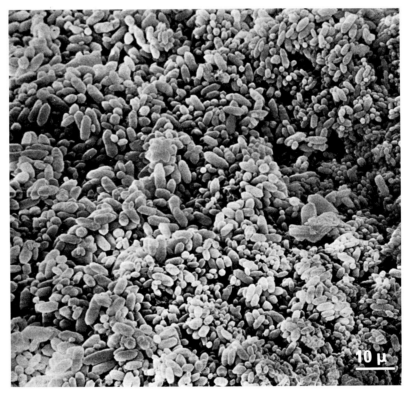

Fig. 5. The statoconia of the statoconium membrane vary considerably in size as illustrated by this scanning electron microscope picture from the guinea pig macula utriculi.

route of the branches found by the axons. A large number of studies have been made to investigate the route of these branches (for references, see Lindeman, 1969). Here only a schematic description of the route of the branches will be given.

The *superior division* of the vestibular ganglion sends peripheral branches to the anterior and lateral ampulla, to the utricle and to the superior anterior part of the saccule.

The *inferior division* supplies the main part of the saccule and the posterior ampulla.

Communicating branches have been demonstrated between the two divisions of the ganglion, between the vestibular and facial nerve and between the vestibular and cochlear nerve. The vestibulo-cochlear anastomosis carries efferent nerve fibres which derive from the superior olive and go via the vestibular nerve through the anastomosis to the cochlea.

Efferent nerve fibres in a limited number pass from nerve cells in the brain stem through the vestibular ganglion and the peripheral branches of the vestibular nerve to the vestibular sensory areas. These fibres are myelinated and of small calibre.

Unmyelinated nerve fibres are to be found in all branches of the vestibular nerve. Many of these fibres stain with the fluorescence method for demonstration of catecholamines. So far they have not been traced into the sensory epithelium.

Structure of the sensory epithelium

The sensory epithelium in all sensory areas of the mammalian vestibular sense organ contains sensory cells and supporting cells. Each sensory area is surrounded by different types of specialized cells, the structure of which indicates a secretory or a reabsorptive function. Large amounts of pigmented cells are found especially in the guinea-pig labyrinth where areas around the ampullar crista and in the utricular wall are heavily pigmented.

The sensory cells. The *sensory cells* are of two types (Figs. 6, 7) (Wersäll, 1956). The *type I sensory cell* is shaped like an amphora. The rounded lower part contains a nearly spherical nucleus. The body of the cell narrows to a thin neck which widens

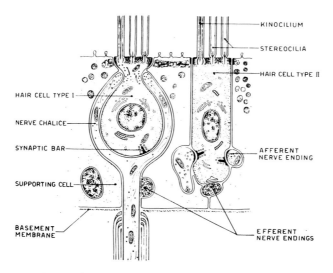

Fig. 6. The sensory cell type I is amphora-shaped and enclosed by a chalice-shaped nerve ending. Scattered synaptic rods are found in the cell in contact with the synaptic membrane. The type II cell is cylindrical in shape with rounded bottom. Several afferent and efferent nerve terminals establish synaptic contact with the cell with nerve endings or en passant synapses. A sensory hair bundle with one kinocilium and around 70 stereocilia protrudes from the cell surface. Schematic drawing.

References pp. 16–17

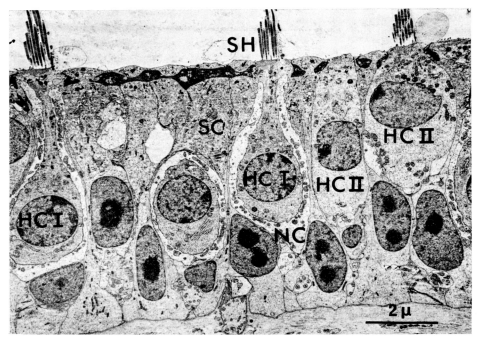

Fig. 7. The nuclei in the type II sensory cells are regularly located closer to the surface than those of the type I cells in the macula utriculi as illustrated in this transmission electron microscopical survey from the guinea pig macula utriculi. In the cristae ampullares the location of the nuclei is usually reversed.

again towards the surface of the epithelium. This part of the cell contains a cuticle from which protrudes a bundle of stereocilia. One side of the cell head lacks a cuticular plate. This part contains a centriole oriented with its triple tubular 9 rods perpendicular to the cell surface (Fig. 8). From the centriole projects a kinocilium. Below this centriole is generally found a second centriole. In some cells two centrioles might be found at the surface and two kinocilia may be found on rare occasions. The body and the neck of the sensory cell type I fits into the chalice-formed nerve endings of an innervating axon from the vestibular nerve (Wersäll, 1956, 1961; Smith, 1956; Wersäll and Flock, 1965).

The *cytoplasmic organization* of the type I sensory cell is often characterized by a high degree of regularity. Thus the neck of the cell contains large numbers of microtubules passing from the head down to the supranuclear portion of the cell body. The Golgi membranes and vesicles are found in a circular zone immediately above the nucleus and the ergastoplasm, that is the basophilic system of ribosome-covered membranes, is often well organized below the nucleus. In some cells it forms a number of communicating flat parallel spaces below the nucleus, closely resembling the Nissl substance of some nerve cells.

The *type II sensory cell* (Figs. 6, 7) differs from the type I cell in shape and innervation. It is irregularly cylindrical in shape. The base of the nucleus varies in different parts of the epithelia, especially in the maculae. The bottom of the cell is in synaptic contact with branches of afferent and efferent nerve fibres, forming nerve endings or en passant contacts with the cell (Wersäll, 1956; Engström, 1958; Engström and Wersäll, 1958; Iurato and Taidelli, 1964). The apical portion of the cell contains a cuticular plate and a pair of centrioles like the type I cell, and a sensory hair bundle with a kinocilium protrudes from the cell surface. The cytoplasm is less regular in structure and the sparse ergastoplasm forms fairly irregular tubes and sacs throughout the cell. Both types of cells contain mitochondria which are often most numerous close to the cuticular plate.

The *supporting cells* surround the sensory cells and the nerve fibres. They reach from the basement membrane to the surface. The base of the cell resting on the basement membrane of the epithelium contains a nucleus with several dense large nucleoli. In the guinea pig some dense large granules are often found in this area. The middle portion of the cell contains sparse mitochondria and the Golgi substance. The apical part contains numerous spherical granules. Close to the surface is found a ring of dense substance forming part of the so-called *reticular laminas* of the epithelium. The surface towards the endolymphatic space is covered with microvilli. Viewing the sensory epithelium from the surface with the light or scanning electron microscope, a fairly regular pattern is seen with rosettes of secretory cells; usually 6 or 7 surround each sensory cell (Lindeman, 1969).

The number of sensory cells of type I and II is not quite equal in all parts of the sensory areas. Thus the central part of the crista has a higher percentage of type I cells than the most peripheral parts (Wersäll, 1956; Spoendlin, 1965; not verified by Lindeman, 1969).

The so-called *striola* of the macula utriculi and macula sacculi is an area resembling a band that runs parallel to the bent lateral border of the macula utriculi and goes along the middle portion of the whole macula sacculi. This area was described by Werner (1940) and carefully analyzed by Lindeman (1969).

The striola contains a larger number of type I sensory cells than the rest of the macular epithelium. The statoconia are small in this region and the layer of statoconia is thinnest in the striola region of the macula utriculi and thicker than anywhere else in the saccular macula (Lindeman, 1969).

The *sensory hairs* protruding from the surface of the sensory cells are observable in the light microscope but most easily studied in the transmission and scanning electron microscope (Fig. 9). Transmission electron microscope studies of the stereocilial sensory hairs reveal the following structure. The axial core of each hair is composed of fine fibrils which condense basally and continue into the cuticle as a rootlet. This rootlet is often surrounded by a less dense channel in the cuticle and might be followed through the cuticle into the cytoplasm of the sensory cell head. The fibrillar core is surrounded by a triple layered plasma membrane which is in continuity with the plasma membrane of the sensory cell.

The *kinocilium* protrudes from the cuticle located at the sensory cell surface outside the cuticular plate (Fig. 8). Whereas the centriole in fishes is often provided with a basal foot, this is not regularly seen in mammals. Serial sections through the centriole

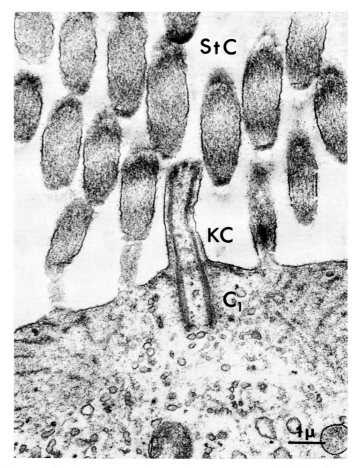

Fig. 8. An oblique section through the apical portion of a sensory cell in the crista ampullaris of a guinea pig illustrates the centriole (C_1) from which protrudes the kinocilium (KC), of which only the basal portion is seen. A number of stereocilia (StC) are visible. Transmission EMG.

of guinea pigs reveal, however, a number of densely stained protrusions which emerge from the triple tubular rods of the centriole towards the surface. The kinocilium proper is longer than the stereocilia. It is more flexible than the stereocilia and has been seen to move in isolated sensory cells suspended in saline.

In frogs, birds and fishes a regular structure is seen in the kinocilia which closely resembles that of moving cilia in the respiratory pathways (Wersäll, 1956; Flock and Duvall, 1965). This bundle is composed of 9 double barreled tubular fibres and is regularly seen surrounded by a triple layered plasma membrane. In mammals this structure is less regular. Thus the tubular structure of the 9 double fibres is less regularly observed and the central double fibre might be missing, single, or without clearly visible tubular structure (Hamilton, 1969). The sensory hair bundle in mammals is also generally more difficult to preserve in fixation than in lower animals.

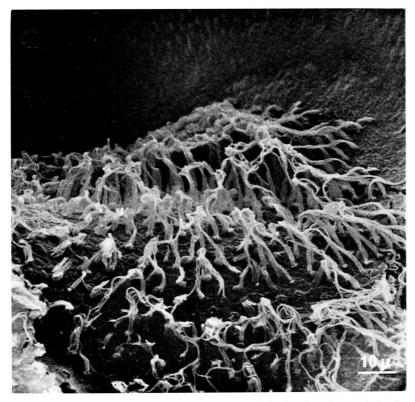

Fig. 9. The hair bundles of the crista ampullaris appear as curled tufts when the cupula has been taken away. Scanning electron microscope picture from a guinea pig crista close to the planum semilunatum. From Wersäll *et al.* (1970).

Cross sections through the sensory hair bundle immediately above the cell surface demonstrate that the hairs are arranged in an extremely regular pattern (Fig. 10). Thus the hairs are arranged in straight crossing rows forming a honeycomb pattern with 6 hairs in a regular hexagonal arrangement surrounding one central hair. The whole bundle has a hexagonal shape. Around 70 hairs are found in each bundle. Cross sections further out in the bundle demonstrate that the number of sensory hairs is rapidly reduced in sections taken further out in the bundle (Fig. 11). This shows that the hairs differ in length. This is even more clearly demonstrated in scanning electron microscope pictures where it is seen that the kinocilium is located on one side of the bundle and that the rows of stereocilia decrease successively in length from the kinocilium.

Orientation of the sensory cells. Electrophysiological studies early indicated a directional sensitivity. A morphological correlate to these physiological findings was found by Loewenstein and Wersäll (1959). They demonstrated that all sensory cells on the lateral semicircular canal crista were oriented with their kinocilia on the utricular side of the sensory hair bundles and on the canal side of the vertical canals. Thus the

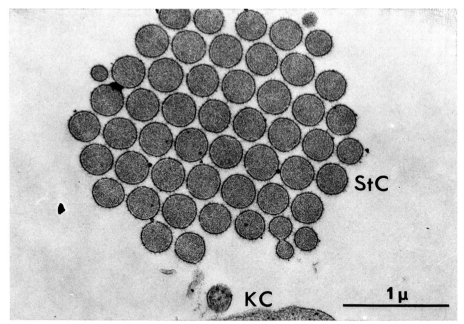

Fig. 10. The extremely regular hexagonal pattern of the stereocilia (StC) in a hair bundle from the macula utriculi of a guinea pig is clearly visible in this section cut close to the cuticle. The kinocilium (KC) is somewhat dislocated from its position in the periphery of the bundle.

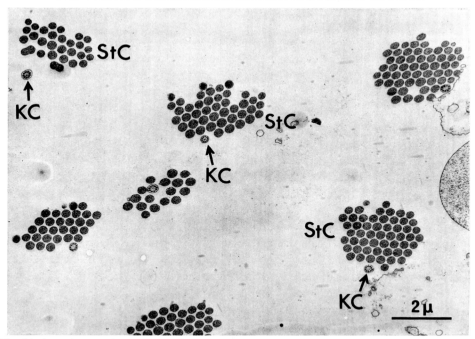

Fig. 11. A section cut through the hair bundle of a macula utriculi epithelium further out from the epithelial surface illustrates a reduced number of sensory hairs due to the varying length of the hairs which decrease in length away from the kinocilium. Although the kinocilium (KC) is located on one side of the bundles, an angular variation is seen in neighbouring bundles illustrating a certain irregularity in the orientation of the bundles.

stimulating direction of displacement of the hairs was found to be towards the kinocilium.

In a series of later work on sensory areas from all parts of the acoustico-lateralis system the orientation of the sensory cells has been shown to follow a characteristic pattern in each sensory area (Loewenstein and Wersäll, 1959; Flock and Wersäll, 1962; Flock, 1964, 1965; Loewenstein *et al.*, 1964; Spoendlin, 1964; Lindeman, 1969). In the mammalian labyrinth the direction of the sensory hair orientation diverges like a fan from a medial marginal area toward a line through the striola. On the opposite side of this imaginative line the orientation turns 180° and the cells along the posterior and lateral border are oriented towards this line. The orientation of the cells on the macula utriculi are thus characterized by an orientation towards a line through the striola. The sensory cells on the macula sacculi are oriented from a line through the striola. Thus the cells on the posterior side of this line are oriented in inferior–

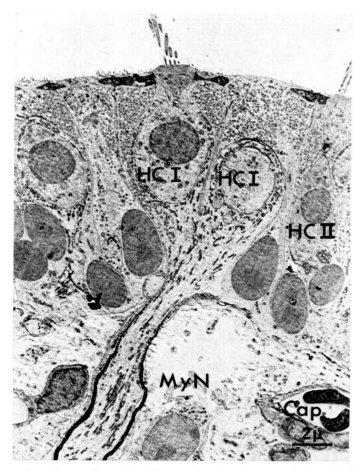

Fig. 12. The myelinated nerve fibres (MyN) innervating the crista ampullaris epithelium lose their myelin sheath when they pass through the basement membrane. HCI, Hair cell type I; HCII, Hair cell type II; Cap, capillary.

superior or posterior–superior direction whereas the cells on the inferior–anterior and superior- anterior side are oriented in inferior– or superior–anterior direction.

Nerve pattern in the epithelia. All myelinated nerve fibres in the labyrinth of mammals loose their myelin sheath when they pass through the basement membrane into the epithelium (Fig. 12). No unmyelinated fibres have so far been traced into the epithelium.

Thicker fibres innervate the centre of the crista and the striolar region of the macula than the periphery. The thicker and some medium sized fibres form nerve chalices around several type I sensory cells. Medium sized nerve fibres form nerve chalices around type I sensory cells and nerve terminals to type II sensory cells and fine nerve fibres form nerve terminals to type II cells and contact the surface of nerve chalices (Figs. 13, 14). Some of the finest fibres are efferent and branch into a large number of

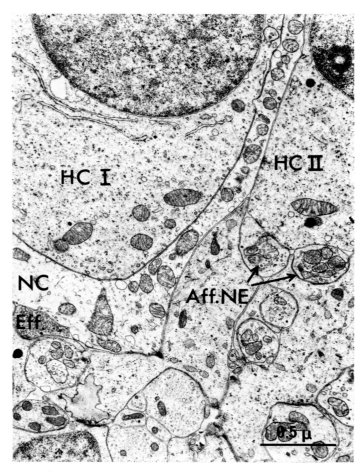

Fig. 13. A nerve chalice (NC) surrounds and encloses a hair cell type I in the guinea pig macula utriculi epithelium but is also in contact with a type II sensory cell which is also innervated by a number of thin terminal branches (Aff. NE). A vesiculated efferent ending (Eff.) lies in contact with the nerve chalice.

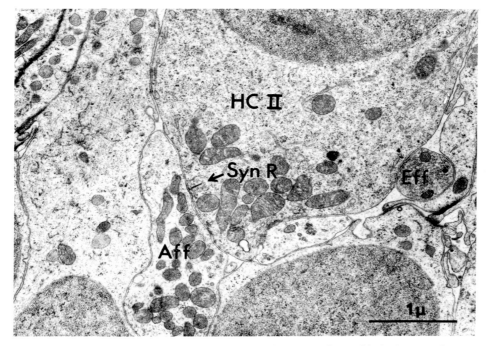

Fig. 14. Synaptic bars in contact with the synaptic membrane are observed in both types of sensory cells. This picture illustrates the bottom of a hair cell type II (HCII) with a synaptic rod (Syn R) in contact with the synaptic surface of an afferent nerve terminal. An efferent nerve terminal (Eff.) forms a synapse on the other side of the cell.

fine terminal branches which form en passant endings and terminal endings on the nerve chalices and on type II sensory cells (Wersäll, 1956; Smith, 1956; Engström, 1958; Dohlman *et al.*, 1958; Engström and Wersäll, 1958; Hilding and Wersäll, 1962; Iurato, 1964; Wersäll and Flock, 1965).

The accumulation of nerve branches of varying calibre in the basal part of the sensory epithelium makes a three-dimensional reconstruction of the distribution of the nerve fibres of varying origin and calibre extremely difficult. The description given is based partly on studies of stained nerve material and partly on studies of serial sections through relatively limited areas of the various sensory areas.

SUMMARY

The following anatomical findings observed and documented by a limited number of scientists during a 15-year period seem to be of major importance for the understanding of the function of the peripheral vestibular sensory areas: the demonstration of two different types of sensory cells; the recognition of a morphological correlate to the physiological polarization of the sensory cells; the demonstration of a double innervation of the vestibular sensory cells, and the finding of a specific organization of the striolar area in the maculae.

References pp. 16–17

It is to be hoped that anatomists and physiologists working on the central nervous system will be able to use these findings for a more elaborate study of the relationship between the peripheral end organ and the central nervous system, the function of the two sensory cell types, the afferent and efferent nerves respectively, and of the various anatomical areas in the peripheral end organs.

ACKNOWLEDGEMENT

This study was supported by the Swedish Medical Research Council, Grant No. 720-05-07.

REFERENCES

CARLSTRÖM, D. AND ENGSTRÖM, H. (1955) The ultrastructure of statoconia. *Acta oto-laryng. (Stockh.)*, **45**, 14–18.

DOHLMAN, G. F. (1965) The mechanism of secretion and absorbtion of endolymph in the vestibular apparatus. *Acta oto-laryng. (Stockh.)*, **54**, 275–288.

DOHLMAN, G. F., FARKASHIDY, J. AND SALOMON, F. (1958) Centrifugal nerve fibres to the sensory epithelium of the vestibular labyrinth. *J. Laryng.*, **72**, 984–991.

ENGSTRÖM, H. (1958) On the double innervation of the inner ear. *Acta oto-laryng. (Stockh.)*, **40**, 5–22.

ENGSTRÖM, H. AND WERSÄLL, J. (1958) The ultrastructural organization of the organ of Corti and of the vestibular sensory epithelia. *Exp. Cell Res.*, **5**, 460–492.

FLOCK, Å. (1964) Structure of the macula utriculi with special reference to directional interplay of sensory response as revealed by morphological polarization. *J. Cell Biol.*, **22**, 413–431.

FLOCK, Å. (1965) Electron microscopic and electrophysiological studies on the lateral line canal organ. *Acta oto-laryng. (Stockh.)*, Suppl. 199, 1–90.

FLOCK, Å. AND DUVALL, A. J. (1965) The ultrastructure of the kinocilium of the sensory cells in the inner ear and lateral line organs. *J. Cell Biol.*, **25**, 1–8.

FLOCK, Å. AND WERSÄLL, J. (1962) A study of the orientation of the sensory hairs of the receptor cells in the lateral line organ fish, with special reference to the function of the receptors. *J. Cell Biol.*, **15**, 19–27.

GACEK, R. R. (1960) Efferent component of the vestibular nerve. In G. L. RASMUSSEN AND W. F. WINDLE (Eds.), *Neural Mechanisms of the Auditory and Vestibular Systems*. Thomas, Springfield, Ill., pp. 276–284.

GACEK, R. R. (1966) The vestibular afferent pathway. In R. J. WOLFSON (Ed.), *The Vestibular System and its Diseases*. Union Pennsylvania Press, Philadelphia, pp. 99–116.

HAMILTON, D. W. (1969) The cilium on mammalian vestibular hair cells. *Anat. Rec.*, **164**, 253–258.

HILDING, D. AND WERSÄLL, J. (1962) Cholinesterase and its relation to the nerve endings of the inner ear. *Acta oto-laryng. (Stockh.)*, **55**, 205–217.

IRELAND, P. E. AND FARKASHIDY, J. (1961) Studies on the efferent innervation of the vestibular end organs. *Ann. Otol. (St. Louis)*, **70**, 490–503.

IURATO, S. AND TAIDELLI, S. (1964) Relationships and structure of the so-called 'much granulated nerve endings' in the crista ampullaris (as studied by means of serial sections). *Electron Microscopy. Proc. Third Europ. Reg. Conf., Prague.* Publishing House of the Czechoslovak Academy of Science, Prague, *Vol. D*, pp. 325–326.

KIMURA, R., LUNDQUIST, P.-G. AND WERSÄLL, J. (1963) Secretory epithelial linings in the ampullae of the guinea pig labyrinth. *Acta oto-laryng. (Stockh.)*, **57**, 517–530.

LINDEMAN, H. H. (1969) Studies on the morphology of the sensory regions of the vestibular apparatus. *Ergebn. Anat. Entwickl.-Gesch.*, **42**, 1–113.

LOEWENSTEIN, O., OSBORNE, M. P. AND WERSÄLL, J. (1964) Structure and innervation of the sensory epithelia of the labyrinth in the thornback ray (Raja Clavata). *Proc. roy. Soc. B*, **160**, 1–12.

LOEWENSTEIN, O. AND WERSÄLL, J. (1959) A functional interpretation of the electron microscopic structure of the sensory hairs in the cristae of the elasmobranch Raja Clavata in terms of directional sensitivity. *Nature (Lond.)*, **184**, 1807.

RASMUSSEN, G. L. AND GACEK, R. (1958) Concerning the question of an efferent fiber component of the vestibular nerve of the cat. *Anat. Rec.*, **130**, 361–362.

SMITH, C. A. (1956) Microscopic structure of the utricle. *Ann. Otol. (St. Louis)*, **65**, 450–469.

SPOENDLIN, H. H. (1964) Organization of the sensory hairs in the gravity receptors in utricle and saccule of the squirrel monkey. *Z. Zellforsch.*, **62**, 701–716.

WERNER, C. F. (1940) *Der Labyrinth.* Thieme, Leipzig.

WERSÄLL, J. (1954) The minute structure of the crista ampullaris in the guinea pig as revealed by the electron microscope. *Acta oto-laryng. (Stockh.)*, **44**, 359–369.

WERSÄLL, J. (1956) Studies on the structure and innervation of the sensory epithelium of the cristae ampullaris in the guinea pig. A light and electron microscopic investigation. *Acta oto-laryng. (Stockh.)*, Suppl. 126, 1–85.

WERSÄLL, J., (1961) Vestibular sensory cell in fish and mammals. *Acta oto-laryng. (Stockh.)*, Suppl. 163, 25–29.

WERSÄLL, J., ENGSTRÖM, H. AND HJORTH, S. (1954) Fine structure of the guinea pig macula utriculi. *Acta oto-laryng. (Stockh.)*, Suppl. 226, 298–303.

WERSÄLL, J. AND FLOCK, Å. (1965) Functional anatomy of the vestibular and lateral line organs. In W. D. NEFF (Ed.), *Contribution to Sensory Physiology.* Academic Press, New York, pp. 39–61.

WERSÄLL, J., FLOCK, Å. AND LUNDQUIST, P.-G. (1966) Structural basis for directional sensitivity in cochlear and vestibular sensory receptors. *Cold Spr. Harb. Symp. quant. Biol.*, **30**, 115–145.

WERSÄLL, J., FLOCK, Å. AND LUNDQUIST, P.-G. (1970) The vestibular sensory areas and the organ of Corti. A scanning electron microscopic study. *Z. Hörgeräteakustik*, **9**, 56–63.

Physiology of the Vestibular Receptors

O. LOWENSTEIN

Department of Zoology and Comparative Physiology, University of Birmingham, Birmingham, Great Britain

Roughly 150 years ago the vestibular organ emerged from the obscurity of its assumed rôle as antechamber to the auditory organ with a possible but ill-defined auditory function into the limelight of recognition of its governorship in the field of control of posture and movement. The names of Flourens and Ewald, Mach, Breuer, Parker, Magnus and de Kleijn are associated with the first pioneering phase in the exploration of the function of the 'non-acoustic' part of the vertebrate labyrinth (for references see Lowenstein, 1936). Their endeavours spanning the second half of the 19th and the first quarter of the 20th century have laid the classical foundation of labyrinth physiology.

With the advent between the two great wars of the oscillographic technique many of the fundamental functional assumptions made chiefly on the basis of the study of the effects of the elimination of the labyrinth as a whole or in part found their final experimental verification or refutation by means especially of single-unit electrophysiological recordings from the endorgan itself and from the vestibular nuclei of the CNS. Theoretical considerations concerning the parameters of the mode of functioning of the semicircular canals on the one hand and the otolith organs on the other were checked, and this led to the direct experimental consideration of quantitative formulations that had previously been inferred from a series of sophisticated otological test procedures such as nystagmography. Insights were gained into the relationship between the continuous electric activity of the various vestibular sense endings and vestibular tonus as well as into the way in which this sensory activity is modulated by mechanical stimulation to provide information to the central nervous system about both the degree and the direction of the displacement of the head in space. The fundamental bidirectionality of semicircular canals and the multi-directionality of the responsiveness of single otolith organs were in this way established and a number of earlier misconceptions concerning the extent of the receptive fields of these endorgans were removed (for references see Lowenstein, 1950).

A new phase of advance was opened up by the electron microscope after the second world war. At last it became possible to collate the electrophysiological picture of the response behaviour of single functional units in semicircular canals and otolith organs with the characteristics of the morphological mechano-receptive unit, the hair cell of the sensory epithelia found in the cristae and maculae of the labyrinth. The topographic arrangement of the distal hair processes with one kinocilium flanked by a population of stereocilia has given substance to the previous physiological findings on the basis of the assumption that mechanical displacement of the hair bundle towards the kinocilium is excitatory and away from it inhibitory. Two-way modulation was found to conform in the case of the canal cristae with the electrophysiological effects of ampullopetal and ampullofugal endolymph displacement during angular acceleration in the plane of the canals. The fact that the hair cells in the cristae were found to be uniformly oriented with the kinocilium pointing towards the interior of the ampulla in the horizontal canal and towards the canal (away from the interior of the ampulla) in the two vertical canals supports the hypothesis that hair cell polarization is responsible for the fact that functional units in the horizontal canal respond with an increase in discharge activity to ampullopetal and with a decrease to ampullofugal endolymph displacement caused by ipsi- and contralateral angular acceleration respectively, and that the response picture in the vertical canals is the diametrically opposite one.

The pleuridirectionality of responsiveness of the maculae of otolith organs is similarly based on the complexity of the directional mapping of the polarized hair cells on the maculae (Lowenstein et al., 1964; Spoendlin, 1965).

It has recently been possible to show how the various sense endings have evolved during the evolution of the vertebrates from an early state still extant in the cyclostome fishes such as Myxine and Lampetra, and also to show how the early embryological development mirrors this sequence of phylogenetic change (Lowenstein et al., 1968).

The arrangement of the polarized hair cells into directional arrays is apparently as old as the labyrinth, whose first origins are of course shrouded in the same mist of uncertainty as the origin of the vertebrates themselves.

After the end of the second world war the science of systems analysis or cybernetics entered the field of biological research, and what better subject could be found for this type of functional analysis than the vestibular system itself and its interaction with the kinesthetic and myotatic mechanisms as well as with vision, responsible for the control of posture and movement. Moreover as Man's activities have now become intricately interlaced with his extrasomatic means of locomotion, the problems of his rôle in vehicle control on land, sea and in the air raise the question of the behaviour of the vestibular sensors and the information transfer from them to the various effector organs involved in postural and movement control under these circumstances. Systems analysis operates with transfer functions, and their interactions in feedback loops invite extensive model making. Models of vestibular function are at present being developed in a number of research centres and some of them have seen the light of day in theses and reports. They all have in common the incorporation of 'black boxes' representing the vestibular sensors. Laplace transforms characteristic for semicircular canal sensors and otolith organs figure within the frame of such black boxes and the question of the physiological basis for the quantification expressed in these transforms is of the highest importance (Young, 1969).

The experimental elucidation of these physiological problems is therefore at present one of the outstanding tasks of vestibular physiology.

Often the contents of one or the other of these black boxes are the results of experiments on human subjects, the most objective indicator phenomena being records of eye elevation, eye counterrolling, or nystagmus. The reflex responses of the extrinsic eye muscles are themselves of course the final output from a 'closed loop' feedback system and the contents of the black box are therefore not necessarily primary data representing the pure transfer activity of the sensor, especially as the receptor process in the sensor — while it resides in the closed loop situation — is most likely adulterated by efferent 'setting' mechanisms converging onto the sensor units by way of efferent nerve terminations closely adjoining to and interacting with the afferent synapses.

Two problems, as I see it, are at present of paramount importance in the intimate functional analysis of our system. The first is a rigorous quantitative re-examination of the behaviour of canal and otolithic sensors in the open-loop situation, *i.e.*, based on recordings gained from different nerve pathways free from interference by efferent setting mechanisms. The second involves an ultrastructural and cytochemical investigation into synaptic transmission from and to the hair cell.

It may be remembered that the original electrophysiological work on the vertebrate labyrinth was in fact carried out on the isolated labyrinth of elasmobranch fishes and of the frog (Lowenstein and Sand, 1936, 1940a, 1940b; Ross, 1936; Ledoux, 1949; Lowenstein and Roberts, 1949, 1950). The results gained with this type of experimental approach form the basis of most of our fundamental conceptions on at least the qualitative mode of function of the sensors in the canal cristae and the maculae. All this is already history. On the quantitative side the experiments on the horizontal semicircular canals of the dogfish and frog furnished data supporting the concept of the cupula–endolymph system as an overdamped torsion pendulum and consequently of the canal as an inertial angular accelerometer whose behaviour in terms of its responses both to sinusoidal and to stepwise stimulation satisfies a differential equation such as

$$\xi'' + \frac{\pi}{\theta} \xi' + \frac{\Delta}{\theta} \xi = 0$$

where π = moment of friction, θ moment of inertia, Δ = cupula restoring couple, and ξ'', ξ', ξ the angular acceleration, velocity and displacement of the cupula–endolymph system relative to the skull. In the elasmobranch experiments π/θ averaged 35, but in closed-loop experiments on human subjects π/θ approximates 10, with Δ/θ near unity (Groen *et al.*, 1952).

We are, however, confronted with the disquieting fact that the mechanical analysis based on dimensional measurements and assessments of endolymph viscosities and other parameters has yielded a postulated value for π/θ a power of 10 higher, namely in the neighbourhood of 200. Various attempts have been made to explain this discrepancy away, and, on the whole, greater credence is given to the values based on experimental findings which appear also to fit in better with the frequency–response range to be postulated on general functional considerations. Be this as it may, it bears out the necessity of looking again more closely at the behaviour of the canal receptors. There are some strange facts that need to be carefully considered before too much weight is placed on formulations derived from the mechanical model concepts. For instance it has not been sufficiently realized that the whole sequence of electrophysio-logical events that can be recorded on rotatory stimulation of a canal preparation (say on a turntable accelerated from rest, then moving at constant speed for a while and finally brought to a stop), *i.e.*, on a steep increase in the rate of discharge of a single unit followed by an exponential decay during constant-speed rotation and finally by inhibition below level of resting discharge with an ultimate exponential return to resting level, can be mimicked by application to the stationary preparation of a D.C. polarizing current routed through the dendrite of the first order neurone. The effect on the discharge activity of the unit under such circumstances is very similar even in its time course to that evoked by cupula displacement on rotatory acceleration and dece-leration. A rigorous quantitative analysis of this parallelism in the endorgan response is at present being carried out in my laboratory. If we assume then for the sake of argument that the two types of stimulation do in fact produce similar time relation-ships, the question arises whether the model based on the assumed mechanical properties of the cupula describes both the necessary and sufficient basis of the func-tion of the system. It must not be overlooked that the gross pendular cupula move-ments described by Steinhausen (1931) and Dohlman (1935) are only indirectly rele-vant to the stimulatory process which is, in effect, supposed to be confined to impart-ing a shearing deformation to the base of the hair bundle of the sensory cell of a magnitude that has been estimated in the case of the hair cells of the cochlea to be at threshold of the order of magnitude of the diameter of the hydrogen atom.

There is yet another circumstance that has recently begun to worry me in the course of my work on the cyclostome labyrinth. Here, especially in Myxine, we have a situa-tion where the crista with its hair cells is certainly not equipped with a cupula closing the endolymphatic space like the blade of a turbine and mechanically rigidly coupled to the endolymph in the semicircular canal. Moreover, in Myxine there just is no such thing as a semicircular canal. The ampulla, 'so-called', opens into a wide endolymph-atic space that does not deserve the name of canalis communis given it on the basis of phylogenetic homology (Lowenstein and Thornhill, 1970).

What then is the possible alternative? It might be argued that the time course of the response of the receptor unit itself may be a function of changes in the liberation and removal of the chemical transmitter system at the synapse of the base of the hair cell and the consequent events affecting the neuronal membrane. What then, one may ask, is the role of the elastic deformation of the hair processes by tangential shear? The answer could be that this may be a gating mechanism opening and closing the synap-tic gate at critical points in the elastic cycle of mechanical displacement of the cupula-endolymph system, which may envelope the basic rhythm of the transmitter release system whose time constants are of the same order of magnitude as those of the ancillary apparatus. I am quite aware that with this tentative hypothesis I have intro-duced a question which might take quite an effort to answer.

In quite a different context I have recently attempted, and not quite successfully as yet, to come to grips with a problem that has been walking with us in the hallowed corridors of vestibular orthodoxy ever since the early days of vestibular electrophysio-logy. The classical division of labour between the semicircular canals as rotary accelerometers and the otolith organs responding to linear accelerations such as gravity, centrifugal acceleration, and vibration has never been wholly satisfactory so far as the otolith organs are concerned. It is obvious that there is no reason why they should not be susceptible to angular accelerations as well. There is experimental evidence that they are, and theoretical models have been designed to show how the central nervous system may deal with such otolithic responses (Mayne, 1966). Obviously their make-up as differential-density accelerometers imposes upon them a frequency response that differs significantly from that of the semicircular canals, although the two may overlap.

The purity of the semicircular canals, whose design has been interpreted as excluding the possibility of response to linear acceleration, has recently been challenged by a number of authors both on geometrical and physiological grounds and this challenge provides us with the problem alluded to above.

Historically the first serious claim of canal susceptibility to linear acceleration dates back to the earliest days of electrophysiological experimentation. Ledoux, recording the integrated response of multifibre pick-ups from the isolated nerve branches of the surviving labyrinth of the frog, fully confirmed the fundamental response mechanism described for the semicircular canals of elasmobranchs (Ledoux, 1949). Ledoux, however, demonstrated that under his experimental conditions semicircular canals, especially the vertical ones, were quite obviously sensitive to the position of the head in space, *i.e.*, to linear gravitational acceleration. His records showed quite clearly that the frequency of the sensory discharge recorded from a certain semicircular canal differed considerably in various positions. Ledoux showed that the resting activity of, *e.g.*, an anterior vertical canal was greatest in nose-down position with a corresponding minimum in the nose-up position. In the horizontal canal the situation was less clear, *i.e.*, maximum activity was in some instances in the nose-up and in others in the nose-down position.

Obviously this could mean that in certain positions the cupula of the given canal was sagging ampullopetally in the horizontal and ampullofugally in the vertical canals. Ledoux pointed out that such displacement could be caused by a difference in density between cupula and endolymph. Such a response should develop relatively slowly after the head has come to rest in a specific position having got there by a constant-speed tilt and should show considerable adaptation in a situation of what is in fact constant gravitational acceleration. This is what Ledoux found and demonstrated.

No mention is made of this type of canal response in the earlier work on elasmobranchs by Lowenstein and Sand (1936, 1940a, 1940b). It is true that the authors observed this to happen, but in contrast to Ledoux, they did not attribute to it a true physiological significance, believing it to be due to deterioration in the elastic properties of the cupula in consequence of the interruption of the blood supply in the isolated preparation.

This is how the matter stood until the description of the continuation of per-rotatory nystagmus during constant-speed rotation of human subjects in the so-called spit position, *i.e.*, around a horizontal sagittal axis of rotation. Naturally under those conditions the subject's position in the gravitational field varies continuously through a cycle of 360°, a movement representing a strong and adequate stimulus to the oto-lith organs. It was chiefly because of the otologists' reluctance to attribute eye nystagmus to otolithic output that the suspicion arose that this per-rotatory nystag-mus might be a canal response to a change in the direction of gravitational linear acceleration. A second type of experiment in which nystagmus was observed to continue during constant-speed rotary movement was designed by Benson *et al.* (1970) in the form of a counter-rotating platform in which the subject's horizontal canals were exposed to a rotating vector of centripetal linear acceleration. Further, it was observed that under conditions of excentric rotation the nystagmic response picture showed a bias attributable to a centripetal linear acceleration depending on the rotatory velocity and the distance from the centre.

Meanwhile analytical work on the physical properties of the perilymph, endolymph and on the cupula showed, in fact, small but significant differences in density. At the same time mathematical models of fluid-filled canals were made to demonstrate that, given an unequal diameter of the system and elasticity of its walls coupled with a possi-bility of the displacement of the whole system within its containing space (in the case of the semicircular canal within the perilymphatic space) the sensory apparatus would in fact be subjected to deformation during linear acceleration (Steer, 1967).

Let us recognise that no closed-loop investigation including the possibility of synaptic interaction between canal and otolith outputs can ever be used as evidence for the receptivity of semicircular canals to linear acceleration. We must open this loop. The isolated preparation represents such an open-loop situation and its beha-viour should therefore give reliable information about the capabilities of the canal system. However, it suffers from two serious disadvantages which could be over-looked only if the result of tests with stimulation by linear acceleration were negative. If, however, the isolated preparation gave a positive response as in the case of Le-doux's findings and my own recent unpublished observations, it must be borne in mind that the result could be due to an artifact caused either by the interruption of the blood supply or by the opening into the perilymphatic space and the consequent disruption of the proper and safe suspension of the organ within that space. Ledoux (1948) rules out the latter possibility, but makes no statement about the degree of interference with vestibular circulation in the work on 'intact' frogs.

Let me now summarize and illustrate some preliminary results obtained by myself and members of my research team on the effect of gravity.

The illustrations (Figs. 1, 2) show beyond any doubt that under the circumstances, the canals, including the horizontal one, are gravity-sensitive. The resting activity of the canals is a function of the head position in space. The important new fact is that this is still the case when the experiment is carried out without opening into the perilymph space of the labyrinth capsule. The horizontal canal shows maximum rest-ing activity near nose up and side up positions provided the ampulla lies below canal level. As in the case of the frog, maxima in the opposite positions have also been observed. The maxima for the anterior vertical canal are in the near nose-down and side-down and for the posterior vertical canal in the near nose-up and side-down positions, when their ampullae lie above the canal level.

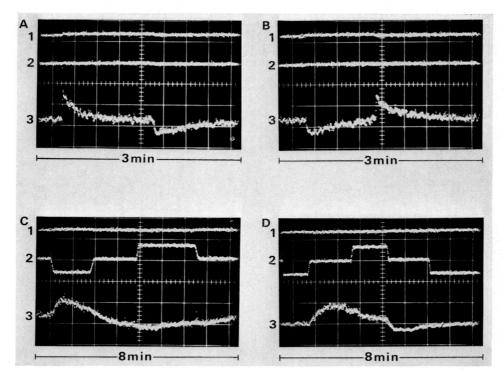

Fig. 1. Responses from an isolated preparation of the horizontal semicircular canal of a dogfish. A, Response to the onset, continuation, and cessation of ipsilateral rotation in a horizontal plane at an angular velocity of 25 rpm = 2.6 rad/sec. B, The same for contralateral rotation at the same angular velocity. Traces 1 and 2 are the output from two accelerometers in antiphase. The acceleration and deceleration happened to be near the response threshold of the accelerometer. Trace 3: The integrated response from a single unit. Upwards deflexion: excitation; downwards deflexion: inhibition. Records A and B demonstrate that the preparation showed the 'classical' response picture of a horizontal semicircular canal unit. Total time 3 min. Ordinate: Relative value of integrated voltage. C, Response of the same preparation to constant-speed tilting from normal to nose-up to upside-down to nose-down to normal and D, From side down to nose-up to side-up to nose-down to side-down, in which positions the preparation was left stationary for some time. Total time: 8 min. It will be seen that the relative integrated voltage of the discharge activity is different in different spatial positions and that the.e is a considerable 'adaptation' during rest in a certain position. These records demonstrate the sensitivity of the horizontal canal to gravitational linear acceleration. In this case maximum activity is shown in near 90° nose-up (downward deflexion of accerelometer trace 1) and minimum activity in near 90° nose-down positions (upward deflection of accelerometer trace 1), with intermediate values in side-up and side-down positions respectively. These, in turn differ from the values attained in the horizontal (normal) and upside-down positions. The accelerometer indicates nose-up position by its lowest level of output.

We still have to take the interruption of blood supply and the consequent aberration in the physical properties of the cupula into account. It is true that in a number of experiments on elasmobranchs that yielded positive results, the first readings were obtained within 15 min from the time of the killing of the animal and the isolation of the labyrinth. But this is not good enough.

We must test this situation in an animal both with unopened labyrinth capsule and

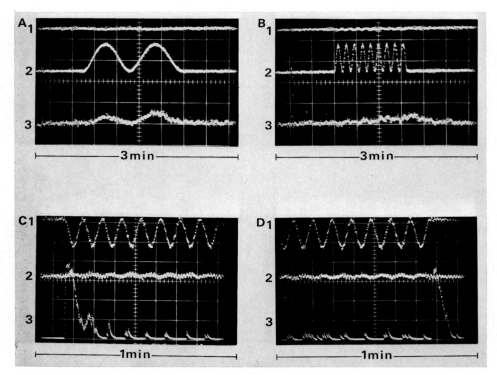

Fig. 2A, B, Same preparation as in Fig. 1. Response to continuous and constant-speed tumbling at 1.5 rpm = 0.16 rad/sec from side-down to nose-up to side-up to nose-down to side-down (A) and at 9 rpm = 0.94 rad/sec in the same direction (B). It will be seen that the gravitational response follows the positional change in A but hardly in B. Total time, 3 min. The traces 1 and 2: two accelerometers monitoring the tumble in antiphase. Upward deflexion in trace 2: 90 °nose-down; downward deflexion 90° nose-up. C, D, Response from the anterior ramus of the eighth nerve in the physiologeously intact unanaesthetized bullfrog (*Rana catesbeiana*) with implanted tungsten electrode. The response has been identified to be derived from a single unit in the crista ampullaris of the anterior vertical canal, and shows that under the physiologically normal condition with unimpaired vestibular blood circulation and uninterrupted afferent and efferent innervation the semicircular canal is position-sensitive and follows constant-speed tumbling at an angular velocity of 10 rpm = 1.05 rad/sec. It shows maximum activity near the nose-down and minimum activity near the nose-up position. The deflexions indicate the occurrence of single impulses registered by the impulse integrator from a spontaneously silent (*i.e.*, unidirectional) canal unit (Trace 3). See the typical response by excitation on ampullo-fugal mechanical impulse at the start (C) and cessation of tumbling movements (D) in opposite directions and the gravitational response during constant-speed rotation. Total time: 1 min. Traces 1 and 2: Two accelerometers monitoring the tumble in antiphase. Upward deflexion in trace 1: 90° nose-down; downward deflexion: 90° nose-up.

with intact and normal blood supply to the labyrinth, recording preferably on the dendritic side of the first-order neurone which lies in the course of the relevant branch of the eighth nerve. This cannot be done in a fish, but is perfectly possible in the frog. My research student, Saunders, has been doing this type of experiment on the bullfrog (*Rana catesbeiana*) using a tungsten electrode pick up from the eighth nerve by a method similar to that described by Gualtierotti and Bailey (1968) (Fig. 2 C, D). However, in this case, for technical reasons, the eighth nerve has not been severed and the efferent nerve supply to the vestibular endings is therefore intact. This means that the open-loop situation is not realized and *indirect* otolith-derived influences via efferent pathways cannot be ruled out.

Accepting now that a semicircular canal is sensitive to gravitational stimulation and that, therefore, its basic activity varies according to spatial position, its fundamental rôle of functioning as an angular accelerometer need not necessarily be affected except for a difference in baseline. This could be compensated for in the central analytical process by the utilization of the concomitant information derived from the otolith organs. So far so good. But what about the observations of continued fluctuations of activity of the horizontal canal during constant-speed rotations about inclined axes?

It will be recalled that the gravitational response establishes itself slowly. It could therefore be expected that rapid rotations about an inclined axis fail to register, because of the inherent time lag of the response. This is in fact the case (Fig. 2A, B).

It is therefore more than likely that the phenomena observed under closed-loop study of the eye responses of human subjects could have been of otolithic origin.

Benson and Barnes (1970) have recently developed a model capable of accounting for all the 'spit' and rotating-vector responses by an otolith stimulation of a special kind superimposed on the shearing deformation of the hair cell processes taking place in response to positional stimuli. We are still far from being able to make a final assessment of this complex situation.

To turn now to the recent findings on otolithic organs, it is undeniably true that our understanding of their mode of functioning is still sketchy and that a lot more work will be necessary before we shall be in a position to give the various 'black boxes' in the systems models their proper and reliable contents. Firstly, the functional rôle of the utriculus, sacculus and the lagena, where present, in the different taxonomic groups of vertebrates and even in different members of one and the same family has not been sufficiently well studied for a critical assessment of the values of the various generalisations made about otolith function as such. They are dual- or even multipurpose sensors whose function ranges from straightforward tonus generation and the sensing of the direction of gravitational pull in static situations to the monitoring of the velocity and degree of rotational changes of head position, *i.e.*, relatively rapid changes in the direction of gravitational acceleration, as well as to linear translational acceleration in the various planes of space, and lastly, in vertebrates lacking an organ of Corti, to vibration reception (reception of rapid phasic linear accelerations) amounting to true hearing in a number of cases. The specific type of function performed by a certain otolith organ or even in certain part of a given otolith organ depends on its exposure to or shielding from a certain type of stimulus. Basically they are best described as differential-density accelerometers, differing from the semicircular canals by the range of their frequency response among other factors. The complex task confronting the central nervous system to process the information simultaneously from semicircular canals and otolith organs is illustrated by any one of the schemata representing an attempt at modelling this complex system (Mayne, 1966; Young, 1969).

The versatility of otolith organs derives from the complexity of the directional

mapping of the hair cells within their maculae which have been analysed ultrastruc-
turally in the recent past (Flock, 1964; Lowenstein *et al.*, 1964; Spoendlin, 1965;
Lowenstein *et al.*, 1968; Lowenstein and Thornhill, 1970) among others. One and the
same macula contains hair cells not only of completely different directional response
but also differing in other response parameters such as frequency response, adaptation,
basic or 'resting' activity, permanent or transient bias, topographic and functional
relationship with the otolith bearing membrane etc.

The simple pressure or traction hypothesis as well as the simple unidirectional
shearing model (von Holst, 1950) are relegated to the lumberroom of Biology. A
complex map-representation somewhere in the central analysers, evaluated by them
with the aid of a system of filters, is the basic situation any interpretation of otolith
function has to envisage if it aims at an understanding of the total rôle of otolith-
generated information on the control of posture and movement in conjunction with
other systems of sensors, such as kinesthetic and myotatic receptors (see de Reuck and
Knight, 1967). All this deals with the analysis of the appropriate function of these
vestibular sensors in the earth's gravitational field in which they have evolved and to
which they are basically adapted.

Man is now venturing beyond this and his excursions into weightlessness or regions
of increased or diminished g have created a new situation. In this context it is eminent-
ly encouraging to note that the question of the behaviour of the otolith organs in
weightlessness is being enterprisingly tackled by Gualtierotti and collaborators with
the farsighted support of NASA and the Italian CNR.

The first launch into space of bullfrogs (*Rana catesbeiana*) with chronic electrodes
implanted into a branch of the eighth nerve of the fully physiologically functioning
animal took place from Wallops Island, Virginia in 1970, and has been fully successful from the biological and space-technological point of view. Recordings of the
behaviour of single utricular units in weightlessness and during and after centrifugal
stimulation are now available and the subject of a detailed computer analysis (Gualtierotti and Bracchi, 1971).

Here I want to mention only one most important preliminary result. It is now absolutely clear that weightlessness does not abolish the basic activity of the hair cells in
the macula. It was believed in some quarters that weightlessness might possibly
result in complete functional deafferentation of the organ. This is not the case (see
also Gualtierotti and Gerathewohl, 1965).

Finally I wish to turn to the problem of neuro-transmission from and to the
vestibular hair cell, by mentioning unpublished results obtained by Osborne and
Thornhill, also members of our vestibular team.

It is now well-known that two different kinds of synapse are found associated with
the hair cell. The afferent synapse is characterized by synaptic electron-dense synaptic
bars surrounded by a halo of synaptic vesicles, whereas the efferent synapse consists
of a bag-like membrane structure opposite the efferent (centrifugal) nerve endings
which themselves are crowded with vesicles. Work in my laboratory by these colleagues
has yielded the following provisional results. Drugs which are known to deplete
indolalkylamine and catecholamine neurotransmitter stores have been injected into

the american bullfrog to note their effects upon the synaptic bar structures in the sensory cells of the labyrinth.

The drugs are: (a) reserpine which depletes both indolalkylamine and catecholamine stores; (b) guanethidine which depletes norepinephrine stores from peripheral but not central nervous tissue; (c) chloramphetamine which produces selective depletion of indolalkylamine stores in neurones.

It has been found that reserpine and guanethidine cause a reduction in electron density of the synaptic bars, whereas chloramphetamine produces little or no such effect.

Both isolated and homogenised lamprey labyrinths when incubated *in vitro* with tritiated DOPA convert some of this DOPA to a catecholamine. Thus the enzyme DOPA-decarboxylase is present in this sense organ.

At present chromatograms are being run in order to identify the specific catecholamines in the radioactive fraction collected from these *in vitro* incubation experiments.

From our present experimental results we strongly suspect that the synaptic bars in the sensory cells are neurotransmitter storage sites which contain a catecholamine, probably norepinephrine or dopamine.

SUMMARY

A number of present-day problems in vestibular physiology are introduced and discussed in the framework of a review of recent developments in the field.

The problems concern a possible revision of our ideas on the range of functions of semicircular canals and otolith organs and their implications for systems analysis.

REFERENCES

BENSON, A. J. AND BARNES, G. R. (1970) Responses to rotating linear acceleration vectors considered in relation to a model of the otolith organs. In *Fifth Symposium on the Role of the Vestibular Organs in Space Exploration. NASA SP*, in press.

BENSON, A. J., GUEDRY, F. E. AND MELVILL JONES, G. (1970) Response of semicircular canal dependent units in vestibular nuclei to rotation of a linear acceleration vector without angular acceleration. *J. Physiol. (Lond.)*, **210**, 475–494.

DOHLMAN, G. (1935) Some practical and theoretical points in labyrinthology. *Proc. roy. Soc. Med.*, **50**, 779–790.

FLOCK, Å. (1964) Structure of the macula utriculi with special reference to directional interplay of sensory responses as revealed by morphological polarization. *J. Cell Biol.*, **22**, 413–431.

GUALTIEROTTI, T. AND BAILEY, P. (1968) A neutral buoyancy micro-electrode for prolonged recording from single nerve units. *Electroenceph. clin. Neurophysiol.*, **25**, 77–81.

GUALTIEROTTI, T. AND BRACCHI, F. (1971) Spontaneous and evoked activity of bullfrogs vestibular statoreceptors in weightlessness. Four units sampled continuously during a six-day orbital flight. *Proc. XXV int. Congr. physiol. Sci.*, Munich, IX, n. 653, 222.

GUALTIEROTTI, T. AND GERATHEWOHL, S. J. (1965) Spontaneous firing and responses to linear acceleration of single otolith units of the frog during short periods of weightlessness during parabolic flight. In *The Role of the Vestibular Organs in the Exploration of Space. NASA SP*-77, 221–229.

HOLST, E., VON (1950) Die Arbeitsweise des Statolithenapparates bei Fischen. *Z. vergl. Physiol.*, **32**, 60–120.

LEDOUX, A. (1949) Activité électrique des nerfs des canaux semicirculaires du saccule et de l'utricule chez la grenouille. *Acta oto-rhino-laryng. belg.*, **3**, 335–349.

LOWENSTEIN, O. (1936) The equilibrium function of the vertebrate labyrinth. *Biol. Rev.*, **11**, 113–145.

LOWENSTEIN, O. (1950) Labyrinth and equilibrium. *Symp. Soc. exp. Biol.*, **4**, 60–82.

LOWENSTEIN, O., OSBORNE, M. P. AND THORNHILL, R. A. (1968) The anatomy and ultrastructure of the labyrinth of the lamprey (*Lampetra fluviatilis L.*). *Proc. roy. Soc. B*, **170**, 113–134.

LOWENSTEIN, O., OSBORNE, M. P. AND WERSÄLL, J. (1964) Structure and innervation of the sensory epithelia of the labyrinth in the thornback ray (*Raja clavata*). *Proc. roy. Soc. B*, **160**, 1–12.

LOWENSTEIN, O. AND ROBERTS, T. D. M. (1949) The equilibrium function of the otolith organs of the thornback ray (*Raja clavata*). *J. Physiol. (Lond.)*, **110**, 392–415.

LOWENSTEIN, O. AND SAND, A. (1936) The activity of the horizontal semicircular canal of the dogfish, *Scyllium cauicula*. *J. exp. Biol.*, **13**, 416–428.

LOWENSTEIN, O. AND SAND, A. (1940a) The individual and integrated activity of the semicircular canals of the elasmobranch labyrinth. *J. Physiol. (Lond.)*, **99**, 89–101.

LOWENSTEIN, O. AND SAND, A. (1940b) The mechanism of the semicircular canal. A study of the responses of single-fibre preparations to angular accelerations and rotation at constant speed. *Proc. roy. Soc. B*, **129**, 256–275.

LOWENSTEIN, O. AND THORNHILL, R. A. (1970) The labyrinth of Myxine: anatomy, ultrastructure and electrophysiology. *Proc. roy. Soc. B*, **176**, 21–42.

MAYNE, R. (1966) The mechanics of the otolith organs. Reports, Manned Spacecraft Center, NASA, Houston, Tex., GERA-112, 1–30.

REUCK, A. V. S., DE AND KNIGHT, J. (1967) *Myotatic, Kinesthetic and Vestibular Mechanisms.* Churchill Ltd., London, pp. xi–331.

ROSS, D. A. (1936) Electrical studies on the frog's labyrinth. *J. Physiol. (Lond.)*, **86**, 117–146.

SPOENDLIN, H. H. (1965) Ultrastructural studies of the labyrinth in squirrel monkeys. In *The Role of the Vestibular Organs in the Exploration of Space. NASA SP*-77, 7–22.

STEER, R. W., JR. (1967) *The Influence of Angular and Linear Acceleration and Thermal Stimulation on the Human Semicircular Canal.* Sc.D. Thesis, M.I.T., pp. XIII–143.

STEINHAUSEN, W. (1931) Über den Nachweis der Bewegung der Cupula in der intakten Bogengangs-ampulle des Labyrinthes bei der natürlichen rotatorischen und calorischen Reizung. *Pflügers Arch. ges. Physiol.*, **228**, 322–328.

YOUNG, L. R. (1969) The current status of vestibular models. *Automatica*, **5**, 369–383.

Some Features in the Anatomical Organization of the Vestibular Nuclear Complex in the Cat

A. BRODAL

Anatomical Institute, University of Oslo, Oslo, Norway

The vast majority of anatomical studies of the vestibular nuclei, especially the experimental ones, have been made in the cat. In spite of certain species differences it appears that the organization of these nuclei is in principle the same in all mammals. Even the vestibular nuclear complex of man appears to be very similar to that of the cat, as can be seen from our study of the architectonics and subdivisions of the human vestibular nuclei (Sadjadpour and Brodal, 1968) and from our study of the vestibulo-spinal projection in man (Løken and Brodal, 1970). The vestibular nuclei of the cat, therefore, are well suited for a consideration of general features in the anatomical organization of this nuclear complex.

The vestibular nuclei may be considered as a mosaic of many small units, each of which has its characteristic anatomical and presumably, therefore, also functional, pattern of organization. In the following I will attempt to document this, by considering the architectonics and subdivisions of the vestibular nuclei, essential points in the organization of their afferent and efferent connections, synaptic relationships and intrinsic organization of the vestibular nuclei.

ARCHITECTURE, SUBDIVISIONS AND NOMENCLATURE OF THE VESTIBULAR NUCLEI

A close study of the cytoarchitectonics of the vestibular region (Brodal and Pompeiano, 1957) shows that in addition to the 4 classical nuclei and the interstitial nucleus of the vestibular nerve of Cajal there are several other cell groups which are topographically closely related to the main nuclei. Furthermore, within each of the latter there are cytoarchitectonically different regions. By themselves such differences tell little. It is a likely assumption, however, that regions which differ with regard to the types of cells present, their orientation, density and distribution, differ in other respects as well, morphologically as well as functionally. On every point where it has been possible to test it, this assumption has turned out to be correct.

I will mention a few data which illustrate the differences between nuclear groups with reference to Fig. 1. This shows our cytoarchitectonic map of the vestibular nuclear complex in the cat as seen in transverse Nissl stained sections. The *superior vestibular nucleus* can be rather clearly outlined as a particular unit. However, the

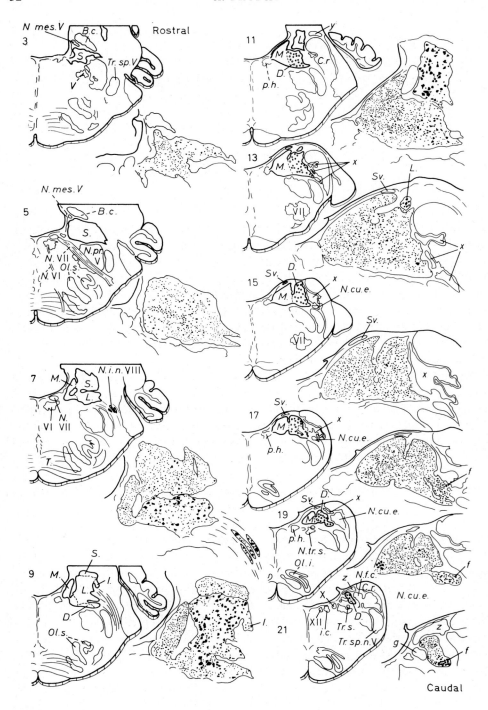

central region differs from the peripheral parts in containing relatively more large and medium sized cells than the latter (drawings 3–9 in Fig. 1). This difference goes parallel to a difference with regard to the sites of terminations of afferents within the nucleus.

Another example is found in the *lateral nucleus of Deiters* (drawings 7–13 in Fig. 1), where the rostroventral part contains chiefly fairly small cells, while the dorsocaudal part harbours most of the well known giant cells. These cellular differences suggest that the two regions are functionally dissimilar as is indeed confirmed by differences in their fibre connections. Corresponding, but less marked regional differences are present within the *medial and descending nucleus*.

Several of the small groups are well characterized and can be easily identified, for example, the *group x* and the minute *group y* (drawings 13–19 and drawing 11, respectively, in Fig. 1). A particularly clear example of a subunit within a greater nucleus is the *group f* (drawings 17–21 in Fig. 1), described first by Meessen and Olszewski (1949) in the rabbit.

The regional differences in cytoarchitecture are recognized also in Golgi sections, as can be seen from the drawing of a sagittal section through the vestibular nuclei in Fig. 2. For example, in the nucleus of Deiters the relatively few giant cells occurring in its rostroventral part have more straight, longer and less amply branching dendrites than those in the dorsocaudal part, and there are differences with regard to their orientation. Other features, visible in Nissl sections, such as the differences between the central and peripheral parts of the superior nucleus, are likewise clearly recognized in Golgi sections.

Some recent authors (Meessen and Olszewski, 1949, in the rabbit; Olszewski and Baxter, 1954, in man; Voogd, 1964, in the cat) have delineated some of the main vestibular nuclei, especially the lateral, in a somewhat different way than done by us (Brodal and Pompeiano, 1957). A subdivision of a nuclear complex on a cytoarchitectonic basis has its primary value by serving as a frame of reference for the description of other observations, morphological and functional. From this point of view any map may be as good as the other. It has been satisfactory to learn in our subse-

---

Fig. 1. A map of a series of drawings of transverse Nissl-stained sections through the vestibular nuclear complex in the cat from rostral to caudal. The inset below to the right of each drawing shows the main cytoarchitectonic features. Note differences within each of the 4 main nuclei and the many small cell groups f, g, l, Sv, x, y, z and the interstitial nucleus of the vestibular nerve (N.i.n. VIII). From Brodal and Pompeiano (1957). Abbreviations: B.c., Brachium conjunctivum (Superior cerebellar peduncle); C.r., Restiform body (Inferior cerebellar peduncle); D, Descending (inferior) vestibular nucleus; f, Cell group f in the descending vestibular nucleus; g, Group rich in glia cells, caudal to the descending vestibular nucleus; i.c., Nucleus intercalatus (Staderini); L, Lateral vestibular nucleus (of Deiters); l, Lateral group (middle-sized cells) of lateral vestibular nucleus; M, Medial vestibular nucleus; N.cu.e., External (accessory) cuneate nucleus; N.f.c., Cuneate nucleus; N.i.n. VIII, Interstitial nucleus of vestibular nerve; N.mes. V, Mesencephalic nucleus of trigeminal nerve; N. VI, VII, Cranial nerves VI and VII; Ol.i., Inferior olive; Ol.s., Superior olive; p.h., Perihypoglossal nuclei; S, Superior vestibular nucleus (of Bechterew); Sv, Supravestibular nucleus; Tr.s., Solitary tract; Tr.sp.n.V, Spinal tract of trigeminal nerve; x, y, z, Small cell groups in the vestibular nuclear complex; V, VI, VII, XII, Cranial motor nerve nuclei; X, Dorsal motor (parasympathetic) nucleus of vagus.

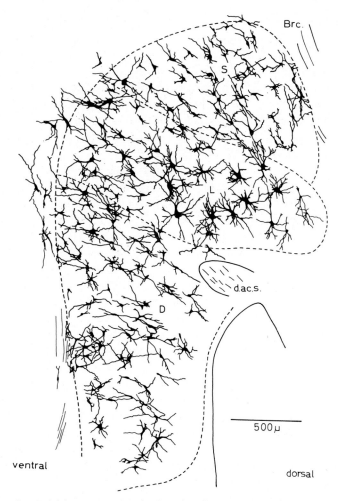

Fig. 2. Drawings of a Golgi-impregnated sagittal section through the vestibular nuclear complex in a 4-day-old kitten to illustrate the main regional differences in cell sizes and dendrite patterns. Note especially the differences in the dorsocaudal (to the right) and the ventrorostral part (to the left) in the lateral vestibular nucleus (L). From Hauglie–Hanssen (1968).

quent investigations that the subdivisions made by us (Brodal and Pompeiano, 1957) are supported by the findings made in experimental anatomical as well as physiological studies.

In our experimental studies it turned out that *within each of the main nuclei there are regions which do not receive fibres* from the labyrinth (Walberg *et al.*, 1958). In a corresponding manner, some of the small groups receive such fibres, while others do not. The restricted termination of primary vestibular fibres, suggested already by Leidler (1914), has been confirmed by other students (Stein and Carpenter, 1967; Gacek, 1969). It follows from this that the *so-called vestibular nuclei are not in their totality directly related to the vestibular apparatus.* However, for practical reasons it is deemed advisable to retain the old terminology (see Brodal *et al.*, 1962, p. 20) and to include the small nuclei, topographically closely related to the four main nuclei, in the concept 'the vestibular nuclear complex'.

The question of delimitation of cell groups by means of cytoarchitectonic criteria requires a few comments. It is well known to anybody who has looked at cell-stained preparations from the central nervous system, for example the brain stem, that some cell groups can be rather easily delimited, while in other instances the transition between cell groups occurs gradually. In the vestibular nuclear complex one meets with various situations. Against the compact fibre bundles the borders are definite, and in some cases the types of cells and their arrangement make it possible to delineate a cell group as a separate structure, such as the group f in the descending nucleus. Where there is a gradual transition the presence of smaller fibre bundles or differences in the course and density of fibres within the region may sometimes serve as guidelines. Careful examination of serial sections is almost always necessary. However, there are instances where the borders between vestibular nuclear units or between these and other regions cannot be clearly indicated.

It is in these situations that the question arises: Is it necessary to indicate borders in these instances? It must be admitted that the drawing of borders here must to some extent be arbitrary. Yet, if one is to use a map as a reference system, borders are essential for orientation. In anatomical representations, especially semidiagrammatic ones, for practical reasons borders must be shown as lines, even if they in fact represent zones of transition. For those making use of these maps, for example in electrophysiological recordings, it is essential to be aware of this. *If a recording point is found to be situated a little outside the border of a nucleus as indicated in an anatomical diagram this does not necessarily mean that there is a real discrepancy between the two sets of observations.* It may be due only to the intermingling of elements of the two neighbouring nuclei in the zone of transition.

To take an example: Nyberg–Hansen (1964), in agreement with Carpenter (1960) and Carpenter *et al.* (1960), studying isolated lesions of the vestibular nuclei in the cat, concluded that all fibres descending to the spinal cord in the medial longitudinal fasciculus are derived from the medial vestibular nucleus. By antidromic stimulation Wilson *et al.* (1967b), however, in addition to cells in the medial nucleus found some spinal projecting cells in the descending nucleus. Presumably these cells functionally belong to the medial nucleus and represent cells displaced at some distance from the majority of the medial nucleus cells. If such aberrant cells are few in number, their degenerating axons can not be recognized in anatomical studies.

In order to avoid false conclusions concerning correspondence or lack of correspondence between anatomical and physiological observations it is important to be aware of the basis on which borders shown in anatomical diagrams are drawn.

AFFERENT CONNECTIONS. PATTERNS OF DISTRIBUTION AND EVALUATION OF FINDINGS

With some exceptions studies of normal preparations, including Golgi sections, are

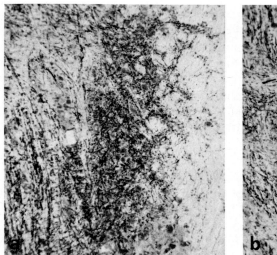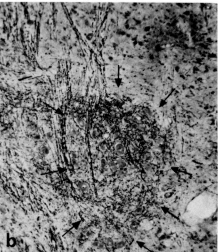

Fig. 3. Photomicrographs of horizontally cut Nauta-stained sections in a cat, killed 8 days after a lesion of one fastigial nucleus. Large numbers of degenerating fibres are seen to end in the group x (a) and the group f (b) with much less degeneration in the adjoining regions of the descending vestibular nucleus (to the left in both photos). The distribution of dense degeneration outlines the two groups as units, in agreement with their delimitation in cell stained sections ($\times$ 100). From Walberg *et al.* (1962).

of restricted value for determinations of the site and distribution within a nucleus of afferents from a particular source. Precise information requires experimental studies with tracing of the fibres which degenerate as a consequence of a lesion of a fibre bundle or its nucleus of origin. In recent years most students have employed one of the many methods for silver impregnation of degenerating axons, most commonly the Nauta (1957) method. Since the staining of normal fibres is suppressed the degenerating elements can be recognized not only by their morphological changes but also by their dark brownish-black colour against a yellow background. The areas containing large numbers of degenerating structures can be recognized even at low powers of the microscope (Figs. 3a, b, 5).

In addition to degenerating fine, unmyelinated axons these methods, and especially the recent modification of Fink and Heimer (1967), impregnate degenerating terminal boutons to a varying degree. The former belief that these methods gave information concerning synaptic relations has turned out to require qualifications. *The great advantage of the silver impregnation methods is that they permit a rather precise mapping of the areas of termination of transected fibres.* The density of degeneration in different nuclear regions may in addition provide information concerning the relative numbers of transected afferents.

By means of these methods it has been shown that *all contingents of afferents to the vestibular nuclei have their particular sites of termination within the nuclear complex.* Reference has already been made to the restricted distribution of the primary vestibular fibres. In a corresponding manner spinal afferents have their main terminal fields

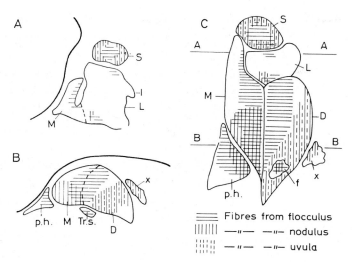

Fig. 4. A diagram of the projection of the vestibulocerebellum onto the vestibular nuclei. The sites of terminations of fibres from the flocculus, nodulus and uvula (see list of Abbreviations in Fig. 1) are shown in drawings of transverse sections (A and B) at two different levels and in the drawing of a horizontal section (C). Differences in density of terminations are not shown. Even if there is considerably more overlapping than can be shown in the diagrams, it is clear that the 'vermal' parts of the vestibulocerebellum (nodulus–uvula) have largely other sites of termination than its 'hemisphereal' part (flocculus). Even the nodulus and uvula do not have entirely similar projection areas. S, D, L, M: superior, descending, lateral and medial vestibular nucleus; l, f, x: small cell groups; p.h.: perihypoglossal nuclei. From Angaut and Brodal (1967).

in the groups x and z (Pompeiano and Brodal, 1957b; Brodal and Angaut, 1967), with a small number of fibres to certain parts of the lateral, descending and medial nucleus. The afferents descending from the interstitial nucleus of Cajal in the mesencephalon appear to end only in the medial nucleus, chiefly its dorsal and caudal parts (Pompeiano and Walberg, 1957). Within the complex cerebellovestibular projections one likewise finds several specific patterns, for example in the fastigiovestibular projection onto the nucleus of Deiters (Walberg et al., 1962). As shown in Fig. 4, even the flocculus and nodulus-uvula have largely separate projection areas within the vestibular nuclear complex (Angaut and Brodal, 1967).

If one studies the sites of ending of transected fibres in a nucleus with one of the silver impregnation methods one usually finds that the terminal areas are not sharply delimited. This is so even if all fibres belonging to a bundle, for example the vestibular nerve, have been transected (Fig. 5). There is an area of transition between the region showing maximum of degeneration and the free regions. Presumably this means that actually fewer fibres terminate in the periphery of the zone of termination. It is of some interest to consider the anatomical basis for this commonly found 'fading off' of degeneration.

The fibres of an afferent system may end in a nucleus by extensively overlapping clusters of axonal branches and collaterals which together cover a fairly large globular or ovoid space (Fig. 6a). If the fibres are interrupted this will produce a gradual

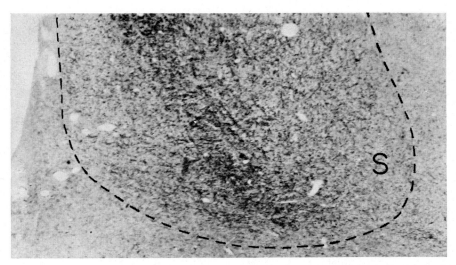

Fig. 5. Photomicrograph of a Nauta-impregnated transverse section through the superior vestibular nucleus in a cat 10 days following transection of the ipsilateral vestibular nerve. Note the central distribution of degeneration (*cf*. Fig. 1), and the somewhat diffuse borders between areas showing degeneration and areas free from degeneration. × 40. From Walberg *et al.* (1958).

decrease of the intensity of degeneration peripherally (Fig. 6b). The same may result, however, if the afferent fibres entering a nucleus diverge more or less in its periphery without overlapping (Fig. 6c), even if the picture seen in the sections through an area of degeneration will be somewhat different (see Figs. 6b, d) with small patches of degeneration outside the central area. A picture like that of the diagram in Fig. 6d can, however, only be recognized if the sections are cut in a favourable direction and when particularly searched for. The occurrence of a tapering off of degeneration in the periphery of a terminal field is, therefore, no conclusive argument that the projection studied is diffusely organized. I will return to this problem in the last section of this paper.

Even if each contingent of afferents has its particular distribution within the vestibular nuclear complex, no region is supplied by one contingent only. The precise determination of the terminal regions of the various groups of afferents may give clues of functional interest. Two or more contingents of fibres coming from different sources and ending in the same region of a nucleus must be assumed to collaborate more intimately than will be the case between fibre contingents which have separate areas of termination. For example, in the superior vestibular nucleus primary vestibular impulses are in a better position to interact with impulses from the flocculus than with those from the nodulus and uvula, since the primary vestibular and floccular fibres both end in the central parts of the nucleus, while those from the nodulus and uvula supply mainly peripheral regions (see Fig. 4). The correctness of these functional implications, made on the basis of anatomical observations, has recently been demonstrated by Ito and his collaborators (Ito *et al.*, 1970; Fukuda *et al.*, 1972). Vestibulo-ocular reflexes mediated by the superior vestibular nucleus are markedly inhibited from the flocculus,

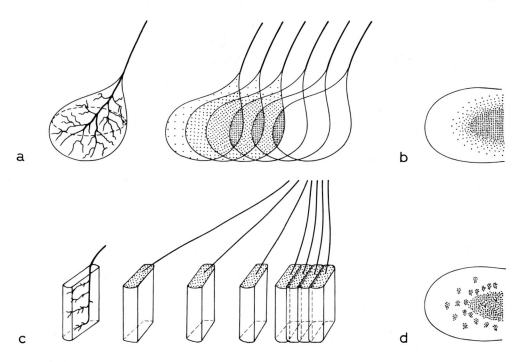

Fig. 6. Diagrams to show how interruption of a bundle of afferent fibres to a nucleus may result in an area of degeneration where the intensity of degeneration (shown by dots) decreases towards its borders. In a each axon with its branches supplies a globular or ovoid volume of tissue, and there is extensive overlapping between axonal branches and collaterals. In sections a picture as shown in b will result. A tapering off of degeneration in the periphery of an area may also result if the fibres end as shown in c. The terminal part of an axon has a straight course and gives off collaterals within a fairly circumscribed lamellar volume of tissue, with only little overlapping between neighbouring lamellae, which are arranged in a strict topographical order. If the lamellae in the peripheral part of the terminal area are farther apart, degeneration here will be less intense. In favourably oriented sections degeneration may be found in patches as shown in d, but usually such details cannot be seen. It follows that diffuse borders of an area of degeneration can not be taken as evidence that the projection in question is diffuse and does not show a topical pattern. (*cf.* Fig. 9 and text).

while no significant inhibition could be produced on stimulation of the nodulus-uvula. However, as is well known, impulses arriving in a particular fibre contingent may influence other nuclear regions than those which are the sites of termination of its fibres. The possible anatomical bases for these phenomena will be considered in a subsequent section of this paper.

EFFERENT CONNECTIONS. PATTERNS OF ORIGIN AND EVALUATION OF FINDINGS

Two approaches may be used for the study of the origin of fibres. One may make a lesion in a nucleus, preferentially stereotactically, and follow the degenerating fibres, or one may transect the efferent fibres and search the nuclei for cells which show retrograde changes. Both methods have their advantages and drawbacks.

When one *traces degenerating fibres following a lesion* in a nuclear complex like the vestibular, there is always considerable risk that fibres other than those which take origin from the destroyed nuclear region have been damaged. Fibres from extravestibular sources, for example the fastigial nucleus, pass through some of the vestibular nuclei, and fibres from one nuclear group often traverse another before leaving the complex. If a lesion is restricted to a part of a unit it is not obvious that the degenerating fibres observed are derived only from this and not from other non-damaged parts of the unit. It follows from this that if conclusions concerning the origin of fibres are to be made in studies of this kind, it is essential to know the course of all contingents of passing fibres which may be damaged. Furthermore, a close microscopical scrutiny of the lesion is essential. The lesion may not be exactly as planned (a rather common occurrence), and there may be secondary damage in the neighbourhood caused by circulatory disturbances. If these sources of error are taken into account reliable conclusions concerning the origin of efferent fibres may often be drawn. The advantage of this approach to the study of efferent connections is that it permits a detailed mapping of the sites of *termination* of efferent fibres. As examples may be mentioned the determination of the endings of the vestibulospinal fibres in the cord (Nyberg–Hansen and Mascitti, 1964) and the mapping within the oculomotor complex of the vestibular fibres ascending in the medial longitudinal fasciculus (Tarlov, 1970).

The other method, the *study of retrograde cellular changes* in a nucleus following interruption of its efferents, can only give crude information as to their sites of ending. On the other hand it usually permits a precise delineation of the areas of origin of efferent fibres. One may either utilize the *acute changes*, occurring within a few days or evaluate the *chronic changes*, the *cell loss* which ensues in the course of some weeks. The most reliable procedure is to use the acute changes. The modified Gudden method (Brodal, 1940) has turned out to be especially favourable since the acute retrograde changes are usually more clear in very young animals than in adult ones (Fig. 7).

Since all affected cells do not react with the same speed to axon transection, there will always be some cells with slighter changes, which may be difficult to distinguish from normal cells. In studies of this kind it is, therefore, *essential to record only cells which show typical changes* (central tigrolysis and peripheral displacement of the nucleus which is often flattened), even if this means that some cells which have actually had their axon transected, are not taken into account. When this criterion is used, however, no area will be erroneously considered as an area of origin of a transected fibre bundle. This method of studying the origin of fibres has another advantage. If a nucleus consists of cells of different types it may often be possible to decide if the retrograde cellular changes involve cells of all types or only a particular type. For example, following lesions of the ipsilateral ventrolateral funiculus cells of all sizes are changed in the lateral vestibular nucleus (Fig. 7) (Pompeiano and Brodal, 1957a). The same is the case in the regions of the vestibular nuclei which send fibres to the cerebellum (Brodal and Torvik, 1957).

It should be noted that negative findings with this method are not conclusive, since in some instances cells do not react in the typical way to transection of their axon. The

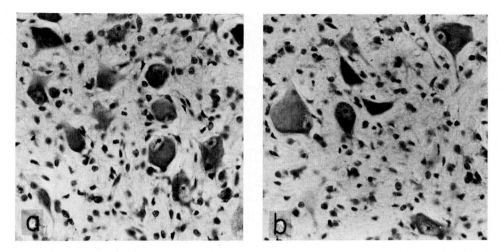

Fig. 7. Photomicrographs ($\times$ 240) showing acute retrograde changes (central tigiolysis and peripheral displacement of nucleus) in cells of the lateral vestibular nucleus in a kitten subjected to transection of the ventrolateral funiculus of the cord between C_2 and C_3 at the age of 8 days and killed 8 days later. Note that changes occur in small (a) as well as in laige and giant cells (b). The cells in a are from the small group 1 of the lateral nucleus (*cf.* Fig. 1). From Pompeiano and Brodal (1957a).

reasons for this are poorly understood. Furthermore, the possibility that the cellular changes may be transneuronal should be considered.

The use of the method described above (discussed in more detail elsewhere, Brodal, 1972) has made it possible to decide with considerable accuracy the sites of origin of several efferent fibre contingents of the vestibular nuclear complex. The results of these studies show that *each efferent contingent has its particular site of origin*. Thus the lateral vestibulospinal tract arises only from the lateral vestibular nucleus, and, as already mentioned, from small as well as large cells (Pompeiano and Brodal, 1957a). This suggests that the axons of this tract are of different calibers, as has been found in anatomical (Nyberg–Hansen and Mascitti, 1964) as well as physiological studies. Furthermore, a somatotopical pattern has been identified in this nucleus (Pompeiano and Brodal, 1957a). This has likewise been confirmed in physiological studies. The fibres ascending to the oculomotor nuclei have been shown to come from the superior nucleus and the rostral part of the medial nucleus (Tarlov, 1960). The fibres to the cerebellum come chiefly from the group x and the ventrolateral part of the descending nucleus (Brodal and Torvik, 1957).

In some instances, for example, as regards the lateral vestibulospinal tract, the sites of origin of the various contingents of vestibular nuclear efferents coincide with particular nuclei. In other cases there appears to be less sharp limits. Thus, in the descending vestibular nucleus the number of cells projecting onto the cerebellum decreases gradually as one passes from caudal to more rostral levels (Brodal and Torvik, 1957).

References pp. 51–53

CORRELATION OF SITES OF TERMINATION OF AFFERENT AND SITES OF ORIGIN
OF EFFERENT CONNECTIONS

Even if there are a number of more or less circumvential routes by which impulses
entering in a particular group of afferents may influence any other part of the vestibular nuclei than its field of termination, it seems a likely assumption that an afferent
fibre contingent will exert its main action in its specific area of termination by monosynaptic contact with its cells. A few examples of anatomical arrangements of this kind
may be mentioned. The superior vestibular nucleus and the rostral part of the medial
nucleus which have been shown to be the sites of origin of the vestibular nuclear
projections to the oculomotor nuclei (see Tarlov, 1970) are the recipients of the primary vestibular fibres from the canals (Stein and Carpenter, 1967; Gacek, 1969). Cells
here accordingly are links in the direct two-neurone vestibulo-oculomotor reflex arc.
The restriction of the terminations of primary vestibular fibres to the rostroventral
part of the nucleus of Deiters (Walberg *et al.*, 1958), furnishes morphological evidence
of a more direct pathway for vestibular impulses to the motoneurones supplying the
forelimb than to those supplying the hindlimb, as agrees with physiological studies.
The regions of the vestibular complex which project onto the cerebellum are the main
sites of ending of spinal afferents (Pompeiano and Brodal, 1957b; Brodal and Angaut,
1967).

*Several specific regions of the vestibular nuclei can thus be outlined as links in fairly
well defined pathways.* Least is known in this respect of the descending nucleus.

Just as there is apparently no region of the vestibular nuclear complex which
receives afferents from one source only, the nuclear regions which can be outlined as
sites of origin of specific projections in addition generally may act on other parts than
the site of termination of their main outflow, since their axons may dichotomize or
give off collaterals. The latter arrangement appears to be the case for most of the
vestibular nuclear efferents to the reticular formation. As to the commissural fibres
(see Ladpli and Brodal, 1968) it appears from the Golgi studies of Hauglie–Hanssen
(1968) that at least some commissural fibres may be collaterals of ascending axons.

The anatomical possibilities for a concomitant influence of different regions of the
brain from several, probably all, parts of the vestibular complex are obviously of
relevance for interpretations of the effects of stimulation of the vestibular nuclei or
their afferents.

INTRINSIC ORGANIZATION AND SYNAPTIC RELATIONS

For a proper understanding of the mode of operation of the vestibular nuclei a knowledge of their intrinsic morphological organization is essential. Some problems to be
tackled are the following: Do afferent fibres from different sources differ with regard
to their terminal patterns of branching and types of synaptic contacts established?
Does each contingent of afferents have synaptic contacts, exclusively or preferentially,
with nerve cells of a specific type? Is there convergence of afferents from different
sources upon individual cells? Do axons of cells in the vestibular nuclei have collaterals

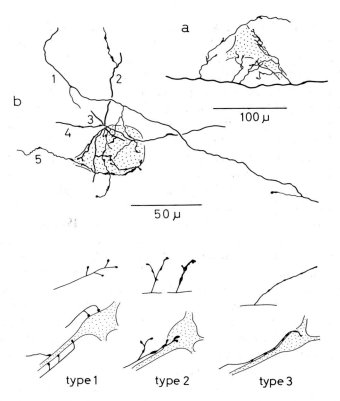

Fig. 8. Drawings from the vestibular nuclei in the cat based on Golgi sections. Above: An afferent fibre may give off a number of collaterals to the same cell (a) and several terminal fibres (1–5), in part from different sources, may converge on a single cell (b). Below drawings of 3 types of afferent terminal fibres which can be distinguished in Golgi sections. Transitional types may be found as well. From Hauglie–Hanssen (1968).

which are distributed to other subdivisions of the complex? Do dendrites of cells of a particular subdivision extend into neighboring subdivisions? Do purely internuncial cells occur in the vestibular nuclei?

To many of these questions final answers cannot yet be given. Information of the intrinsic organization can be obtained mainly by studies of Golgi preparations and in electron microscopical studies of normal and experimental material. Investigations of the latter type have so far been published only as concerns the lateral vestibular nucleus of Deiters.

It is possible here to consider briefly only some of the problems listed above (for more complete discussions see Hauglie–Hanssen, 1968; Brodal, 1972). Following a presentation of some selected anatomical data an attempt will be made to evaluate their functional implications.

(i) The course, types of branching and types of synaptic contacts of afferent fibres to the vestibular nuclei are as yet only imperfectly known. In Golgi studies the terminal fibres of the afferents can be seen to differ. Hauglie–Hanssen (1968) distinguishes 3

types (Fig. 8, below). Some fibres (type 1) are thin and give off short side branches with relatively small terminal boutons. Other fibres (type II) in addition to terminal boutons, have boutons en passage and are often found to climb along soma or dendrites. Type III fibres are characterized by being thin, having small boutons en passage and to 'climb' along soma or dendrites for considerable distances. Further subdivisions of types of afferents have been suggested by Mugnaini, Walberg and Hauglie–Hanssen (1967b). An afferent fibre often gives off several collaterals to a single cell (a in Fig. 8 above). A single fibre usually contacts more than one neurone. Collaterals from different sources can be seen to converge on one cell (b in Fig. 8 above). In the nucleus of Deiters, collaterals and terminal fibres often form so-called pericellular baskets as first described by Cajal (1896). According to Hauglie–Hanssen (1968) particularly the cerebellovestibular afferents participate in the formation of baskets.

Electron microscopic studies in the cat (Mugnaini *et al.*, 1967a) have confirmed the presence (in the nucleus of Deiters) of different kinds of synaptic endings (for a corresponding study in the rat see Sotelo and Palay, 1968, 1970). Complete correlations are not possible, but in addition to globular terminal boutons, slender as well as larger (sausage-like) boutons of passage have been identified, probably representing fibres of type III and type II, respectively. In further agreement with the Golgi studies, electron micrographs have shown that synaptic contacts are established with dendrites as well as somata. However, while the perikarya of large cells are amply beset with terminal boutons, the small cells have only few boutons on their soma. The same is the case in the nucleus of Deiters in the rat (Sotelo and Palay, 1970) and in the superior vestibular nucleus of the cat (unpublished observations). There are considerable variations in the ultrastructure of the terminal boutons, for example with regard to types of vesicles present. Some contain only round vesicles, others round as well as elongated ones. A classification of boutons according to their fine structure is, however, difficult. Axoaxonic synapses were not found in the nucleus of Deiters in the cat (but are abundant in the same nucleus in the rat according to Sotelo and Palay, 1970). Spines are common on dendrites as well as on perikarya in all vestibular nuclei (Hauglie–Hanssen, 1968).

Regarding the distribution of the terminal branches and their collaterals some findings deserve mention. Hauglie–Hanssen (1968), extending previous observations with the Golgi method of Cajal (1896, 1909–11) and Lorente de Nó (1933), noted that the main contingents of afferents to the vestibular complex run parallel to its longitudinal axis. The collaterals of these fibres generally enter the areas of terminations in planes oriented nearly transversely to this axis. The collaterals and their short side branches are distributed within elongated zones, having the shape of cylinders or lamellae (Fig. 9) with only little overlapping.

(ii) The *dendrites* of most cells in the main vestibular nuclei are rather long and straight, but there are some variations among cells in different groups (see Fig. 2). The cells thus belong to the isodendritic type of Ramón–Moliner and Nauta (1966). In the superior, lateral and descending nuclei the dendrites tend to be oriented in planes transverse to the longitudinal axis of the complex, and hence parallel to the main contingents of afferents.

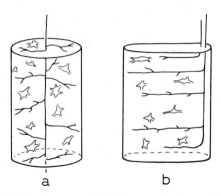

a   b

Fig. 9. Schematic drawings which illustrate principal features in the distribution of terminal fibres and collaterals of afferents in the vestibular nuclei. The terminal fibres and collaterals may be arranged so as to occupy a cylinder-like (a) or a lamellar (b) volume of tissue with only little overlapping. Type a is found in the terminations of the ipsilateral (probably cortical) vestibulocerebellar fibres, while type b is found in the terminations of primary vestibular fibres and fibres from the fastigial nucleus (*cf*. text and Fig. 6). From Hauglie–Hanssen (1968).

Of particular interest is the question whether dendrites extend beyond the borders of the nuclei of their parent cells. Based on a study of the dendritic spheres of the cells, *i.e.*, the space covered by all dendrites of a cell (Fig. 10) Hauglie–Hanssen (1968) found that the dendritic spheres of most cells are distributed within the parent nucleus. However, cells situated close to the border may often extend their dendrites into a neighbouring nucleus. This is most marked at the transition between the medial and descending nucleus.

(iii) Concerning the question whether there are pure *internuncial cells* in the vestibular nuclei it appears from Golgi studies of various authors that most cells in the vestibular nuclei give off long axons. Typical Golgi II type cells with short amply branching axons have not been found. Pure internuncial cells thus appear to be absent. However, some axons give off a few simple collaterals within the subdivision where the soma is located. In addition there are cells which give off thin, relatively richly branching axon collaterals distributed in the neighbourhood of the parent cell. The situation appears to be similar to that found in the reticular formation (Scheibel and Scheibel, 1958; Valverde, 1961) and in the spinal cord (Scheibel and Scheibel, 1966). It seems a likely assumption that cells of this kind in addition to being projection neurons may function as internuncials.

(iv) The observations described above are of relevance for our views on *the functional organization of the vestibular nuclei*. Only some points can be discussed here. One of these concerns the *anatomical possibilities for impulses entering in a particular afferent fibre system to influence other regions of the vestibular complex than its site of termination*. This question is of relevance, for example, for the influences of impulses from the labyrinth on spinal motoneurons for the hindlimb, since primary vestibular afferents are restricted to the forelimb region of the lateral vestibular nucleus, and the spinal projection from the medial vestibular nucleus reaches only the upper thoracic cord. There is thus little anatomical evidence for a direct monosynaptic pathway from

References pp. 51–53

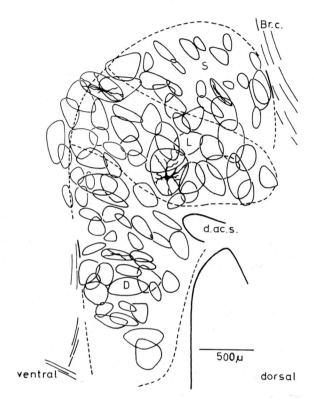

Fig. 10. Outlines of dendrite spheres in the vestibular nuclei of a 4-day-old kitten as seen in a sagittal Golgi impregnated section. Note differences in dendrite spheres and also that the spheres of most cells do not exceed the borders of the nucleus where the perikarya are situated. From Hauglie–Hanssen (1968).

the labyrinth via the vestibular nuclei to the lumbar motoneurons. In agreement with this, cells in the nucleus of Deiters projecting to the cervical cord are driven mono-synaptically by stimulation of the ipsilateral labyrinth, while those projecting to the lumbosacral cord are driven mainly polysynaptically (Precht *et al.*, 1967; Wilson *et al.*, 1967a; Ito *et al.*, 1969). Possible anatomical routes by which impulses from the labyrinth may reach the hindlimb region of Deiters' nucleus are depicted in Fig. 11. The possibility shown in A, extension of dendrites of cells in the hindlimb region into the forelimb region, does not appear very likely, on account of the restricted distribution of dendritic spheres of the cells (*cf*. Fig. 10). Since true internuncial cells appear to be absent, the possibility shown in B is unlikely. Recurrent collaterals, suggested in C, have been observed in Golgi preparations by several authors, but it has not been possible to follow them far enough to decide where they end. The amply branching collaterals given off by some axons close to the perikarya will probably influence cells in their immediate vicinity only. A final possibility, shown in D, is that axons or collaterals of vestibular nuclear cells establish synaptic contact with cells in another vestibular cell group or in an extravestibular cell group. These cells may send axons

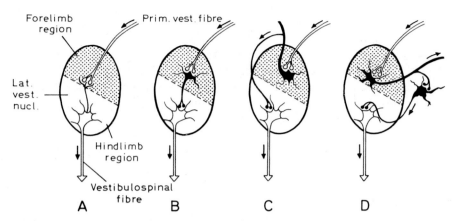

Fig. 11. Diagram to illustrate possible anatomical routes by which impulses from the labyrinth entering in primary vestibular fibres, restricted to the forelimb region of the lateral vestibular nucleus, may be imagined to influence the cells of its hindlimb region. The possibilities shown in A and B are rather unlikely to exist (*cf*. text).

back to another part of the vestibular complex than the one which receives the particular afferent contingent. Among extravestibular cell groups the reticular formation presents itself as a likely candidate. However, the organization of the reticulovestibular projections is not sufficiently known to permit definite conclusions as to whether such neuronal circuits may operate in situations like those discussed above with reference to the spread of labyrinthine impulses to the hindlimb part of the lateral vestibular nucleus. This is only one of several situations where impulses entering in a particular afferent component may act outside the sites of ending of its fibres.

Another problem concerns the *existence of internuncial cells operating within the territory of a main afferent distribution area*. Physiological evidence for the existence of internuncial cells of this kind has been brought forward concerning especially the medial nucleus (Shimazu and Precht, 1966; Wilson *et al.*, 1968, and others). Even if, as mentioned above, no cells of the Golgi II type have been found in the vestibular nuclei, their presence cannot be entirely excluded on the basis of negative evidence in Golgi sections. It appears extremely likely, however, that long axon cells giving off collaterals to the vicinity of the parent cell body may function as internuncials in these cases. Such cells have been found in all the main nuclei, except the lateral (Hauglie-Hanssen, 1968) and may be particularly common in the medial nucleus. In the case of the commissural connections, for example, such internuncials may be situated in a nucleus on the side of stimulation, in the nucleus receiving the commissural fibres, or in both.

As concerns the *terminations of afferents within the vestibular nuclei* there are several unsolved problems. One of these concerns their *mode of termination*, another their *patterns of distribution*.

It seems a likely assumption that fibres ending as type I, II or III or any other type, are derived from different sources. However, according to the Golgi studies of Hauglie–Hanssen (1968) fibres belonging to a particular contingent of afferents are not always uniform. While it appears that the fastigiovestibular fibres have endings of type III only (slender climbing fibres with small boutons, see Fig. 8), terminals of types I and II occur together in several afferent contingents. It appears extremely likely that the differences among the terminations reflect functional differences. In the case of the primary vestibular fibres it may be conjectured that the two kinds of terminals are related to fibres coming from different kinds of receptor cells (the bottle-shaped and cylindrical ones), but it is not known whether this is so. (Other correlations may also be thought of, such as to tonic and kinetic neurones, respectively, or to macular and cristae receptors, respectively.) Electron microscopical studies (Mugnaini et al., 1967a), however, have not given convincing evidence for differences among boutons degenerating in the lateral nucleus as a consequence of transection of the vestibular nerve. Preliminary studies (unpublished) suggest that the boutons degenerating in the superior vestibular nucleus following transection of the vestibular nerve are of the same kind as in the lateral nucleus.

The presence of more than one type of termination as seen in Golgi preparations in other afferent systems may suggest that there are functional differences between their fibres. In electron microscopical studies of the cerebellar cortical fibres to the lateral vestibular nucleus Mugnaini and Walberg (1967) found some degenerating boutons to be of the terminal type, but most are of the en passage type with coarse swellings, and appear to correspond approximately to the type II in Fig. 8. These differences may be of relevance to the question whether all Purkinje cells are actually functionally uniform and inhibitory.

Indications that there may be differences between terminals from different sources is provided by the observation that the primary vestibular fibres to the lateral nucleus when transected show degenerating boutons of the 'dark type' (Mugnaini et al., 1967a) while those coming from the cerebellar cortex show the 'filamentous type' of degeneration (Mugnaini and Walberg, 1967). These two types of afferents further differ with regard to the time course of degeneration.

Much remains to be done in the study of the terminations of afferents. Experimental electron microscopical studies may be of value in solving some of these problems, for example, whether fibres from different sources establish synaptic contact with the same cells. According to Walberg and Mugnaini (1969) some cells in the lateral nucleus receive primary vestibular as well as cortical cerebellar fibres. Other questions which lend themselves for studies of this kind are whether the fibres of an afferent contingent establish synaptic contact with one type of cell only in a nucleus composed of cells of different types, and whether contacts are established with soma or dendrites or both. In the lateral nucleus it appears from our studies that primary vestibular and cortico-vestibular fibres both end on somas as well as on large and small dendrites. A vast amount of technically difficult experimental electron microscopical work is needed to clarify the anatomy of the synaptic relationships in the vestibular nuclei. An additional promising approach to these problems is the use of microchemical analyses of minute, anatomically defined regions of the nuclear complex, as exemplified by the recent study of Fonnum, Storm–Mathisen and Walberg (1970) on the contents of GABA in the lateral vestibular nucleus following degeneration of the cortical cerebellovestibular fibres.

In preceding sections of this paper reference has been made to the *question of borders between subdivisions of the nuclei* and of the delimitation of areas giving off or receiving particular fibre contingents. As we have seen, in neither case are there sharp limits if the word sharp is taken in the strict sense. However, as touched upon previously, this does not mean that there is a diffuse pattern of organization within the vestibular nuclei, and that there are no clear topical relations between certain parts of the vestibular nuclei and the regions with which they are connected.

A strong argument for the presence of *precise topical relations* is furnished by the fact that the fibres of several main contingents of afferents have been found by Hauglie–Hanssen (1968) and others to be distributed in the form of cylinders or lamellae with only little overlapping (see Fig. 6 and 9). In some instances there is direct experimental evidence for a precise topical arrangement, for example, the restricted but mutually somewhat differently located degeneration in the superior nucleus following destruction of fibres from the 3 canals (Stein and Carpenter, 1967; Gacek, 1969). The segmental pattern of distribution of spinal afferents in the group x (Pompeiano and Brodal, 1957b; Brodal and Angaut, 1967) is another example. Supporting evidence is also provided by the observation that following partial interruptions of the vestibular nerve, terminal degeneration in the nuclei is often found in clusters, lying rather far apart (Walberg *et al.*, 1958). In other instances a clear-cut experimental demonstration of a topical pattern is difficult, for example in the cerebellovestibular projections. The areas of degeneration in the vestibular nuclei following lesions of the fastigial nucleus and the cerebellar vermis are never sharply circumscribed, but have diffuse borders (Walberg *et al.*, 1962, and Walberg and Jansen, 1961, respectively). Several circumstances may contribute to this. If, as suggested in Fig. 6, there is some divergence of the afferents in the periphery of the zone of termination, this would tend to produce gradual transitions even if the fibres end in circumscribed lamellar areas without much overlapping. Furthermore, it is impossible to produce lesions which destroy selectively only a few cerebellar folia, involving those from the summit to the depths of the sulci and to make circumscribed lesions of the fastigial nucleus which do not interrupt fibres from neighbouring regions of the nucleus. In situations like these experimental anatomical methods usually can show only the general trends in the patterns, such as obvious differences in location of terminal fields according to lesions of, for example, fore- and hindlimb regions. The *unsharp borders of terminal areas in these and some other instances, therefore, do not argue against the view that these projections are organized in a rather strict topical pattern.* This conclusion is strongly supported by the physiological observations of Pompeiano and Cotti (1959) since in single unit recordings from the nucleus of Deiters, 48 out of 76 units were influenced by threshold polarization of a single folium only of the anterior lobe.

There is reason to believe that other projections are likewise very precisely organized, even if the anatomical details have not yet been worked out. Some examples in support of this have been given elsewhere in this text (see, for example, Fig. 4). This necessitates that *great attention is devoted to the topography and anatomical situation of*

regions destroyed, stimulated or recorded from, in physiological investigations. Many
studies from recent years in different fields of research bear evidence of the presence of
extremely intricate patterns of organization of the vestibular nuclei. Every step forward
appears to make our picture of this organization more complex. For fruitful progress it
becomes more and more important that anatomical and physiological observations
are correlated. It is encouraging to see how well observations in the two fields are in
agreement when they are performed with sufficient care.

SUMMARY

The vestibular nuclei may be considered as a mosaic of many small units, each of which
has its particular anatomical organization. This appears from studies of their cytoarchitectonics as seen in Nissl-stained sections as well in Golgi sections.

Even if certain parts of the main nuclei as well as some of the smaller cell groups do
not receive primary vestibular afferents, it is deemed appropriate to retain the name
'vestibular nuclei' for the entire complex.

The problem of delimiting cell groups and drawing borders between them is discussed, likewise the methods for studies of afferent and efferent connections.

The afferent fibre contingents to the vestibular nuclei all have their particular sites
of termination, but no region of the nuclei receives fibres from one source only. Close
collaboration may be expected between impulses from different sources whose efferent
fibres have common terminal regions.

The various contingents of efferent vestibular connections have their particular sites
of origin. In some instances these coincide with certain nuclear subdivisions. To some
extent the site of origin of an efferent system coincides with the site of terminations of
a particular contingent of afferents, suggesting a direct, monosynaptic, impulse passage through the region in question. However, such regions appear always to influence
in addition other stations in the nervous system.

The problems of the intrinsic organization of the vestibular nuclei are discussed,
mainly on the basis of Golgi and electron microscopical observations. Pure internuncial cells appear to be absent in the vestibular nuclei, but many cells give off collaterals from their long axons and thus may serve as internuncials. These data are of
relevance for the explanations of how impulses reaching a particular unit of the
vestibular complex may influence another unit or area.

The afferent fibres differ morphologically and can be subdivided into 3 or more
types. It appears that usually more than one type is found within a group of afferents,
suggesting that the afferents from a particular source may differ functionally. In
electron microscopical studies it has been found that cerebellar corticovestibular as
well as primary vestibular fibres establish synaptic contact with cell somata as well as
thin and thick dendrites.

Most, if not all, afferents to the vestibular nuclei have terminal branches and collaterals which cover a cylindrical or a lamellar shaped space, with only little overlapping.
This, as well as some experimental data, show that there is a high degree of topo-

graphical precision in the anatomical organization of the nuclei and in their connections with other parts of the brain.

It is to be expected that experimental electron microscopical studies as well as microchemical studies will in future bring forth important new data on the fine organization of the vestibular nuclei.

REFERENCES

ANGAUT, P. AND BRODAL, A. (1967) The projection of the 'vestibulocerebellum' onto the vestibular nuclei in the cat. *Arch. ital. Biol.*, **105**, 441–479.

BRODAL, A. (1940) Modification of Gudden method for study of cerebral localization, *Arch.Neurol. (Chicago)*, **43**, 46–58.

BRODAL, A. (1972) Anatomy of the vestibular nuclei and their connections. In H. H. KORNHUBER (Ed.), *Handbook of Sensory Physiology. Vol. VI. Vestibular System.* Springer, Berlin, in press.

BRODAL, A. AND ANGAUT, P. (1967) The termination of spinovestibular fibres in the cat. *Brain Res.*, **5**, 494–500.

BRODAL, A. AND POMPEIANO, O. (1957) The vestibular nuclei in the cat. *J. Anat. (Lond.)*, **91**, 438–454.

BRODAL, A., POMPEIANO, O. AND WALBERG, F. (1962) *The Vestibular Nuclei and their Connections. Anatomy and Functional Correlations*, Oliver and Boyd, Edinburgh, London, pp. viii–193.

BRODAL, A. AND TORVIK, A. (1957) Über den Ursprung der sekundären vestibulo-cerebellaren Fasern bei der Katze. Eine experimentell-anatomische Studie. *Arch. Psychiat. Nervenkr.*, **195**, 550–567.

CAJAL, S., RAMÓN Y (1896) *Beitrag zum Studium der Medulla oblongata des Kleinhirns und des Ursprungs der Gehirnnerven.* Johann Ambrosius Barth, Leipzig, pp. 139.

CAJAL, S., RAMÓN Y (1909–1911) *Histologie du Système Nerveux de l'Homme et des Vertébrés.* Maloine, Paris.

CARPENTER, M. B. (1960) Fiber projections from the descending and lateral vestibular nuclei in the cat. *Amer. J. Anat.*, **107**, 1–22.

CARPENTER, M. B., ALLING, F. A. AND BARD, D. S. (1960) Lesions of the descending vestibular nucleus in the cat. *J. comp. Neurol.*, **114**, 39–50.

FINK, R. P. AND HEIMER, L. (1967) Two methods for selective silver impregnation of degenerating axons and their synaptic endings in the central nervous system. *Brain Res.* **4**, 369–374.

FONNUM, F., STORM–MATHISEN, J. AND WALBERG, F. (1970) Glutamate decarboxylase in inhibitory neurons. A study of the enzyme in Purkinje cell axons and boutons in the cat. *Brain Res.* **20**, 259–275.

FUKUDA, J., HIGHSTEIN, S. M. AND ITO, M. (1972) Cerebellar inhibitory control of the vestibulo-ocular reflex investigated in rabbit IIIrd nucleus. *Exp. Brain Res.*, **14**, 511–526.

GACEK, R. R. (1969) The course and central termination of first order neurons supplying vestibular endorgans in the cat. *Acta oto-laryng. (Stockh.)*, Suppl. 254, 1–66.

HAUGLIE–HANSSEN, E. (1968) Intrinsic neuronal organization of the vestibular nuclear complex in the cat. A Golgi study. *Ergebn. Anat. Entwickl.-Gesch.*, **40**/5, 1–105.

ITO, M., HIGHSTEIN, S. M. AND FUKUDA, J. (1970) Cerebellar inhibition of the vestibulo-ocular reflex in rabbit and cat and its blockage by picrotoxin. *Brain Res.*, **17**, 524–526.

ITO, M., HONGO, T. AND OKADA, Y. (1969) Vestibular-evoked postsynaptic potentials in Deiters' neurones. *Exp. Brain Res.*, **7**, 214–230.

LADPLI, R. AND BRODAL, A. (1968) Experimental studies of commissural and reticular formation projections from the vestibular nuclei in the cat. *Brain Res.*, **8**, 65–96.

LEIDLER, R. (1914) Experimentelle Untersuchungen über das Endigungsgebiet des Nervus vestibularis. 2. Mitteilung. *Arb. neurol. Inst. Univ. Wien*, **21**, 151–212.

LORENTE DE NÓ, R. (1933) Anatomy of the eighth nerve. I. The central projection of the nerve endings of the internal ear. *Laryngoscope (St. Louis)*, **43**, 1–38.

LØKEN, A. C. AND BRODAL, A. (1970) A somatotopical pattern in the human lateral vestibular nucleus. *Arch. Neurol. (Chicago)*, **23**, 350–357.

MEESSEN, H. AND OLSZEWSKI, J. (1949) *A Cytoarchitectonic Atlas of the Rhombencephalon of the Rabbit.* Karger, Basel, pp. 52.

MUGNAINI, E. AND WALBERG, F. (1967) An experimental electron microscopical study on the mode of

52 A. BRODAL

termination of cerebellar corticovestibular fibres in the cat lateral vestibular nucleus (Deiters' nucleus). *Exp. Brain Res.*, **4**, 212–236.

MUGNAINI, E., WALBERG, F. AND BRODAL, A. (1967a) Mode of termination of primary vestibular fibres in the lateral vestibular nucleus. An experimental electron microscopical study in the cat. *Exp. Brain Res.*, **4**, 187–211.

MUGNAINI, E., WALBERG, F. AND HAUGLIE–HANSSEN, E. (1967b) Observations on the fine structure of the lateral vestibular nucleus (Deiters' nucleus) in the cat. *Exp. Brain Res.*, **4**, 146–186.

NAUTA, W. J. H. (1957) Silver impregnation of degenerating axons. In W. F. WINDLE (Ed.), *New Research Techniques of Neuroanatomy*. Thomas, Springfield, Ill., pp. 16–27.

NYBERG–HANSEN, R. (1964) Origin and termination of fibers from the vestibular nuclei descending in the medial longitudinal fasciculus. An experimental study with silver impregnation methods in the cat. *J. comp. Neurol.*, **122**, 355–367.

NYBERG–HANSEN, R. AND MASCITTI, T. (1964) Sites and mode of termination of fibers of the vestibulospinal tract in the cat. An experimental study with silver impregnation methods. *J. comp. Neurol.*, **122**, 369–387.

OLSZEWSKI, J. AND BAXTER, D. (1954) *Cytoarchitecture of the Human Brain Stem*. Karger, Basel, 1954, pp. 199.

POMPEIANO, O. AND BRODAL, A. (1957a) The origin of vestibulospinal fibres in the cat. An experimental–anatomical study, with comments on the descending medial longitudinal fasciculus. *Arch. ital. Biol.*, **95**, 166–195.

POMPEIANO, O. AND BRODAL, A. (1957b) Spino-vestibular fibers in the cat. An experimental study. *J. comp. Neurol.*, **108**, 353–382.

POMPEIANO, O. E COTTI, E. (1959) Analisi microelettrodica delle proiezioni cerebello-deitersiane. *Arch. Sci. biol. (Bologna)*, **43**, 57–101.

POMPEIANO, O. AND WALBERG, F. (1957) Descending connections to the vestibular nuclei. An experimental study in the cat. *J. comp. Neurol.*, **108**, 465–504.

PRECHT, W., GRIPPO, J. AND WAGNER, A. (1967) Contributions of different types of central vestibular neurons to the vestibulospinal system. *Brain Res.*, **4**, 119–123.

RAMÓN–MOLINER, E. AND NAUTA, W. J. H. (1966) The isodendritic core of the brain stem. *J. comp. Neurol.*, **126**, 311–335.

SADJADPOUR, K. AND BRODAL, A. (1968) The vestibular nuclei in man. A morphological study in the light of experimental findings in the cat. *J. Hirnforsch.*, **10**, 299–323.

SCHEIBEL, M. E. AND SCHEIBEL, A. B. (1958) Structural substrates for integrative patterns in the brain stem reticular core. In H. H. JASPER, L. D. PROCTOR, R. S. KNIGHTON, W. C. NOSHAY AND R. T. COSTELLO (Eds.), *Reticular Formation of the Brain*. Henry Ford Hosp. Symp., Little Brown and Co., Boston, Mass., pp. 31–55.

SCHEIBEL, M. E. AND SCHEIBEL, A. B. (1966) Spinal motoneurons, interneurons and Renshaw cells. A Golgi study. *Arch. ital. Biol.*, **104**, 328–353.

SHIMAZU, H. AND PRECHT, W. (1966) Inhibition of central vestibular neurons from the contralateral labyrinth and its mediating pathway. *J. Neurophysiol.*, **29**, 467–492.

SOTELO, C. AND PALAY, S. L. (1968) The fine structure of the lateral vestibular nucleus in the rat. I. Neurons and neuroglial cells. *J. Cell Biol.*, **36**, 151–179.

SOTELO, C. AND PALAY, S. L. (1970) The fine structure of the lateral vestibular nucleus in the rat. II. Synaptic organization. *Brain Res.*, **18**, 93–115.

STEIN, B. M. AND CARPENTER, M. B. (1967) Central projections of portions of the vestibular ganglia innervating specific parts of the labyrinth in the rhesus monkey. *Amer. J. Anat.*, **120**, 281–318.

TARLOV, E. (1970) Organization of vestibulo-oculomotor projections in the cat. *Brain Res.*, **20**, 159–179.

VALVERDE, F. (1961) A new type of cell in the lateral reticular formation of the brain stem. *J. comp. Neurol.*, **117**, 189–195.

VOOGD, J. (1964) *The Cerebellum of the Cat. Structure and Fibre Connexions*. Van Gorcum and Co., Leiden, pp. 215.

WALBERG, F., BOWSHER, D. AND BRODAL, A. (1958) The termination of primary vestibular fibers in the vestibular nuclei in the cat. An experimental study with silver methods. *J. comp. Neurol.*, **110**, 391–419.

WALBERG, F. AND JANSEN, J. (1961) Cerebellar corticovestibular fibers in the cat. *Exp. Neurol.*, **3**, 32–52.

WALBERG, F. AND MUGNAINI, E. (1969) Distinction of degenerating fibres and boutons of cerebellar and peripheral origin in the Deiters' nucleus of the same animal. *Brain Res.*, **14**, 67–75.

WALBERG, R., POMPEIANO, O., BRODAL, A. AND JANSEN, J. (1962) The fastigio-vestibular projection in the cat. An experimental study with silver impregnation methods. *J. comp. Neurol.*, **118**, 49–76.

WILSON, V. J., KATO, M., PETERSON, B. W. AND WYLIE, R. M. (1967a) A single-unit analysis of the organization of Deiters' nucleus. *J. Neurophysiol.*, **30**, 603–619.

WILSON, V. J., WYLIE, R. M. AND MARCO, L. A. (1967b) Projection to the spinal cord from the medial and descending vestibular nuclei of the cat. *Nature (Lond.)*, **215**, 429–430.

WILSON, V. J., WYLIE, R. M. AND MARCO, L. A. (1968) Synaptic inputs to cells in the medial vestibular nucleus. *J. Neurophysiol.*, **31**, 176–185.

Comparative Anatomy of the Vestibular Nuclear Complex in Submammalian Vertebrates

W. R. MEHLER

Experimental Pathology Branch, NASA, Ames Research Center, Moffett Field, California, U.S.A.

There is a complex of cell groups in the brain stem of most vertebrates that receives the centripetal axon terminals of cells located in the vestibular ganglion of Scarpa. Functionally, the cell groups that receive these primary vestibular fibers constitute the true vestibular nuclei. Together with several interspersed cell groups they form the vestibular nuclear complex (VNC).

The sense organs of the labyrinth arise from the same anlage as the lateral line organs in aquatic vertebrates. It is not surprising, therefore, that there are basic similarities in the morphology of the cells in the respective peripheral ampullae and that there is some apparent overlap in the central distribution of their primary afferent fibers (Herrick, 1948; Dijkgraaf, 1962; Flock, 1967). Ariens Kappers, who contributed much to our knowledge about the brains of fishes, postulated that the vestibular nuclei were among the first supraspinal cell groups to evolve out of the reticular formation (Kappers *et al.*, 1936). Ramón–Moliner and Nauta's (1966) classification of the chief VNC cell types as 'iso-dendritic,' based on the dendritic architectural similarities of vestibular and reticular neurons, adds continuing support to Kappers' notion. Phylogenetically the vestibular system evolved before the auditory system, and embryologically vestibular neurons differentiate before acoustic cells (Windle, 1970). Viewed together these facts reinforce again notions contained in the old adage 'ontogeny recapitulates phylogeny' and demonstrate the phyletic age and fundamental neurologic importance of the vestibular system.

Cyclostomes

Although cyclostomes are close relatives of the most primitive fossil vertebrates they already have well developed labyrinths in addition to a separate lateral-line system. Centrally, however, there appears to be considerable overlap in the termination of the primary axons of these two systems that terminate in the brain stem nuclei or 'neuropil' which constitutes the vestibular nuclear complex in the lamprey, for example. Two nuclei have been described as generally discernible in cyclostomes, a dorsal and a ventral. According to Kappers *et al.*, (1936) these nuclei are composed of small granular type cells and large spindle shaped cells with richly branched dendrites. Steffanelli (1937) also found some small cells interspersed among the incoming VIII nerve fibers and suggested that these cells represented the tangential nucleus. This vestibular cell group is more prominent in teleosts and birds. Cajal (1908a, b), who studied brains of these classes of vertebrates and applied the name tangential nucleus, considered these cells homologous to the interstitial nucleus of the VIII nerve of mammals.

Larsell's (1967) more recent review, brought to final publication by the editorial efforts of Professor J. Jansen, updates and clarifies the literature on the vestibular area in submammals. This extensive review indicates, however, that even at the level of the lamprey some other vestibular nuclear subdivisions can be discerned. Thus, it appears that while various authors cannot fully agree on the actual number of individual nuclei or subdivisions in the vestibular complex of cyclostomes, the fundamental vestibular cell groups appear to be present even at this primitive level of brain development.

Elasmobranchs and teleosts

Some refinements are found in the development of the peripheral vestibular organs in elasmobranchs, but centrally it is chiefly developments in the lateral-line and the acoustico-lateral systems and the cerebellum that overshadow any apparent significant morphological changes in the vestibular nuclear complex. The connections of the vestibular nerve in elasmobranchs are reportedly analogous to those found in cyclostomes (Kappers *et al.*, 1936). Heier (1948) and Larsell (1967) review what is known about the VIII nerve fibers. In teleosts similar trends in development continue to appear, especially in relation to special adaptations and structural enlargements in the lateral-line system in the higher fishes. Primary lateral-line and vestibular fibers from multiple roots of both nerves reportedly overlap in their central connections. Most of our present understanding about the organization of the acoustico-lateral region in nonmammalian species, however, has been gained from neuroembryological and adult normal fiber studies. This situation raises the question: how precise are the existing data on the vestibular nuclear complex in fishes based on normal fiber studies alone?

While there has been some renewed interest in the brain of fishes (Llinás, 1969; Bernstein, 1970) anatomical studies have dealt chiefly with classical questions about forebrain organization or the cerebellum in a classical manner (*e.g.*, Nieuwenhuys, 1969). Ebbesson, however, recently initiated more experimentally oriented studies of the optic system employing new Nauta method variations on elasmobranch (Ebbesson and Ramsey, 1968) and teleost (Ebbesson, 1968) species. New experimental investigations of other cranial nerves in fishes also have begun. For example, Maler's (1971) initial report on a Nauta method experimental study on the projections of the lateral-line nerves in *Gnathonemus petersii*, a mormyrid or 'low voltage' electric fish, confirms that there is some overlap in the central connections of the anterior and posterior lateral-line nerves but he has not yet indicated the latter's central relationships with vestibular fibers of the VIII nerve.

Two vestibular nuclei are identified in teleosts, a small-celled tangential nucleus and a large-celled Deiters' nucleus, based on VIII nerve fiber connections in normal fiber studies according to Kappers *et al.* (1936). Four nuclei, however, were initially described by Cajal (1908b), a dorsal small-celled zone, dorsal to Deiters', and a small-celled descending nucleus in addition to the tangential and Deiters' nuclei.

In these species, as in most of the submammalian orders, these nuclei are not cell rich. They contain relatively few cells and are composed chiefly of the pervading neuropil that C. J. Herrick sought to decipher. We are beginning to understand now from electron microscopy studies that much of the neuropil is composed of just such cellular processes which are not readily visible in light microscopy preparations. The large cells predominate in the ventral nucleus and Kappers *et al.* (1936) speculated on the possibility that some of these large cells might be the precursors of the Mauthner cells of higher fishes.

Based upon a more functional notion that the vestibular nuclear complex is composed of those cells that receive primary vestibular fibers, a definition that we will follow throughout this treatise, the giant cells of Mauthner also should be included in the vestibular nuclear complex in fish. Mauthner cells receive primary as well as secondary vestibular connections (Retzlaff and Fontaine, 1960). Mauthner cells, however, also receive spinal and trigeminal projections as well, therefore they are more reticular-like than truly vestibular.

Unique cap or spoonlike endings of VIII nerve fibers synapse on tangential cells in fishes and in birds that also possess a large tangential nucleus. These large synapses should be of particular interest to the electron microscopist interested in peculiar synapses (see Sotelo and Palay, 1968). The interstitial nucleus, to which the tangential nucleus is compared, projects its axons into the medial longitudinal fasciculus leading to the suggestion that these cells are aberrant Deiters' cells (Brodal *et al.*, 1962). Experimental studies of this nucleus in fish or birds could verify some of these notions. Connectional studies, for example, even those based on normal fibers, indicate that some of these 'vestibular' nuclei are auditory relay nuclei and suggest that others belong to that part of the lateral-line that does not have VIII nerve overlap (Larsell, 1967).

Urodeles

According to Herrick (1930) the vestibular area in necturus is an obscure group of cells although the VIII nerve is formidable in size. It is not much more clearly differentiated in Amblystoma. As Herrick (1948) later pointed out, however, there is physiological evidence that salamanders exhibit vestibular control of posture and locomotion that implies an organized central apparatus that is selective for the specialized peripheral endorgans of the internal ear. The VIII nerve reportedly is undifferentiated into even primitive auditory and vestibular components but it is known that it contains fibers of different calibers. The VIII nerve fibers all make T-form divisions upon entering the brain stem. The distal end of the ascending division Herrick described seemed to invade the neuropil of the superior trigeminal nucleus as well as that of the lateral-line and the lateral cerebellar lobule. The descending branch of the VIII nerve, according to Herrick, merges imperceptively with the spinal trigeminal tract and dorsal funicular anlage.

Extremely primitive 'open-like' (Mannen, 1960) vestibular and trigeminal sensory regions were conceived by Herrick based on his observations that dendrites of cells in both regions overlap with each other and with their respective fiber tracts. A vestibular or 'VIII nucleus' (Herrick, 1930) composed of large and small cells can be discerned in several species of Salamanders in the acoustico-lateral area. Herrick (1948), however, believed that VIII nerve fibers terminated also in the lateral-line neuropil as well as the vestibular. He reported some decussating VIII nerve fibers coursing in the so-called acoustico-lateral commissure that terminate in the molecular layer on both sides of the midline of the cerebellum and other fibers that continue to the contralateral lateral lobule. Herrick described the terminals of these vestibulo-cerebellar fibers only as fine branches. He did not mention any comparison of these elements with either mossy or climbing fiber types found in mammals. Vestibulo-cerebellar fibers in the cat, it should be noted, end as mossy fibers (Brodal and Høivik, 1964) but there is no general agreement on the type of endings found in mammals.

Later studies of the tractus solitarius led Herrick (1944) to recognize a fascicle of fibers he identified as tract *b* related to the VIII nerve. This 'tract' is composed of fibers located between the VIII nerve divisions and the dorsally situated fiber group related to the lateral-line. One questions the primary vestibular fiber nature of these axons, however, because of the reported extent of their connections with both sides of the brain stem and with the spinal cord. Herrick (1948) himself later reconsidered that these fibers were probably secondary vestibular cell projections because some could be followed into the MLF. Larsell (1967) similarly concluded that those 'tract *b*' fibers are secondary vestibular axons and he speculated that those elements that reach the spinal cord probably are homologous with the vestibulospinal tract of higher vertebrates. Experimental methods of investigation, however, have not yet been applied to the connections of the vestibular complex in tailed amphibians. Only the Anura have begun to be so examined and they are the subject of the next section.

Anurans

We have examined the vestibular nerve fiber distribution in some frogs with complete VIII nerve interruptions proximal to the ganglia. Concomitant studies of the location of the primary neurons or 'ganglia' relative to the nerve and its branches, in these cases, and in 8 other nerves serially sectioned specifically for this purpose (Carpenter and Mehler, unpublished), revealed no aberrant cells located in the main trunk proximal to the fusion of the anterior and posterior nerve branches. In these animals (*Rana catesbeiana*) the ganglia were concentrated chiefly in the two branches at or near the point of fusion, and aberrant cells were only occasionally seen in branch twigs distal to the major ganglia as Geisler *et al.* (1964) reported. Neurotomies of the VIII nerve proximal to the brain stem in the frog, therefore, should interrupt all afferent vestibular fibers.

Following the functional anatomical definition that the vestibular nuclear complex is that medullary region outlined by the distribution of vestibular fibers, Fig. 1 depicts the complex in the frog and the related vestibulo-cerebellum that receive primary

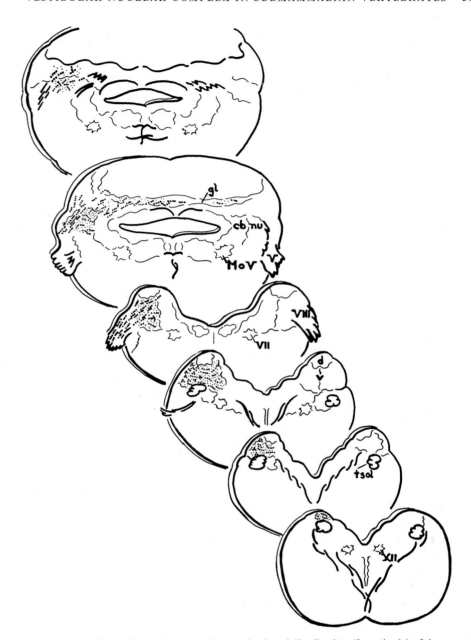

Fig. 1. Coronal sections depicting the course (heavy dots) and distribution (fine stipple) of degenerating anterior or vestibular root fibers of the VIII nerve of the frog (see text). cb nu, cerebellar nucleus; d, dorsal acoustic nucleus; gl, granular layer; Mo V, trigeminal motor nucleus; t. sol., tractus solitarius; v, ventral vestibular nucleus; V, trigeminal nerve; VII, facial nucleus; VIII, eighth cranial nerve; XII, hypoglossal nucleus.

vestibular fibers. These data confirm the findings of Gregory (1972) but differ in certain details with the distributions reported by Hillman (1969).

In complete nerve section cases of 12 or 20 days postoperative survival time under 20° C conditions, the descending degenerating VIII nerve fibers outline the acoustico-lateral area of the ipsilateral side down to the level of the oral pole of the XII nucleus. In the absence of brain stem involvement, no fibers cross to the contralateral side of the medulla oblongata as Wallenberg (1907b) reported in an early Marchi method investigation. In addition to the lack of decussating fibers in our material, or in Hillman's (1969) or Gregory's (1972), there also is no evidence to support the notion of direct 'VIII nerve-spinal' connections in adult frogs as Wallenberg (1907a) also reported. Gregory (1972) has called attention to a centripetal blood vessel in the frog that frequently accompanies the VIII nerve into the brain stem. Damage to this vessel in neurotomies in frogs or, as we have found, to a similar vessel in mammals, can lead to intrinsic vestibular cell changes or extrinsic fiber projections such as Wallenberg described.

Nuclear subdivisions are not much more evident in Nauta material, even with Nissl counterstains, but the acousticolateral area can be objectively delineated from adjacent regions by the selective impregnation of the degenerating VIII nerve fibers. Differential destructions of the anterior or vestibular root alone, according to Gregory (1972), produce degeneration restricted to the ventral vestibular nucleus, separating the ventral nucleus from the dorsally located acoustic nucleus. The degenerating primary vestibular fibers descend in the lateral part of the acousticolateral region forming an area fasciculata similar to that found in mammals. Some neurons which appear to receive terminals can be observed intercalated in the descending root. The descending fibers issue collaterals medially into the more cell populated, large-celled part of this primitive vestibular complex (Fig. 1). A nonterminal region, as found in Deiters' nucleus in mammals, is not evident in the frog.

Degenerating fibers ascend into the granule cell layer of the marginal zone of the auricular lobe of the cerebellum and some fibers decussate to the contralateral side. Only a few collateral-like offsets appear to issue into the vestibulo-cerebellar nucleus. Golgi preparations, however, suggest that the dendrites of the latter cells extend out into the afferent cerebellar peduncle in an 'open' (Mannen, 1960) type of synaptic arrangement (Larsell, 1967; Gregory, 1972).

Hillman (1969) whose study was chiefly concerned with the frog vestibulo-cerebellum, found that VIII nerve fibers descend in the brain stem only to the level of entrance of the IX nerve. He described degenerating vestibulo-cerebellar fibers that ascended into the molecular layer as well as the granular layer of the cerebellum. Both mossy and climbing fiber types of cerebellar afferents were identified in light microscopy studies as vestibular in origin by Hillman. He noted that the majority of fibers, however, appear to terminate in the vaguely delimited, less cellular, lateral region of the cerebellar nucleus. Gregory (1972), on the basis of Golgi observations, believes this region is composed chiefly of dendrites of cerebellar nucleus cells that extend laterally into this neuropil-like region. While we have observed some degenerating pre-terminal fibers enter what we would call the granule cell layer and a few decussate to the contralateral side, evidence to support the notion of climbing fibers of vestibular origin that project into the molecular layer cannot be found in our material. Dark impregnating, beaded and varicosed fibers frequently appear and cells containing argyrophilic granules also are disconcerting in this type of sub-mammalian material. Hillman (1969) utilized shorter survival times than we have studied and he states that the vestibular fiber degeneration in the molecular layer proceeds more rapidly. He notes that such fibers at the 3-day stage are 'beaded.' To date, however, Gregory (1972) also is unable to confirm any vestibular fibers in the molecular layer even in short survival experiments of two days.

Extended survival times are required in these cold-blooded animals to reach acceptable levels of fiber degeneration. Two to four weeks are generally required according to Riss *et al.* (1963) who pioneered in the application of the Nauta method to amphibian material. Mention of these extended survival times leads us to a precautionary note concerning the necessity of complete interruptive destruction of VIII nerve fibers, preferably by crushing, since functional regeneration can be established in opposed axons in as short a time as 8 days in the frog (Sperry, 1945).

Kosareva (1964) appears to have been the first to experimentally demonstrate cerebello-vestibular connections in anurans. He confirmed the existence of such connections in Nauta series of hemicerebellectomized toads and frogs. He found their distribution to be restricted to the magnocellular part of the vestibular complex, but Hillman (1969) indicated that cerebellofugal connections distribute throughout the vestibular complex similar to the VIII nerve afferent pattern. Neither of these authors appear to have had sufficient differential lesions to distinguish whether these cerebello-vestibular connections originate as long corticofugal fibers from the Purkinje cells or from deep cerebellar nuclei or from both neuronal sources. Senn and Goodman (1969), on the other hand, have recently demonstrated that long corticofugal fibers of Purkinje cell origin exist in reptiles.

Reptiles

Much interest has been shown in the vestibular complex of reptiles from the time since Holmes (1903) and Beccari (1912) studied it up through Weston's (1936) analysis to Larsell's (1967) resynthesis. Even the phylogenetically old vestibular system, like a number of other fundamental brain regions, shows considerable advances in anatomical differentiation in the reptilian brain. What is known of the vestibular nuclei and their connections based upon normal histology has recently been synopsized in Larsell's (1967) monograph and Ebbesson (personal communication) has begun an experimental investigation of the region, so we will not belabor the subject beyond essential comparisons.

Weston (1936) recognized 6 nuclei in reptiles. A tangential nucleus intercalated in the entering VIII nerve fibers, which is maximally developed in birds, is considered to be homologous with the interstitial nucleus of Cajal found in mammals. It is more of an entity in lizards than in turtles. The latter nucleus receives primary fiber connections in mammalian species qualifying it as a vestibular nucleus and it appears such connections also exist in reptiles (Larsell, 1967). A predominantly large-celled Deiters' or ventrolateral nucleus can be discerned. According to Weston (1936), some of these cells are larger but fewer in snakes than in other reptilian species, but the nucleus reaches its highest development in the quadrupedal alligator. Subdivisions of Deiters' nucleus that vary in position and cellular composition in different reptilian species also were described by Weston. An ill-defined but typical small-celled medial or 'ventro-medialis' nucleus is present and there is a mixed, medium and small-cell populated descending nucleus whose cell bodies are more distinctly intercalated in the descending root of the VIII nerve. Both of the latter nuclei are more clearly differentiated in the reptilian brain than they are in the brains of teleosts or anurans. Questions exist in the descriptive literature concerning the actual existence of a superior vestibular nucleus based upon cytoarchitectural evidence alone. Weston (1936) states that a superior vestibular nucleus is distinct only in the turtle. Experimental studies of vestibulo-oculomotor connections in reptilian species might resolve this question.

The sixth 'vestibular' nucleus is the dorsolateralis nucleus, according to Weston (1936), who distinguishes it as a separate entity from the small-celled divisions of Deiters' nucleus. This mixed, often cell-rich nucleus varies somewhat in position from species to species in Weston's description but it appears to generally occupy a position dorsolateral to Deiters' and ventral to the auditory nucleus laminaris. Based on its relationship to the ascending division of the vestibular nerve, it also has been labeled as a 'superior' nucleus. This suggestion of primary vestibular fiber connections allows us to agree with Weston and include this nucleus dorsolateralis as a probable component of the vestibular nuclear complex of reptiles. Positionally, subnucleus Deiters' δ (Pl.X, Meessen and Olszewski, 1949) or cell group 'y' (Brodal and Pompeiano, 1957) might be the mammalian vestige of this dorsolateral nucleus since the latter mentioned vestibular region cell group reportedly receives direct VIII nerve connections in the cat (Brodal and Høivik, 1964).

Information on connections of the VIII nerve in reptiles are based chiefly on normal fiber studies. Differential distributions of fibers originating in various branches have been described (Larsell, 1967). Direct primary vestibular neuron projections into the reticular formation (Weston, 1936) or the spinal cord (Herrick, 1948) also have been reported. The functional organization of the reptilian vestibular nuclear complex, however, needs to be clarified and these extra-vestibular connections experimentally verified.

Long cerebellar corticofugal fiber connections distributing throughout the vestibular complex have been verified as previously mentioned. Senn and Goodman (1969) also confirmed that these long corticofugal fiber connections originate from Purkinje cells in reptiles (*i.e.*, *Caiman sclerops*) similar to their mode of origin in mammals. Cerebello-vestibular projections that originate from the deep cerebellar nuclei also exist but there are no data on their distribution. Reticulo-vestibular relationships in reptiles have been suggested mainly on the basis of dendritic overlap in Golgi preparations (Weston, 1936).

Ebbesson (1967) has demonstrated a limited 'spino-vestibular' projection in the Tegu lizard associated with the dorsal spino-cerebellar tract that connects with both large and small cells in the ventral third of Deiters' nucleus. Another possible spino-vestibular connection described by this author were connections with a small-celled component near the dorsal funicular nuclei and cells ventro-medial to Deiters' which lay close to the ventricle throughout vestibular nuclear levels up to the level of the VIII nerve entrance. These projections appear to be derived from the so-called spinal lemniscus (Herrick, 1948). The latter ascends through the medial reticular formation similar in its course to the medial spino-reticular system in mammals that also issues terminal fibers into a comparably located vestibular nucleus in such animals as the opossum and rat (Mehler, 1969). Initial studies of Nissl sections of differential level spinal lesions in these cases (Ebbesson, personal communication) suggest that somato-topic organizational differences might exist in the intranuclear location of the cells of origin of vestibulospinal projections to the 'leg' in Tegu comparable to the organization found in most mammals.

In another species of lizard (*Lacerta viridis*), Jacobs (1967) reported finding a more profuse spino-vestibular connection than that reported by Ebbesson (1967) but these studies have not been published in detail. A pilot study series of ascending spinal fiber degeneration in the Caiman (Mehler, unpublished) suggests a comparable (*i.e.*, ventral part of Deiters' nucleus) small but definite spino-vestibular connection also exists in a crocodilian. Further studies in these species are needed to confirm these connections and establish the somatotopy of their respective fore- and hindleg VNC regions. Such information, coupled with Goodman's (1969) functional data on the Caiman might provide a simpler or less complex model of vestibular organization for physiological studies of a primitive quadruped. In the cat the spino-vestibular connec-tion appears to constitute a feedback system that originates from the lumbosacral region and distributes chiefly to that part of Deiters' nucleus that sends vestibulo-spinal projections to the lumbosacral levels (Pompeiano and Brodal, 1957a, b). Studies by Robinson (1969) have confirmed chiefly that there is a vestibulospinal tract in the lizard comparable to the mammalian that runs in the anterior funiculus in *Lacerta viridis*. No somatotopic organization in the Deitersospinal projections, however, could be deduced from the cases in this study because the anterior funiculi were unaffected in the lower spinal lesion cases. This author also raises some unresolved questions about the crossed and uncrossed nature of vestibulospinal projections that should be re-examined.

Aves

The VNC of birds has interested a large number of anatomical investigators including Ramón y Cajal (1908a, b) who identified the large nucleus tangentialis of birds which is intercalated in the VIII nerve at its point of entry into the brain stem. Subsequent extensive comparative studies of Bartels (1925), Sanders (1929) and others have led to the recognition of a variety of nuclei and subdivisions, some of which are difficult to homologize with respective nuclei in reptiles or mammals according to Stingelin (1965) who measured the volumes of vestibular nuclei in various species of birds.

To be comprehensive our review should contain a lengthy commentary on the vestibular nuclei of birds, which have been thoroughly analyzed in a number of avian species. However, Stingelin (1965) has recently reviewed the subject and Larsell (1967) devotes 6 full pages to what has been written about the VNC and its connections in avian species; discussion here without new data would therefore be unnecessarily redundant. In this regard it should be noted that Karten and Boord (personal communication) have new experimental data based on recently completed analyses of primary vestibular fiber connections in the pigeon that they are preparing for publication. Since they are more familiar with the bird brain (Karten and Hodos, 1967; Boord, 1968), and they will again review the literature within the context of their new findings, we shall not discuss the VNC in birds.

SUMMARY

This synopsis of the literature was undertaken in an effort to assess what is known about the natural history of the vestibular nuclear complex (VNC) in lower vertebrates. Our review disclosed that there is considerable descriptive information but it is widely dispersed in the literature. Larsell (1967) provides a detailed review and a complete bibliography of the more pertinent literature. The present survey, therefore, is intended to serve only as a key or critical introduction to the subject chiefly for those interested in initiating experimental studies on the functional organization of the VNC's afferent and efferent connections. Such data are needed to help establish structural homologies and perhaps discover in some species a new, more simple functional model for physiological investigation of vestibular function.

An increased complexity is found in the general level of organization of the brain in amphibians over that observed in fishes. Intra-, and interspecific adaptations and changes that have evolved in the peripheral vestibular organs, however, appear to be reflected very slowly in the elaboration and differentiation of the central nuclei that constitute the VNC in lower vertebrates. In the amphibian brain stem, for example, there appear to be only minor modifications in the primitive central vestibular nuclei and other parts of the acousticolateral region in comparison with a wide variety of morphological changes in the peripheral organs and the lateral-line system. The differentiation of auditory mechanisms in amphibians and reptiles also overshadows morphological changes in the vestibular system but there is little actually known about the central connections of either system in these classes of animals.

The lack of perceptible central anatomical changes in some cases is not too surprising when we recall Larsell's (1967) observation that neurons in the acousticolateral area of the brain stem in the tadpole that lose their lateral-line hair cell connections in the adult frog subsequently receive fibers from the auditory apparatus hair cells. It is important to remember here that while peripheral receptor organs might show adaptations to the various functional needs of the species, the cells forming the secondary central neural system are fundamentally designed to receive and transfer nerve impulses originating from exteroceptive hair cells which develop from the same anlage either before or after metamorphosis. This lack of central change might be considered as another example of the stability of organization in established central nervous system mechanisms like that shown to exist in the regeneration of vestibular and optic connections in amphibians (Sperry, 1945). Our impressions of the phyletic continuity of spinal connections are noted in another context (Mehler, 1969).

Excepting for a few early Marchi method investigations there have been few anatomical studies of the vestibular nerve utilizing newer experimental methods. Hillman (1969) and Gregory's (1972) studies with the Nauta method are the first that provide complete data on the areal distribution of the primary fibers of the vestibulo-acoustic nerve in the frog. Primary fiber connection data on other species are incomplete and the existence of cerebello-vestibular afferents has been confirmed only in a few amphibian and reptile species. Vestibulospinal projections appear in the 'lowest' vertebrates but it is unclear at what phyletic level vestibulo-oculomotor connections first appear.

There is a strong thread of correspondence in the basic mode of distribution of primary vestibular fibers in vertebrates that suggests phylogenetic continuity and homology. However, information about the topology, number and cellular composition of the cell groups that compose the VNC is sketchy, and we would concur with Larsell (1967) that there is little agreement in the literature on the secondary connections of these nuclei in lower vertebrates. Therefore, while data supporting an ontogenetic basis of homology exist, considerable cytological and hodological information is still needed to establish which parts of the VNC actually are homologous (Campbell and Hodos, 1970). The complete natural history of the VNC has yet to be written.

REFERENCES

BARTELS, M. (1925) Über die Gegend des Deiters und Bechterewskernes der Vögeln. *Z. Anat. Entwickl-Gesch.*, **77**, 726–784.

BECCARI, N. (1912) La costituzione, i nuclei terminali e le vie di connessione del nervo acustico nella Lacerta muralis. *Arch. ital. Anat. Embriol.*, **10**, 646–698.

BERNSTEIN, J. (1970) Anatomy and physiology of the central nervous system. *Fish physiol.*, **4**, 1–90.

BOORD, R. L. (1968) Ascending projections of the primary cochlear nuclei and nucleus laminaris in the pigeon. *J. comp. Neurol.*, **133**, 523–542.

BRODAL, A. AND HØIVIK, B. (1964) Site and mode of termination of primary vestibulocerebellar fibres in the cat. An experimental study with silver impregnation methods. *Arch. ital. Biol.*, **102**, 1–21.

BRODAL, A. AND POMPEIANO, O. (1957) The vestibular nuclei in the cat. *J. Anat. (Lond.)*, **91**, 438–454.

BRODAL, A., POMPEIANO, O. AND WALBERG, F. (1962) *The Vestibular Nuclei and their Connections. Anatomy and Functional Correlations*. Thomas, Springfield, Ill., pp. VIII–193.

CAMPBELL, C. B. G. AND HODOS, W. (1970) The concept of homology and the evolution of the nervous system. *Brain Behav. Evol.*, **3**, 353–367.

DIJKGRAAF, S. (1962) The functioning and significance of the lateral-line organs. *Biol. Rev.*, **38**, 51–105.

EBBESSON, S. O. E. (1967) Ascending axon degeneration following hemisection of the spinal cord in the Tegu lizard (*Tupinambis nigropunctatus*). *Brain Res.*, **5**, 178–206.

EBBESSON, S. O. E. (1968) Retinal projections in two teleost fishes (*Opsanus tau* and *Gymnothorax funebris*): An experimental study with silver impregnation methods. *Brain Behav. Evol.*, **1**, 134–154.

EBBESSON, S. O. E. AND RAMSEY, J. S. (1968) The optic tracts of two species of sharks (*Galeocerdo cuvier* and *Ginglymostoma cirratum*). *Brain Res.*, **8**, 36–53.

FLOCK, Å. (1967) Ultrastructure and function in the lateral line organs. In P. CAHN (Ed.), *Lateral Line Detectors*. Indiana University Press, Bloomington, pp. 163–197.

GEISLER, C. D., BERGEIJK, W. A. VAN AND FRISHKOPF, L. S. (1964) The inner ear of the bullfrog. *J. Morph.*, **114**, 43–58.

GOODMAN, D. C. (1969) Behavioral aspects of cerebellar stimulation and ablation in the frog and alligator and their relationship to cerebellar evolution. In R. LLINÁS (Ed.), *Neurobiology of Cerebellar Evolution and Development*. Amer. Med. Ass., Chicago, pp. 467–473.

GREGORY, K. M. (1972) Central projections of the eight nerve in frogs. *Brain, Behav. Evol.*, **5**, 70-88.

HEIER, P. (1948) Fundamental principles in the structure of the brain. A study of the brain of Petromyzon fluviatilis. *Acta anat. (Basel)*, Suppl. VIII, 1–213.

HERRICK, C. J. (1930) The medulla oblongata of necturus. *J. comp. Neurol.*, **50**, 1–96.

HERRICK, C. J. (1944) The fasciculus solitarius and its connections in amphibians and fishes. *J. comp. Neurol.*, **81**, 307–331.

HERRICK, C. J. (1948) *The Brain of the Tiger Salamander*. Univ. of Chicago Press, Chicago, pp. viii–409.

HILLMAN, D. E. (1969) Light and electron microscopical study of the relationships between the cerebellum and vestibular organ of the frog. *Exp. Brain Res.*, **9**, 1–15.

HOLMES, G. (1903) On the comparative anatomy of the nervus acusticus. *Trans. roy. irish Acad.*, **32**, 101–144.

JACOBS, V. L. (1967) A spinovestibular component of the dorsal funiculus in a lizard (*Lacerta viridis*). *Anat. Rec.*, **157**, 264–265.

KAPPERS, C. U. A., HUBER, G. C. AND CROSBY, E. C. (1936) *The Comparative Anatomy of the Nervous System of Vertebrates, Including Man*. MacMillan, New York.

KARTEN, H. J. AND HODOS, W. (1966) *A Stereotaxic Atlas of the Brain of the Pigeon (Columba livia)*. The Johns Hopkins Press, Baltimore, pp. IX–193.

KOSAREVA, A. A. (1964) Efferent connections of cerebellum in amphibia and mammals. In L. A. ORBELI (Ed.), *Evolution of Functions. Symp. in the Memory of the 80th Anniv. of the Acad.*, Publ. USSR Acad. Sci., Moscow, Leningrad, pp. 264–272.

LARSELL, O. (1967) *The Comparative Anatomy and Histology of the Cerebellum from Myxinoids through Birds*. Univ. of Minnesota Press, Minneapolis, pp. VIII–291.

LLINÁS, R. (1969) *Neurobiology of Cerebellar Evolution and Development*. Amer. Med. Ass., Chicago, pp. X–931.

MALER, L. (1971) Projections of the lateral line nerves of Gnathonemus petersii. *Anat. Rec.*, **169**, 374.

MANNEN, H. (1960) 'Noyau fermé' et 'noyau ouvert'. *Arch. ital. Biol.*, **98**, 333–350.

MEESSEN, H. AND OLSZEWSKI, J. (1949) *A Cytoarchitectonic Atlas of the Rhombencephalon of the Rabbit*. Karger, Basel, pp. 52.

MEHLER, W. R. (1969) Some neurological species differences — *a posteriori*. *Ann. N.Y. Acad. Sci.*, **167**, 424–468.

NIEUWENHUYS, R. (1969) A survey of the structure of the forebrain in higher bony fishes (osteichthyes). *Ann. N.Y. Acad. Sci.*, **167**, 31–64.

POMPEIANO, O. AND BRODAL, A. (1957a) The origin of vestibulospinal fibers in the cat. An experimental-anatomical study, with comments on the descending medial longitudinal fasciculus. *Arch. ital. Biol.*, **95**, 166–195.

POMPEIANO, O. AND BRODAL, A. (1957b) Spino-vestibular fibers in the cat. An experimental study. *J. comp. Neurol.*, **108**, 353–381.

RAMÓN–MOLINER, E. AND NAUTA, W. J. H. (1966) The isodendritic core of the brain stem. *J. comp. Neurol.*, **126**, 311–336.

RAMÓN Y CAJAL, S. (1908a) Los ganglios centrales del cerebelo de las aves. *Trab. Lab. Invest. biol. Univ. Madrid*, **6**, 177–194.

RAMÓN Y CAJAL, S. (1908b) Sur un noyau spécial du nerf vestibulaire des poissons et des oiseaux. *Trab. Lab. Invest. biol. Univ. Madrid*, **6**, 1–20.

RETZLAFF, E. AND FONTAINE, J. (1960) Reciprocal inhibition as indicated by a differential staining reaction. *Science*, **131**, 104–105.

RISS, W., KNAPP, H. D. AND SCALIA, F. (1963) Optic pathways in *Cryptobranchus allegheniensis* as revealed by the Nauta technique. *J. comp. Neurol.*, **121**, 31–43.

ROBINSON, L. R. (1969) Bulbospinal fibres and their nuclei of origin in *Lacerta viridis* demonstrated by axonal degeneration and chromatolysis respectively. *J. Anat. (Lond.)*, **105**, 59–88.

SANDERS, E. B. (1929) A consideration of certain bulbar, midbrain and cerebellar centers and fiber tracts in birds. *J. comp. Neurol.*, **49**, 155–222.

SENN, D. AND GOODMAN, D. C. (1969) Patterns of localization in the cerebellar corticofugal projections of the alligator (*Caiman sclerops*). In R. LLINÁS (Ed.), *Neurobiology of Cerebellar Evolution and Development*. Amer. Med. Ass., Chicago, pp. 475–479.

SOTELO, C. AND PALAY, S. L. (1968) The fine structure of the lateral vestibular nucleus in the rat. *J. Cell Biol.*, **36**, 151–179.

SPERRY, R. (1945) Centripetal regeneration of the 8th cranial nerve root with systemic restoration of vestibular reflexes. *Amer. J. Physiol.*, **144**, 735–741.

STEFFANELLI, A. (1937) Il sistema statico dei Petromizonti (sistema laterale, sistema vestibolare, cervelletto). *Arch. zool. ital.*, **24**, 209–273.

STINGELIN, W. (1965) Qualitative und quantitative Untersuchungen an Kerngebiete der Medulla oblongata bei Vögeln. *Bibl. anat. (Basel)*, **6**, 1–116.

WALLENBERG, A. (1907a) Die kaudale Endigung der bulbo-spinalen Wurzeln des Trigeminus, Vestibularis und Vagus beim Frosche. *Anat. Anz.*, **30**, 564–568.

WALLENBERG, A. (1907b) Beiträge zur Kenntnis des Gehirns der Teleostier und Selachier. *Anat. Anz.*, **31**, 369–399.

WESTON, J. K. (1936) The reptilian vestibular and cerebellar gray with fiber connections. *J. comp. Neurol.*, **65**, 93–199.

WINDLE, W. F. (1970) Development of neural elements in human embryos of four to seven weeks gestation. *Exp. Neurol.*, Suppl. 5, 44–83.

Observations on Morphological Features and Mechanical Properties of the Peripheral Vestibular Receptor System in the Frog

D. E. HILLMAN

Division of Neurobiology, Department of Physiology and Biophysics, University of Iowa, Iowa City, Iowa, U.S.A.

Breuer (1891) noted that tuft-like structures projected from the surface of the receptor epithelium. He attributed the receptor function to the shearing motion of these hair-like masses. With electron microscopy two types of cilia are found in the tuft (Wersäll, 1956): (*i*) numerous stereocilia which are positioned over a relatively ridged cuticular plate that is placed at the luminal end of the cell and (*ii*) a single kinocilium which stands over a notch in this plate (Flock and Wersäll, 1962; Spoendlin, 1965; Hillman, 1969) (Figs. 1, 2). Since all the kinocilia are on the same side of the tuft Lowenstein and Wersäll (1959) were able to relate this morphological polarity to the activity within the vestibular nerve. A force which was directed toward the kinocilium caused an increase in the activity of the vestibular nerve while a decrease in activity was seen when the force was directed away from the kinociliary side of the cell.

The action of the ciliary hairs in the otolithic organs following a positional change shows that the sterocilia have a sliding motion at their distal ends (Hillman and Lewis, 1971) (Fig. 3B–D). The kinocilia, however, are different in that the distal portion of the kinocilium, at least in the case of the frog, is attached to the adjacent stereocilia (Figs. 2, 3A). For this reason the kinocilium cannot slide at its distal end but is displaced at its base (Figs. 2, 4). When a force is directed toward the kinociliary side of the cell, a plunging motion results on the kinocilium which produces a deformation of the cell membrane at the kinociliary base (Fig. 4A, B). At the same time a distension of the remaining membrane over the cuticular notch occurs as a protrusion of the cell in the notch region (Fig. 4A, B).

When a force is applied in the opposite direction (toward the stereociliary side of the cell) the base of the kinocilium is raised while the stereocilia, which stand on the ridged cuticle, slide at their distal ends (Figs. 3B, 4C, D). This results in a rounding of the surface membrane of the cell over the notch region and thereby reduces the distension of the membrane at this active site (Fig. 4C, D). The result is a directional mechanism which is postulated to produce the conductive changes necessary for modulation of transmitter release and the activation of afferent fibers.

The relationship between the ciliary apparatus and the otolithic membrane is compatible with the plunging motion of the kinocilium. In the case of the sacculus in

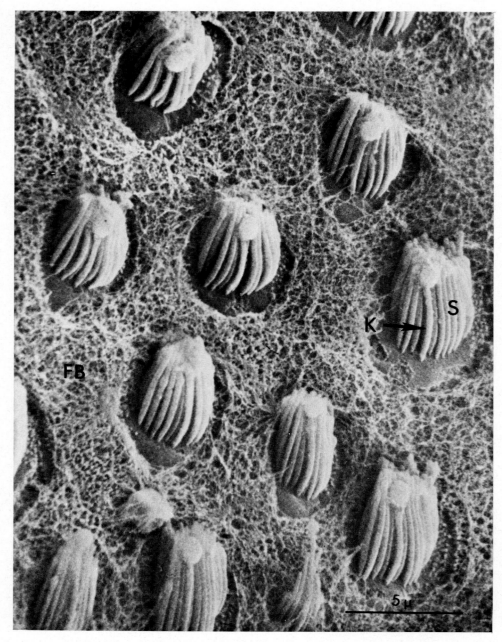

Fig. 1. Scanning electron micrograph showing the ciliary tufts on the saccular macula of the frog. The ciliary tuft is composed of stereocilia (S) and a single kinocilium (K) which has a bulb at its apex. The ciliary tufts are bent away from the kinociliary side of the cell. A filamentous mat (FB) which is over the supporting cells delineates the luminal surface of the receptor cells.

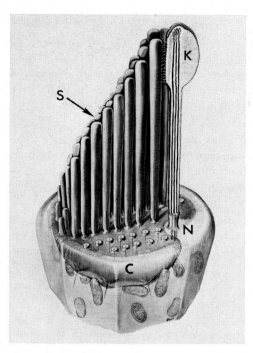

Fig. 2. Diagram to show the vestibular ciliary apparatus and its relationship to the apical end of the receptor cell in the frog. The stereocilia (S) stand on the cuticular plate (C) which is in the apical end of the receptor cell. The kinocilium (K) is positioned over a notch (N) in the cuticle where its base is in contact with the cell cytoplasm. Due to a filamentous attachment of the kinociliary bulb to adjacent stereocilia the pliable region in the area of the cuticular notch can yield to axial motion of the kinocilium. Two rows of stereocilia are cut at their base.

the frog, the bulb at the apex of the kinocilium (Figs. 1–3) is attached to the rim of a port in the otolithic membrane (Hillman and Lewis, 1971). In the utricle where the kinocilium is 3 to 4 times longer than the longest stereocilia the apical part of the kinocilium is embedded in the otolithic membrane. The otolithic membrane is attached to supporting cells by filament-like structures (Figs. 1, 3B–D) which cross the sub-membranous base to become part of the otolithic membrane (Hillman and Lewis, 1971). This submembranous zone is the shearing site for displacement between the supporting cells and the otolithic membranes (Hillman, in preparation). A displacement of the otolithic membrane draws the kinocilium and the adjacent stereocilia in the direction of its motion and thereby produces the axial motion in the kinociliary shaft which is related to the direction of the motion (Fig. 4).

In the canal system the ciliary processes are 50 μm or more in length. A row of stereocilia, 5 or 6, accompanies the kinocilium across the subcupular space where the kinocilium enters and is embedded in the cupula. Like the otolithic membrane, the subcupular space is crossed by fine filaments which anchor the cupula to the supporting cell (Dohlman, 1971).

The action of the cupula is the subject of much controversy since varied opinions and observations exist (Steinhausen, 1934; Trincker, 1962; Zalin, 1967; Dohlman, 1969). It has been commonly accepted that the cupula acts as a swinging door with its axis on the crista. Numerous factors, however, indicate that such a movement is incompatible with the properties of such a structure. An alternative possibility is an elastic diaphragm which has a resiliency that would return it to the original position. The small displacement volume which Oman and Young (1972) calculated for physiological movement indicates that under the conditions of their study, the movement of the hairs would be negligible. An elastic diaphragm which is bound circumferentially to the ampullary wall, except for the crista where it is loosely bound by filaments which cross the wide subcupular space, would have its greatest displacement near the crista somewhat like the pendulum proposed by Zalin (1967) (Fig. 4E). This would result in the greatest amount of ciliary displacement for a given volume of endolymph. The cupular zone near the center of the crista would have minimal resistance and could allow for responses to small movements. On the other hand, during large endolymph changes (possibly non-physiological), attachment of a cupula to the crista through the kinocilia and filaments holds the cupular base to this structure while the apex breaks away (Hillman and Llinás, unpublished observation) and thereby gives the classical swinging door appearance seen by Steinhausen (1934), Dohlman (1969) and other investigators.

To amplify the small movement which appears to be present during small angular deviations, the ciliary apparatus itself may bend in an arching manner which physically amplifies the axial motion of the kinocilium over and above that of straight processes (Fig. 4F). This arching may be due in part to the pipe organ arrangement of the stereocilia which have a graded resistance so that bending away from the kinocilium produces a pulley-like arch for the kinocilium (Fig. 3B). With motion toward the kinociliary side of the cell, the longer stereocilia have the least resistance so that bending occurs near the distal end of the kinocilium as a distal arch of the ciliary apparatus. Arching which results over a small length of the kinocilium can greatly enhance the displacement seen at the base of the kinocilium. In a model of a 50 μm long kino-stereociliary tuft which has a contoured bend the displacement at the base as significant with a 3 μm apical displacement (Fig. 4F). This movement is in the realm

---

Fig. 3. Transmission and scanning electron micrographs from the frog to show the relationship between the stereocilia and kinocilium due to displacement during fixation of the sacculus. A, Transmission electron micrograph showing the filaments which bind the apical end of the kinocilium (K) to an adjacent stereocilium (S). Small filamentous processes arise from a dense zone on the kinociliary membrane and traverse a cleft to join the membrane of the stereocilium. B, Scanning electron micrograph showing the ciliary tuft of the kinocilium (K) and numerous stereocilia which are bent away from the kinociliary side of the receptor cell (RC). A filamentous mat (FB) overlies the supporting cells. C, Scanning electron micrograph from the region of the striola of the saccular macula showing the opposed orientation of the ciliary tufts. D, A scanning electron micrograph showing two directionally opposed ciliary tufts which have been fixed while the gravitational force on the otolithic mass was changed by 180°. The top stereociliary tuft is bent away from the kinociliary side of the cell while the lower tuft is bent toward the kinociliary side of the cell. The sliding between the stereocilia is obvious in this preparation. At the arrow the raised cell membrane over the cuticular notch is evident. B and D from Hillman and Lewis (1971).

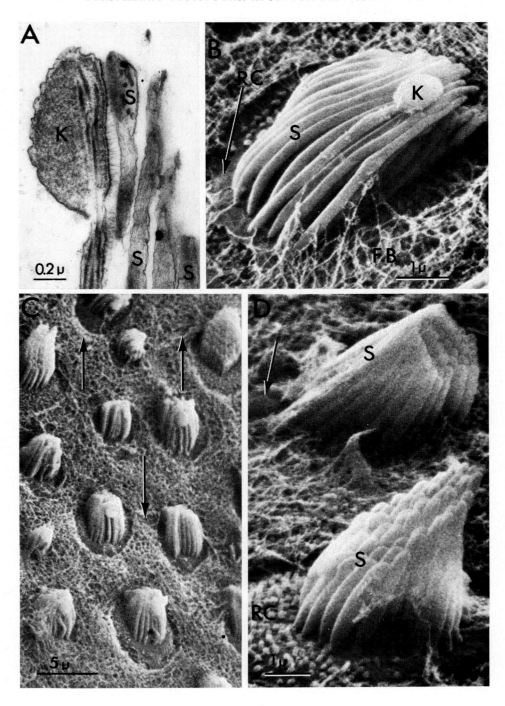

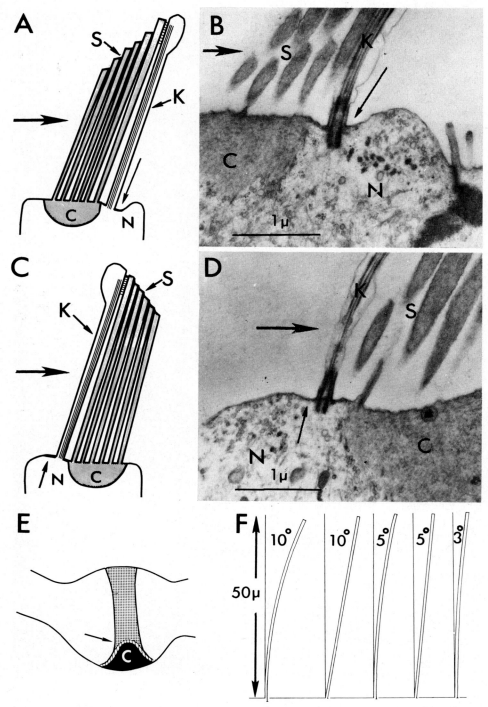

Fig. 4. Diagrams and transmission electron micrographs to show the axial motion of the kinocilium
due to directional displacement of the ciliary tuft. A and B, Motion toward the kinociliary side of the
cell causes the kinocilium (K) to plunge into the cuticular notch (N) which results in a deformation and
distention of the membrane in this region. C and D, Displacement away from the kinociliary side of
the cell raises the base of the kinocilium causing the membrane over the cuticular notch to round and
thereby reduce the distention. E, Motion of the cupula is possibly the greatest near the crista (C)
because of the wide subcupular space where the cupula is loosely attached. F, A contour head of the
ciliary apparatus results in amplification of the axial displacement of the kinocilium as seen when
comparing the paired models at 5 or 10°. Even at 3°, where the displacement is 3 μm, the change at the
base of the kinocilium is significant.

of central cupular displacement given by Oman and Young (1972) for a cupula which swings as a door so that displacement is in the shape of a wedge. On the other hand, their results correlate very closely to the cupular movement which would obtain if the volume displacement given by the authors were applied to an elastic diaphragm that has its greatest displacement near the crista at midpoint of its length.

REFERENCES

BREUER, J. (1891) Über die Function der Otolithen-Apparate. *Pflügers Arch. ges. Physiol.*, **48**, 195 306.

DOHLMAN, G. F. (1969) The shape and function of the cupula. *J. Laryng.*, **83**, 43–53.

DOHLMAN, G. F. (1971) The attachment of the cupulae, otolith and tectorial membranes to the sensory cell areas. *Acta oto-laryng. (Stockh.)*, **71**, 89–105.

FLOCK, Å. AND WERSÄLL, J. (1962) A study of the orientation of the sensory hairs of the receptor cells inthe lateral line organ of fish, with special reference to the function of the receptors. *J. Cell Biol.*, **15**, 19–27.

HILLMAN, D. E. (1969) New ultrastructural findings regarding a vestibular ciliary apparatus and its possible functional significance. *Brain Res.*, **13**, 407–412.

HILLMAN, D. E. AND LEWIS, E. R. (1971) Morphological basis for a mechanical linkage in otolithic receptor transduction in the frog. *Science*, **174**, 416–419.

LOWENSTEIN, O. AND WERSÄLL, J. (1959) A functional interpretation of the electronmicroscopic structure of the sensory hairs in the cristae of the elasmobranch *Raja clavata* in terms of directional sensitivity. *Nature (Lond.)*, **184**, 1807–1808.

OMAN, C. M. AND YOUNG, L. R. (1972) Physiological range of pressure difference and cupula deflections in the human semicircular canal: theoretical considerations. In A. BRODAL AND O. POMPEIANO (Eds.), *Progress in Brain Research. Vol. 37. Basic aspects of central vestibular mechanisms.* Elsevier, Amsterdam, pp. 529–539.

SPOENDLIN, H. H. (1965) Ultrastructural studies of the labyrinth in squirrel monkeys. In *The Role of the Vestibular Organs in the Exploration of Space. NASA SP*-77, 7–22.

STEINHAUSEN, W. (1934) Über die direkte Beobachtung der Sinnes-Endstellen des inneren Ohres (mit Film). *Zool. Anz.*, **36**, 85–91.

TRINCKER, D., (1962) The transformation of mechanical stimulus into nervous excitation by the labyrinthine receptors. *Symp. Soc. exp. Biol., Biological Receptor Mechanisms*, **16**, 289–316.

WERSÄLL, J. (1956) Studies on the structure and innervation of the sensory epithelium of the cristae ampullares in the guinea pig. *Acta oto-laryng. (Stockh.)*, **126**, 1–85.

ZALIN, A. (1967) On the function of the kinocilia and stereocilia with special reference to the phenomenon of directional preponderance. *J. Laryng.*, **81**, 119–135.

II. LABYRINTHINE INPUT TO THE VESTIBULAR NUCLEI

Light and Electron Microscopical Data on the Distribution and Termination of Primary Vestibular Fibers

F. WALBERG

Anatomical Institute, University of Oslo, Oslo, Norway

The primary vestibular fibers are generally said to be distributed to the whole vestibular complex. This, however, is not the case. Leidler (1914) in an experimental study in the rabbit noted that after transection of the vestibular nerve in the descending nucleus degeneration was found only ventromedially. Furthermore, he found that what appears to be the dorsal part of the nucleus of Deiters was free from degeneration. In a recent study (Walberg *et al.*, 1958) this distribution was confirmed, and additional data were obtained. The study, which was made by means of the Glees (1946) and the Nauta (1957) methods in the cat, revealed that while all four main nuclei receive primary vestibular fibers, there are within all nuclei regions which do not receive primary afferents (Fig. 1). In the superior nucleus the fibers supply the central area. In the lateral nucleus, the ventral part receives primary afferents, especially the rostral abundant distribution caudally, and in the descending nucleus the degeneration is, although widespread, less intense ventrolaterally than dorsomedially. The dorsal medial region is the main target for the fibers. An interesting observation is that the small cell group f, which lies within the descending vestibular nucleus, is free from degeneration although there is heavy degeneration in the immediate surroundings of this group. The primary vestibular fibers also reach the interstitial nucleus of Cajal, while the groups x and z of Brodal and Pompeiano (1957) are free. Brodal and Høivik (1964) later noted that the small cell group y receives primary vestibular fibers.

Although borders between regions receiving primary vestibular fibers and regions not receiving such fibers, are not sharp, the selective distribution is nevertheless clear. Transverse sections through the nuclear complex give a very good demonstration of this specific distribution of the primary vestibular fibers. One of the important conclusions emerging from this finding, is that in the lateral vestibular nucleus primary vestibular fibers supply chiefly the forelimb region.

The restricted distribution of primary vestibular fibers in the cat has been confirmed by Carpenter (1960). Carpenter (1960) and Stein and Carpenter (1967) found the same distribution in the monkey, but they describe the number of fibers to the lateral nucleus as being modest. Golgi studies are also in agreement with these findings (Lorente de Nó, 1933; Hauglie–Hanssen, 1968).

The experimental studies with silver impregnation techniques have not given evi-

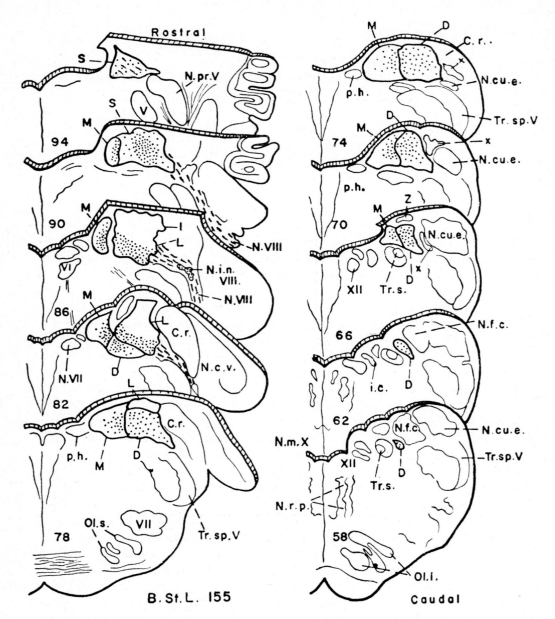

Fig. 1. Diagram showing the distribution of the primary vestibular fibers as seen in a series of transverse sections through the brain stem. From Walberg *et al.* (1958). Abbreviations: C.r., corpus restiforme; D, descending vestibular nucleus; D.A.S., dorsal acoustic stria; D.V.N., descending vestibular nucleus; i.c., nucleus intercalatus; L, lateral vestibular nucleus; L.V.N., lateral vestibular nucleus; l, small-celled group 1; M, medial vestibular nucleus; M.V.N., medial vestibular nucleus; N.c.v., ventral cochlear nucleus; N.cu.e., external cuneate nucleus; N.f.c., cuneate nucleus; N.i.n. VIII, interstitial nucleus of vestibular nerve; N.I.V., interstitial nucleus of vestibular nerve; N.pr.V, principal sensory nucleus of fifth nerve; N.VII, seventh nerve; N.VIII, vestibular nerve; O.C.B., olivo-cochlear bundle (efferent); Ol. i., inferior olive; Ol.s., oliva superior; P.C.N., posterior canal nerve fibers; p.h., nucleus praepositus hypoglossi; S.V.N., superior vestibular nucleus; Sacc. N., saccular nerve; Tr.s., tractus solitarius; Tr.sp. V, spinal tract of fifth nerve; Utric. N., utricular nerve; x, cell group x; z, cell group z; VII, nucleus of seventh nerve; XII, nucleus of twelfth nerve.

dence for primary vestibular fibers crossing the midline (Walberg *et al.*, 1958; Carpenter, 1960). Previous descriptions of such fibers (Leidler, 1914; Ingvar, 1918) are based on studies where additional damage to the vestibular nuclei appears to have occurred. The negative observations made in silver stained material agree with the findings made by Rasmussen (1932) in Marchi material. The physiological study by Shimazu and Precht (1966) supports these findings. The authors found no evidence for impulse transmission via primary fibers to the contralateral vestibular nuclei.

Although collaterals from the primary vestibular fibers to the reticular formation have been observed by Lorente de Nó (1933) and Hauglie–Hanssen (1968) in Golgi material, no evidence for such fibers was found experimentally (Walberg *et al.*, 1958). Carpenter (1960) claims that such fibers exist in the cat, and he describes primary vestibular fibers passing into and around the solitary fasciculus and its nucleus. His study on monkeys (1960) likewise gave evidence for degeneration in the solitary fasciculus, but the author suggests that this degeneration may be caused by interruption of fibers in the intermediate nerve. This can obviously explain his findings also in the cat. Carpenter (1960) found, however, no evidence that primary vestibular fibers ascend in the medial longitudinal fasciculus.

Since there are two types of receptor cells in the vestibular sensory epithelia (see Wersäll, 1972) the question may be raised whether the primary afferent fibers contacting them differ morphologically with regard to their mode of termination in the vestibular nuclei. Furthermore, it seems a likely assumption that fibers coming from different receptor areas may differ in their distribution within the vestibular nuclei. While little is known concerning the first subject, recent studies have brought forward some information concerning the second.

Lorente de Nó (1931) was the first to give a detailed description of the distribution of the primary vestibular fibers from the various cristae and maculae. His observations were based on Golgi sections, and he was able to identify the location of the ganglion cells related to the fibers from the various cristae and maculae. In a subsequent paper Lorente de Nó (1933) analyzed the distribution of the fibers derived from the various parts of the vestibular ganglion, and showed details in their distribution within the vestibular complex. Lorente de Nó's findings were made in the mouse. A correlation of his observations with the situation in the cat is difficult, since there are differences in the limitation of the nuclei in various species, and in nomenclature. However, it appears from Lorente de Nó's studies that fibers from the cristae terminate in the superior vestibular nucleus, the lateralmost part of the descending nucleus, and probably in the medial nucleus. The lateral vestibular nucleus appears to be free from such fibers. This nucleus receives fibers from the utricular macula, and these fibers are distributed to the ventral region of the nucleus. The fibers from the utricular macula in addition appear to supply the descending nucleus, and this region also receives fibers from the saccular macula. The conclusion emerging from these findings is, it appears, that even if fibers from the maculae and cristae in part have different representations within the vestibular complex, there is no clear selective distribution among the primary fibers.

The first experimental study where the problem of a selective distribution of the

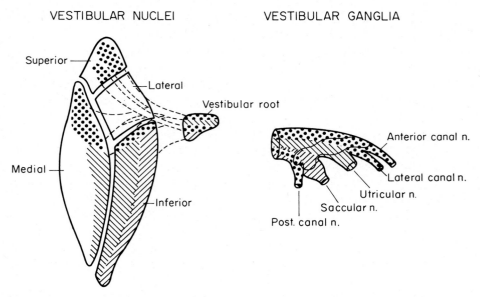

Fig. 2. Diagram showing the relationships between portions of the vestibular nerve and the various regions of the vestibular complex. For details, see text. Redrawn from Stein and Carpenter (1967).

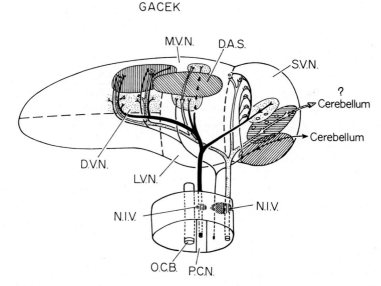

Fig. 3. Diagram showing the distribution of the nerve fibers from the semicircular canals to the various parts of the vestibular nuclei. Cp. text. Abbreviations, see Fig. 1. From Gacek (1969).

primary vestibular fibers has been attacked, is that by Stein and Carpenter (1967). They made small lesions in different parts of the vestibular ganglia in the monkey. and mapped the ensuing degeneration in the vestibular complex. They found that the fibers from the 3 cristae appear to terminate in the same regions, but that the fibers from the crista of the posterior canal pass in another branch of the nerve than do the fibers from the other canals. The fibers coming from the cristae of the semi-circular canals project primarily to the superior vestibular nucleus and to the rostral parts of the medial vestibular nucleus (Fig. 2). The findings indicate that there is a partially different distribution of the fibers from the individual canals within the total area, especially within the superior nucleus. The fibers from the macula of the utricle project primarily to parts of the medial and descending vestibular nucleus, and fibers from the saccular macula project preferentially to the dorsolateral part of the descending vestibular nucleus. The authors had difficulties in finding a projection to the lateral vestibular nucleus. They found, however, that some fibers from the utricle gave off collaterals to the ventral part of Deiters' nucleus. They stress that it is difficult to make a lesion of the utricular part of the ganglion, and that this may explain the scanty projection to the lateral nucleus. They also refer to the previous study (Carpenter, 1960), in which it was shown that medial fibers of the vestibular root projected to the medial and ventral part of the lateral vestibular nucleus. An additional reason for the scanty distribution to the lateral nucleus, may be the fact that there are species differences, and that fibers to the nucleus of Deiters are sparse in the monkey. It is of interest that Stein and Carpenter (1967) found that all receptor regions project to the interstitial nucleus of the vestibular nerve, and that there appears to be a differential distribution within this small cell group. This nucleus may thus be the only part of the vestibular complex which receives fibers from all receptor regions.

Gacek (1969) recently made a study of the course and central termination of the fibers coming from different parts of the vestibular apparatus in the cat following small, isolated lesions of various parts of the vestibular ganglion. Gacek's study is of considerable interest, since it is the most detailed investigation of this problem hitherto done.

Gacek finds that the neurons supplying the cristae have their fibers in the rostral two-thirds of the vestibular nerve, those coming from the maculae occupy the caudal portion. Furthermore, the neurons from the *cristae* after giving off collaterals to the interstitial nucleus of Cajal, proceed into the brain stem where the axons bifurcate into an ascending and a descending branch. The ascending branch terminates in the superior vestibular nucleus and in the cerebellum, while the descending branch passes medially into the lateral, medial and descending vestibular nucleus (Fig. 3).

The ascending branches of the *utricular* neurons terminate in the rostroventral part of the lateral vestibular nucleus, and in the rostral part of the medial vestibular nucleus. Their descending branches give off collaterals to the caudal part of the medial vestibular nucleus and the rostral part of the descending vestibular nucleus. The author found no projection from the maculae to the interstitial nucleus of Cajal or to the superior vestibular nucleus. The fibers coming from the saccular macula projected mainly to the cell-group y and to a lesser extent to the lateral and descending vestibular nuclei (Fig. 4).

Large and small diameter nerve fibers were found in all vestibular nerve branches, but a separate central localization in the nerve was found for neurons supplying the posterior canal crista, as opposed to those supplying the cristae of the superior and

GACEK

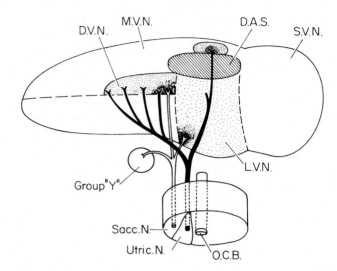

Fig. 4. Diagram showing the distribution of the nerve fibers from the macular regions to the various parts of the vestibular nuclei. Cp. text. Abbreviations, see Fig. 1. From Gacek (1969).

horizontal canals. Gacek found, furthermore, that in Nauta sections the large calibre fibers terminating in the superior vestibular nucleus were distributed around large cells in the centre of the nucleus, while the small diameter fibers ended more peripherally in the same nucleus, where small cells predominate. He suggests that such findings indicate different functional properties for type I and type II vestibular hair cells.

The findings referred to here are partly at variance with those made by Stein and Carpenter (1967) in the monkey. The details given by Gacek are very interesting, and it would be of great importance to study this projection with the electron microscope. Such studies will be necessary before definite conclusions concerning details in the synaptological arrangements of the fibers from the vestibular ganglion can be drawn. Such studies would likewise be of great interest for physiological investigations.

Our experimental light microscopical study (Walberg et al., 1958) revealed that following lesions of the entire nerve in the cat in the Nauta sections, argyrophilic particles were aggregated in small clusters, often lying far apart. This finding led us to the conclusion that the spatial distribution of a single axon is rather restricted. This fits well with the results of a later Golgi study (Hauglie–Hanssen, 1968), in which it was shown that the ascending and descending branches of the primary vestibular fibers give off collaterals directed medially. These collaterals again give off numerous short side branches. Each side branch shows small thickenings, presumably boutons, along its course and its ends, and tiny varicosities are also seen along the collaterals. Due to the parallel course of the collaterals and the side branches the terminal fields of these fibers will be rather narrow zones extending from lateral to medial. This arrangement would favour a spatially precise transmission of impulses from the vestibular receptors to the vestibular nuclei. Details in this arrangement have been considered by Brodal (1972).

The Golgi study of Hauglie–Hanssen (1968) revealed further details. The terminal and preterminal branches of afferent fibers to the nuclear complex were shown to differ morphologically, and they were divided into 3 types. Fibers of types 2 and 3 were often found to climb along the soma and dendrites of the cells. However, Hauglie–Hanssen was not able to find that one contingent of afferents was provided with only one type of terminals. Cajal (1896, 1909) concluded that the pericellular baskets in the nucleus of Deiters were formed by collaterals of primary vestibular fibers. The findings made by Hauglie–Hanssen (1968), however, show that this view is scarcely tenable. His findings indicate that particularly the cerebello-vestibular fibers partici-pate in the formation of the baskets. His observations thus make it clear, that the baskets seen in Golgi preparations in the vestibular nuclei probably represent a generalized mode of organization of terminal axons related to proximal dendrites and the soma of cells.

Although Walberg et al. (1958) made a detailed mapping of the distribution of argyrophilic particles and fragmented fibers as this appears in the light microscope, electron microscopy is necessary before final conclusions can be drawn concerning synaptic relationships. The experimental electron microscopical study by Mugnaini et al. (1967) confirmed the distribution of the primary vestibular fibers observed in the light microscope and in addition gave ultrastructural details of synaptology. The study was limited to the lateral vestibular nucleus, and revealed that the de-

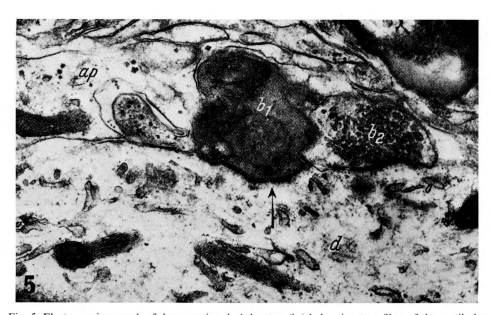

Fig. 5. Electron micrograph of degenerating dark bouton (b_1) belonging to a fiber of the vestibular nerve. The degenerating bouton has at the arrow a synapse with a dendrite (d) of a small cell. A normal bouton (b_2) is present adjacent to the degenerating one. ap, astrocytic process. The survival time for this cat was 3 days. $\times$ 28 000. From Mugnaini et al. (1967).

generating primary vestibular fibers react with the dark type of degeneration, that is, the fibers and boutons are electron dense from the onset of degeneration (Fig. 5). The reaction can be recognized as early as two days following transection of the nerve. The degenerating boutons are very characteristic. The matrix has a dark granular appearance, in which the fragmenting mitochondria and synaptic vesicles gradually become invisible. The changes proceed very rapidly, and practically all degenerating boutons are removed after 9 to 11 days of survival. The astroglial and microglial cells take part in the process of removal, and it is interesting that only the microglial cells appear to digest the included material. The speed of the process is in great contrast to what has been found for the speed of degeneration of the cerebellovestibular fibers (see below). A correlation with normal ultrastructure was difficult, but the degenerating boutons appeared to belong to the round type of boutons present in normal material (Mugnaini *et al.*, 1967).

This experimental electron microscopical study revealed furthermore, that the primary vestibular fibers contact cell bodies as well as thick and thin dendrites. An important conclusion was also that some giant cells as well as smaller cells received afferent fibers. This conclusion was in contrast to what had been said in the previous light microscopical study (Walberg *et al.*, 1958), and is a good example of the previously mentioned fact that electron microscopy is essential for decisive conclusions concerning synaptical contacts. Since no quantitative estimates were done in the experimental electron microscopical study it could not be decided whether small or giant cells are most amply supplied with primary vestibular fibers. Furthermore, since parent cells of thin dendritic profiles can not be identified in electron micrographs, we were unable to make conclusions as regards such dendrites. Small dendritic profiles were amply contacted by boutons of primary vestibular fibers.

I will not here enter upon a discussion about the probable significance of rounded versus flattened or cylindrical synaptic vesicles (for a recent review, see Walberg, 1968). Nevertheless, it is important to stress that where synaptic vesicles could be identified in degenerating boutons, these were often of the flattened type. However, it has been shown (see, for example Holländer *et al.*, 1969) that round synaptic vesicles may acquire a flattened shape in degenerating boutons. No functional implications can therefore be made from the finding that degenerating axon terminals of primary vestibular fibers can have flattened vesicles. Another finding to be mentioned, is that the synapses established by the boutons of the fibers were of the symmetrical as well as of the asymmetrical type, and that spines as well as smooth parts of the cell surface were contacted by terminals of the afferent fibers.

Physiological studies are in good agreement with the anatomical observations as regards the distribution of primary vestibular fibers, but they will not be considered here. However, it is remarkable and comforting, that the physiological observations agree so well with the morphological ones. The important contributions by Wilson and co-workers, by Ito and collaborators, and by Shimazu and Precht, are good examples of this. Peterson has lately added new knowledge to a detailed understanding of the function of the vestibular receptors in systematic studies, where tilting of the animals has been the physiological stimulus. These and other physiological studies represent a challenge for anatomists to reveal further details in morphology, especially concerning the intrinsic organization of the nuclear complex. One important question to reconsider would be the eventual distribution of internuncial cells of the Golgi II type in the various nuclei. Although Hauglie–Hanssen (1968) found little evidence for their existence, modifications of the Golgi method might in the future give the student a greater possibility to map short-axon cells. Negative findings in Golgi material obviously do not allow decisive statements.

SUMMARY

A review is given of the distribution and termination of the primary vestibular fibers. Light microscopical studies with silver methods have shown that the fibers of the nerve are not given off to the entire territory of each single nucleus, but that they terminate only in circumscribed areas of the various regions of the complex. Experimental electron microscopical investigations have, furthermore, revealed that the fibers of the nerve reach large as well as small cells in the nuclei, and that synaptic contacts are established with all parts of the postsynaptic neurons. Reference is also made to recent Golgi studies which show that the spatial distribution of a single axon is rather restricted. Such an arrangement would favor a precise transmission of impulses from the vestibular receptors to the vestibular nuclei. Other details in the distribution of the nerve fibers are also considered.

REFERENCES

BRODAL, A. (1972) Some features in the anatomical organization of the vestibular nuclear complex in the cat. In A. BRODAL AND O. POMPEIANO (Eds.), *Progress in Brain Research. Vol. 37. Basic aspects of central vestibular mechanisms*. Elsevier, Amsterdam, pp. 31–53.

BRODAL, A. AND HØIVIK, B. (1964) Site and mode of termination of primary vestibulocerebellar fibres in the cat. An experimental study with silver impregnation methods. *Arch. ital. Biol.*, **102**, 1–21.

CAJAL, RAMON Y, S. (1896) *Beitrag zum Studium der Medulla oblongata, des Kleinhirns und des Ursprungs der Gehirnnerven*. Barth, Leipzig, pp. 139.

CAJAL, RAMON Y, S. (1909) *Histologie du Système Nerveux de l'Homme et des Vertébrés*. Maloine, Paris.

CARPENTER, M. B. (1960) Experimental anatomical–physiological studies of the vestibular nerve and cerebellar connections. In G. L. RASMUSSEN AND W. WINDLE (Eds.), *Neural Mechanisms of the Auditory and Vestibular Systems*. Thomas, Springfield, Ill., pp. 297–323.

GACEK, R. (1969) The course and central termination of first order neurons supplying vestibular end organs in the cat. *Acta oto-laryng. (Stockh.)*, Suppl. 254, 1–66.

GLEES, P. (1946) Terminal degeneration within the central nervous system as studied by a new silver method. *J. Neuropath. exp. Neurol.*, **5**, 54–59.

HAUGLIE–HANSSEN, E. (1968) Intrinsic neuronal organization of the vestibular nuclear complex in the cat. A Golgi study. *Ergebn. Anat. Entwickl.-Gesch.*, **40/5**, 1–105.

HOLLÄNDER, H., BRODAL, P. AND WALBERG, F. (1969) Electronmicroscopic observations on the structure of the pontine nuclei and the mode of termination of the corticopontine fibres. An experimental study in the cat. *Exp. Brain Res.*, **7**, 95–110.

INGVAR, S. (1918) Zur Phylo- und Ontogenese des Kleinhirns nebst einem Versuche zu einheitlicher Erklärung der zerebellaren Funktion und Lokalisation. *Folia neuro-biol. (Lpz.)*, **11**, 205–495.

LEIDLER, R. (1914) Experimentelle Untersuchungen über das Endigungsgebiet des Nervus vestibularis. 2. Mitteilung. *Arb. neurol. Inst. Univ. Wien*, **21**, 151–212.

LORENTE DE NÓ, R. (1931) Ausgewählte Kapitel aus der vergleichenden Physiologie des Labyrinthes. Die Augenmuskelreflexe beim Kaninchen und ihre Grundlage. *Ergebn. Physiol.*, **32**, 73–242.

LORENTE DE NÓ, R. (1933) Anatomy of the eighth nerve. The central projection of the nerve endings of the internal ear. *Laryngoscope (St. Louis)*, **43**, 1–38.

MUGNAINI, E. AND WALBERG, F. (1967) An experimental electron microscopical study on the mode of termination of cerebellar corticovestibular fibres in the cat lateral vestibular nucleus (Deiters' nucleus). *Exp. Brain Res.*, **4**, 212–236.

MUGNAINI, E., WALBERG, F. AND BRODAL, A. (1967) Mode of termination of primary vestibular fibres in the lateral vestibular nucleus. An experimental electron microscopical study in the cat, *Exp. Brain Res.*, **4**, 187–211.

NAUTA, W. J. H. (1957) Silver impregnation of degenerating axons. In W. F. WINDLE (Ed.), *New Research Techniques of Neuroanatomy*. Thomas, Springfield, Ill., pp. 17–26.

RASMUSSEN, A. T. (1932) Secondary vestibular tracts in the cat. *J. comp. Neurol.*, **54**, 143–171.

SHIMAZU, H. AND PRECHT, W. (1966) Inhibition of central vestibular neurons from the contralateral labyrinth and its mediating pathway. *J. Neurophysiol.*, **29**, 467–492.

STEIN, B. M. AND CARPENTER, M. B. (1967) Central projections of portions of the vestibular ganglia innervating specific parts of the labyrinth in the rhesus monkey. *Amer. J. Anat.*, **120**, 281–318.

WALBERG, F. (1968) Morphological correlates of postsynaptic inhibitory processes. In C. VON EULER, S. SKOGLUND AND U. SÖDERBERG (Eds.), *Structure and Function of Inhibitory Neuronal Mechanisms*. Pergamon Press, Oxford, pp. 7–14.

WALBERG, F., BOWSHER, D. AND BRODAL, A. (1958) The termination of primary vestibular fibers in the vestibular nuclei in the cat. An experimental study with silver methods. *J. comp. Neurol.*, **110**, 391–419.

WERSÄLL, J., (1972) Morphology of the vestibular receptors in mammals. In A. BRODAL AND O. POMPEIANO (Eds.), *Progress in Brain Research. Vol. 37. Basic aspects of central vestibular mechanisms*, Elsevier, Amsterdam, pp. 3–17.

Responses of Vestibular Nuclear Neurons to Ampullar Input

W. PRECHT AND R. LLINÁS

Max-Planck-Institute for Brain Research, Frankfurt a.M., G.F.R. and Division of Neurobiology,
Department of Physiology and Biophysics, University of Iowa, Iowa City, Iowa, U.S.A.

In all vertebrates 3 semicircular canals are present in each labyrinth. They are oriented in such a way that they approximately represent the 3 dimensions of space. Receptor cells—the sensory hair cells—are located in the ampulla of each canal and their cilia are embedded in a gelatinous structure, the cupula, which follows the movement of the endolymph thereby causing the cilia of the receptor cells to deviate in one or the other direction depending on the direction of the angular acceleration. It has been shown that the primary vestibular fibers of fish which supply the sensory hair cells of the semicircular canals are bidirectionally sensitive to rotation provided that they show spontaneous activity (Lowenstein and Sand, 1940a, b). In the case of the horizontal semicircular canal, by far the best studied canal system, the frequency of firing increases during ipsilateral angular acceleration (utriculopetal cupula movement) and decreases during opposite rotation (utriculofugal deviation) (Lowenstein and Sand, 1940 a, b). The converse, *i.e.*, an increase in firing frequency on utriculofugal cupula movement and a decrease in utriculopetal deviation is found in the vertical canals (Lowenstein, 1956; Trincker, 1957). These electrophysiological data were consistent with the conclusions obtained by direct stimulation of the semicircular canals (Ewald, 1892; Szentágothai, 1950) and were found in general to be in agreement with the torsion pendulum theory of the cupula–endolymph system (Steinhausen, 1931, 1933; van Egmond *et al.*, 1949; Groen *et al.*, 1952). Recent studies on the frog have confirmed and expanded the earlier data obtained in fish and have added to the knowledge of the dynamic characteristics of horizontal canal fibers (Precht *et al.*, 1971). Unfortunately, in no species has there been done a complete study of both the responses of the primary fibers and the response characteristics of vestibular neurons which would allow us to compare first and second order systems. Since the study of the frog vestibular nerve fibers has been performed using similar stimulating procedures as in the case of the second order vestibular neurons of the cat (Shimazu and Precht, 1965) a brief description of their response characteristics will, therefore, precede the description of the response patterns of the second order vestibular neurons.

MODULATION OF THE DISCHARGE FREQUENCY OF FROG'S VESTIBULAR NERVE FIBERS IN RESPONSE TO ACCELERATION AND VELOCITY STEPS

The microelectrode recordings to be described here were obtained for the most part

from the anterior branch of the VIII nerve or its proximal continuation, where
many fibers were found to respond to horizontal angular accelerations. Stimulating
and recording techniques are fully described elsewhere (Precht *et al.*, 1971). The
overwhelming majority of the units which showed a distinct response to rotation
increased their discharge frequencies during angular acceleration to the side of the
recording electrode (ipsilateral rotation) and/or following a sudden arrest of the turntable after it has been rotating in the contralateral direction at constant angular
velocity for some time. Contralateral angular acceleration or sudden arrest after
ipsilateral rotation at constant velocity produced a cessation of the resting discharge,
provided that such form of firing was present in the unit under study. Nerve fibers that
showed responses different from the ones described above are described in the paper
on the efferent vestibular system (see Llinás and Precht, 1972).

The problem of vestibular adaptation. Since angular acceleration is regarded as an
adequate stimulus for semicircular canal receptors, a protracted period of constant
acceleration should be applied in order to determine whether there is any frequency
adaptation. In the present experiment it was found that approximately 35% of the
fibers from the horizontal canal did not show any significant adaptation. This is
exemplified by the frequency plots of a primary fiber illustrated in Fig. 1. In each of
the diagrams the frequency of discharge increased along an approximately exponential
time course and reached maximal values whose levels were dependent on the rate of
acceleration applied. The maximum level of discharge was maintained constant during
the remainder of the acceleration. On termination of the acceleration, *i.e.*, after the

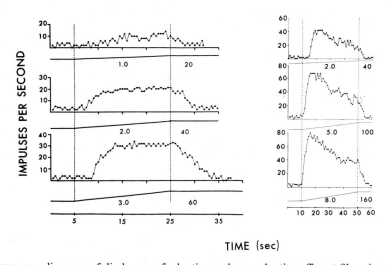

TIME (sec)

Fig. 1. Frequency diagrams of discharges of adapting and non-adapting afferent fibers in response to
ipsilateral constant angular accelerations. In each diagram the ordinate represents spikes per sec of
single unit discharges measured in each half-second. Onset of acceleration is indicated by left vertical
broken line, and cessation of acceleration (or beginning of constant velocity rotation) by the right
vertical broken line. The line below each frequency diagram indicates velocity of rotation. The left-
hand number in each diagram indicates the acceleration rate, and the right-hand number the velocity
of constant rotation. From Precht *et al.* (1971).

onset of constant velocity of rotation, the discharge frequencies returned to control levels. The presence of a considerable number of non-adapting fibers in the frog VIII nerve should be emphasized, particularly since Ledoux's (1949, 1961) data would tend to suggest the opposite.

In approximately 65% of the afferent fibers studied a distinct frequency adaptation during constant angular acceleration was noted. This kind of response pattern is illustrated by the frequency plots of the right-hand diagram in Fig. 1. In each of the frequency diagrams of this figure, a frequency decline was noted in response to different rates of accelerations applied for periods of 20 sec. The magnitude of the response decline varied from unit to unit, ranging from barely visible adaptation to complete return to the level of resting discharge. Adapting and non-adapting units have further been tested by applying two acceleration steps sequentially. Linear addition of the responses was observed in non-adapting units whereas the adapting units were characterized by lack of summation of superimposed acceleration steps (Precht et al., 1971). It is important, however, to emphasize that the linearity of the response which relates to the monotonic relationship between the amplitude of the stimulus and the magnitude of the response, does not seem to be correlated with the presence or absence of adaptation.

Frequency increase and magnitude of stimulation. As illustrated in Fig. 1 a relationship exists between the magnitude of acceleration and maximal frequency increase of a given fiber. A total of 49 horizontal canal fibers was individually tested with 4–6 different rates of acceleration (varying from $0.2–10°/sec^2$). The average resting discharge was determined before the onset of each stimulation and was subtracted from the average of the peak frequency value produced by a given acceleration step. This value was plotted against the acceleration of 49 fibers studied in that manner, 30 units showed a non-linear relationship between frequency increase and acceleration. Examples of 4 of such fibers are illustrated in the right-hand diagram of Fig. 2 where the frequency increases are plotted against the logarithmic scale of acceleration. In 19 units, on the other hand, an approximately linear relation has been obtained between frequency increase and rate of acceleration. Examples of 3 such fibers are illustrated

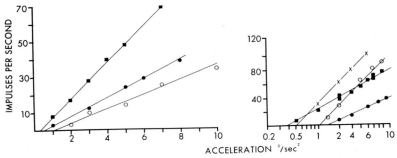

Fig. 2. Relation between angular acceleration and maximum frequency increase of afferent fibers. In each of the diagrams, regression lines connect the points obtained from a single fiber by subtracting the resting discharge from the average of the maximum frequency increase. Note semilogarithmic plot of right-hand diagram. From Precht *et al.* (1971).

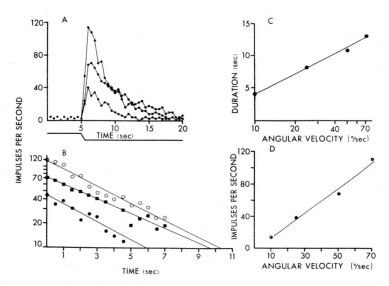

Fig. 3. Frequency diagrams of linear afferent fiber in response to velocity steps and relation between rate of velocity and duration of responses. A ,Responses of single fiber to velocity steps ('impulses') of varying magnitudes (25°/sec, 50°/sec, 70°/sec). Onset of cessation of rotation is indicated by deflection of curve below the diagram. B, Semilogarithmic plot of impulse frequencies of falling phases of the curves shown in A. Filled circles refer to the lower, square symbols to the middle, and open circles to the upper curve shown in A. C, Semilogarithmic plot of duration of responses against velocity steps of various magnitudes. D, Relation between rate of angular velocity and maximum increase of frequency of single unit discharge. From Precht *et al.* (1971).

in the left-hand diagram of Fig. 2 where the frequency increase was plotted against the linear scale of acceleration. Input–output diagrams of single afferent fibers were also obtained by applying velocity steps. Examples of such diagrams are shown for a linear unit in Fig. 3D. The gradients of the regression lines of the units shown in Fig. 2 varied over a relatively wide range, indicating that the responsiveness of afferent fibers to acceleration of the same magnitude shows considerable differences. No clear relationship existed between the level of resting discharge and the gradient of the regression lines as it was the case for second order vestibular neurons of the cat (see below).

The points where the regression lines cross the abscissae in Fig. 2 approximately indicate the threshold for the frequency increase in each fiber. Threshold values for afferent fibers ranged from 0.3 to 2.5°/sec^2 with a peak between 0.5 and 1.5°/sec^2. These values are well within the range found in central vestibular neurons of higher vertebrates (see below).

TIME COURSE OF RESPONSES OF FIBERS TO ACCELERATION AND VELOCITY STEPS

At resting condition, many vestibular afferents showed spontaneous firing that varied between 2 and 35 impulses/sec. The majority of these units, however, were firing with a rate below 15/sec. Some units remained silent over the whole period studied. Since it is obviously much more difficult to detect silent neurons, a numerical comparison between tonic and silent fibers does not appear to be a reliable index of the true population of these two types. This study has not revealed any significant differences between these two types of fibers as far as their response characteristics to rotation are concerned (compare, however, the differences found in second order neurons as described below). They will, therefore, be treated as one group in this section.

The linear unit in Fig. 1 (left hand diagram) illustrates plots of the afferent fiber impulse frequencies during different rates of ipsilateral horizontal angular acceleration. As shown in each of these diagrams, the discharge frequencies increase along an approximately exponential time course to a peak value. Generally, the time interval between onset of rotation and commencement of frequency increase is directly related to the magnitude of acceleration, although exceptions to this rule are seen (Fig. 1, middle and lower diagrams). After attaining constant velocity of rotation, the discharge frequency decayed along an approximately exponential time course (Fig. 1). The time constants of the increasing (Fig. 5B) and decreasing phase in response to acceleration steps of various magnitudes and those of the decaying phase following velocity steps were approximately the same for a given linear unit (Precht *et al.*, 1971). Similarly, the time constants of the falling phase of the frequency plots of a given unit after velocity step stimulation (Fig. 3A) of various magnitudes were similar (3.7, 4.0, and 3.3 sec from the top to the bottom in the plots of Fig. 3B). As one would expect from previous investigations (Ledoux, 1958), the durations of the responses of single fibers to velocity steps of different magnitudes are proportional to the logarithm of the angular velocity as shown in Fig. 3C.

In Fig. 4 are shown the frequency diagrams of an afferent fiber that is characterized by a non-linear acceleration frequency relationship. There is a marked difference in the time course of the rising phases of the frequency increases to constant acceleration as compared to linear units. In order to allow a comparison between the properly determined time constants of linear units, in non-linear units the time that was necessary to reach 63% of the average peak frequencies was measured in the linear range and the values were adopted as a rough approximation of the time constant. These values are combined with the time constants of linear units in the histogram of Fig. 5A. The majority of the fibers have a time constant of about 3 sec. Fig. 5B compares the time constants of linear units with the apparent 'time constants' of non-linear units beyond their linear range. As expected, the time constants of linear units did not change with different rates of acceleration (broken lines), whereas the apparent 'time constants' of the non-linear units showed considerably smaller values with increasing stimulation (Fig. 5B).

The experimental finding that the time constants of vestibular nerve fibers of the frog show considerable variations (Fig. 5A) indicates that this variation in the dynamic properties of vestibular fibers is either caused by different receptor properties in the semicircular canal or by different electrophysiological properties of the peripheral afferent terminals. Since morphologically only one type of hair cell has been found in the frog (Hillman, 1969) it is more likely that differences in the transduction–encoder

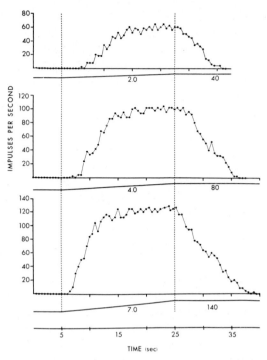

Fig. 4. Frequency diagrams of afferent fiber in response to horizontal angular accelerations showing decrease of 'time constant' with increasing acceleration. Arrangement of diagrammatic representation is the same as in Fig. 1. From Precht *et al.* (1971).

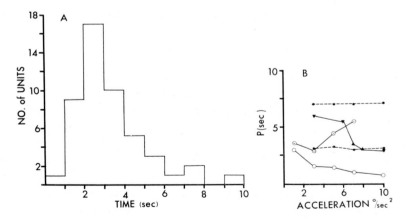

Fig. 5. Time constants of frequency responses of afferent fibers to ipsilateral horizontal angular acceleration. A, Histogram of time constants of responses of fibers to constant horizontal angular acceleration measured in the linear range of the units. B, Relation between acceleration rate and time constants for different fibers. Broken lines connect points obtained from two linear units. Open circles and triangles represent measurement of time constants of rising phases obtained from two non-linear units. Note decrease of 'time constant' as acceleration rate increases. Dotted circles show the time constant of the falling phase of same unit whose time constant of the rising phase is illustrated by open circles. From Precht *et al.* (1971).

system of the terminals account for the variation in time constants of different afferents. As for the functional meaning of such variations it has been suggested that fibers having rather short time constants to a step input may simulate acceleration channels, while fibers characterized by long time constants represent velocity channels (Precht *et al.*, 1971). The disparities of afferent fibers in the frog horizontal canal system and the second order vestibular neurons of cat (see below) can be so significant that the mechanical properties of a torsion pendulum model cannot be derived from their activity. All models of the cupula–endolymph system, however, are based either on single or mass activity recordings from the VIII nerve (Groen *et al.*, 1952; Ledoux, 1958) or on recordings of vestibular evoked eye movements (Young, 1969).

RESPONSES OF CAT'S SECOND ORDER VESTIBULAR NEURONS TO ANGULAR ACCELERATION AND ELECTRICAL STIMULATION

Numerous anatomical studies have contributed to the present knowledge of the histological organization of the vestibular nuclei and the distribution of primary fibers in various subdivisions of this voluminous nuclear complex in the brain stem (for details, see Brodal *et al.* (1962) and Walberg (1972). Similarly, physiological studies of the vestibular input to the vestibular nuclei during the last few decades have greatly advanced our knowledge of the functional aspects of the vestibular nuclei and their neurons. In this paper we shall briefly summarize the data that have been obtained from single vestibular units on natural and electrical stimulation of the semicircular canals. Their responses to natural stimulation will be described first and this description will be followed by a brief review of the synaptology of the vestibular neurons as revealed by electrical stimulation of the VIII nerve.

Responses of single vestibular neurons to angular acceleration. Adrian (1943) was the first to record from individual neurons in the vestibular nuclei of the cat, *i.e.*, from secondary vestibular units. Moreover, his experiments were the first ones to be performed on central vestibular neurons. The majority of the neurons responding to rotation give persistent low-frequency discharges when the head is at rest (Fig. 6), while a smaller number of neurons is characterized by a complete lack of resting discharge (Fig. 6). With the horizontal canal in plane of rotation, ipsilateral rotation (utriculopetal endolymph movement) increases the discharge frequency of the vestibular unit whereas contralateral angular acceleration (utriculofugal endolymph movement) decreases its resting discharge. Thus, the second order neurons respond qualitatively the same way as has been described for primary vestibular neurons of the horizontal canal in the earlier part of this paper. This response pattern will be called type-I as designated by Gernandt (1949) and Duensing and Schaefer (1958). Their studies on central vestibular neurons of the horizontal canal system have confirmed Adrian's (1943) observation that the majority of the units showed type-I responses.

However, it was found that in addition to type-I responses several other response patterns could be recorded. Among them are the type-II neurons originally described by Duensing and Schaefer (1958) which increase and decrease their firing rate in a way just opposite to type-I, *i.e.*, a decrease in firing occurs on ipsilateral rotation and an

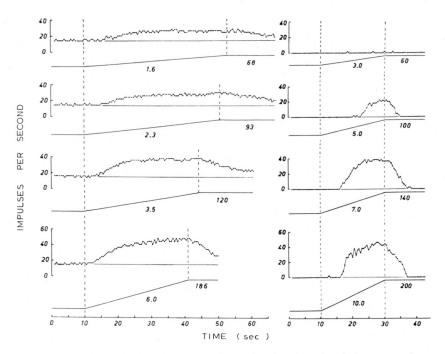

Fig. 6. Frequency diagrams of discharges of a tonic and a kinetic type-I vestibular neuron in response to ipsilateral, horizontal, constant angular accelerations. The plane of the stereotaxic frame was inclined 30° upward from the horizontal position, such that the horizontal semicircular canals are approximately in a horizontal position. In each diagram, the ordinate represents spike per sec of single unit discharges measured in each half-second. The horizontal line in each diagram represents the average frequency over 10 sec before rotation. Onset of rotation is indicated by the left vertical broken line in each diagram, and cessation of acceleration (or beginning of constant velocity rotation) by the right vertical broken line. Curve below each frequency diagram indicates the velocity of rotation. The left-hand number in each diagram indicates the acceleration rate (degree/sec²) and the right-hand number indicates the velocity (degree/sec). From Shimazu and Precht (1965).

increase in discharge frequency is observed on contralateral rotation. Fig. 7 illustrates the time course of a type-II vestibular neuron in response to ipsilateral (A) and contra-lateral (B) acceleration and deceleration. It has been shown by Shimazu and Precht (1966) that type-II neurons receive their input exclusively from the contralateral laby-rinth via the commissural fiber system. This finding easily explains their response pattern. Details of this commissural system and its functional implications are des-cribed by Shimazu (1972) in this volume. Parenthetically, it should be mentioned that some of the type-II responses persisted even after the contralateral labyrinth had been destroyed. Although the functional organization leading to this kind of type-II response is not known yet, it may be tentatively suggested that the horizontal semi-circular canal input—the only one being stimulated in the present situation—activates some inhibitory interneurons which in turn would cause the suppression of the type-II neuron on ipsilateral rotation. This hypothesis would imply that type-II represents a second order neuron of an end organ other than the horizontal canal. Its suppression

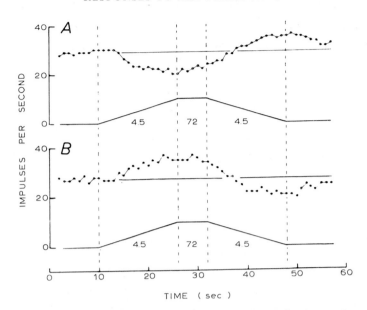

Fig. 7. Frequency diagrams of discharges of a type-II vestibular neuron in response to constant angular acceleration and deceleration in unanesthetized, decerebrate cat. A, Ipsilateral rotation. B, Contralateral rotation. Ordinate represents spikes per sec. The horizontal line in each diagram represents the average frequency before rotation. Broken vertical lines indicate, from left to right, the onset and cessation of acceleration and those of deceleration. Acceleration and deceleration rates were 4.5°/sec² and constant speed of rotation after acceleration was 72°/sec.

during ipsilateral rotation may be functionally related to a mechanism known as lateral inhibition as suggested by Shimazu and Precht (1966). Besides type-I and type-II vestibular neurons which are the frequently found units, several investigators have observed neurons that increase their firing rate on ipsi- and contralateral acceleration (type-III) and others which cease to fire on rotation in both directions (type IV) (Gernandt, 1949; Eckel, 1954; Duensing and Schaefer, 1958; Shimazu and Precht, 1965). At present, no further data are available on the functional mechanisms causing these response patterns. It is interesting to note that type-III neurons are also activated by stimuli other than labyrinthine (somato-sensory and occasionally acoustical stimulation) and they may, therefore, be of importance for sensory convergence in the vestibular nuclei. As for their projection the only region known so far is the spinal cord (Precht et al., 1967). There is a possibility that some of the type-III neurons may be efferent vestibular neurons projecting to the hair-cells since in the frog such kind of responses have been recorded in the eighth nerve (Precht et al., 1971).

Unlike the horizontal canal influences, the effects of vertical canal stimulation on vestibular neurons have not been studied in great detail. As mentioned above, in the vertical semicircular canals utriculofugal endolymph movements are accompanied by an increase in discharge frequency of primary afferents whereas utriculopetal deviation of the cupula causes a decrease of the resting discharge. Thus, the vertical canals show just the opposite polarity, as compared to the horizontal canals. Corresponding frequency changes of neurons on vertical canal stimulation have been observed by Adrian (1943) and Duensing and Schaefer (1959). Markham (1968) has studied the effect of angular acceleration on central vestibular neurons when the vertical canals were in the plane of rotation. Since the anterior canal on one side is approximately in the same plane as the posterior canal on the other side, any attempt to bring one of them in the plane of a horizontally rotating table will result in placing both of them in this plane. By recording from the side where the anterior canal was in plane of rotation, it was found that most units increased their resting discharge during utriculofugal endolymph flow in this canal and decreased by utriculopetal flow. These neurons may represent the second order neurons of the anterior canal. Similar to the horizontal canal system, adequate stimulation of the anterior canal reveals a group of neurons responding in a way opposite to the one just described. It is very likely that these neurons receive their main excitatory input from the contralateral posterior canal which is also in plane of rotation (Markham, 1968). Thus, they are similar to the type-II neurons of the horizontal canals which receive their input from the opposite side (Shimazu and Precht, 1966) and which exert an inhibitory action on the main second order neurons. Neurons increasing their discharge rate to rotation in both directions have also been recorded (Markham, 1968). It was noted that vertical units in general have higher thresholds for frequency increase during angular acceleration, as compared to the horizontal canal units, a finding which is in agreement with the higher threshold of vertical nystagmus reported by Decher (1963). Furthermore, it appears that the number of units responding to vertical canal stimulation is smaller than the one responding to excitation of the horizontal canals (type-I neurons). This may be related to the finding that the muscle tension developed by stimulation of the anterior canal nerve is smaller, as in the case of stimulation of the horizontal canal nerve (Suzuki and Cohen, 1966). Histological checking of the recording points showed that the second order neurons of the semicircular canals are mainly found in the superior and medial vestibular nuclei (Shimazu and Precht, 1965; Markham, 1968). This location is in good agreement with anatomical studies showing the differential projection of the various labyrinthine receptor organs in the vestibular nuclei (Lorente de Nó, 1933; Stein and Carpenter, 1967; Gazek, 1969).

Mode of increase and decrease in discharge frequency. At present a quantitative description of the response characteristics of central vestibular neurons can only be presented for type I neurons of the horizontal canal system. A detailed description of their dynamic characteristics has been given by Shimazu and Precht (1965) and, therefore, only a brief review will be presented here. In Fig. 6 (left column) are plotted the serial changes of impulse frequencies of a tonic type-I vestibular neuron caused by ipsilateral rotations at different rates of accelerations. When the turntable was rotated in the ipsilateral direction with long-lasting constant angular acceleration, the discharge frequency initially increased along an approximately exponential time course and then maintained a fairly constant value during the remainder of the acceleration. After reaching constant velocity of rotation, the frequency decreased gradually to the level of the resting discharge. Nystagmic modulation of the frequency was rarely observed in decerebrate, unanesthetized animals, but it was present in intact animals under light ether anesthesia (Duensing and Schaefer, 1958).

Besides the tonically active type-I neurons, there is another group of type-I units which shows no resting discharge, the kinetic type-I neuron according to Shimazu and Precht (1965). As shown in Fig. 6 (right-hand diagrams) this type of neuron responds to ipsilateral rotation along an exponential time course after a remarkable long latency and rapidly reaches its maximum frequency. The decay in frequency after reaching constant velocity of rotation is equally steep. In comparing the time constants of tonic and kinetic neurons it was found that the former have significantly longer time constants (8.1 ± 1.6 sec) as compared to the latter (3.7 ± 0.8 sec).

Frequency increase and magnitude of stimulation. As can be seen in Fig. 6, there is a relationship between rates of acceleration and the peak frequencies. In Fig. 8 (right-hand diagram), the maximum frequency increases at different rates of accelerations are plotted for several units against the logarithm of angular acceleration. Each series of points, calculated from records of a given type-I neuron during various rates of acceleration, appears to be distributed along a straight line within a range of 0.5–$10°/$ sec^2 of acceleration. Thus, for most of the second order vestibular (44 out of 46) neurons a non-linear input–output relationship has been observed. This finding is somewhat different from the ratio of non-linear versus linear in the primary neuron of the frog (see above).

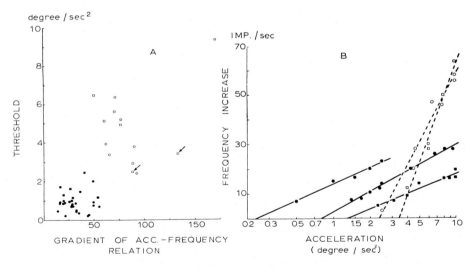

Fig. 8. A, Diagram showing the thresholds and gradients of acceleration–frequency curves (shown in B) in tonic and kinetic vestibular neurons of unanesthetized, decerebrate cat. Filled symbols represent tonic neurons; open symbols represent kinetic neurons (except those indicated by arrows). B, Relation between acceleration rate and frequency increase at its maximum level in tonic and kinetic type-I vestibular neurons. Each solid (tonic neurons) or broken (kinetic neurons) line indicates the regression line of points obtained from a single neuron tested with different acceleration rates. Abscissa is in logarithmic scale.

References pp. 105–107

The points where the regression lines cross the abscissa indicate the threshold of each unit for frequency increase (Shimazu and Precht, 1965). The mean threshold of tonic vestibular neurons was $0.65 \pm 0.25°/sec^2$, which is significantly lower than the mean value for kinetic type-I neurons ($4.65 \pm 1.84°/sec^2$). It appears, therefore, that the low thresholds of tonic neurons best reflect the high sensitivity of the vestibular system to angular acceleration.

If one measures the gradients of the regression lines of tonic and kinetic neurons characterizing the acceleration-frequency relationship (Fig. 8) one finds that the former have distinctly lower values (31.6 ± 11.8) as compared to the latter (85 ± 30.5). The relationship between threshold for frequency increase and gradients of tonic and kinetic vestibular neurons is shown in the left hand diagram of Fig. 8.

It appears, therefore, that under decerebrate unanesthetized conditions, the type-I vestibular neurons are divided into two distinct groups when tested with adequate stimulation of the horizontal semicircular canals. The *kinetic* neurons are characterized by lack of resting discharge, a high threshold for frequency increase, a rapid time course of frequency changes, and a steep gradient of the acceleration-frequency relationship, the *tonic* neurons showing the opposite of these characteristics. The precise response of the central vestibular system to horizontal head movement or rotation of the whole body in the horizontal plane seems to be secured with the help of a double safety mechanism. The low threshold of tonic neurons assures the sensitivity of the responses, and their resting activity provides part of the vestibular tone which is important for the musculature of the trunk, limbs and eyes. The high threshold kinetic neurons respond with high frequency discharge and rapid changes in impulse frequency at higher acceleration rates and may be a second factor essential for the precision of the vestibular responses in particular as far as eye movements are concerned. These characteristics may complement those of tonic neurons such as, slow responsiveness and frequency saturation at higher acceleration rates.

Adaptation of central vestibular neurons. As described in the first part of this paper about 65% of the primary vestibular fibers of the frog showed a distinct frequency adaptation during constant angular acceleration. Using the same kind of stimulation, *i.e.*, a protracted period of constant horizontal angular acceleration, most of the second order vestibular neurons showed no significant frequency adaptation as may be seen in Fig. 6 (Shimazu and Precht, 1965). Similar suggestions were made by Ross (1936) and Adrian (1943). As shown in Fig. 9, a small number of type-I neurons show a slight decrease in frequency after attaining their peak value (Fig. 9A). All these neurons, however, showed a clear undershoot of discharge frequency when the turntable was stopped after constant speed rotation (Fig. 9B and C). In some cases the frequency returned from this undershoot and still increased beyond the basic rate, *i.e.*, damped oscillatory changes were observed (Fig. 9C, D). None of the neurons which maintained their constant impulse rate during acceleration showed these oscillatory changes in frequency. This may indicate that the drop in frequency of some neurons is not a true adaptation but only an initial part of the frequency oscillation. At present, it is impossible to decide whether the oscillation is produced by peripheral or central mechanisms. Undershoots of impulse frequency have also been observed in the

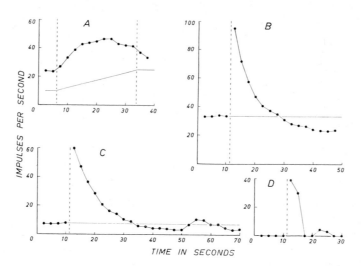

Fig. 9. Various response patterns of discharge frequencies of single vestibular neurons to horizontal rotation. A–C represent tonic neurons, and D, a kinetic neuron. A, Response to ipsilateral constant angular acceleration ($7°/sec^2$). The left- and right-hand vertical lines indicate the onset and cessation of acceleration, respectively. The constant speed of rotation after acceleration was $195°/sec$. B–D, responses to sudden arrest after constant speed ($100°/sec$ in B, $65°/sec$ in C, and $150°/sec$ in D) of contralateral rotation. Horizontal lines in B and C indicate average frequencies during constant rotation. Vertical broken lines in B–D indicate the time when the turntable was stopped. A and B were obtained from an animal in which the contralateral labyrinth was destroyed. All records were obtained from unanesthetized, decerebrate cats. From Shimazu and Precht (1965).

peripheral neuron (Groen *et al.*, 1952; Ledoux, 1961; Precht *et al.*, 1971). In this case it may be partially caused by the efferent vestibular system. In comparing the primary vestibular fibers of the frog with the second order vestibular neurons of cat significant differences become apparent as far as adaptation is concerned. Obviously, it remains to be studied whether primary fibers of cat show similar adaptation phenomena as in the frog and whether second order neurons of the frog reveal any sign of adaptation.

Synaptology of vestibular neurons. In using natural, rotatory stimulation no information can be obtained regarding the number of synapses involved in a particular pathway. Electrical stimulation of the vestibular nerve, therefore, is an essential prerequisite for any attempt to study the synaptic arrangement of vestibular neurons. In this paragraph a brief review will be given of the synaptology of type-I vestibular neurons. All of these neurons were first identified by their responses to natural stimulation whereupon their responses to electrical stimulation of the VIII nerve have been studied. Since both natural and electrical stimulation have been employed with each neuron the recordings were necessarily of extracellular character.

When a microelectrode is inserted into the vestibular nuclei, a characteristic field potential is evoked by a single electrical shock of the ipsilateral VIII nerve (Fig. 10). A detailed description of this field potential complex has been given by Precht and Shimazu (1965) part of which will be repeated here since recording of the vestibular field potential has proven to be a helpful guide in studying the synaptology of the

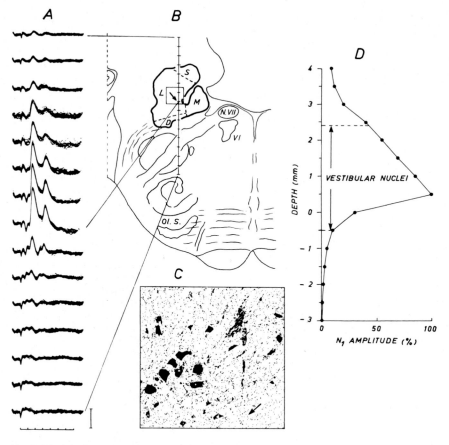

Fig. 10. Field potentials generated by stimulation of the vestibular nerve and recorded by a micro-electrode in the ipsilateral vestibular nuclei of unanesthetized, decerebrate cat. A, Potential fields evoked by single shocks of the vestibular nerve (the first downward deflection indicates stimulation artifact). Upward deflection indicates negativity of the microelectrode. Each record is composed of about 20 superimposed traces and was obtained from the site indicated by the scale in B. Time: 1 msec; voltage calibration: 0.5 mV. B, Line drawing of histological section of the brain stem. The vertical line shows the insertion of the recording electrode. Scales on this line indicate 500 μm. Arrow indicates the site where coagulation was made with the microelectrode. S, superior nucleus; L, lateral nucleus: M, medial nucleus; D, descending nucleus; Ol.s., superior olive; N.VII, seventh cranial nerve; VI, sixth cranial motor nucleus. C, Microphotograph of the part surrounded by a square in B. Arrow indicates the position of the tip of the electrode. D, Diagram showing relative amplitude of N_1 potential in A, correlated with the location of the electrode. Zero millimeters in the depth scale corresponds to the level of the surface in the midline of the fourth ventricle. Upper and lower borders of the vestibular nuclei are indicated by the two vertical arrows. Note the sharp decrease in amplitude of N_1 as the electrode approaches the ventral border of the vestibular nuclei. From Shimazu and Precht (1965)

vestibular nuclei. As shown in Fig. 10 the field potential is restricted to the vestibular nuclei provided that the stimulus strength does not exceed two times the N_1 threshold. When the microelectrode moved through the ventral border of the vestibular nuclei, N_1 potential amplitude decreased with fairly sharp gradients (Fig. 10A, D). The field potential consists of 3 components: (1) an initial positive–negative deflection (P-wave) followed by a large sharp negative (N_1) wave and a delayed small negative (N_2) potential. It was shown that the P-potential (latency: 0.66 ± 0.14 msec) represents the action currents of primary vestibular fibers supplying the vestibular nuclei. The N_1 potential (latency: 1.06 ± 0.22 msec) is composed of the action currents and synaptic currents produced monosynaptically in vestibular neurons by the excitatory action of primary vestibular fibers. Finally, the N_2 potential (latency: 2.46 ± 0.26 msec) is composed of the excitatory synaptic currents and action currents generated in vestibular neurons through polysynaptic paths. Possible anatomical substrates for multisynaptic excitation of vestibular neurons may be either internuncial neurons in the vestibular nuclei or collaterals of the axons leaving the nuclei. It is interesting to note that the double activation of vestibular neurons by single shock stimulation has also been seen when recordings are obtained from the axons of vestibular neurons in the medial longitudinal fascicle (Cook *et al.*, 1969; Precht and Baker, 1972). The field potential complex is of similar configuration in all vestibular nuclei, although differences in the size of the amplitudes of the various components can be seen in different recording positions. Thus, the P-wave is larger the more lateral the recording electrode is placed and the N_2 wave appears to be relatively larger in the ventro-medial part of the medial nucleus, whereas N_1 potential is larger in the ventro-lateral part of this nucleus. The latter part is known to receive primary afferent fibers whereas the former seems to be free of primary terminals (Brodal *et al.*, 1962).

Single unit recordings in the region where the vestibular field potentials can be found, have shown that many of them respond to adequate stimulation of the semicircular canals as well as to electrical stimulation of the VIII nerve. Tonic and kinetic type-I vestibular neurons have been tested with electrical single pulse stimulation of the vestibular nerve and their latencies of activation have been correlated with the N_1 and N_2 potentials (Precht and Shimazu, 1965). Most of the kinetic neurons are excited by weak VIII nerve stimulation with fairly fixed latencies, and the spikes are superimposed on the N_1 peak of the field potential (Fig. 11A). With stronger stimulation, the units are evoked with delays of 0.4–0.8 msec after arrival of presynaptic activity. This and other characteristics (Precht and Shimazu, 1965) suggest that kinetic neurons are mainly monosynaptically activated by primary fibers.

Tonic type-I neurons responded in a completely different manner. Stimulation of the VIII nerve excites the neurons with long and widely fluctuating latencies (Fig. 11B). As the stimulus strength is increased from top to bottom of Fig. 11B, the latencies are gradually shortened but still remain in the N_2 range even with strong stimulation. In half of the type-I neurons tested, these clear differences in latencies between tonic and kinetic neurons were obscured when the stimulation was very strong. Under this condition, kinetic neurons show double activation, the second spike falling on N_2, and tonic neurons are also repetitively activated with the first spike riding on N_1 potential. Even in these neurons, however, clear differences were found when tested with weak stimulation. The responses occurring in conjunction with the N_2 potential were effectively blocked by pentobarbital administration. Multisynaptic pathways in the vestibular nuclei, therefore, best explain the long latency activation of tonic

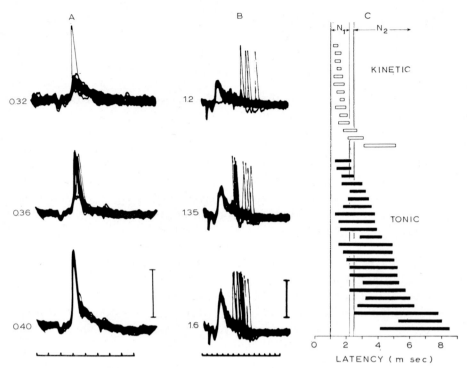

Fig. 11. Responses of kinetic (A) and tonic (B) type-I vestibular neurons to electrical stimulation of the ipsilateral VIII nerve. All records were obtained from unanesthetized, decerebrate cat. A, B, 3/sec stimulation. Each record is composed of about 20 superimposed traces. The numerals on the left of each record indicate stimulation voltage. The first downward deflection indicates the stimulus artifact. N_1 field potential is seen in all records except the one at the bottom of A. Time: 1 msec; amplitude calibration: 1mV. C, Latency distribution of kinetic and tonic neurons. The horizontal extent of open oblongs (kinetic neurons) and filled oblongs (tonic neurons) indicates that latencies of the earliest spikes of each neuron evoked by weak stimulation of the ipsilateral vestibular nerve were distributed within these ranges. These results were obtained from 30 to 40 serial trials at 2–3/sec. N_1 and N_2, indicated by vertical lines, represent the ranges of N_1 and N_2 field potentials. From Precht and Shimazu (1965).

neurons with weak stimulation (Precht and Shimazu, 1965). In Fig. 11C the latencies of a larger number of tonic and kinetic type-I neurons are shown in correlation with the range of N_1 and N_2 potentials. The tendency of kinetic and tonic neurons being related to N_1 and N_2 field potential respectively can clearly be recognized. Recent intracellular recordings from vestibular neurons in cat have further supported the interpretation of the field potential waves and the unitary potentials by showing that monosynaptic and polysynaptic excitatory synaptic potentials (EPSPs) can be recorded from vestibular neurons (Kawai et al., 1969; Ito et al., 1969) following single shock stimulation of the vestibular nerve.

Although in this paper the influence of the semicircular canals on vestibular neurons was to be described, it is important to emphasize that second order neurons are not to be considered only as simple relay neurons carrying the labyrinthine message to higher vestibular centers or to various output levels. There is evidence for considerable convergence of labyrinthine receptors on single vestibular neurons (Duensing and Schaefer, 1959). Furthermore, other sources such as the cerebellar cortex, the cerebellar nuclei, the spinal cord, the reticular formation and the contralateral vestibular nuclei via the commissural fiber system act in various combinations on second order vestibular neurons. Thus, the vestibular nuclei and their neurons have to be considered as a highly integrative functional system where various other systems combine with the vestibular input in order to assure high precision for the adjustment of the body in space. This is finally achieved by the efferent projections of the vestibular nuclei to the spinal cord, the ocular motor nuclei, the reticular formation and the cerebellum. Recent studies have shown that this output is also partly inhibitory in nature. Thus, inhibitory axons originating from second order vestibular neurons project to the spinal cord (Wilson and Yoshida, 1969), the abducens nuclei (Richter and Precht, 1968; Baker et al., 1969) and the trochlear nuclei (Precht and Baker, 1972). This is important to emphasize since the vestibular nuclei have long been considered as being purely excitatory in nature (Sherrington, 1898; Magnus, 1924; Fulton et al., 1930; Bach and Magoun, 1947).

SUMMARY

The responses of single vestibular nerve fibers of the frog to horizontal angular acceleration (acceleration and velocity steps) are described and compared with the responses obtained from cat's second order vestibular neurons.

Of the afferent fibers the majority showed frequency adaptation (65%) to prolonged constant angular acceleration. Second order neurons, however, showed no significant adaptation.

The majority of both afferent fibers and second order neurons showed a non-linear relation between frequency increase and angular acceleration. The lowest thresholds for frequency increase were similar in both groups (ca. $0.3°/sec^2$).

Time constants of the majority of nerve fibers were about 3 sec (range 1–10 sec). It is suggested that fibers having short time constants represent acceleration sensitive units whereas those having long time constants monitor angular velocity. Time constants of second order neurons were distinctly different for tonic (resting discharge) and kinetic (no resting discharge) type-I neurons (8.1 ± 1.6 sec and 3.7 ± 0.8 sec, respectively). Functional implications of these two groups of neurons are discussed.

The synaptology and location of second order vestibular neurons of the semicircular canals are described.

REFERENCES

ADRIAN, E. D. (1943) Discharges from vestibular receptors in the cat. *J. Physiol. (Lond.)*, **101** 389–407.

BACH, L. M. N. AND MAGOUN, H. W. (1947) The vestibular nuclei as an excitatory mechanism for the cord. *J. Neurophysiol.*, **10**, 331–337.

BAKER, R. G., MANO, N. AND SHIMAZU, H. (1969) Postsynaptic potentials in abducens motoneurons induced by vestibular stimulation. *Brain Res.*, **15**, 577–580.

BRODAL, A., POMPEIANO, O. AND WALBERG, F. (1962) *The Vestibular Nuclei and Their Connections. Anatomy and Functional Correlations*, Oliver and Boyd, Edinburgh, London, pp. 193.

COOK, JR., W. A., CANGIANO, A. AND POMPEIANO, O. (1969) An electrical investigation of the efferent pathways from the vestibular nuclei. *Arch. ital. Biol.*, **107**, 235–274.

DECHER, D. (1963) Neues zur Labyrinthphysiologie. Die Drehreiz-Schwellen der verticalen Bogengänge. *Arch. Ohr.-Nas.-u. Kehlk.-Heilk.*, **181**, 395–407.

DUENSING, F. UND SCHAEFER, K. P. (1958) Die Aktivität einzelner Neurone im Bereich der Vestibulariskerne bei Horizontalbeschleunigungen unter besonderer Berücksichtigung des vestibulären Nystagmus. *Arch. Psychiat. Nervenkr.*, **198**, 225–252.

DUENSING, F. UND SCHAEFER, K. P. (1959) Über die Konvergenz verschiedener labyrinthärer Afferenzen auf einzelne Neurone des Vestibulariskerngebietes. *Arch. Psychiat. Nervenkr.*, **199**, 345–371.

ECKEL, W. (1954) Elektrophysiologische und histologische Untersuchungen im Vestibulariskerngebiet bei Drehreizen. *Arch. Ohr.-, Nas.-, u. Kehlk.-Heilk.*, **164**, 487–513.

EWALD, J. R. (1892) *Physiologische Untersuchungen über das Endorgan des N. Oktavus*. Bergmann, Wiesbaden, pp. 324.

FULTON, J. F., LIDDELL, E. G. T. AND RIOCH, D. McK. (1930) The influence of unilateral destruction of vestibular nuclei upon posture and knee-jerk. *J. Physiol. (Lond.)*, **70**, XXII.

GACEK, R. R. (1969) The course and central termination of first order neurons supplying vestibular endorgans in the cat. *Acta oto-laryng. (Stockh.)*, **254**, 1–66.

GERNANDT, B. E. (1949) Response of mammalian vestibular neurons to horizontal rotation and caloric stimulation. *J. Neurophysiol.*, **12**, 173–184.

GROEN, J. J., LOWENSTEIN, O. AND VENDRIK, A. J. H. (1952) The mechanical analysis of the responses from the end organs of the horizontal semicircular canal in the isolated elasmobranch labyrinth. *J. Physiol. (Lond.)*, **117**, 329–346.

HILLMAN, D. E. (1969) Light and electron microscopical study of the relationships between the cerebellum and the vestibular organ of the frog. *Exp. Brain Res.*, **9**, 1–15.

ITO, M., HONGO, T. AND OKADA, Y. (1969) Vestibular-evoked postsynaptic potentials in Deiters' neurones. *Exp. Brain Res.*, **7**, 214–230.

KAWAI, N., ITO, M. AND NOZUE, M. (1969) Postsynaptic influences on the vestibular non-Deiters' nuclei from primary vestibular nerve. *Exp. Brain Res.*, **8**, 190–200.

LEDOUX, A. (1949) Activité électrique des nerfs des canaux semicirculaires du saccule et de l'utricle chez la grenouille. *Acta oto-rhino-laryng. belg.*, **3**, 335–349.

LEDOUX, A. (1958) Les canaux semi-circulaires. Etude électrophysiologique. Contribution à l'effort d'uniformisation des épreuves vestibulaires. Essai d'interprétation de la sémiologie vestibulaire. *Acta oto-rhino-laryng. belg.*, **12**, 109–348.

LEDOUX, A. (1961) L'adaptation du système vestibulaire périphérique. *Acta oto-laryng. (Stockh.)*, **53**, 307–316.

LLINÁS, R. AND PRECHT, W. (1972) Vestibulocerebellar input: physiology. In A. BRODAL AND O. POMPEIANO (Eds.), *Progress in Brain Research. Vol. 37. Basic aspects of central vestibular mechanisms*. Elsevier, Amsterdam, pp. 341–359.

LORENTE DE NÓ, R. (1933) Anatomy of the eighth nerve. The central projection of the nerve endings of the internal ear. *Laryngoscope*, **43**, 1–38.

LOWENSTEIN, O. (1956) Peripheral mechanisms of equilibrium. *Brit. med. Bull.*, **12**, 114–118.

LOWENSTEIN, O. AND SAND, A. (1940a) The mechanism of the semicircular canal. A study of the responses of single-fibre preparations to angular accelerations and rotation at constant speed. *Proc. roy. Soc. B*, **129**, 256–275.

LOWENSTEIN, O. AND SAND, A. (1940b) The individual and integrated activity of the semicircular canals of the elasmobranch labyrinth. *J. Physiol. (Lond.)*, **99**, 89–101.

MAGNUS, R. (1924) *Körperstellung*. Springer, Berlin, pp. XIII–740.

MARKHAM, C. H. (1968) Midbrain and contralateral labyrinth influences on brainstem vestibular neurons in the cat. *Brain Res.*, **9**, 312–333.

PRECHT, W. AND BAKER, R. (1972) Synaptic organization of the vestibulo-trochlear pathway. *Exp. Brain Res.*, **14**, 158–184.

PRECHT, W., GRIPPO, J. AND WAGNER, A. (1967) Contribution of different types of central vestibular neurons to the vestibulo-spinal system. *Brain Res.*, **4**, 119–123.

PRECHT, W., LLINÁS, R. AND CLARKE, M. (1971) Physiological responses of frog vestibular fibers to horizontal angular rotation. *Exp. Brain Res.*, **13**, 378–407.

PRECHT, W. AND SHIMAZU, H. (1965) Functional connections of tonic and kinetic vestibular neurons with primary vestibular afferents. *J. Neurophysiol.*, **28**, 1014–1028.

RICHTER, A. AND PRECHT, W. (1968) Inhibition of abducens motoneurones by vestibular nerve stimulation. *Brain Res.*, **11**, 701–705.

ROSS, J. A. (1936) Electrical studies on the frog's labyrinth. *J. Physiol. (Lond.)*, **86**, 117–146.

SHERRINGTON, C. S. (1898) Decerebrate rigidity and reflex cooidination of movements. *J. Physiol. (Lond.)*, **22**, 319–332.

SHIMAZU, H. (1972) Organization of the commissural connections: physiology. In A. BRODAL AND O. POMPEIANO (Eds.), *Progress in Brain Research. Vol. 37. Basic aspects of central vestibular mechanisms*. Elsevier, Amsterdam, pp. 177–190.

SHIMAZU, H. AND PRECHT, W. (1965) Tonic and kinetic responses of cat's vestibular neurons to horizontal angular acceleration. *J. Neurophysiol.*, **28**, 991–1013.

SHIMAZU, H. AND PRECHT, W. (1966) Inhibition of central vestibular neurons from the contralateral labyrinth and its mediating pathway. *J. Neurophysiol.*, **29**, 467–492.

STEIN, B. M. AND CARPENTER, M. B. (1967) Central projections of portions of the vestibular ganglia innervating specific parts of the labyrinth in the rhesus monkey. *Amer. J. Anat.*, **120**, 281–318.

STEINHAUSEN, W. (1931) Über den Nachweis der Bewegung der Cupula in der intakten Bogengangs-ampulle des Labyrinthes bei der natürlichen rotatorischen und calorischen Reizung. *Pflügers Arch. ges. Physiol.*, **228**, 322–328.

STEINHAUSEN, W. (1933) Über die Beobachtung der Cupula in den Bogengangsampullen des lebenden Hechts. *Pflügers Arch. ges. Physiol.*, **232**, 500–512.

SUZUKI, J. I. AND COHEN, B. (1966) Integration of semicircular canal activity. *J. Neurophysiol.*, **29**, 981–995.

SZENTÁGOTHAI, J. (1950) The elementary vestibulo-ocular reflex arc. *J. Neurophysiol.*, **13**, 395–407.

TRINCKER, D. (1957) Bestandspotentiale im Bogengangssystem des Meerschweinchens und ihre Änderung bei experimentellen Cupula Ablenkungen. *Pflügers Arch. ges Physiol.*, **264**, 351–382.

VAN EGMOND, A. A. J., GROEN, J. J. AND JONGKEES, L. B. W. (1949) The mechanism of the semi-circular canal. *J. Physiol. (Lond.)*, **110**, 1–17.

WALBERG, F., (1972) Light and electron microscopical data on the distribution and termination of primary vestibular fibers. In A. BRODAL AND O. POMPEIANO (Eds.), *Progress in Brain Research. Vol. 37. Basic aspects of central vestibular mechanisms*. Elsevier, Amsterdam, pp. 79–88.

WILSON, V. J. AND YOSHIDA, M. (1969) Monosynaptic inhibition of neck motoneurons by the medial vestibular nucleus. *Exp. Brain Res.*, **9**, 365–380.

YOUNG, L. R. (1969) Biocybernetics of the vestibular system. In L. D. PROCTOR (Ed.), *Biocybernetics of the Central Vestibular System*. Little, Brown and Co., Boston, pp. 79–117.

Responses of Vestibular Nuclear Neurons to Macular Input

B. W. PETERSON

The Rockefeller University, New York, N.Y., U.S.A.

Primary vestibular afferent fibers innervating the maculae of the utriculus and sacculus are known from anatomical studies to terminate in 3 of the 4 major vestibular nuclei: the lateral, medial and descending nuclei (Lorente de Nó, 1926, 1933; Stein and Carpenter, 1967; Gacek, 1969). The physiological properties of this macular input can be studied from two points of view. A number of investigators have described the characteristics of the responses of vestibular neurons to natural stimuli that activate macular afferent fibers and have attempted to relate these responses to properties of the receptors and afferent pathways. I will begin my discussion of macular responses with a review of some work of this kind. As more has become known about the anatomical structure of the vestibular nuclei and their projections, it has also become possible to relate responses to macular input to the anatomical organization of the vestibular complex and to determine the type of macular activity that is relayed to motor centers. In the second part of this paper I will discuss several aspects of data I have obtained in studying the macular input to the lateral vestibular nucleus from this point of view.

Investigators studying the macular input to the vestibular nuclei have employed inclination of the head with respect to gravity as a means of modulating afferent activity reaching the vestibular nuclei from the utricular and saccular maculae. Tilting of the head produces both a transient and a tonic change in activity of afferent fibers from otolith organs (Lowenstein and Roberts, 1949), but produces only a transient increase or decrease in activity of semicircular canal afferents (Lowenstein and Sand, 1940). Therefore, if sufficient time is allowed after tilting, any change in vestibular activity mediated by the labyrinth must be due to the otolith organs. Because the saccular macula is oriented vertically and the utricular macula horizontally, tilting the head within 10–20° of the horizontal position will produce a significant change in shearing force and hence in afferent discharge only in the utriculus. Since most investigators have employed tilts within this range, I will assume that responses to tilting are produced primarily by modulation of the activity of utricular afferents.

RESPONSES OF VESTIBULAR NEURONS TO TILTING

Changes in discharge rates of mammalian vestibular neurons in response to steady inclination of the head were first observed by Adrian (1943) and have been described by a number of others (Duensing and Schaefer, 1959; Fujita *et al.*, 1968; Hiebert and

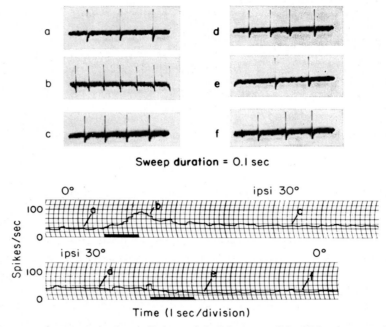

Fig. 1. Response of a neuron in the vestibular nuclei of the cat to tilting. Inkwriter records in lower part of figure indicate discharge rate averaged over 1 sec intervals. During period indicated by heavy line in first record the animal was tilted 30° toward the right (ipsilateral) side. After adaptation of rate, animal was tilted back to horizontal position during time indicated in lower record. Oscilloscope sweeps in upper part of figure illustrate firing of neuron at points indicated on inkwriter records. From Peterson (1970).

Fernandez, 1965; Peterson, 1970). Fig. 1 is an example of such a response recorded in the lateral vestibular nucleus of the cat. Tilting of the recording (ipsilateral) side downward gave rise to both transient and maintained excitation of this neuron. When the animal was returned to the horizontal position the neuron exhibited a transient depression of discharge rate after which the rate returned to its original value. The first exhaustive study of the types of responses evoked by sideways and forward–backward tilting was performed by Duensing and Schaefer (1959) who classified the responses as shown in Table I. All of the response types listed have been observed physiologically (Duensing and Schaefer, 1959; Peterson, 1970).

A recent quantitative study (Fujita *et al.*, 1968) of the responses of vestibular neurons in the cat to tilting within 10° of horizontal has emphasized the non-stationarity of the position transduction process. Two effects were described that gave rise to different discharge rates in successive trials at the same position. The first, termed 'looping', resulted in a different rate depending upon the direction of approach to the final position. This kind of behavior may result from viscous properties of the otolith membrane of the utriculus. A second form of non-stationary behavior, characterized by a steady increase or decrease in the discharge rate corresponding to a given position over a series of trials, was named 'creep'. This effect also appears to involve the recep-

TABLE I

TYPES OF NEURAL RESPONSES TO TILTING

Responses to lateral tilting

Response type	Direction of tilting	
	Ipsilateral side down	Contralateral side down
Type α	+	—
Type β	—	+
Type γ	+	+
Type δ	—	—

Responses to forward–backward tilting

Response type	Direction of tilting	
	Nose down	Tail down
Type 1	—	+
Type 2	+	—
Type 3	+	+
Type 4	—	—

Nomenclature introduced by Duensing and Schaefer (1959) to describe neural responses to tilting. The symbol + represents an increase in discharge rate; the symbol — represents a decrease.

tor since discharge rates were stable in each position between movements. The lack of stationarity poses difficulties for investigators seeking to analyze information transfer in the otolith system. It is not certain, for instance, whether errors produced by looping and creep are randomly distributed in the vestibular neuron pool such that they can be compensated for by averaging responses over large populations, or whether they represent macro properties of the otolith organ and may effect entire groups of neurons simultaneously. Under many circumstances, however, these errors may become small relative to the responses of neurons to tilting. In my study of responses of vestibular neurons in the cat, for instance, I used 20° tilts and found that whereas variations in discharge rate at a given position seldom exceeded 10° of the average rate, many responses to tilt increased or decreased the discharge rate by 30% or more. It is therefore possible when using relatively large tilts to study and compare single neuron responses to tilting in the vestibular nuclei.

I have recently completed a series of experiments designed to obtain information about the distribution of responses to tilt within the vestibular nuclei and about the relation between these responses and afferent input from the labyrinth (Peterson, 1970). Experiments were performed on anesthetized cats in which the cerebellum was removed, thereby eliminating several indirect pathways by which otolith activity may reach vestibular neurons. Extracellular recordings were made in all 4 vestibular nuclei

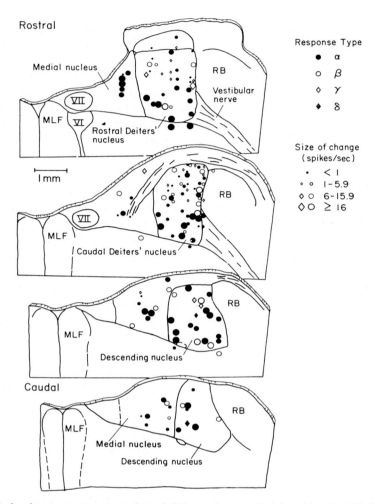

Fig. 3. Relation between responses to lateral tilting and anatomical location of vestibular neurons. Locations of neurons whose responses to 20° lateral tilting were measured have been superimposed on a series of typical cross sections of the vestibular nuclei. Type of symbol used for each neuron indicates its response type as shown in legend (see Table I for definitions of types). Size of symbol indicates magnitude of response in impulses/sec. From Peterson (1970).

Neurons exhibiting the various types of responses described by Duensing and Schaefer (1959) were distributed throughout the nuclei without any apparent pattern. The greatest number of large responses were encountered in the descending nucleus and the ventral part of the lateral nucleus. These regions contained many second order (MONO) cells with a high sensitivity to tilting. Small responses were concentrated in the dorsal part of the lateral (Deiters') nucleus, which lacks MONO cells, and in the superior nucleus where most neurons of all classes had low sensitivity to tilting. POLY and NON cells with medium to large responses contributed to the response pattern in the medial and descending nuclei. The distribution is, therefore, a composite of effects produced by direct, monosynaptic connections and by less direct, polysynaptic pathways. Responses of neurons receiving direct labyrinthine input agreed with anatomical information on distribution of utricular afferents. Not enough is known about pathways transmitting activity from MONO cells to higher order neurons to permit a neuroanatomical interpretation of the response patterns of POLY and NON cells.

RESPONSES OF VESTIBULOSPINAL NEURONS TO TILTING

The remainder of this paper will be devoted to the responses of vestibulospinal neurons to tilting.

I will begin by discussing the relation of these responses to the cellular organization of Deiters' nucleus from which the lateral vestibulospinal tract originates and then attempt to relate my results to known properties of labyrinthine reflexes. Studies of retrograde degeneration following spinal section (Pompeiano and Brodal, 1957) and of antidromic activation from different spinal levels (Wilson et al., 1967) have shown that Deiters' nucleus is somatotopically organized with neurons projecting to caudal parts of the spinal cord lying more dorsocaudally than neurons projecting to more rostral parts. In my experiments I identified two categories of vestibulospinal neurons: cells whose axons could be activated by stimulation at the third lumbar level (L cells) and cells whose axons could be activated by stimulation at the third cervical but not the third lumbar level (C cells). The distribution of these two types of cells, illustrated in Fig. 4, follows the general somatotopic pattern described by Wilson et al. (1967). The labyrinthine input to Deiters' nucleus is also anatomically organized in that primary afferent fibers terminate only within the ventral part of the nucleus (Walberg et al., 1958). The result of this distribution, as first described by Wilson et al. (1967), is that numerous MONO cells can be found in ventral Deiters' nucleus whereas most cells encountered in dorsal Deiters' nucleus are POLY or NON cells. Since responses to tilting are quite different for these 3 classes of cells, we might expect to see a distribution of responses to tilting within Deiters' nucleus related to the distribution of MONO, POLY, and NON cells. Fig. 4b shows the distribution of these 3 classes of cells and also lists the mean responses of all cells in each of 4 dorsal–ventral zones to lateral tilting in two directions. Average responses to tilting the ipsilateral side downward (left number in each pair) became larger when going from dorsal to ventral; average responses to tilting in the opposite direction (right number) changed from small positive to larger negative values. Responses in dorsal Deiters' nucleus therefore resembled the averaged responses of NON cells, listed in Fig. 4c, whereas the responses in the most ventral zone resembled those of MONO cells. A shift in response sizes and types with depth is also apparent in Fig. 3.

Because of the shift in responses to tilting with dorsal–ventral location, it might be expected that L and C cells would also exhibit different responses, those of L cells resembling the small, positive responses in dorsal Deiters' nucleus (where most L cells were located) and those of C cells resembling the larger, positive–negative responses found in ventral Deiters' nucleus (which contained the majority of C cells). The

a   Distribution of Spinal Projection

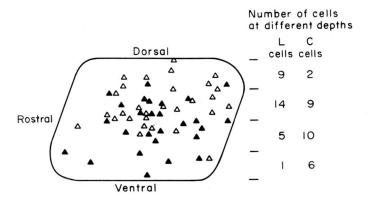

b   Distribution of Labyrinthine Input

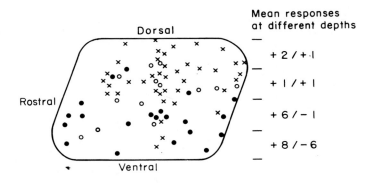

c   Symbols and Mean Responses

Projection	Mean response	Labyrinthine input	Mean response
△ L cells	+2/+2	● MONO cells	+9/−7
▲ C cells	+4/−3	○ POLY cells	+4/−1
N cells	+5/−1	× NON cells	+1/+1

Fig. 4. Relation between anatomical organization of Deiters' nucleus and responses of Deiters' neurons to tilting. a, Distribution of vestibulospinal neurons projecting to lumbosacral (L cells) or cervicothoracic (C cells) spinal cord. Locations of cells are shown superimposed on a schematic lateral projection of Deiters' nucleus. Numbers of L and C cells in 4 dorsal–ventral segments of the nucleus are given at the right of the diagram. b, Distribution of neurons classified as MONO, POLY or NON cells according to their response to an electrical shock to the labyrinth. Locations are plotted as in part a. Mean responses to lateral tilting of cells in 4 dorsal–ventral segments of the nucleus are indicated at the right of the diagram by two values separated by a slash. Values on left of slash are mean responses to 20° ipsilateral tilting; those on right, mean responses to 20° contralateral tilting. c, Symbols used in plotting locations of various types of neurons are shown together with mean responses of those neuron types to lateral tilting, expressed as in part b. From Peterson (1970).

averaged responses of C and L cells, listed in Fig. 4c, are in agreement with this prediction. Calculations based on the data in Fig. 4 indicated that the difference between the locations of C and L cells was sufficient to account for the difference in their mean responses to tilting (Peterson, 1970). Although data of this kind cannot establish the existence of a causal link between anatomical organization and response to tilting, it is clear that there is a strong relationship between the spatial distribution of Deiters' neurons and the patterns of macular activity transmitted to different regions of the spinal cord by the lateral vestibulospinal tract.

Before discussing the possible significance of the average responses of C and L cells to tilting, it is important to consider the wide variability of responses to the same tilting stimulus. Fig. 5 contains plots summarizing the responses of 6 groups of Deiters' neurons to lateral tilting. The plot in the upper left depicts the responses of the 21

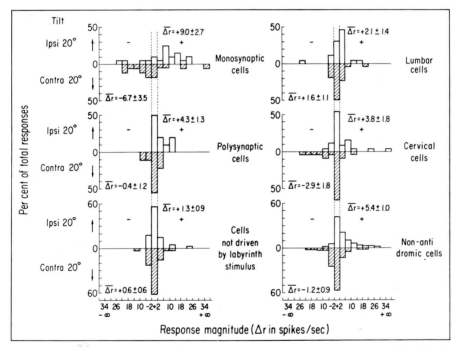

Fig. 5. Frequency of occurrence of various rate changes in response to 20° lateral tilting. Each of 6 plots contains two histograms which describe the distribution of firing rate changes in response to a specified angle of tilt. In each case the distribution of rate changes evoked by 20° ipsilateral tilt is plotted in the upward direction by unshaded bars. The abscissa is divided into categories of firing rate change: —2 to +2, +2 to +6, +6 to +10, etc. The height of each upward bar indicates the frequency (calibrated in percent on the ordinate) with which responses in a given range occurred during 20° ipsilateral tilt. The figure labeled $\overline{\Delta r}$ at the upper right of each plot gives the mean response to 20° ipsilateral tilting plus or minus the standard error. In a similar way the frequency of occurrence of the various rate changes in response to 20° contralateral tilt are plotted by the downward-extending shaded bars and mean contralateral response is indicated by the $\overline{\Delta r}$ at the lower left of each plot. Rate changes smaller than 2 spikes/sec were included in the central bar with zero responses because in many cells with discharge rates above 20 spikes/sec, random rate fluctuations masked any changes less than 2 spikes/sec. From Peterson (1970).

MONO cells encountered in Deiters' nucleus. As shown by the upward-extending (unshaded) bars most of these cells tended to increase their discharge rate during a 20° tilt towards the ipsilateral side. There were, however, several responses in the opposite direction, given by MONO cells with a β type response pattern. Similarly the downward-extending (shaded) bars show that although most MONO cells decreased their discharge rate during 20° tilt towards the contralateral side, several β type cells increased their firing rates. As mentioned earlier these opposing responses are probably the result of input from oppositely polarized hair cells in the utricular macula.

The question then arises: why does the utricular system have this pattern of opposite responses which is not present in the semicircular canal system? We have already seen in Fig. 3 that neurons exhibiting both α and β type responses are found intermingled in the vestibular nuclei. It could still be possible, however, for synaptic pathways to relay one type of activity to a given functional group of neurons such as vestibulo-spinal or vestibulo-extraocular neurons while the other type is directed to other neuron groups. This is not the case with respect to vestibulospinal neurons, however. The two plots on the upper right of Fig. 5 show that both L and C cells can give either a rate increase or decrease in response to either direction of tilt. Cells that could not be excited by stimulation at the third cervical segment exhibited a similar variety of responses. A further possibility is that vestibulospinal neurons with opposite response patterns produce different actions at the spinal level. This possibility can only be tested when techniques become available to determine the effect of a single, identified vestibular neuron upon spinal interneurons and motoneurons. In the absence of a demonstrated differential effect of oppositely responding neurons at the spinal level, we must assume that the mean responses of all C and L cells are an accurate measure of the activity reaching different parts of the spinal cord. Under this assumption we are forced to conclude that the unique organization of the utriculus confuses rather than enhances information about head position transmitted by the lateral vestibulospinal tract.

When mean responses to tilting are considered, a good correspondence between neuronal data and reflex behavior is obtained. Activation of fibers in the lateral vestibulospinal tract produces increased activity in extensor muscles of the ipsilateral fore and hindlimbs (Lund and Pompeiano, 1968; Wilson and Yoshida, 1969; Grillner et al., 1970). Assuming that many C cells terminate in the cervical enlargement and act on ipsilateral forelimb muscles, we predict that extension of the ipsilateral forelimb should increase when that side is tilted downward and decrease when the opposite side is tilted downward. Experimental studies (Nagaki, 1967; Roberts, 1967) show that this pattern of responses is obtained when care is taken to eliminate neck and cutaneous reflexes. If L cells act upon hindlimb motoneurons, a slight increase in activity of hindlimb extensors should be produced by both directions of tilt. In a recent detailed study of hindlimb responses to changes in head position, Erhardt and Wagner (1970) found that tilt toward the ipsilateral side increased hindlimb extensor activity whereas tilt in the opposite direction produced either a smaller increase or a decrease in extension activity. The contrast between these results and the clear reciprocal changes in forelimb extension are in agreement with the single neuron data. The variability of lumbar responses may in part be due to the cerebellum (removed in vestibular experiments) which acts most strongly upon the region of Deiters' nucleus containing the majority of L cells.

The results summarized here represent only the beginning of an understanding of macular input to the vestibular system. With respect to afferent pathways that mediate vestibular responses to head tilt we need information about responses to tilts in the range of 90° from the horizontal in which the sacculus may play a role. We also need studies similar to those described here but with the cerebellum intact to determine the role of cerebellar pathways in vestibular responses to tilt. Studies of afferent pathways are also handicapped by a lack of detailed information on vestibulo-vestibular connections that are involved in all polysynaptic responses. With respect to macular input to vestibular efferent systems, information similar to that discussed above is needed for the vestibulo-extraocular systems and for the crossed vestibular projections. Finally, before the relevance of macular input to efferent neuron groups can be evaluated we need more detailed information about the action of individual vestibular efferent neurons on reflex systems. A great deal of important research lies ahead in this area.

SUMMARY

Changes in afferent input from macular receptors, produced by tilting the head with respect to gravity, can modulate discharge rates of neurons in all of the 4 major vestibular nuclei. All second-order vestibular neurons studied in a recent investigation were found to respond to tilting in opposite directions with rate changes of opposite sign. More complex responses, including all possible combinations of rate increases and decreases, were obtained from higher-order neurons. The largest responses to tilting were exhibited by second-order neurons in Deiters' nucleus and the descending nucleus, indicating that these neurons receive extensive input from macular afferent fibers.

In agreement with known patterns of reflex responses to tilting, the average discharge rate of vestibulospinal tract neurons projecting to the cervicothoracic spinal cord has been found to increase during tilt toward the ipsilateral side and decrease during tilt toward the opposite side, whereas the average discharge rate of neurons projecting to the lumbo-sacral spinal cord increased during tilt in both directions. Analysis of this data has shown that the difference in response between the two neuronal populations is related to the anatomical organization of Deiters' nucleus but has failed to reveal the significance of the large variability of responses evoked by the same tilt stimulus.

REFERENCES

ADRIAN, E. D. (1943) Discharges from vestibular receptors in the cat. *J. Physiol. (Lond.)*, **101**, 389–407.

DUENSING, F. AND SCHAEFER, K. P. (1959) Über die Konvergenz verschiedener labyrinthärer Afferenzen auf einzelne Neurone des Vestibulariskerngebietes. *Arch. Psychiat. Nervenkr.*, **199**, 345–371.

ERHARDT, K. J. AND WAGNER, A. (1970) Labyrinthine and neck reflexes recorded from single spinal motoneurons in the cat. *Brain Res.*, **19**, 87–104.

FLOCK, A. (1964) Structure of the macula utriculi with special reference to the directional interplay of sensory receptors as revealed by morphological polarization. *J. Cell Biol.*, **22**, 413–431.

FUJITA, Y., ROSENBERG, J. AND SEGUNDO, J. P. (1968) Activity of cells in the lateral vestibular nucleus as a function of head position. *J. Physiol. (Lond.)*, **196**, 1–18.

GACEK, R. (1969) The course and central termination of first order neurons supplying vestibular endorgans in the cat. *Acta oto-laryng. (Stockh.)*, Suppl. 254, 1–66.

GRILLNER, S., HONGO, T. AND LUND, S. (1970) The vestibulospinal tract. Effects on alpha-motoneurons in the lumbosacral spinal cord in the cat. *Exp. Brain Res.*, **10**, 94–120.

HIEBERT, T. G. AND FERNANDEZ, C. (1965) Deitersian response to tilt. *Acta oto-laryng. (Stockh.)*, **60**, 180–190.

LORENTE DE NÓ, R. (1926) Etudes sur l'anatomie et la physiologie du labyrinthe de l'oreille. II. *Trab. Lab. Invest. biol. Univ. Madr.*, **24**, 53–153.

LORENTE DE NÓ, R. (1933) Anatomy of the eighth nerve. The central projection of the nerve endings of the internal ear. *Laryngoscope (St. Louis)*, **43**, 1–38.

LÖWENSTEIN, O. AND ROBERTS, T. D. M. (1949) The equilibrium function of the otolith organs of the thornback ray (*Raja clavata*). *J. Physiol. (Lond.)*, **110**, 392–415.

LÖWENSTEIN, O. AND SAND, A. (1940) The mechanism of the semicircular canal. A study of the responses of single-fiber preparations to angular acceleration and rotation at constant speed. *Proc. roy. Soc. B*, **129**, 256–275.

LUND, S. AND POMPEIANO, O. (1968) Monosynaptic excitation of alpha extensor motoneurons from supraspinal structures in the cat. *Acta physiol. scand.*, **73**, 1–21.

NAGAKI, J. (1967) Effects of natural vestibular stimulation on alpha extensor motoneurons of the cat. *Kumamoto med. J.*, **20**, 102–111.

PETERSON, B. W. (1970) Distribution of neural responses to tilting within vestibular nuclei of the cat. *J. Neurophysiol.*, **33**, 750–767.

POMPEIANO, O. AND BRODAL, A. (1957) The origin of vestibulospinal fibers in the cat. An experimental-anatomical study, with comments on the descending medial longitudinal fasciculus. *Arch. ital. Biol.*, **95**, 166–195.

ROBERTS, T. D. M. (1967) Labyrinthine control of the postural muscles. In *Third Symposium on the Role of the Vestibular Organs in Space Exploration. NASA SP*-152, 169–180.

STEIN, B. M. AND CARPENTER, M. B. (1967) Central projections of portions of the vestibular ganglia innervating specific parts of the labyrinth in the rhesus monkey. *Amer. J. Anat.*, **120**, 281–317.

WALBERG, F., BOWSHER, D. AND BRODAL, A. (1958) The termination of primary vestibular fibers in the vestibular nuclei of the cat. An experimental study with silver methods. *J. comp. Neurol.*, **110**, 391–419.

WILSON, V. J., KATO, M., PETERSON, B. W. AND WYLIE, R. M. (1967) A single unit analysis of the organization of Deiters' nucleus. *J. Neurophysiol.*, **30**, 603–619.

WILSON, V. J. AND YOSHIDA, M. (1969) Comparison of the effects of stimulation of Deiters' nucleus and medial longitudinal fasciculus on neck, forelimb and hindlimb motoneurons. *J. Neurophysiol.*, **32**, 743–758.

Labyrinthine Convergence on Vestibular Nuclear Neurons Using Natural and Electrical Stimulation

C. H. MARKHAM AND I. S. CURTHOYS

Department of Neurology, School of Medicine, University of California, Los Angeles, California U.S.A.

Sensory input from the several angular and linear acceleration detectors of the labyrinth contributes heavily to eyeball stability and accuracy of eye movement. While powerful neural connections with few synapses exist between each semicircular canal and two eye muscles (Szentágothai, 1943), they are inadequate to explain the observed precision of conjugate eye control. A number of possibilities exist for offering such control. One of them, the subject of this paper, is convergence of labyrinthine input at the level of the vestibular nucleus.

Convergence on single brain stem vestibular neurons was first demonstrated by Duensing and Schaefer (1959) by means of angular acceleration and tilting in several planes. Desole and Pallestrini (1969) warmed or cooled individual canal ampullae and showed several patterns of convergence on lateral vestibular nucleus neurons. The present study, dealing with natural and with electrical labyrinthine stimulation, shows there is extensive convergence on second order vestibular neurons, and defines some of the patterns of convergence (Curthoys and Markham, 1971).

NATURAL STIMULATION

Data were obtained from 27 cats. After ether anesthesia, a tracheostomy was done, followed by high cervical cord transsection. The midline cerebellum was sucked off and the fourth ventricle exposed. In 16 cats, the midline of the brain stem was cut to a depth of 2–3 mm from aqueduct to obex. The animal was maintained on artificial respiration. Local anesthetic was infiltrated into wound edges and pressure points initially and several times during the experiment. The animal's head was held in a stereotaxic frame and was mounted with stereotaxic zero precisely in the center of a servo-controlled rotating table and gimbal.

The gimbal-turntable was used to deliver angular acceleration or constant angular velocity in 3 orthogonal planes: yaw, pitch and roll. In order to place the 3 canals approximately parallel to a plane of stimulation, the cat's head was rotated 45° to the left (placing the left posterior canal and right anterior canal parallel to the pitch plane of the gimbal; and the left anterior and right posterior canals parallel to the gimbal's roll plane). In order to bring the horizontal canals into the plane of the horizontal turntable, the head was tipped nose down 21°. It was then rotated 21° left, ear down

References pp. 136–137

to again bring the horizontal canals into the plane of the turntable. This final position was termed the 'standard position,' and it was used for the natural stimulation portion of this paper. The Appendix discusses a misalignment in this 'standard position,'

Regarding otolith stimulation, it should be noted that the 'standard position' above resulted in gravitational linear acceleration acting on the head placed 45° to the naso-occipital and interaural tipping usually used for otolith experiments (Adrian, 1943; Peterson, 1967; Fujita *et al.*, 1968).

The units were recorded extracellularly with glass microelectrodes filled with 2 M NaCl and fast green FCF dye. The D.C. resistance of the electrodes was 0.9–4 MΩ. The action potentials were led off to a cathode follower, amplified and recorded on film or tape. The electrodes were passed into the vestibular nuclei from above, using visual control.

The units were initially tested with angular acceleration in the horizontal plane. Type-I units were facilitated by ipsilateral rotation and inhibited by contralateral rotation (Gernandt, 1949; Duensing and Schaefer, 1958). Type-II neurons had the opposite response (Duensing and Schaefer, 1958). The infrequent type-III units which were facilitated with accelerations in both directions were discarded. Units were also classif-

TABLE I

THE ORDER AND TYPE OF STIMULATION GIVEN TO EACH UNIT WHICH HAD BEEN FOUND TO RESPOND TO HORIZONTAL CANAL STIMULATION

Head in standard position				
Pitch otolithic tests	1.	Constant velocity tilt in pitch,	in a tail down direction,	for 20° extent
	2.	Stop		
	3.	Constant velocity tilt in pitch,	in a tail up direction,	for 20° extent
	4.	Stop		
Head in standard position				
Roll otolithic tests	5.	Constant velocity tilt in roll,	in a right ear downward direction,	for 20° extent
	6.	Stop		
	7.	Constant velocity tilt in roll,	in a left ear downward direction,	for 20° extent
	8.	Stop		
Head in standard position				
Pitch acceleration tests	9.	Angular acceleration in pitch,	in a tail down direction,	for 20° extent
	10.	Stop		
	11.	Angular acceleration in pitch,	in a tail up direction,	for 20° extent
	12.	Stop		
Head in standard position				
Roll acceleration tests	13.	Angular acceleration in roll,	in a right ear downward direction,	for 20° extent
	14.	Stop		
	15.	Angular acceleration in roll,	in a left ear downward direction,	for 20° extent
	16.	Stop		
Head in standard position				

ied as being 'kinetic' if their firing rate was about 1/sec or less (Shimazu and Precht, 1965), or 'tonic' if it was greater.

After units were classified as type-I or type-II, tonic or kinetic, the stimulation sequence in Table I was carried out, returning to the 'standard position' between each series. After each acceleration, and at the end of each otolith stimulation, there was a

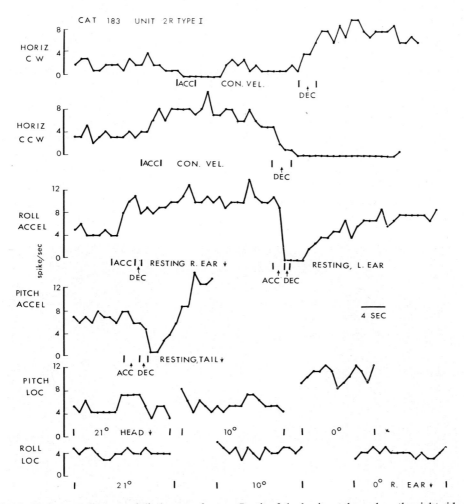

Fig. 1. Frequency diagram of discharges of a type-I unit of the horizontal canal on the right side of the brain stem. For each row, the ordinate is spikes per sec measured each half-second, and the abscissa is time in sec. Row 1 shows that with clockwise (CW) horizontal acceleration, the firing rate fell to zero. On deceleration, the unit was facilitated and then the resting rate stabilized at a new, higher level for about a minute (not shown). Row 2 shows the inverse of Row 1. Row 3 shows unit facilitation by 'roll' plane acceleration, toward the right ear. A new resting level of discharge continues while the cat remains right ear down, even though there is no otolithic response to roll (Row 6). On accelerating left ear down, there is unit inhibition. Row 4 shows a modest increase followed by marked decrease in unit firing on 'pitch' acceleration. At rest in a tail-down position, the unit frequency rises and stabilizes at 12–14/sec (only 3 sec of this new resting level are shown). This last response is due to the otolith stimulus as shown in Row 5.

pause of 20–30 sec. The acceleration used on the turntable and on the two arcs of the gimbal was 4°/sec². If we could not detect an obvious change in unit firing, the unit was discarded. The otolithic-induced responses were noted both during slow (0.5°/sec) velocity tilts and during steps at the ends and occasionally at one or more points during the 20° excursions. If there were any ambiguities in the unit's response, the tests were repeated. If the uncertainty remained, the unit was discarded.

Lesions were made using 20–30 μA current for 5 min, the brains were fixed in formalin, and later the brain stems were serially sectioned and stained with a Nissl stain or by the Klüver technique. On examination, if the cat had a midline section of the brain stem and it was less than 2.5 mm for the whole length of the vestibular nuclei, the data from that experiment were discarded.

A total of 469 units responded to horizontal canal stimulation. Of these, 304 were studied completely and had unambiguous responses. Of the 304, 144 were from animals with histologically verified midline sections of the brain stem, and 160 were from non-sectioned cats.

The resting rate of the units varied from 0 to 60/sec, with an average of about 15–20/sec. Most showed a fluctuation in resting rate of 2–3/sec over a minute's time, and tended to oscillate about a mean. On natural stimulation the majority of units changed their firing rate in a symmetrical, or mirror image fashion, to the same kind of

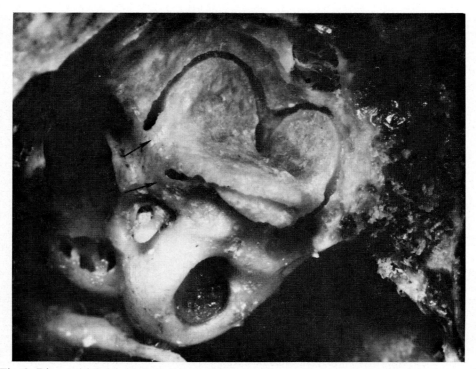

Fig. 2. Dissected left labyrinth, looking medially, parallel to the horizontal stereotaxic plane and perpendicular to the sagittal plane. The upper arrow shows the usual electrode placement for stimulating the anterior canal nerve; and the lower shows the site for stimulating the horizontal canal nerve.

stimulus delivered in opposite directions. Such a response may be seen in Fig. 1, line 2. Some neurons, after an acceleration and/or deceleration in the horizontal plane ended up with a new resting rate for some minutes (see Fig. 2, line 1). This was often more marked on the roll and pitch accelerations, sometimes because the cat's head ended up in a position where utricular convergence would contribute to the new resting rate. For an example of this, note line 4, Fig. 1, showing an increased resting rate in a tail-down position, which was also a position causing otolithic facilitation, as shown in line 5. On still other occasions, units would fail to return to their former firing rate after canal or otolithic stimulation, even after some minutes. These are similar to Crampton's (1965) canal 'memory' units, or the utricular units showing 'multivaluedness' observed by Fujita *et al.* (1968).

Type-I neurons numbered 128 (80%) in the nonsectioned, and 115 (79.9%) in the

TABLE II

THE CONVERGENCE PATTERNS OF HORIZONTAL CANAL NEURONS IN SECTIONED AND NON-SECTIONED ANIMALS

		Type-I		Type-II		Total	
		Non-sectioned	Sectioned	Non-sectioned	Sectioned	Non-sectioned	Sectioned
All units	No.	128	115	32	29	160	144
	%	(80)	(79.9)	(20)	(20.1)	(100)	(100)
Horizontal canal only	No.	42	46	8	6	50	52
	%	(26.2)	(31.9)	(5.0)	(4.2)	(31.2)	(36.1)
Horizontal canal plus otolith	No.	29	28	9	14	38	42
	%	(18.1)	(19.5)	(5.6)	(9.7)	(23.7)	(29.2)
Pitch	No.	10	9	1	0		
Roll	No.	10	7	3	6		
Pitch + Roll	No.	9	12	5	8		
Horizontal canal plus other canals	No.	17	19	8	3	25	22
	%	(10.6)	(13.2)	(5.0)	(2.1)	(15.6)	(15.3)
Anterior canal	No.	7	5	5	0		
Posterior canal	No.	7	13	2	3		
Anterior + posterior canal	No.	3	1	1	0		
Horizontal canal plus other canals plus otoliths	No.	40	22	7	6	47	28
	%	(25.0)	(15.3)	(4.4)	(4.2)	(29.4)	(19.5)
Anterior + otolith	No.	5	10	5	1		
Posterior + otolith	No.	31	11	2	5		
Anterior + posterior + otolith	No.	4	1	0	0		

The non-italicized figures in brackets are percentages of the total number of units recorded in non-sectioned animals (160). The italicized figures in brackets are percentages of the total number of units recorded in sectioned animals (144).

sectioned animals. There were 32 (20%) type-II's in the non-sectioned animals and 29 (20.1%) in the sectioned cats. The virtually identical percentages between the sectioned and non-sectioned preparations is surprising, specially for the type II's, and will be considered further in the Discussion.

The main patterns of convergence are: (*i*) As may be seen in Table II, there is little difference between individual groups of neurons from the animals with vestibular commissural fibers intact, and those with them sectioned. This suggests, as in the case of type-I and type-II categories, that none of these subdivisions receive their primary drive via the commissural fibers from the contralateral labyrinth. (*ii*) Table II shows for the non-sectioned animals 31.2% of the total (50 units) and 36.1% of the total (52 units) for the sectioned ones had labyrinthine connections with the horizontal canal only. These figures are too low for reasons given in the Appendix. Recalculation of the data leads to the following approximations. About 40% of the horizontal canal neurons showed no convergence at all; about 35% had convergence only from otolithic receptors; about 10% from one or both vertical canals; and about 10% from the otolith plus one or two canals. (*iii*) There are 6 type-II's in animals with the vestibular commissural fibers which responded only to horizontal acceleration. Since the entire midline cerebellum was sucked off, they could derive their input either from the ipsilateral horizontal canal, or from the opposite labyrinth by pathways passing deep in the reticular formation. (*iv*) Tonic and kinetic units have distinct patterns of convergence. Of the 304 fully studied neurons, 12% are comparable to those kinetic neurons found by others (Adrian, 1943; Shimazu and Precht, 1965; Melvill Jones and Milsum, 1970). In the non-sectioned cats, 25% (34/136) of tonic neurons and 66.7% (16/24) of kinetic neurons responded only to horizontal canal acceleration. For the non-sectioned animals, 32.3% (42/150) of tonic neurons, and 71.5% (10/14) of kinetic neurons responded to horizontal canal stimulation only. Thus, tonic units receive convergence information about twice as often as do the kinetic neurons.

ELECTRICAL STIMULATION

The initial operating procedures were like those described in the natural stimulation part of this paper, except that the midline brain stem was not sectioned. Bipolar steel teflon coated 40 μm wires were gently inserted into the perilymphatic space of the ampullae, or close to the nerves of the horizontal semicircular canal and the anterior canal. Less frequently electrodes were inserted into the ipsilateral posterior canal, and on two occasions into the ampullae of both the anterior and posterior canals. The positions of the electrode tips were adjusted so that on stimulation with 0.1 msec pulses at 100–200/sec, characteristic eye movements (Cohen and Suzuki, 1963; Cohen *et al.*, 1964; Tokumasu *et al.*, 1971) were evoked at the lowest possible thresholds. This stimulus was referenced against a silver–silver chloride electrode placed in adjacent temporalis muscle. The eye movements were checked throughout the experiment and, if the eye movements or their thresholds changed significantly, no further recording was done. A ball-shaped silver–silver chloride electrode was placed in the contralateral round window for contralateral whole nerve stimulation.

Brain stem vestibular neurons were recorded extracellularly. As in the section on natural stimulation in this paper, neurons were selected for study which responded to natural stimulation as type-I or II neurons of the horizontal canal. Electrical stimulation at 1 or 2/sec of the canals and the contralateral whole labyrinth was then performed.

During the individual trials of electrical stimulation, the cat was tested with horizontal angular acceleration to make sure the unit was functioning as before. After the electrical stimulation was completed, the cat was occasionally tested with angular acceleration in the plane of a vertical canal, or by tipping with respect to gravity.

The characteristic eye movements were elicited from the stimulation of the horizontal canal at a threshold value of 9.9 V $\pm$ 3.7 (mean $\pm$ S.D.) (n = 17); from the anterior canal 9.0 $\pm$ 3.7 (n = 25); and from the posterior canal 10.0 $\pm$ 5.2 (n = 25).

The field potentials, as shown in Figs. 3, 4 and 5, varied in size and shape when recorded from a given location, depending on which canal was stimulated. These differences were regularly observed and may reflect differences in fiber projection from each vestibular sensory region to the vestibular nucleus (Stein and Carpenter, 1967; Kasahara and Uchino, 1971). The N_1 portion of the field potential has thresholds on horizontal canal stimulation of 8.3 $\pm$ 4.3 (n = 17), the anterior canal, 6.8 $\pm$ 4.0 (n = 25); and the posterior canal 6.0 $\pm$ 3.4 (n = 10). Although these values are not significantly different from the eye movement thresholds, in almost every cat the voltage required to elicit an N_1 potential was smaller than that required to produce a threshold eye movement.

Determination of convergence, or lack of it, with the extracellular technique we used depended on several factors. First, we recorded neural responses in relation to the N_1 thresholds produced with single shocks at 1 or 2/sec + 0.1 msec duration (Precht and Shimazu, 1965). We rarely stimulated above 2 times N_1 threshold. The instances we are inclined to consider as convergence first occurred at 1.0 to 1.3 $\times$ N_1 threshold. (It should be noted we found clear instances of 'spread' at 1.8 $\times$ N_1 threshold and above from anterior to horizontal canal nerve and *vice versa*.) Second, we considered convergence likely *only* if there was a latency difference of 0.3 msec or more between the responses from two canal ampullae (while true convergence might take place on single neurons from two receptor sites with the same latency, we could not detect this extracellularly, and had to rely on latency differences which might be accounted for by smaller fiber diameter or extra synapses in one path). Thirdly, if the character of the responses were also different, such as firing in couplets on stimulating one receptor site, we considered this supportive evidence of convergence and not spread.

The relationship between the horizontal and anterior canal nerves was best studied. Horizontal canal type-II neurons, some of which may be considered to be activated from a vertical canal on other grounds (Shimazu and Precht, 1966), showed the following responses to horizontal and anterior canal nerve stimulations. Of 27 such neurons, 15 were not affected by stimulation of the ipsilateral horizontal canal at voltages up to 2 $\times$ N_1 threshold. (On stimulating the anterior canal, 6 of these showed no response, and 9 were facilitated at 1.1 to 6.0 msec latencies.) Of the original 27, 12 were facilitated by stimulating the horizontal canal nerve, having latencies ranging from 1.3 to 8.0

msec and thresholds of no more than $1.3 \times N_1$. Of these 12, 7 were also facilitated on anterior canal nerve stimulation at latencies ranging from 1.0 to 3.0 msec. These responses were obtained at thresholds ranging from 1.0 to $1.3 \times N_1$. Of these 7, while true convergence might account for the responses of them all, only 4 (4/27 = 15%) showed clear differences in latency and other criteria noted above, and thus represent convincing examples of convergence (see Figs. 3 and 4). The neurons in both these figures show a distinctly shorter latency for the paths from anterior canal ampulla to

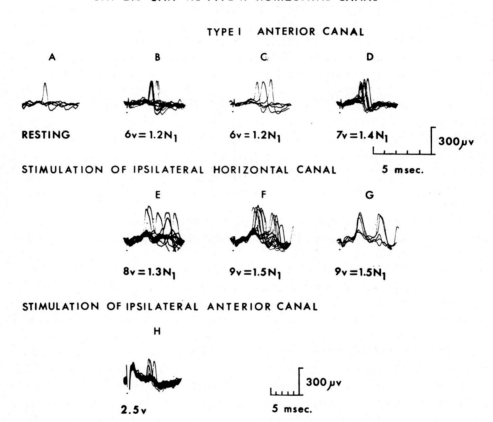

CAT 216 UNIT 11L TYPE II HORIZONTAL CANAL

TYPE I ANTERIOR CANAL

A   B   C   D

RESTING $6v = 1.2N_1$ $6v = 1.2N_1$ $7v = 1.4N_1$ 300μv

STIMULATION OF IPSILATERAL HORIZONTAL CANAL   5 msec.

E   F   G

$8v = 1.3N_1$ $9v = 1.5N_1$ $9v = 1.5N_1$

STIMULATION OF IPSILATERAL ANTERIOR CANAL

H

300μv

2.5v   5 msec.

STIMULATION OF CONTRALATERAL VIII NERVE

Fig. 3. Shows a tonic type-II neuron of the horizontal canal. On stimulation of the ipsilateral horizontal nerve, the latency was 1.8 msec at 1.2 times N_1 (B and C) and shortened to 1.5 at 1.4 times N_1 (D). This unit was then tested to angular acceleration in the planes of the vertical canals and was shown to be a type-I unit of the anterior canal. In E–G, it is the same neuron and still quite sensitive to angular acceleration in spite of the changed waveform. On stimulating the ipsilateral anterior canal nerve the latency was 1.2 msec at 1.3 and 1.5 times N_1 threshold (E–G), but at the higher stimulation level (F and G) the unit fired in couplets. On stimulating the contralateral vestibular nerve, the neuron was facilitated at a shortest latency of 3.4 msec. 15 sweeps were used on B, D–F and H; and 5 for A, C and G.

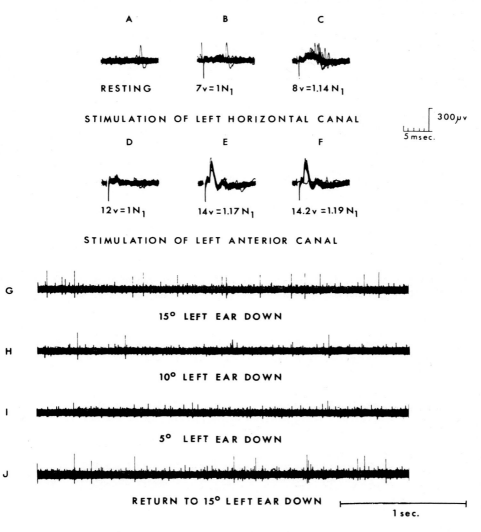

Fig. 4. Type-II unit of the horizontal canal. B and C show response to stimulating ipsilateral horizontal canal nerve; the shortest latency is 3.2 msec, shown in C (there is another lower amplitude unit with a shorter latency which is not our unit). On stimulating the ipsilateral anterior canal nerve with gradually increasing voltage, the unit started firing with great security at a voltage of 1.17 times N_1 at 1.0 msec latency (E and F). The unitary response falls on top of a small N_1. There were about 15 sweeps per frame, A–F. In G–J, the unit's response to ipsilateral otolithic stimulation is shown.

brain stem type-II neuron. However, in other instances, not shown, the horizontal canal ampulla to brain stem neuron had the shorter latency.

On contralateral nerve stimulation, 90% of type-II's (17/19) showed facilitation. In Fig. 4, note also the convergence from otolith receptors as shown by natural stimulation.

Type-I neurons of the horizontal canal (as determined by natural stimulation) had the following relations on electrical stimulation of the horizontal and anterior canal nerves. Of 42 type-I neurons, 38 were facilitated by horizontal canal nerve stimulation at thresholds of less than $2.0 \times N_1$ and 4 were unaffected. The latencies ranged from 1.0 to 7.0 msec. Of the 38, 19 were unaffected by anterior canal nerve stimulation up to $2 \times N_1$, 15 showed possible spread of current to other sensory regions, and 4 (4/38 = 10%) showed convergence. Fig. 5 shows one such unit. The latencies from the horizontal canal ranged from 1.2 to 2.0 msec, while values from the anterior canal were from 1.3 to 2.3 msec. In most instances the horizontal canal to brain stem path had the shorter latency. It should be noted that all the units showing convergence on electrical stimulation were tonic. The thresholds of convergence responses ranged from 1.0 to $1.3 \times N_1$ on both horizontal and anterior canal nerve stimulation. In all instances the threshold of the horizontal canal response was slightly less $(0.1 \text{ or } 0.2 \times N_1)$ than that from the anterior canal. Lastly, of the type-I's tested, 67% (14/21) were inhibited on contralateral whole nerve stimulation.

CAT 217 UNIT 4L TYPE I HORIZONTAL CANAL

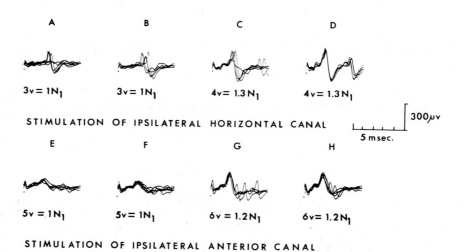

Fig. 5. Shows a tonic type-I unit of the horizontal canal on stimulating the ipsilateral horizontal canal nerve (A–D). In A and B, unit fires at N_1 threshold at 2.0 msec latency, shortening to 1.4 msec on being stimulated at 1.3 times N_1 threshold (C and D). On stimulating the anterior canal nerve, an incrementally growing N_1 may be seen in E–G. In G and H, at 1.2 times N_1 threshold, the unit first fires, falling between N_1 and N_2 with a fluctuating latency, the shortest being 2.2 msec.

Convergence from the posterior canal nerve onto horizontal canal brain stem neurons was looked into, but not as extensively as the anterior canal path. However, because the posterior canal ampulla is much further away from the horizontal canal receptor the data is worth noting. Type-I and type-II horizontal canal nerves showed facilitation on posterior canal stimulation at thresholds of $1.5 \times N_1 \pm 0.13$ (n = 3) and $1.39 \times N_1 \pm 0.35$ (n = 7) respectively. The latencies of facilitatory response on posterior canal nerve stimulation were from 1.1 to 6.0 msec with most of the responses showing a fluctuating latency and falling on N_2. Only tonic neurons were facilitated. Eight percent (3/38) of type-I neurons, and 14% (7/50) of type-II's showed facilitation on posterior canal electrical stimulation, these figures thus being similar to the anterior canal convergence patterns (Fig. 6).

One other type of canal–canal interaction was found: inhibition of horizontal canal type-I and II neurons was noted in a few instances on stimulating the vertical canals. See Fig. 6, bottom two rows, for an example of a unit which showed a combination of both inhibition and facilitation on stimulation of the ipsilateral posterior canal. However, because of problems of interpreting inhibition using extracellular recording, and the possibility of current spread, we cannot be definite about the mechanism of

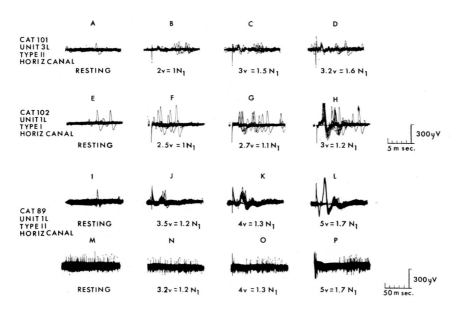

STIMULATION OF IPSILATERAL POSTERIOR CANAL

Fig. 6. Shows two type-II and one type-I unit which respond to ipsilateral posterior canal nerve stimulation. The neuron in A to D is facilitated at N_1 threshold (B) with fluctuating latency. The latency shortens from 5 to 4 msec on increased stimulus strength (D). The type-I unit in the second row is also facilitated at N_1 threshold (F), fires in couplets at 1.1 and 1.2 times N_1 (G, H). In H the earliest latency is 1.1 msec. The type-II unit in the third and fourth rows is both facilitated (I–L) with the spike falling on the falling phase of N_1 (J and K); and is also inhibited at the same stimulus strengths (O and P). All stimulations including M–P were done at 2/sec with 0.1 msec duration pulse. A–L consist of about 15, and M–P, 50 superimposed sweeps.

References pp. 136–137

this effect. It should be noted that Ito *et al.* (1969) have found with intracellular record-ing disynaptic inhibition in Deiters' neurons on labyrinthine stimulation.

Thirty-eight units from the natural stimulation and electrical stimulation studies were located histologically. In the medial nucleus there were 28, 8 in the superior, one in the lateral and one in the descending nucleus. Type-I's tended to cluster in the rostral part of the medial nucleus, while type-II's were usually found in the rostral, inferior part of the medial nucleus and the inferior part of the superior nucleus. There was no clustering of units connected with a particular receptor, but this negative result is not particularly important since this study was not designed to analyze this point.

DISCUSSION

Convergence of vestibular receptor activity onto brain stem units has been studied in this paper by natural stimulation and electrical stimulation. While there are problems in experimentation and interpretation with both approaches which should be discussed, we feel we can conclude that two or more vestibular receptors may show convergence on single second order vestibular units.

The problems with natural stimulation include: (*i*) Not positioning the animal in such a way that the angular acceleration stimulus is parallel or nearly parallel to the plane of the canal being stimulated. During the course of this experiment we perform-ed precise measurements on the canal planes in relation to the stereotaxic planes, and concluded that while most of the stimuli were being delivered correctly, the data obtained from our roll plane was suspect. When this was dealt with as explained in the Appendix, the percentages were not markedly different from the original findings. The Appendix data, incidentally, should allow other investigators to precisely position their experimental cats for angular acceleration. (*ii*) If there is a significant angular accelera-tion component during linear acceleration, canal stimulation may occur and confuse the results. However, the position changes with respect to gravity were very slow (0.5°/sec) and the pauses between movement long (20–30 sec). So we can rule out this possible artifact. (*iii*) It has been claimed that the vertical canals have a broad response range and can respond to angular accelerations widely removed from their own plane (Lowenstein and Sand, 1940; Ross, 1936; Vilstrup, 1951; Ledoux, 1958). We are now investigating this possibility. Type-II responses have also been explained by invoking a broad vertical canal response range (Crampton, 1965). Our finding of some type-II's of the horizontal canal which were not affected by natural stimulation of other canals, and the discovery that this broad response mode may be limited to the dogfish (Lowenstein, 1970), casts some doubt on using the broad vertical canal effect as an explanation for type-II responses.

In the present experiment, the main hurdle to overcome with electrical stimulation was that of stimulus spread. Tokumasu *et al.* (1971) concluded that stimulus spread to neighboring vestibular receptors with electrical stimulation by bipolar electrodes simi-lar to ours did not become a problem until voltages 2.5 to 3 times the threshold needed to produce a characteristic eye movement were reached. During the unit stimulation procedures we rarely got up to 2 times eye movement threshold. However, we used the

N_1 field threshold, which was obtained slightly below the eye movement threshold as our main guide. None of the responses we concluded as showing convergence were obtained at initial values higher than $1.3 \times N_1$, although we often increased the stimulus strength up to $2 \times N_1$. Further, we often found second order horizontal canal units which were unaffected by $2 \times N_1$ threshold stimulation of a vertical canal were found immediately adjacent to other similar units which were facilitated by electrical stimulation at or just above N_1 threshold.

Differences in the waveform of the field potential evoked by electrical stimulation of two receptor sites suggests that the current spread, if any, is small. Also, finding the same type of interaction from stimulating the posterior canal nerve as the anterior canal nerve makes stimulus spread unlikely in view of the relatively long distance of the posterior ampulla from the horizontal canal ampulla. Another point in favor of a functional converging path is the finding of convergence on a single unit by both electrical and natural stimulation techniques as was shown in Fig. 4.

Convergence tended to occur on tonic vestibular units in the majority of instances in the natural stimulation study, and in all of those studied with electrical stimulation. The paucity of phasic units may be significant. Kasahara and Uchino (1971) found little evidence of convergence, but they were doing intracellular recording under barbiturate anesthesia with labyrinthine polarization from vestibular units with distinctly shorter latencies than ours. These several factors suggest they were examining phasic neurons for the most part, while we were looking mostly at tonic units.

From a functional standpoint, there seems to be good a priori grounds for expecting convergence of vestibular inputs. 'The functional value of complementary sensory inputs from the otoliths and canals should not be overlooked. The canals alone cannot indicate the axis of rotation relative to gravity by classical concepts of cupula mechanics. Theoretically, the same pattern of canal input could be produced by rotation around any of a variety of axes. Hence, interplay between canals and otoliths is necessary for accurate perception and appropriate compensatory reactions to various movements relative to the earth' (Guedry, 1966). Our results show that extensive integration of vestibular information is evident at the second order neuron level in the vestibular system.

Lastly, an interesting ancillary finding should be noted. The 80 : 20 ratio (120/160 to 32/160) of type-I to type-II units was not altered by histologically verified sections (115/144 to 29/144) of the floor of the fourth ventricle to a depth of 2–3 mm. These incisions were deep enough and long enough to cut the vestibular commissural fibers (Gray, 1926; Rasmussen, 1932; Ferraro et al., 1940; Ladpli and Brodal, 1968). We might have seen a drop in the number of type-II neurons in the sectioned preparations since Shimazu and Precht (1966) found 95% (40/42) type-II neurons were facilitated by electrical stimulation of the contralateral whole vestibular nerve; and in looking at another group of type-II neurons they found about half (31/61) were not influenced by stimulation of the ipsilateral vestibular nerve, even at stimulus strengths of 4 to 5 times N_1 threshold. Our own similar experiments (Markham, 1968) bear out the thesis that contralateral labyrinthine drive is important for some type-II neurons, as is the finding that type-II neurons may be easily found in the vestibular nucleus on the side of an acute labyrinthectomy, at a time and place where type-I neurons are very difficult to find (Precht *et al.*, 1966). Yet, the present experiment suggests the commissural fibers do not carry the paramount vestibular driving force for a significant number of type-II neurons. The most likely explanation is that a number of type-II's derive their influence from the contralateral labyrinth via pathways passing deep via the reticular formation rather than, or in addition to, the commissural pathway. We are now looking into this possibility.

SUMMARY

Neurons in the vestibular nuclei were examined by extracellular recording in cats with cervical cord transections and were physiologically identified by their response to angular acceleration in the plane of the horizontal canal. They were then tested with natural and/or electrical labyrinthine stimulation.

On natural stimulation of otolith receptors and the anterior and posterior canals, approximately 40% of type I and II horizontal canal neurons showed no convergence at all; about 35% had convergence only from otolith receptors; about 10% from one or both vertical canals and about 10% from the otolith plus one or two canals. Tonic neurons received convergence information about twice as often as did kinetic neurons. Section of the brain stem vestibular commissural fibers did not alter these figures significantly.

Single shock electrical stimulation of individual horizontal and anterior canal nerves and, less frequently, posterior canal nerves was performed while recording from neurons naturally responsive to horizontal canal stimulation. Unit thresholds were compared to eye movement and N_1 field thresholds. Convergence, principally determined by differences in latency, from single vertical canals was shown to take place on a minority of tonic I and II neurons, thus confirming the natural stimulation findings. No electrical stimulation was performed on the otolith receptors, those receptors which showed the most frequent convergence on natural stimulation.

APPENDIX

Because we found we could not specify precisely the planes of the canals relative to the planes of stimulation, the following measurements were taken. In the skulls of 7 cats, a number of points were determined along each canal, planes were fitted to these points using a component analysis technique, and the angles between these planes were computed. These measures and their analysis are the subject of a forthcoming paper (Blanks *et al.*, 1972); see Table III for some of these measures. Then, a mathematical rotation of axes equivalent to the physical rotations used to orient the skull to the 'standard position' were performed and the values of these angles are given in Table IV. The means and cosine of each mean (in parentheses) are presented. The latter is given since it appears that as the canal is moved out of a plane of angular acceleration, endolymph flow should decrease by a cosine function. Ideally, each canal should have been parallel (*viz.*, made an angle of 0°, cosine = 1.0) with one plane, and

TABLE III

ANGLES IN DEGREES BETWEEN THE SEMICIRCULAR CANAL PLANES AND OTHER MAJOR PLANES

Angle between the plane of the	And the plane of the	Mean	N	S.D.	95% Confidence Limits	
					Lower	Upper
Horizontal canal	Anterior canal	89.61	14	8.70	84.59	94.64
Anterior canal	Posterior canal	90.21	14	4.04	87.87	92.54
Horizontal canal	Posterior canal	94.23	14	3.84	92.01	96.45
Left anterior canal	Right posterior canal	14.49	7	4.52	10.31	18.67
Right anterior canal	Left posterior canal	13.92	7	3.99	10.23	17.61
Right horizontal canal	Left horizontal canal	12.49	7	9.21	3.97	21.00

TABLE IV

ANGLES (IN DEGREES) BETWEEN THE SEMICIRCULAR CANAL PLANES AND THE PLANES OF THE ANGULAR ACCELERATION STIMULI WITH THE CAT'S HEAD IN THE STANDARD POSITION

Angle between the plane of the	And the					
	Horizontal plane		'Roll' plane		'Pitch' plane	
	Actual	Ideal	Actual	Ideal	Actual	Ideal
Left horizontal canal	15.44 (0.96)	0	57.86 (0.53)	90	79.52 (0.18)	90
Left anterior canal	73.41 (0.29)	90	32.83 (0.84)	0	86.94 (0.05)	90
Left posterior canal	84.80 (0.09)	90	81.02 (0.16)	90	9.16 (0.99)	0
Right horizontal canal	27.27 (0.89)	0	49.89 (0.64)	90	71.88 (0.31)	90
Right anterior canal	76.16 (0.24)	90	86.11 (0.07)	90	14.54 (0.97)	0
Right posterior canal	67.78 (0.39)	90	39.20 (0.77)	0	80.42 (0.17)	90

have been at 90° (cosine $= 0.0$) with the other planes. Because of the orientation of the canals in the skull and the restrictions of our apparatus, this was not the case. If we figure 2°/sec² is enough above threshold for the acceleration response to be easily detected by ear with most units; and since we used test accelerations of 4°/sec², canals thought to be well out of plane of the servo-motor driven arc, but actually intersecting it with cosines of 0.5 or more, might unintentionally activate units (figuring $4° \times 0.5 = 2.0°$/sec²). Figuring this way, the left and right horizontal canals would intersect with the roll planes with angles (57.86° and 49.89° respectively) which almost certainly

References pp. 136–137

resulted in more canal-to-canal convergence than is correct.

On the other side of the coin, there were no canals sufficiently far out of the plane they were supposed to be in to render them insensitive at $4°/sec^2$.

The data were recalculated as follows: The pitch plane *was* fairly well aligned with its target canals, and so the total amount of intercanal convergence was estimated from those neurons which responded to horizontal plane and *pitch plane* stimulation. This estimation required reallocation of some probably misclassified neurons to other categories. Estimation of this kind, and correction of probable misclassification can only provide very general approximations. Considering sectioned and non-sectioned units together, approximately 40% of horizontal canal units showed no convergence at all; about 35% had convergence only from otolithic receptors; about 10% from one or both vertical canals; and about 10% from the otoliths plus one or two canals.

REFERENCES

ADRIAN, E. D. (1943) Discharges from vestibular receptors in the cat. *J. Physiol. (Lond.)*, **101**, 389–407.

BLANKS, R. H. I., CURTHOYS, I. S. AND MARKHAM, C. H. (1972) Planar relationships of the semicircular canals in the cat. *Amer. J. Physiol.*, in press.

COHEN, B. AND SUZUKI, J.-I. (1963) Eye movements induced by ampullary nerve stimulation. *Amer. J. Physiol.*, **204**, 347–351.

COHEN, B., SUZUKI, J.-I. AND BENDER, M. B. (1964) Eye movements from semicircular canal nerve stimulation in the cat. *Ann. Otol. (St. Louis)*, **73**, 153–169.

CRAMPTON, G. H. (1965) Response of single cells in cat brain stem to angular acceleration in the horizontal plane. In *The Role of the Vestibular Organs in the Exploration of Space. NASA SP*-77, 85–96.

CURTHOYS, I. S. AND MARKHAM, C. H., (1971) Convergence of labyrinthine influences on units in the vestibular nuclei of the cat. I. Natural stimulation. *Brain Res.*, **35**, 469–490.

DESOLE, C. AND PALLESTRINI, E. A. (1969) Responses of vestibular units to stimulation of individual semicircular canals. *Exp. Neurol.*, **24**, 310–324.

DUENSING, F. UND SCHAEFER, K.-P. (1958) Die Aktivität einzelner Neurone im Bereich der Vestibulariskerne bei Horizontalbeschleunigungen unter besonderer Berücksichtigung des vestibulären Nystagmus. *Arch. Psychiat. Nervenkr.*, **198**, 225–252.

DUENSING, F. UND SCHAEFER, K.-P. (1959) Über die Konvergenz verschiedener labyrinthärer Afferenzen auf einzelne Neurone des Vestibulariskerngebietes. *Arch. Psychiat. Nervenkr.*, **199**, 345–371.

FERRARO, A., PACELLA, B. L. AND BARRERA, S. E. (1940) Effects of lesions of the medial vestibular nucleus. An anatomical and physiological study in macacus rhesus monkeys. *J. comp. Neurol.*, **73**, 7–36.

FUJITA, Y., ROSENBERG, J. AND SEGUNDO, J. P. (1968) Activity of cells in the lateral vestibular nucleus as a function of head position. *J. Physiol. (Lond.)*, **196**, 1–18.

GERNANDT, B. E, (1949) Response of mammalian vestibular neurons to horizontal rotation and caloric stimulation. *J. Neurophysiol.*, **12**, 173–184.

GRAY, L. P. (1926) Some experimental evidence on the connections of the vestibular mechanism in the cat. *J. comp. Neurol.*, **41**, 319–364.

GUEDRY, F. E. (1966) Modification of vestibular responses induced by unnatural patterns of vestibular stimulation. In R. J. WOLFSON (Ed.), *The Vestibular System and Its Diseases*. Univ. of Pennsylvania Press, Philadelphia, pp. 242–266.

ITO, M., HONGO, T.AND OKADA, Y. (1969) Vestibular-evoked postsynaptic potentials in Deiters' neurones. *Exp. Brain Res.*, **7**, 214–230.

KASAHARA, M. AND UCHINO, Y. (1971) Selective mode of commissural inhibition induced by semicircular canal afferents on secondary vestibular neurons in the cat. *Brain Res.*, **34**, 366–369.

LADPLI, R. AND BRODAL, A. (1968) Experimental studies of commissural and reticular formation projections from the vestibular nuclei in the cat. *Brain Res.*, **8**, 65–96.

LEDOUX, A. (1958) Les canaux semi-circulaires. Etude électrophysiologique. Contribution à l'effort d'uniformisation des épreuves vestibulaires. Essai d'interprétation de la sémiologie vestibulaire. *Acta oto-rhino-laryng. belg.*, **12**, 109–346.

LOWENSTEIN, O. (1970) The electrophysiological study of the responses of the isolated labyrinth of the lamprey (*Lampetra fluviatilis*) to angular acceleration, tilting and mechanical vibration. *Proc. roy. Soc. B*, **174**, 419–434.

LOWENSTEIN, O. AND SAND, A. (1940) The individual and integrated activity of the semicircular canals of the elasmobranch labyrinth. *J. Physiol. (Lond.)*, **99**, 89–101.

MARKHAM, C. H. (1968) Midbrain and contralateral labyrinth influences on brain stem vestibular nerves in the cat. *Brain Res.*, **9**, 312–333.

MELVILL JONES, G. AND MILSUM, J. H. (1970) Characteristics of neural transmission from the semicircular canal to the vestibular nuclei of cats. *J. Physiol. (Lond.)*, **209**, 295–316.

PETERSON, B. W. (1967) Effect of tilting on the activity of neurons in the vestibular nuclei of the cat. *Brain Res.*, **6**, 606–609.

PRECHT, W. AND SHIMAZU, H. (1965) Functional connections of tonic and kinetic vestibular neurons with primary vestibular afferents. *J. Neurophysiol.*, **28**, 1014–1028.

PRECHT, W., SHIMAZU, H. AND MARKHAM, C. H. (1966) A mechanism of central compensation of vestibular function following hemilabyrinthectomy. *J. Neurophysiol.*, **29**, 996–1010.

RASMUSSEN, A. T. (1932) Secondary vestibular tracts in the cat. *J. comp. Neurol.*, **54**, 143–171.

ROSS, D. A. (1936) Electrical studies on the frog's labyrinth. *J. Physiol. (Lond.)*, **86**, 117–146.

SHIMAZU, H. AND PRECHT, W. (1965) Tonic and kinetic responses of cat's vestibular neurons to horizontal angular acceleration. *J. Neurophysiol.*, **28**, 991–1013.

SHIMAZU, H. AND PRECHT, W. (1966) Inhibition of central vestibular neurons from the contralateral labyrinth and its mediating pathway. *J. Neurophysiol.*, **29**, 467–492.

STEIN, B. M. AND CARPENTER, M. B. (1967) Central projections of portions of the vestibular ganglia innervating specific parts of the labyrinth in the rhesus monkey. *Amer. J. Anat.*, **120**, 281–318.

SZENTÁGOTHAI, J. (1943) Die zentrale Innervation der Augenbewegungen. *Arch. Psychiat. Nervenkr.*, **116**, 721–760.

TOKUMASU, K. SUZUKI, J.-I. AND GOTO, K. (1971) A study of the current spread on electric stimulation of the individual utricular and ampullary nerves. *Acta oto-laryng. (Stockh.)*, **71**, 313–318.

VILSTRUP, G. (1951) On the eye reflexes induced by the semicircular canals. *Acta ophthal. (Kbh.)*, **29**, 163–167.

Transfer Function of Labyrinthine Volleys Through the Vestibular Nuclei

G. MELVILL JONES

Canadian Defence Research Board, Aviation Medical Research Unit, Department of Physiology, McGill University, Montreal, Quebec, Canada

In order to control the movement of a body in 3-dimensional space, it is necessary to know the separate components of movement in 3 translational and 3 rotational degrees of freedom. One of the basic means of obtaining such information derives from inertial forces generated by the body's accelerations in those degrees of freedom. These forces, being dependent only upon acceleration relative to stellar, or inertial, space yield information about absolute movement. The principle has become familiar through the method of inertial guidance in man-made space vehicles.

However, living systems evolved inertial guidance mechanisms long before Newton! The principle is used very early in the phylogenetic scale. Thus grains of starch in plant cells may transmit gravitational stimuli to the surrounding protoplasm, and Protozoan vacuoles may function in a similar way (Lowenstein, 1956a). Certainly, inertia-dependent statocysts are common in the Metazoa, and combined rotational and translational sensing endorgans are evident as early as the cyclostomes, where in Myxine two vertical ampullae share a single canal and a single undivided otolith-bearing macula (Lowenstein, 1956b). In the fully developed vestibular system of vertebrates, all 6 degrees of freedom are represented in the mechanical endorgan. The endorgan in turn generates afferent neural signals bearing systematic relationships with both rotational and linear accelerative movements of the head. However, a key word here is 'systematic'. The relation is seldom a direct one, and indeed the meaningful content of the neural signal may be quite different from that of acceleration; and yet it must always bear a systematic relation to the imposed acceleration since this is the basic adequate stimulus to the inertia-dependent sensory elements. This statement may appear at first sight to be paradoxical. Hopefully, its implications may be clarified by more detailed attention to the physical characteristics of the semicircular canals.

PHYSICAL CHARACTERISTICS OF THE SEMICIRCULAR CANALS

The basic inertia-sensing properties of the semicircular canals have been appreciated for many years. For example, Breuer (1874) and later Stefani (1876) demonstrated the inertia-dependent movement of fluids in primitive models of the canals. Gaede (1922) appears to be the first to have recorded in the literature a proper physical analysis of the fluid dynamics in a small closed circular tube. As so often happens, at about the same time several other authors arrived at similar analytical derivations of probable physical response characteristics (Masuda, 1922; Rohrer, 1922; Schmaltz, 1925, 1931; Rohrer and Masuda, 1926). Broadly, these authors attempted to calculate the likely relative movement of fluid in the endolymphatic canal as a result of angular acceleration of the head in a plane parallel to that canal. However, they were not in a position to appreciate the significance of forces introduced by deviation of the cupula in the ampulla, since at that time it was not certain whether such an organ existed. Steinhausen (1927–39) added the effects of a water-tight elastic cupular mechanism and derived a second order differential equation in an attempt to establish a quantitative relation between the angle of cupular deflection relative to its zero position and the angular acceleration of the head. The concept of a water-tight elastic cupula received support from the experimental work of Dohlman (1935). Various authors have developed the theme from this point to generate experimental investigations of the validity of Steinhausen's conclusions. Thus, van Egmond et al. (1949) developed the method of cupulometry in an attempt to make rational measurements of clinical impairment in human subjects. At about the same time, Mayne (1950) using the relatively new methodology of systems analysis, inferred hydrodynamic response characteristics similar to those implicit in the differential equation formulated by Steinhausen. Later investigators have attempted to extend the observations of earlier workers using measurable manifestations of efferent reflex response to controlled rotational stimulation of the canals. Thus, Hallpike and Hood (1953), and subsequently Hixson and Niven (1961, 1962), used various measures of reflexly induced compensatory eye movement consequent to excitation of the vestibulo-ocular reflex arc.

Others have used the information content of trains of unit action potentials in primary (Ross, 1936; Lowenstein and Sand, 1940; Groen et al., 1952; Rupert et al., 1962; Sala, 1965; Klinke, 1970; Goldberg and Fernández, 1971; Fernández and Goldberg, 1971) and subsequent neural locations in the brain stem (Adrian, 1943; Gernandt, 1949; Duensing and Schaefer, 1958; Wilson et al., 1965; Shimazu and Precht, 1965; Wilson et al., 1968; Ryu et al., 1969; Melvill Jones and Milsum, 1970, 1971). The present article describes some results of a series of experiments in which the informational content of unit responses in the brain stem of cat vestibular nuclei has been examined as a function of various patterns of rotational stimulation of the endorgan.

The endorgan response

In order to appreciate the rationale for the methods of data analysis employed, it is first appropriate to examine the physical characteristics of the assumed endorgan response. Fig. 1 illustrates a simplified system comprising a thin circular tube containing a water-tight but freely moving piston, the movement of which faithfully follows fluid displacement round the circuit of the canal. To simulate the elastic characteristics of the cupular mechanism, the hypothetical piston is located between

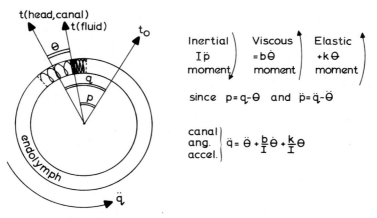

Fig. 1. Simple model of hydrodynamic components of the canal.

two springs in the circular tube of Fig. 1, in such a way that the spring mechanisms and their supports are supposed not to interfere with the fluid movement.

Consider now the whole system commencing to rotate at time t_0 in the direction indicated and at an angular acceleration $\ddot{q}$. In the figure, the arrow labelled t_0 indicates the angular position at which the undeviated piston was located at the commencement of the acceleration. After a given time (t), the whole system has rotated to the position marked by the arrow labelled t (head, canal). However, owing to the inertia of the fluid (*i.e.*, due to its mass), the fluid has been left behind relative to the tube so that the piston has only reached the position marked by the arrow labelled t (fluid). In doing so the movement of the piston has compressed the hypothetical spring as shown.

Using this simple analogy of the real canal, we may now equate moments generated in opposite directions. Thus, since the fluid has moved through an angle p, then the fluid's actual angular acceleration is given by $\ddot{p}$. Hence, a clockwise moment is established due to the inertial response of the fluid to its own angular acceleration. The value of this moment is given by $I\ddot{p}$, where I = moment of inertia of the contained fluid. This moment is represented on the left-hand side of the equation in Fig. 1. However, as soon as fluid flow occurs as a result of this moment, there is an opposing viscous moment. Significantly, owing to the very small diameter, and hence Reynold's number, of the fluid system, such flow as occurs must be *strictly laminar*. Under these specific conditions, the moment due to viscous forces must be strictly proportional to the *rate* of relative fluid flow. The viscous moment in the equation of Fig. 1 is therefore given as $b\dot{\Theta}$, where $\dot{\Theta}$ = the relative angular velocity of fluid flow and b = the viscous coefficient. Notice that the direction of this moment is opposite to the inertial moment. The viscous moment is represented in the first term on the right-hand side of the equation. Acting in the same direction as the viscous moment, there will also be an elastic moment, this time proportional to the relative displacement of fluid in the tube, and in the equation this is represented by $k\Theta$, where Θ = the relative

References pp. 154–156

angular displacement of the fluid and k = spring constant. Since these are the only moments exerted on the fluid, we may write

$$I\ddot{p} = b\dot{\Theta} + k\Theta \tag{1}$$

As indicated in Fig. 1, we may rearrange this equation in the form

$$\ddot{q} = \ddot{\Theta} + \frac{b}{I}\dot{\Theta} + \frac{k}{I}\Theta \tag{2}$$

Thus a second order differential equation emerges in which the left-hand side gives the forcing function, namely, canal angular acceleration, and the right-hand side describes the response, Θ, expressed here as the relative angle of fluid displacement in the canal. Of course, in the real canal, this would be equivalent to the angular deviation of the cupula in the ampulla, when a constant of proportionality, a, must be introduced to account for the proportionate relationship between cupular angle in the ampulla and the angle of relative fluid displacement round the canal circuit. Jones and Spells (1963), using the expression $a = \pi^2 r^2 R/V$ found a mean value of $a = 0.50$ from measurements made on 44 different species. In this expression $r =$ internal radius of the endolymphatic canal, $R =$ radius of curvature of the canal and $V =$ the volume of the ampulla. Equation (2) is essentially similar to that derived by Steinhausen and used in the formulation of the classical experimental study of van Egmond et al. (1949) referred to above.

   Providing this equation remains linear, it may conveniently be restated as a transfer function of the form proposed by Jones and Milsum (1965),

$$\frac{\Theta}{\ddot{q}}(s) = \frac{1}{s^2 + (b/I)\,s + (k/I)} \tag{3}$$

Owing to the heavy viscous damping term (b), the denominator may be restated in the form,

$$\frac{\Theta}{\ddot{q}}(s) = \frac{I/k}{(T_1 s + 1)(T_2 s + 1)} \tag{4}$$

where $\qquad T_1 T_2 = I/k \ \text{and} \ T_1 + T_2 = b/k.$

Since it can be shown that T_1 is probably more than two orders of magnitude greater than T_2, we may write to a close approximation,

$$T_1 = b/k.$$

Substituting this value of T_1 we may write

$$T_2 = I/b.$$

   We now see the functional implication of this relationship is that two time-constants, T_1 and T_2 emerge, having numerical values closely equal to identifiable ratios of coefficients in the equation.

   What does this imply in the context of the present theme? Probably the most useful, and functionally meaningful, way of illustrating the outcome of these observations

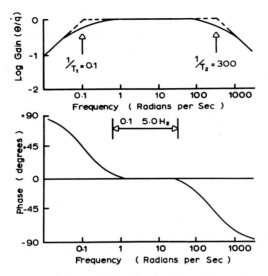

Fig. 2. Frequency response of the model in Fig. 1. Adapted from Jones and Milsum (1965).

is by means of a Bode plot of the form shown in Fig. 2. First, it is helpful to rewrite the transfer function of equation (4) in the form

$$\frac{\Theta}{\dot{q}}(s) = \frac{(I/k)s}{(T_1s + 1)(T_2s + 1)} \qquad (5)$$

From this we may draw a frequency response diagram as in Fig. 2. Here the upper curve is a conventional amplitude ratio plot in which the log of the gain (in this case, cupular angle/head angular velocity) is plotted as ordinate, against a logarithmic frequency scale plotted in radians per sec (rad/sec $= 2\pi$Hz) as abscissa. Under this is plotted the conventional phase diagram in which the ordinate gives the phase of cupular response relative to that of stimulus head angular velocity. The plus sign indicates phase advancement of the response; the minus sign, phase lag.

In a diagram such as this, the two time constants, T_1 and T_2, emerge as the reciprocal of the frequencies (in rad/sec) at which the asymptotic projections of the gain curve produce 'break-off' points indicated by the two vertical arrows. Thus choosing $T_1 = 0.1$ sec and $T_2 = 1/300$ sec (Jones and Milsum, 1965), a curve emerges which is flat over a frequency range extending from about 0.1–5.0 Hz, as indicated between the two short vertical lines in the figure. Particularly noteworthy is the fact that over this range the response would be approximately in phase with the stimulus head angular velocity. However, with the extension of the frequency range below the 0.1 Hz level, both the amplitude and the phase begin to change rapidly with decreasing frequency. Similarly in the upper range of frequencies the response of the transfer function in equation (5), namely, the displacement of cupula per unit head angular velocity, decreases with increasing frequency; but here a phase lag would begin to develop.

References pp. 154–156

Thus, we may say from this relatively simple analysis that the hydrodynamic characteristics of the tube in Fig. 1 would be expected to perform one integration on the imposed angular acceleration, so that the relative fluid displacement would provide a measure of angular velocity at every instant, but only over a limited frequency range as indicated by the 'flat' region in Fig. 2. Specifically, the system in Fig. 1 would act as an angular speedometer, but only over the middle frequency range determined by the actual values of $T_1 = b/k$ and $T_2 = I/b$.

Two additional features may be emphasized at this point. First, these conclusions only hold so long as the pattern of fluid flow in the tube is always strictly laminar, *i.e.*, obeys the Hagen–Poiseuille law of laminar flow in small tubes of circular cross section. Of particular relevance is the fact that this feature is ensured in the endolymphatic canal by its very small internal diameter, about 0.3 mm in man. Secondly, the speed registered is that of the head relative to inertial space. The vestibular system 'sees' the absolute velocity independently of all the other complex physiological variables such as neck and body rotation and limb movement.

Critical dependence of canal response upon physical dimensions

The critical dependence of the canal response upon its physical dimension may be further understood by examining the derivation of the coefficients in equation (5). Van Egmond *et al.* (1949) give the coefficients I and b as,

$$I = 2\pi^2 \varrho r^2 R^3 \qquad (6)$$

and

$$b = 8\pi^2 \eta R^3 \qquad (7)$$

Whilst Jones and Spells (1963) give

$$k = \pi r^2 \mu R \qquad (8)$$

where R = radius of curvature of endolymphatic canal
  r = internal radius of the thin endolymphatic tube
  ϱ = fluid density
  η = fluid viscosity
  μ = the pressure exerted by the cupula per unit angular deflection of fluid round the circuit.

There are certain reservations attached to some of these relations, but it is not appropriate to enter into these details in this article. They are considered at greater length in another article (Melvill Jones, 1972). In that article and from the work of Jones and Spells (1963), the results of dimensional analysis predict that if the canal is to continue to measure head angular velocity during head movements, then these dimensions, particularly r and R, should increase with animal size according to the slower head movements to be expected from larger animals. However such increase would only be very gradual indeed, roughly 10 log cycles increase in weight being required for one log cycle increase in canal radius of curvature. Moreover, it was predicted that r^2, and R and R^2/r^2 should all vary in proportion to one another, maintaining the ratio r^2/R constant.

Now it can be seen from equations (6) and (7) that the value of T_2 ($= I/b$) is proportional to r^2. Moreover, the longer time-constant, T_1 ($= b/k$), is proportional to R^2/r^2. Thus, from the previous paragraph it emerges that if the above criteria are maintained, then the two break frequencies in Fig. 2 ($1/T_1$ and $1/T_2$ rad/sec) would move proportionately up and down the frequency scale (abscissa) according to animal size. In effect, therefore, the frequency range of angular velocity transduction would be increased or decreased to match the likely frequency content of natural head movement. As Jones and Spells (1963) showed, for this to occur it is only necessary that the two variable r^2 and R, and hence also R^2/r^2, should vary according to a power relationship to body mass, such that

$$r^2, \text{ R and } R^2/r^2 \propto (\text{body mass})^n$$

The prediction was that n should be close to 0.1.

In view of these analytical conclusions, it was particularly intriguing to find from a survey of canal dimensions in 93 specimens from 87 different species ranging from mouse to horse (about 0.04 kg to 450 kg), that this general relation was rather closely maintained, since a statistically reliable value of $n = 0.095 \pm 0.05$ emerged from these data. The detailed dimensional analysis of cat canals made by Fernández and Valentinuzzi (1968) conforms closely with this general conclusion.

NEURAL RESPONSE

These two analytical approaches suggest rather strongly that evolution has favoured very particular physical characteristics for the semicircular canal such that, over the range of natural head movement, the hydrodynamics of the system should perform one accurate integration on the angular acceleration of the head relative to inertial space. It therefore becomes of special interest to investigate the extent to which this conclusion is realized in the information content of the afferent neural signal received by the brain. A series of experiments was therefore performed with this end in view (Milsum and Melvill Jones, 1969; Melvill Jones and Milsum, 1969, 1970, 1971).

Fig. 3 illustrates diagramatically the system of experimental equipment employed in these experiments. Decerebrate cats were located in a stereotaxic device mounted on a multi-degree of freedom platform capable of being fixed coaxially to a horizontal velocity-servo-controlled turntable. The platform could be suspended either from 4 parallel springs or 4 parallel inextensible wires, permitting multi-degree of freedom of movement. The usual procedure was to advance an extra-cellular steel microelectrode through the floor of the fourth ventricle at approximately the anteroposterior level of the medial vestibular nucleus, whilst maintaining gentle multidegree freedom of movement. Relevant units were then subjected to sequential movement excitation in the separate rotational and translational degrees of freedom. Only units responding specifically to rotational movement in the plane of one pair of canals were retained for measurement of their response to angular movements. Cells selected

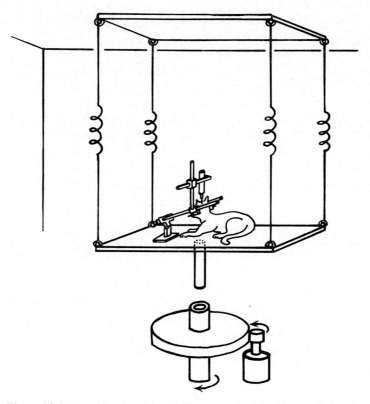

Fig. 3. The multi-degree of freedom stimulus system. From Melvill Jones and Milsum (1970).

were therefore specifically sensitive to rotational stimulation in the plane of one pair of canals. With these canals oriented in the plane of turntable rotation, the neural responses to sinusoidal and transient rotational stimuli were examined systematically. Fig. 4 illustrates a sample of spike responses to sinusoidal rotational stimulation within the frequency range presumed to be associated with angular velocity trans- duction in the canal of the cat. Evidently, at least when the cell was firing actively, the spike frequency was modulated approximately in phase with the stimulus record, which in all records was derived from a tachometer registering turntable *angular velocity*.

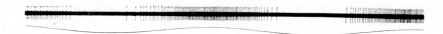

Fig. 4. Extract from an original train of action potentials (upper trace) related to the sinusoidal angular velocity of rotational stimulation (lower trace). Period, 4.0 sec; Amplitude, 32°/sec. From Milsum and Melvill Jones (1969).

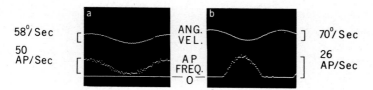

Fig. 5. Averaged stimulus angular velocity and neural response (action potential frequency) from two canal-dependent units in the medial vestibular nuclei of decerebrate cats during sinusoidal rotation in the plane of the lateral canals. (a) Period, 1.4 sec; (b) Period, 4.0 sec. From Melvill Jones and Milsum (1970).

Computer analysis of records such as these can be made to yield averaged responses in the form shown in Fig. 5. In both halves of this figure, the upper trace gives averaged turntable angular velocity during a typical cycle of the sinusoidal stimulus and the dotted trace gives the computer-averaged spike frequency associated with every point in the stimulus cycle. Again, it seems that the spike frequency tends to be modulated in an approximately sinusoidal fashion in phase with the sinusoidal stimulus angular velocity. In a detailed investigation, Melvill Jones and Milsum (1970) concluded that this general relation was representative of the information content of the neural signal received in the brain stem during sinusoidal rotational

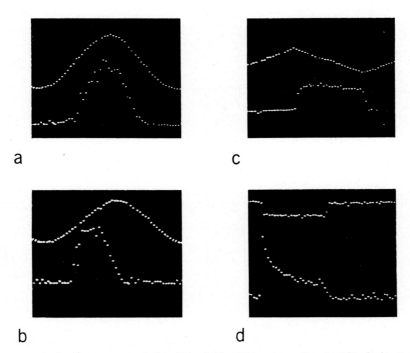

Fig. 6. Averaged stimulus response relationships obtained from one unit assessed to be located in the left medial vestibular nucleus. (a) Period, 4 sec; (b) Period, 64 sec; (c) Triangular velocity ramps of period 128 sec; (d) Square wave changes in angular velocity of period 64 sec. From Melvill Jones (1968).

stimuli in the frequency range about 0.25–1.0 Hz; a conclusion which is closely in line with the predictions made on the analytical and dimensional bases discussed above.

Low frequency and transient responses

If the neural signal were to maintain a faithful representation of the endorgan mechanical response, then it would be expected from the transfer function of equation (5) that at low frequencies the response, rather than being tied to the stimulus angular velocity, would progressively phase advance with respect to it as the frequency of stimulus decreased. Fig. 6a,b shows two responses recorded at frequencies of 1/4 and 1/64 Hz respectively. Marked phase advancement is evident in this second (low frequency) response.

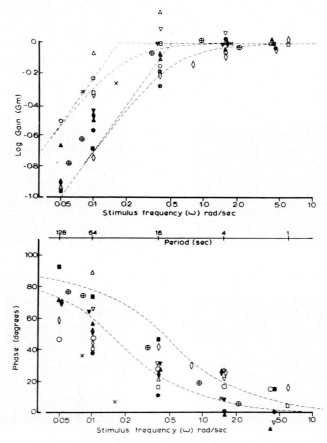

Fig. 7. Bode plot of normalised gain and phase from twelve single units retained sufficiently long to examine their frequency response over a wide frequency range of sinusoidal rotational stimulation. Normalisation of gain based on the mean gain in the frequency range 0.25 Hz–1.0 Hz. The intermittent lines give the response of equation (5), with $T_1 = 2.0$ and 6.0 sec. Individual cells are represented by separate symbols. From Melvill Jones and Milsum (1971).

Fig. 7 gives the Bode plot of accumulated data reported by Melvill Jones and Milsum (1971) and examines this feature in terms of the curves in Fig. 2. The results only examine response characteristics across the low frequency half of the curves in Fig. 2. Bearing in mind that the two sets of data in the upper and lower curves are essentially tied to one another, it is remarkable to see how closely the data points obtained conform with the predictions of the simple linear transfer function for the *mechanical* response of the canal, as shown in equation (5). Not only does the gain, expressed here as the ratio of change in firing frequency per unit change in angular velocity, decrease rapidly with decreasing stimulus frequency (note the logarithmic ordinate) but also an appropriate phase advancement occurs over the two decades of frequency employed.

The same transfer function predicts specific patterns of response to transient or step changes in both angular velocity and angular acceleration of stimulus. The systematic nature of the neural responses to such stimuli can be seen in Fig. 6d and c respectively. A sudden change in stimulus angular velocity (Fig. 6d) leads to a correspondingly sudden change in firing frequency followed by an exponential decay towards the steady state value. A sudden change in angular acceleration (Fig. 6c) shows the predicted exponential rise to a plateau level which in the absence of non-linearity would be maintained indefinitely. Thus, at least from the records discussed here, it seems that the neural signal received in the brain stem does indeed tend to follow the hydrodynamical response of the endorgan with generally good fidelity, even during movements extending well beyond the natural evolutionary experience.

Non-linearities

If the neural response to rotational canal stimulation were to follow accurately the simple transfer function of equation (5), linearity would have to obtain throughout. However, various forms of non-linearity have been described in the literature and it is therefore important to examine their influence on the system's response. For example, Melvill Jones and Milsum (1970), investigating the dependence of neural gain (change of firing frequency per unit change in angular velocity) upon stimulus amplitude (angular velocity) at a given sinusoidal frequency, found a power relationship such that

$$\text{Gain} \propto (\text{angular velocity})^{-0.28}$$

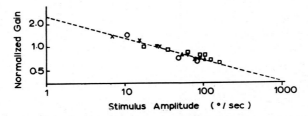

Fig. 8. Dependence of gain upon stimulus amplitude. Individual cells are represented by separate symbols. From Melvill Jones and Milsum (1970).

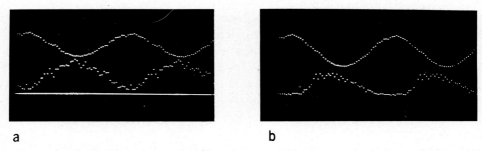

a   b

Fig. 9. Transition from all-round firing to threshold cut-off in a single unit, to illustrate the asymmetric pattern of firing associated with the cut-off pattern. From Milsum and Melvill Jones (1969).

Fig. 8 illustrates the normalized data from 5 units and indicates a rather consistent relationship in which the slope of —0.28 is clearly statistically significant. An intriguing point is that such a small index would lead to but a small divergence from linearity over a considerable range of stimulus magnitudes.

Fig. 9 illustrates a further form of non-linearity (Milsum and Melvill Jones, 1969) such that there appears to be a tendency for units exhibiting 'threshold cut-off' to respond with a more rapidly changing leading, than trailing, edge in their response waveform. Interestingly, this finding was statistically significant in units cut off at one point in their cycle by their threshold of firing, but not evident, even in the same unit, when firing was maintained throughout the cycle due to either a high spontaneous firing frequency or because of a relatively low stimulus amplitude or both. Possibly this phenomenon is one manifestation of the 'kinetic' response patterns seen by Shimazu and Precht (1965). In any case, presumably both these phenomena would contribute to the changes in upper frequency response characteristics reported by Goldberg and Fernández (1971). Examining neural unit responses in primary afferent fibres of the monkey, they have shown a marked tendency for phase advancement and gain increase of the response to occur as the frequency of sinusoidal stimulation increases above about 1.0 Hz. Moreover, their results conform well with those of Benson (1970) who investigated the gain of vestibulo-ocular response in man at high frequencies. It seems therefore that the upper frequency range of Fig. 2 may not be as representative of the real system's response as is the middle frequency range.

In the lower frequency range, an adaptive term becomes significant. Although some units, both in the primary (Goldberg and Fernández, 1971) and subsequent (Shimazu and Precht, 1965; Melvill Jones and Milsum, 1971) neural pathways appear to be essentially non-adapting, others show consistent adaptation. A relatively non-adaptive pattern is seen in the response to a step change of angular acceleration in Fig. 6c, whilst a relatively adaptive response is seen in the corresponding record at the top right hand corner of Fig. 10 obtained from another cell.

Moreover an adaptive term has been shown to account for the systematic response of subjective sensation (Oman, 1968; Young, 1969) and compensatory nystagmus (Oman, 1968; Malcolm and Melvill Jones, 1970) during low frequency rotational stimulation of man. The latter authors, for example, showed that a transfer function of the form

$$\frac{\dot{\psi}}{\dot{q}}(s) = \varrho \left\{ \frac{(I/k)s}{(T_1s + 1)} - \frac{(I/k)s}{(T_1s + 1)(T_3s + 1)} \right\} \qquad (9)$$

stimulated the observed nystagmoid response of human subjects very closely, where

$\dot{\psi}$ = angular velocity of slow phase eye movement relative to the head

T_3 = an adaptive time constant

ϱ = a proportionality constant

I, k, $\dot{q}$ and T_1 are as in equation (5).

The similarity of equations (9) and (5) becomes evident when it is appreciated that compensatory slow phase eye angular velocity ($\dot{\psi}$) is functionally related to cupular angle (Θ), and that at low frequencies the influence of the short (inertia/viscous) time constant (T_2) becomes negligible. Malcolm and Melvill Jones (1970) found the adaptive time constant (T_3) to be 82 sec (S.E. $\pm$ 6.5) in man, and this is the same order of magnitude as the estimates of Oman (1968) and Goldberg and Fernández (1971). In the present context an important conclusion is that the great length of this adaptive time constant excludes its significant influence upon the system's response in the middle and upper frequency ranges of Fig. 2.

It is, of course, well known that habituation can in the long term substantially influence the transfer of information from sensory endorgan to efferent response. Indeed it has very recently been shown that, with an appropriate long term experimental procedure, it is even possible to effect retained reversal of the adult human vestibulo-ocular reflex (Gonshor, 1971; Gonshor and Melvill Jones, 1971).

But it is not yet possible to predict with assurance how effects such as these may modify the transfer function of labyrinthine volley through the vestibular nuclei.

Interactions between rotational and linear accelerative stimuli

An additional complication associated with real natural movement stems from interactions between linear and accelerative stimuli. Fig. 10 illustrates one aspect of this feature. The upper 3 computer-averaged records from this single cell show that its response derived essentially from mechanical stimulation of the semicircular canal. Thus, decreasing frequency of sinusoidal stimulation produced the substantial phase advancement to be expected from the transfer function of equation (5). Moreover, transient accelerative stimuli produced the response characteristic of exponential rise to a plateau as discussed above. Furthermore, the unit was non-responsive to linear accelerative stimuli imposed in straight lines by means of the parallel swing suspension of Fig. 3.

However, when the whole parallel swing system was moved in such a way that its centre of gravity described a circular path without there being rotational movement of the platform (sometimes referred to as counter rotational stimulation), the spontaneous activity of this cell (lower left-hand record of Fig. 10) was systematically increased (lower middle record of Fig. 10) during movement of the platform round

References pp. 154–156

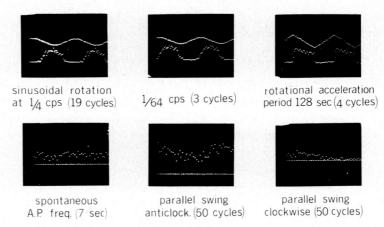

sinusoidal rotation   1/64 cps (3 cycles)   rotational acceleration
at 1/4 cps (19 cycles)   period 128 sec (4 cycles)

spontaneous   parallel swing   parallel swing
A.P. freq. (7 sec)   anticlock. (50 cycles)   clockwise (50 cycles)

Fig. 10. Series of averaged responses to rotational stimulation (upper series) and counter rotating stimuli (lower series), to illustrate interaction between rotational and linear accelerative stimulations. From Melvill Jones (1968).

a circle in the same direction as that of excitatory endolymphatic fluid flow. In contrast to this, during counter rotation in the opposite direction, the maintained firing frequency of this cell was suppressed well below that during counter rotation in the excitatory direction (lower right-hand record of Fig. 10), and even below that associated with 'spontaneous' neural activity shown in the lower left figure.

This counter rotating movement imposes a rotating, radially oriented, linear acceleration vector without introducing real rotation of the animal. Thus, it is quite possible to complicate the pattern of response in a specifically semicircular canal-dependent unit by imposing changes of direction in a linear acceleration vector. This feature has been systematically explored by Benson *et al.* (1970) who concluded that possibly the interference was due to alteration of the mechanical response in the end-organ, although neural interaction between canal and otolithic afferent signals could not be excluded.

DISCUSSION

The combined outcome of these analytical, anatomical and neurophysiological studies leads the author to the general conclusion that evolutionary pressures have strongly favoured a canal 'design' such that its hydrodynamical response to rotation accurately registers instantaneous head angular velocity during much natural head movement, *i.e.*, in the middle frequency range of Fig. 2. Not only do the directly observed patterns of neural signals dispatched from the brain stem of cats favour this view: but associated analytical and anatomical studies indicate that, with very specifically appropriate changes of canal dimensions with animal size, head angular velocityco ntinues to be the relevant informational content of the canal signal generated by natural head movements over a wide range of animal species of varying size.

Of course, the neurophysiological findings from a single series of experiments must always be treated with caution until further results become available in the literature. But the recent comprehensive investigation of response in primary afferent neurones of the squirrel monkey by Goldberg and Fernández (1971) and Fernández and Goldberg (1971), and the earlier investigation of cat brain stem units by Shimazu and Precht (1965) together with the results summarised above (Melvill Jones and Milsum, 1970, 1971) substantially support the view that many neurones carry informational content broadly described by the transfer function of equation (5), at least in the middle frequency range of Fig. 2.

This general conclusion in turn leads one to enquire into the potential functional advantage of accurate rate-dependent feedback from head rotation. In this connection, it is noteworthy that the dynamic response of the purely visual tracking system associated with optokinetic following of a moving visible object when the head is still, is rather poor (Young, 1962; Young and Stark, 1963); particularly so when the target movement is relatively random in nature (Michael and Melvill Jones, 1966). However, it seems that the rate-dependent vestibular signal from the canals is entirely appropriate for establishing neuromuscular damping of such head movement *relative to space*, through vestibulo-collic stabilising reflexes (Outerbridge, 1969; Outerbridge and Melvill Jones, 1971) which have recently been shown to exhibit extremely rapid neural response characteristics (Wilson and Yoshida, 1969a,b). In addition, such residual head movement relative to space as remains after vestibulo-collic reflex stabilisation of the head, would seem to be most appropriately compensated by a velocity driven vestibulo-ocular reflex system (Melvill Jones, 1971).

An additional important feature to which attention has been drawn by Roberts (1967) is the close functional link established between canal afferents and motor responses in the limbs. Thus, nose-down rotation of the head of the cat activates forelimb extensors, so that velocity-modulated canal afferents would automatically induce an appropriate damping term in these, and presumably other, postural muscles as a consequence of unintended changes in body attitude. One might well ask how such automatic stabilising responses would be suppressed in order to permit intended voluntary changes in attitude. Perhaps the remarkable observations of Klinke (1970) will go far towards answering this question. Apparently the attempt of a paralysed fish to follow a rotating visual target substantially modified the *primary afferent* vestibular signal in such a way that *voluntary* angular movements would be associated with automatic nulling of the induced vestibular response, presumably through the efferent innervation of the vestibular organ (Gacek, 1960).

SUMMARY

Simple analysis of canal hydrodynamics yields a second order linear differential equation which is restated as a transfer function.

An experimental study of action potential frequencies induced in central vestibular units by rotational stimulation of the canals yields a similar transfer function.

It is inferred that the nervous system transfers the canal response signal to the brain stem with generally good fidelity. In particular it is shown that, over a middle range of frequencies, probably corresponding to those encountered in natural life, the informational content of this signal essentially corresponds to that of head angular velocity. Adjustment of canal frequency response according to animal size is apparently brought about by precise, but very small, changes in canal dimension from one species to another.

Attention is drawn to various non-linearities in the whole system. These include a form of dynamic asymmetry in the neural signal, a power relation between input and output amplitudes, neural adaptation to prolonged unidirectional stimuli and habituation to repeated stimuli which conflict with other sensory information.

The potential influence of these non-linearities calls for caution in the utilisation of a simple transfer function to predict the overall physiological response to canal stimulation.

REFERENCES

ADRIAN, E. D. (1943) Discharges from vestibular receptors in the cat. *J. Physiol. (Lond.)*, **101**, 389–407.

BENSON, A. J. (1970) Interactions between semicircular canals and gravireceptors. In D. E. BUSBY (Ed.), *Proc. XVIII int. Congr. Aviation and Space Med.*, Reidel Publishing Co., Dordrecht, Holland, pp. 249–261.

BENSON, A. J., GUEDRY, F. E. AND MELVILL JONES, G. (1970) Response of semicircular canal dependent units in vestibular nuclei to rotation of a linear acceleration vector without angular acceleration. *J. Physiol. (Lond.)*, **210**, 475–494.

BREUER, J. (1874) Über die Funktion der Bogengänge des Ohrlabyrinthes. *Wien. med. Jahrb.*, **4**, 72–124.

DOHLMAN, G. (1935) Some practical and theoretical points in labyrinthology. *Proc. roy. Soc. Med.*, **28**, 1371–1380.

DUENSING, F. UND SCHAEFER, K. P. (1958) Die Aktivität einzelner Neurone im Bereich der Vestibulariskerne bei Horizontalbeschleunigungen unter besonderer Berücksichtigung des vestibulären Nystagmus. *Arch. Psychiat. Nervenkr.*, **198**, 225–252.

FERNÁNDEZ, C. AND GOLDBERG, J. M. (1971) Physiology of peripheral neurons innervating the semicircular canals of the squirrel monkey. II. The response to sinusoidal stimulation and the dynamics of the peripheral vestibular system. *J. Neurophysiol*, **34**, 661–675.

FERNÁNDEZ, C. AND VALENTINUZZI, M. (1968) A study on the biophysical characteristics of the cat labyrinth. *Acta oto-laryng. (Stockh.)*, **65**, 293–310.

GACEK, R. R. (1960) Efferent component of the vestibular nerve. In G. L. RASMUSSEN AND W. F. WINDLE (Eds.), *Neural Mechanisms of the Auditory and Vestibular Systems*. Thomas, Springfield, Ill., pp. 276–284.

GAEDE, W. (1922) Über die Bewegungen der Flüssigkeit in einem rotierenden Hohlring. *Arch. Ohr.-, Nas.- u. Kehlk.-Heilk.*, **110**, 6–14.

GERNANDT, B. E. (1949) Response of mammalian vestibular neurons to horizontal rotation and caloric stimulation. *J. Neurophysiol.*, **12**, 173–184.

GOLDBERG, J. M. AND FERNÁNDEZ, C. (1971) Physiology of peripheral neurons innervating the semicircular canals of the squirrel monkey. I. The resting discharge and the response to constant angular accelerations. *J. Neurophysiol.*, **34**, 635–660.

GONSHOR, A. (1971) Habituation of natural head movement in man. *Proc. XXV int. Congr. physiol. Sci.*, Munich, IX, n. 619, 211.

GONSHOR, A. AND MELVILL JONES, C. (1971) Plasticity in the adult human vestibulo-ocular reflex arc. *Proc. Can. Fed. Biol. Soc.*. **14**, 25.

GROEN, J. J., LOWENSTEIN, O. AND VENDRIK, A. J. H. (1952) The mechanical analysis of the responses from the end-organ of the horizontal semicircular canal in the isolated elasmobranch labyrinth. *J. Physiol. (Lond.)*, **117**, 54–62.

HALLPIKE, G. S. AND HOOD, J. D. (1953) The speed of the slow component of ocular nystagmus induced by angular acceleration of the head: its experimental determination and application to the physical theory of the cupular mechanism. *Proc. roy. Soc. B*, **141**, 216–230.

HIXSON, W. C. AND NIVEN, J. I. (1961) Application of system transfer function concept to a mathematical description of the labyrinth. I. Steady state nystagmus response to semicircular canal stimulation by angular acceleration. *NASA SR*-57, 1–21.

HIXSON, W. C. AND NIVEN, J. I. (1962) Frequency response of the human semicircular canals. II. Nystagmus phase shift as a measure of nonlinearities. *NASA SR*-73, 1–17.

JONES, G. M. AND MILSUM, J. H. (1965) Spatial and dynamic aspects of visual fixation. *IEEE Trans. Bio-med. Eng.*, **12**, 54–62.

JONES, G. M. AND SPELLS, K. E. (1963) A theoretical and comparative study of the functional dependence of the semicircular canal upon its physical dimensions. *Proc. roy. Soc. B*, **157**, 403–419.

KLINKE, R. (1970) Efferent influence on the vestibular organ during active movements of the body. *Pflügers Arch. ges. Physiol.*, **318**, 325–332.

LOWENSTEIN, O. (1956a) Peripheral mechanisms of equilibrium. *Brit. med. Bull.*, **12**, 114–118.

LOWENSTEIN, O. (1956b) Comparative physiology of the otolith organs. *Brit. med. Bull.*, **12**, 110–113.

LOWENSTEIN, O. AND SAND, A. (1940) The mechanism of the semicircular canal. A study of responses of single fibre preparations to angular accelerations and to rotation at constant speed. *Proc. roy. Soc. B*, **129**, 256–275.

MALCOLM, R. AND MELVILL JONES, G. (1970) A quantitative study of vestibular adaptation in humans. *Acta oto-laryng. (Stockh.)*, **70**, 126–135.

MASUDA, T. (1922) Beitrag zur Physiologie des Drehnystagmus. *Pflügers Arch. ges. Physiol.*, **197**, 1–65.

MAYNE, R. (1950) The dynamic characteristics of the semicircular canals. *J. comp. physiol. Psychol.*, **43**, 304–319.

MELVILL JONES, G. (1968) From land to space in a generation: an evolutionary challenge. *Aerospace Med.*, **39**, 1271–1283.

MELVILL JONES, G. (1971) Organization of neural control in the vestibulo-ocular reflex arc. In P. BACH-Y-RITA, C. C. COLLINS AND I. E. HYDE (Eds.), *The Control of Eye Movements*. Academic Press, New York, pp. 497–518.

MELVILL JONES, G. (1972) Functional significance of semicircular canal size. In H. H. KORNHUBER (Ed.), *Handbook of Sensory Physiology. Vol. VI. Vestibular System*. Springer, Berlin, in press.

MELVILL JONES, G. AND MILSUM, J. H. (1969) Fidelity of information transfer in a vestibular afferent pathway. *J. Physiol. (Lond.)*, **205**, 29P.

MELVILL JONES, G. AND MILSUM, J. H. (1970) Characteristics of neural transmission from the semicircular canal to the vestibular nuclei of cats. *J. Physiol. (Lond.)*, **209**, 295–316.

MELVILL JONES, G. AND MILSUM, J. H. (1971) Frequency response analysis of central vestibular unit activity resulting from rotational stimulation of the semicircular canals. *J. Physiol. (Lond.)*, **219**, 191–215.

MICHAEL, J. A. AND MELVILL JONES, G. (1966) Dependence of visual tracking capability upon stimulus predictability. *Vision Res.*, **6**, 707–716.

MILSUM, J. H. AND MELVILL JONES, G. (1969) Dynamic asymmetry in neural components of the vestibular system. *Ann. N.Y. Acad. Sci.*, **156**, 851–871.

OMAN, C. M. (1968) *Influence of Adaptation on the Human Semicircular Canals and the Role of Subjective Angular Velocity Cues in Spatial Orientation*. Sc.M. Thesis, M.I.T., Cambridge, Mass., pp. 179.

OUTERBRIDGE, J. S. (1969) *Experimental and Theoretical Investigation of Vestibularly-Driven Head and Eye Movement*. Ph. D. Thesis, Department of Physiology, McGill University, Montreal, pp. 216.

OUTERBRIDGE, J. S. AND MELVILL JONES, G. (1971) Reflex vestibular control of head movement in man. *Aerospace Med.*, **42**, 935–940.

ROBERTS, T. D. M. (1967) *Neurophysiology of Postural Mechanisms*. Butterworths, London, pp. XVII–354.

ROHRER, F. (1922) Zur Theorie der Drehreizung des Bogengangsapparates. *Schweiz. med. Wschr.*, **3**, 669–674.

ROHRER, F. AND MASUDA, T., (1926) Bogengangsapparat und Statolithenapparat. In A. BETHE *et al.* (Eds.), *Handbuch der normalen und pathologischen Physiologie. Vol. 2*. Springer, Berlin, pp. 985–1001.

ROSS, D. A. (1936) Electrical studies on the frog's labyrinth. *J. Physiol. (Lond.)*, **86**, 117–146.

RUPERT, A., MOUSHEGIAN, G. AND GALAMBOS, R. (1962) Microelectrode studies of primary vestibular neurones in cat. *Exp. Neurol.*, **5**, 100–109.

RYU, J. H., MCCABE, B. F. AND FUNASAKA, S. (1969) Types of neuronal activity in the medial vestibular nucleus. *Acta oto-laryng. (Stockh.).* **68**, 137–141.

SALA, O. (1965) The efferent vestibular system. *Acta oto-laryng. (Stockh.).* Suppl. 197, 1–34.

SCHMALTZ, G. (1925) Versuche zu einer Theorie des Erregungsvorganges im Ohrlabyrinth. *Pflügers Arch. ges Physiol.,* **207**, 125–128.

SCHMALTZ, G. (1931) The physical phenomena occurring in the semicircular canals during rotary and thermic stimulation. *Proc. roy. Soc. Med.,* **25**, 359–381.

SHIMAZU, H. AND PRECHT, W. (1965) Tonic and kinetic responses of cat's vestibular neurones to horizontal angular acceleration. *J. Neurophysiol.,* **28**, 991–1013.

SHIMAZU, H. AND PRECHT, W. (1966) Inhibition of central vestibular neurones from the contralateral labyrinth and its mediating pathway. *J. Neurophysiol.,* **29**, 467–492.

STEFANI, A. (1876) Studi sulla funzione dei canali semicircolari e sui rapporti fra essi ed il cervelletto. *Accad. di Ferrara.* Cited by M. Camis, *La Fisiologia dell'Apparato Vestibolare,* Zanichelli, Bologna, 1928, pp. VII–358.

STEINHAUSEN, W. (1927) Über Sichtbarmachung und Funktionsprüfung der Cupula terminalis in den Bogengangsampullen des Labyrinthes. *Pflügers Arch. ges. Physiol.,* **217**, 747–755.

STEINHAUSEN, W. (1928) Über die histologische Struktur der Cupula terminalis in den Bogengangen des Labyrinthes. *Z. Zellforsch.,* **7**, 513–518.

STEINHAUSEN, W. (1931) Über den Nachweis der Bewegung der Cupula in der intakten Bogengangsampulle des Labyrinthes bei der natürlichen rotatorischen und calorischen Reizung. *Pflügers Arch. ges. Physiol.,* **228**, 322–328.

STEINHAUSEN, W. (1933) Über die Funktion der Cupula in den Bogengangsampullen des Labyrinths. *Z. Hals.-, Nas.- u. Ohrenheilk.,* **34**, 301–211.

STEINHAUSEN, W. (1933) Über die Beobachtung der Cupula in den Bogengangsampullen des Labyrinths des lebenden Hechts. *Pflügers Arch. ges. Physiol.,* **232**, 500–512.

STEINHAUSEN, W. (1939) Das Bogengangssystem des inneren Ohres als Wahrnehmungsorgan für Drehungen. *Hochschulfilm,* C323, Berlin.

STEINHAUSEN, W. (1939) Über Modellversuche zur Physiologie des Labyrinthes und über ein neues Bogengangsmodell. *Acta oto-laryng. (Stockh.),* **27**, 107–122.

VAN EGMOND, A. A. J., GROEN, J. J. AND JONGKEES, L. B. W. (1949) The mechanics of the semicircular canal. *J. Physiol. (Lond.),* **110**, 1–17.

WILSON, V. J., KATO, M., PETERSON, B. W. AND WYLIE, R. M. (1965) A single unit analysis of the organization of Deiters' nucleus. *J. Neurophysiol.,* **30**, 603–619.

WILSON, V. J., WYLIE, R. M. AND MARCO, L. A. (1968) Synaptic inputs to cells in the medial vestibular nucleus. *J. Neurophysiol.,* **31**, 176–185.

WILSON, V. J. AND YOSHIDA, M. (1969a) Comparison of effects of stimulation on Deiters' nucleus and medial longitudinal fasciculus on neck, forelimb, and hindlimb motoneurones. *J. Neurophysiol.,* **32**, 743–758.

WILSON, V. J. AND YOSHIDA, M. (1969b) Monosynaptic inhibition of neck motoneurons by the medial vestibular nucleus. *Exp. Brain Res.,* **9**, 365–380.

YOUNG, L. R. (1962) *A Sampled Data Model for Eye Tracking Movements.* Sc.D. Thesis, MIT, Cambridge, Mass., pp. 1–204.

YOUNG, L. R. (1969) A control model of the vestibular system. *Automatica,* **5**, 369–383.

YOUNG, L. R. AND STARK, L. (1963) Variable feedback experiments testing a sampled data model for eye tracking movements. *IEEE Trans. on Human Factors in Electronics,* **4**, 38–51.

Semicircular Canal Inputs to Vestibular Nuclear Neurons in the Pigeon

V. J. WILSON AND L. P. FELPEL*

The Rockefeller University, New York, N.Y., U.S.A.

In order to understand the manner in which the vestibular nuclei process afferent input, it is necessary to know the pattern of input from different receptors in the labyrinth to second and third order neurons. Natural stimulation has shown that the same neuron in mammalian vestibular nuclei may be influenced by both acceleration and tilt (for example Duensing and Schaefer, 1969; Curthoys and Markham, 1971), and sometimes by acceleration in the plane of two or more canals (Curthoys and Markham, 1971). The pathways responsible for such convergence are not known. They may be short mono- or disynaptic links; on the other hand they may be more complex, involving the reticular formation or cerebellum. We have approached this question by means of electrical stimulation of individual ampullae in the pigeon, an animal whose accessible labyrinth makes it suitable for such investigation. This paper presents some aspects of the findings described in more detail elsewhere (Wilson and Felpel, 1972).

In early experiments animals were anesthetized with Equithesin (Jensen–Salsbery Labs), 4 cc/kg, i.m.; more recently with urethane in Ringer's solution, 1.5 g/kg, i.p. The trachea was cannulated and the left abdominal air sac opened. The bird was paralyzed by i.m. injection of Flaxedil (American Cyanamid Co.) and ventilated by blowing through it a mixture of O_2 and CO_2 (95 : 5) at 250 ml/min. After the head was mounted in a holder similar to that of Karten and Hodos (1967) the bone overlying the labyrinth on one side was removed and the ampullae of the semicircular canals exposed. Bipolar electrodes made from 130 μm, insulated, stainless steel wire (total diameter 170 μm) were inserted into two holes 0.5–1.0 mm apart in each ampulla (*cf.* Cohen and Suzuki, 1963). After insertion the area was sealed with a vaseline–mineral oil mixture to prevent leakage of endolymph, and the electrodes were fixed in place with acrylic dental cement. The animals were then mounted and prepared as described by Wilson and Wylie (1970) and maintained at 41–42° C. The brain stem was approached from the ventral surface with micro-electrodes filled with 2 M NaCl saturated with Fast Green FCF. Conventional circuits were used for stimulating and recording. The location of all cells was estimated in serial sections from the positions of dye marks made in each track (Thomas and Wilson, 1965), and was identified

---

* Special Fellow of the National Institutes of Health (2 F11 NS 2108-02).

References pp. 162–163

by referring to the atlas of Karten and Hodos (1962). Localization is only approximate as the boundaries of the nuclei are not clear. In addition, the plane of our sections is not the same as that of the sections of Karten and Hodos: our headholder was mounted with an angle of only 30–35° to the horizontal, to facilitate tracking in the more rostral areas of the nuclei.

FIELD POTENTIALS IN THE VESTIBULAR NUCLEI

Before the study of single units could begin it was necessary to determine whether the 3 stimulating electrodes were functional and stimulus spread minimal. This was achieved by study of the field potentials evoked by stimulation of the individual ampullae. In areas of the nuclei where there is substantial labyrinthine input the fields, previously described briefly (Wilson and Wylie, 1970), are as illustrated in the inset of Fig. 1. The P wave represents the arrival of afferent volleys. When the recording electrode is situated in the midst of or near vestibular afferent fibers, the N_1 potential is probably made up of both afferent and monosynaptic activity (Wilson and Wylie, 1970). The N_2 wave consists entirely of polysynaptic activity. More dorsally the appearance of the fields may change (Fig. 2). The P wave becomes less distinct, the slope of the N_1 less steep and the potential is then probably entirely postsynaptic. In general, except for their shorter latency and briefer time course, the fields resemble those described for the vestibular nuclei of the cat (Precht and Shimazu, 1965).

When the strength of the stimulus to one ampulla was increased from threshold (T) the P-N_1 complex grew to a plateau that was often reached near 3 T, as illustrated in Fig. 1. At strengths of stimulation that varied (2.5 to 16 T, or more) the plateau was interrupted by a new growth, sometimes substantial and sometimes small as in Fig. 1. In some cases there were no such sudden breaks in the growth curve, in others two

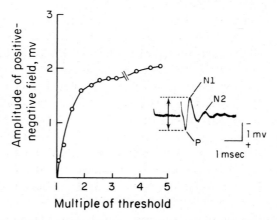

Fig. 1. Amplitude of the field potential evoked by stimulation of the posterior canal ampulla as a function of stimulus strength. At a strength between 3.2 and 3.9 times threshold there is a break in the curve, which had previously reached a plateau. The position of the break, known only approximately, is indicated by the slanted lines. Inset shows the field, and indicates how measurement was made. Description of P, N_1 and N_2 components in text.

were seen. We suggest that these breaks in the curve relating field amplitude to stimulus strength are due to stimulus spread to another nerve in the labyrinth. In agreement with this interpretation, when two ampullae were stimulated at or near simultaneity with stimuli below threshold for breaks, the two fields summed completely. Above break threshold occlusion was often seen: in such cases the stimulus spread to another canal nerve. At other times there was no occlusion, even above break threshold. The stimulus may then have been spreading to a nerve not available for stimulation, perhaps the nerve from one of the maculae. It could be suggested that the break represents activity due to the recruitment of smaller fibers in the ampullary nerve. There are arguments against such an interpretation. (*i*) From the distribution of fiber diameters in pigeon ampullary nerves there is no reason to expect two fiber populations with a clear threshold division (Boord, 1964, and personal communication); (*ii*) the threshold of the break was very variable; (*iii*) there were sometimes no breaks, and sometimes two. We therefore believe the break in the growth curve is due to stimulus spread, and results with single units will be interpreted accordingly.

In searching for single units we have investigated the superior, descending and Deiters' nuclei, as well as the area medial to the tangential nucleus and ventral to Deiters' nucleus, partly occupied by vestibular nerve fibers (from P 0.50 rostral in Karten and Hodos, 1962). Following Bartels (1925) we call the latter area ventral

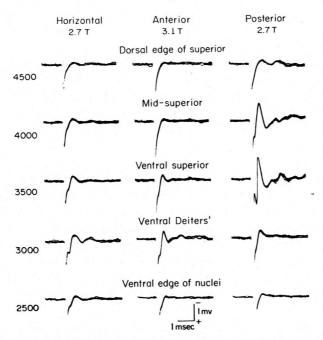

Fig. 2. Appearance of the field potentials produced by stimulation of the 3 ampullae at different depths in a track through the vestibular nuclei at approximately AP 0. Numbers at the left show depth from the ventral surface of the brain stem. The 3 ampullae were stimulated at the multiples of threshold indicated. The stimuli were strong enough so that the amplitude of the fields was close to maximal, but too weak to cause a break in the growth curve.

References pp. 162–163

Deiters' nucleus. There was a general tendency for the 3 stimulating electrode pairs to evoke fields that differed in amplitude and appearance and reached maximal size in different locations (Fig. 2). In some regions stimulation of the 3 ampullae evoked fields of similar amplitude (depth of 3000 in Fig. 2), in others one ampullary input clearly predominated (depths of 3500, 4000 in Fig. 2). In every track in which units were studied fields were recorded at different depths, so that input to the cells could be related to the amplitude of the fields produced by stimulation of the different ampullae.

UNIT RESPONSES

Firing behavior

We have recorded extracellulary from 114 units, most of which were located in the superior, descending and ventral Deiters' nuclei. Unit discharges were usually predominantly negative and ranged in amplitude from 150 μV to more than 1 mV. Cells were found by tracking through the nuclei while stimulating the 3 ampullae simultaneously with strong shocks at the rate of 5/sec. The units selected were fired by stimulation of an ampulla at low threshold. Expressed in terms of the threshold, T, at which a field could be detected in the nuclei on stimulation of that ampulla, firing was first observed with a stimulus strength of 1.7 ± 0.5 T (mean $\pm$ SD, n $=$ 113); the earliest latency was achieved with shocks 2.6 ± 0.8 T (n $=$ 105). Units that responded only to much stronger stimuli were discarded, because the origin of the afferent input to these cells could not be identified with certainty. The nature of the firing was classified as mono- or polysynaptic mainly on the basis of the position of the earliest-latency firing on fields such as those of Fig. 2. Spikes on the N_1 were monosynaptic, those on or after the N_2 polysynaptic (for further details see Wilson and Felpel, 1972). For analysis of the data on convergence it is sufficient to consider all cells as belonging to one population.

Studies of convergence

These experiments were carried out on six pigeons in which stimulation of each ampulla evoked fields and fired units, and in which there was no spread of stimulus below approximately 3T. Ninety-five units were studied that were easily identifiable from the appearance of their action potential and that were tested with stimulation of all 3 canals.

Eighty-nine cells were fired preferentially by stimulation of one ampulla, the 'active' ampulla, with single shocks delivered at the rate of 1–5/sec. This group included 36 cells fired by stimulation of the anterior ampulla, 28 by the horizontal and 27 by the posterior. The cells were distributed throughout the superior, ventral Deiters' and descending nuclei. Further details about their location are discussed elsewhere (Wilson and Felpel, 1972). Six cells showed clear convergence. The total of 95 cells can be subdivided as follows.

Group A, 48 cells (50%). These cells were fired only by stimulation of one ampulla, even though the others were tested with shocks usually in the range 5–15 T. Such shocks are not only considerably stronger than the average threshold for firing from an active ampulla (1.7 T, see firing behavior above), but are also above the strength required to evoke the response with the shortest latency from that ampulla (2.6 T).

Group B, 29 cells (31%). These cells were fired not only from the active ampulla but also from a second one. Firing from the second ampulla, however, was evoked only by stimuli at or above a strength that produced a break in the growth curve of the field potential evoked from that ampulla (usually 3.5 T and up). There was occlusion between the field potentials produced by stimulation of the second ampulla at this strength and of the active ampulla by shocks about 3 T. Apparently the input to the cells in this group was specifically from the active ampulla, and firing from the second ampulla was due to stimulus spread to the active. In 28/29 cells the two ampullae that fired the cell were the anterior and horizontal, i.e., the two located next to each other.

Group C, 12 cells (13%). In addition to being fired from the active ampulla, these cells were fired by stimulation of a second ampulla. The stimulus to the second ampulla was above the strength producing a break in the growth curve, but there was either no occlusion between the fields evoked by stimulation of the active and second ampulla, or no information of occlusion. In some cases firing from the second ampulla could be due to stimulus spread to the active. In others it is not, but may be due to spread to a nerve from one of the maculae. This group involved various combinations of the 3 ampullae.

Group D, 6 cells (6%). Five of these cells displayed convergence from two ampullae, one from three. Threshold stimuli were always under 3 T for each ampulla, in two cells they were under 2 T. In all cases the stimuli were below the level of stimulus spread, indicating that convergence was real. Where convergence was from two ampullae these were the anterior and posterior, or anterior and horizontal.

DISCUSSION

These brief remarks will be limited to the matter of specificity of ampullar input to neurons in the pigeon vestibular nuclei. There is in fact great specificity, as 81% of the cells (groups A and B, above) receive afferent input from only one ampulla. From that ampulla, the input is often both mono- and polysynaptic. Of course the results do not rule out subthreshold convergence, with secondary inputs too weak to fire the cell. In 31 cells, however, ampullae other than the active one were tested not only with single but also with triple shocks (2–3 msec intervals), with no significant change in the results. This argues against subthreshold convergence, as do preliminary findings with intracellular recording. The possibilities that the specificity is due in part to damage resulting from electrode implantation, or to selective depression by the anesthetic of weak converging pathways, must be considered. Both, however, are unlikely since stimulation of each ampulla fired cells in every experiment and activation was poly- as well as monosynaptic.

The specificity we have found in the superior, descending and ventral Deiters' nuclei does not result from sampling only areas in which input from one ampulla was dominant. Of the cells fired from only one ampulla, half were in areas where fields evoked from the 3 ampullae were approximately equivalent (for example a cell driven from the horizontal, another from the anterior ampulla at a depth of about 3000 in the track illustrated in Fig. 2). Some cells were in locations where the active ampulla was better represented than the others (a cell fired from the posterior ampulla, at a depth of 3500–4000, Fig. 2), but the opposite was true for a greater number of neurons. Although few cells were found in Deiters' nucleus, the nucleus was studied often and field evidence indicates that ampullary projection to this group of large neurons is scant, except perhaps for the posterior ampulla. Deiters' is therefore unlikely to be an area where extensive canal convergence takes place, and recent experiments suggest the same is true of the medial nucleus.

While some of our results (group C) indirectly suggest possible convergence between ampullary and macular input, true convergence between ampullae by means of simple mono- or polysynaptic pathways seems negligible. Unfortunately there are no data on the behavior of pigeon vestibular neurons to natural stimulation activating different labyrinthine receptors, such as there are for mammals (*e.g.*, Duensing and Schaefer, 1959; Curthoys and Markham, 1971). Our results suggest that the convergence observed in the cat may take place predominantly by way of complex pathways, but the pattern of input may differ in birds and mammals.

Pigeon head movements, like those of mammals, usually will activate more than one canal. It may be advantageous to have pathways carrying specific information to different areas of target neurons, extraocular or spinal, with integration of inputs taking place at these neurons. It seems certain that convergence and integration of information must also be taking place more centrally, and the cerebellum is a possible site of such convergence.

SUMMARY

Bipolar stimulating electrodes were inserted into the 3 semicircular canal ampullae in the pigeon labyrinth. The effect of stimulation of the 3 ampullae on single neurons in the vestibular nuclei was tested in experiments which met the following criteria: all 3 electrode pairs functioned; there was no evidence of stimulus spread between the electrodes with moderate stimuli; when spread did occur the stimulus strengths at which it appeared, and the ampullae to which it spread, were identified. In such experiments a large fraction (81%) of units received afferent input, mono- and/or polysynaptic, from only one ampulla, while only 6% showed unequivocal convergence. Some indirect evidence suggests there may be convergence between ampullary and macular inputs.

ACKNOWLEDGEMENT

Supported in part by N.I.H. Grants NS 02619 and NS 05463.

REFERENCES

BARTELS, M. (1925) Über die Gegend des Deiters' und Bechterewskernes bei Vögeln. *Z. Anat. Ent wickl.-Gesch.*, **77**, 726–784.

BOORD, R. L. (1964) The number and diameter of myelinated fibers in the statoacoustic nerve of the adult pigeon. *Amer. Zool.*, **4**, 101.

COHEN, B. AND SUZUKI, J.-I. (1963) Eye movements induced by ampullary nerve stimulation. *Amer. J. Physiol.*, **204**, 347–351.

CURTHOYS, I. S. AND MARKHAM, C. H. (1971) Convergence of labyrinthine influences on units in the vestibular nuclei of the cat. I. Natural stimulation. *Brain Res.*, **35**, 469–490.

DUENSING, F. UND SCHAEFER, K. P. (1959) Über die Konvergenz verschiedener labyrinthären Afferenzen auf einzelne Neurone des Vestibulariskerngebietes. *Arch. Psychiat. Nervenkr.*, **199**, 345–371.

KARTEN, H. J. AND HODOS, W. (1962) *A Stereotaxic Atlas of the Brain of the Pigeon.* Johns Hopkins Press, Baltimore, pp. IX–193.

PRECHT, W. AND SHIMAZU, H. (1965) Functional connections of tonic and kinetic vestibular neurons with primary vestibular afferents. *J. Neurophysiol.*, **28**, 1014–1028.

THOMAS, R. C. AND WILSON, V. J. (1965) Precise localization of Renshaw cells with a new marking technique. *Nature (Lond.)*, **206**, 211–213.

WILSON, V. J. AND FELPEL, L. P. (1972) Specificity of the semicircular canal input to neurons in the pigeon vestibular nuclei, *J. Neurophysiol.*, **35**, 253–264.

WILSON, V. J. AND WYLIE, R. M. (1970) A short-latency labyrinthine input to the vestibular nuclei in the pigeon. *Science*, **168**, 124–127.

·III. ORGANIZATION OF THE COMMISSURAL CONNECTIONS

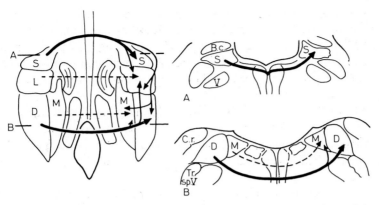

Fig. 4. To the left a schematic diagram summarizing the commissural connections of the vestibular nuclei in the cat as determined experimentally. A and B represent transverse sections at levels indicated. Broken lines indicate commissural connections which are either scanty (between the lateral vestibular nuclei), or whose origin has not been definitely established (between medial vestibular nuclei). From Ladpli and Brodal (1968).

fibres are distributed to the ventral and lateral parts of the descending nucleus. In addition there is some degeneration in the ventralmost areas of the three other main nuclei, very few in the superior.

Since lesions of the *medial vestibular nucleus* will interrupt commissural fibres from the descending nucleus, the precise area of termination of commissural fibres from the medial nucleus cannot be determined. It may be concluded only that the commissural fibres from the medial nucleus, which appear to be rather abundant, must terminate within the same regions as do the commissural fibres from the descending nucleus.

It is seen from this brief survey that *the four main vestibular nuclei differ markedly with regard to their commissural connections*. Fig. 4 shows the main points. As to the lateral nucleus the anatomical possibilities for an influence on the contralateral vestibular nucleus seem to be very restricted since the lateral nucleus gives off only very few commissural fibres, mainly to the lateral nucleus of the other side (some also to the descending nucleus, not shown in Fig. 4). It appears that authors who advocate ample interconnections between the two lateral nuclei have used lesions which encroached upon the descending nucleus.

The two superior and the two descending nuclei on the other hand, are amply interconnected by commissural fibres. The commissural fibres from these nuclei pursue a different course (Fig. 4, drawings A and B), a point of some interest in physiological studies. Furthermore, these two nuclei are capable of acting on all four contralateral main nuclei (the small contingent from the descending to the contralateral superior nucleus is not shown in the diagram of Fig. 4), but their main action is obviously on their partner on the opposite side. A final point of interest is that while the commissural fibres from the superior nucleus supply the entire contralateral superior nucleus, all other commissural contingents end only in the ventral parts of the contralateral nuclei. It appears thus that among the main vestibular nuclei the superior is particularly well equipped for a collaboration with its partner on the other side. The medial nucleus probably also has rather abundant connections with its counterpart on the other side. No information could be obtained concerning the origin of possible commissural connections from the small groups of the vestibular complex, but following certain lesions, degeneration was found in the contralateral groups x and f (see Ladpli and Brodal, 1968, for details),

In a study of efferent fibres from the vestibular nuclei in the macaque, baboon and chimpanzee, Tarlov (1969) made observations which agree with our findings on the terminations of the commissural fibres in the cat, even if his making use of fairly large lesions prevented detailed conclusions concerning the sites of origin of the commissural fibres.

Even if the pattern of commissural connections found in our study is rather specific there are certainly further details which have so far not been brought out.

Physiological data concerning the commissural relations are in good accord with the anatomical. Midline incisions of the brain stem in the region where the commissural fibres pass, abolish the inhibition of type-I neurons as well as the excitation of type-II neurons which can be evoked by stimulation of the contralateral vestibular nerve (Shimazu and Precht, 1966). Most of the cells influenced by stimulation of the contralateral labyrinth have been found in the superior nucleus, especially ventromedially, and in the rostral part of the medial nucleus (Shimazu and Precht, 1966; Markham, 1968; Wilson et al., 1968), that is in regions which receive many commissural fibres (see Figs. 2 and 3). Concerning the origin of the commissural fibres involved, there is positive evidence for those situated in the medial nucleus (Mano, Oshima and Shimazu, 1968), while the other nuclei have apparently not been studied from this point of view.

According to physiological observations the synaptic relationships may be different for different kinds of neurons. Since the latency for the contralateral inhibition of kinetic type-I neurons is shorter than for the tonic ones the former appear to be influenced by a more direct commissural pathway than the latter. It may consist of an inhibitory neuron (excited from the ipsilateral labyrinth) and sending its axon to the contralateral nucleus (Kasahara et al., 1968). The longer latencies for the inhibition of contralateral tonic type-I neurons and the even longer ones for the excitation of type-II neurons (Shimazu and Precht, 1966; Markham, 1968) suggest that there may be intercalated neurons in these commissural pathways. Different views on possible arrangements of this kind have been set forth on the basis of physiological observations, mainly on the medial nucleus (see Shimazu and Precht, 1966; Markham, 1968; Wilson et al., 1968). The available anatomical data do not permit specific conclusions concerning such arrangements. According to Cajal (1909), Lorente de Nó (1933) and Hauglie-Hanssen (1968) true Golgi II type cells appear not to be common in the vestibular nuclei. A few have been found only in the medial and descending nuclei. However, cells sending their axons out of the medial nucleus have been found to give off amply branching collaterals distributed in the immediate neighbourhood of the parent cells (Hauglie-Hanssen,1968). These cells may presumably function as interneurons within their own nucleus in the transmission of impulses from the ipsilateral labyrinth to commissural neurons. They may also be imagined to serve as internuncials for impulses arriving in commissural fibres.

As to the other *anatomical possibilities for mutual interactions between the impulses from the two labyrinths*, mentioned in the introduction, our knowledge is incomplete. An action by cells of the reticular formation, receiving *primary* vestibular fibres and projecting to the vestibular nuclei on the other side, appears to be unlikely, since only very few primary vestibular afferents reach the reticular formation (in the region close to the nuclei). The available Golgi studies give no information as to whether axons of cells in this part of the reticular formation cross the midline and reach the contralateral vestibular nuclei.

However, there are anatomical possibilities for another pathway. Cells in those parts of the reticular formation (mainly the nucleus reticularis gigantocellularis and pontis caudalis) which receive fibres from the vestibular nuclei may send axons or collaterals back to these. This necessitates the presence of crossing fibres in one of the two links. A certain part of the vestibuloreticular projections are crossed (see Fig. 5, and Table I in Brodal, 1972a), namely fibres from the descending vestibular nucleus to the nucleus reticularis gigantocellularis and some fibres from the superior and lateral vestibular nucleus to the reticularis pontis caudalis. Reticulovestibular connections able to mediate an influence on the contralateral vestibular nuclei would therefore have to be uncrossed. Cells with such axonal trajectories have been observed in Golgi preparations, for example by Scheibel and Scheibel (1958), but information concerning their numbers, particular location and the sites of ending of their axons is not available. The uncrossed vestibuloreticular projections (see Fig. 5) would have to act via reticular cells whose axons cross the midline (see for example, Scheibel and

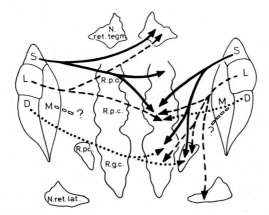

Fig. 5. A diagram of the main projections from the vestibular nuclei onto the reticular formation as determined experimentally in the cat by Ladpli and Brodal (1968). The projections from the medial vestibular nucleus could not be determined, but their terminations are within the territory covered by the fibres from the descending nucleus. N. ret. lat. and N. ret. tegm.: Nucleus reticularis lateralis and tegmenti pontis, respectively. R.g.c.: Nucleus reticularis gigantocellularis in the medulla. R.pc.: Nucleus reticularis parvicellularis. R.p.c. and R.p.o.: Nucleus reticularis pontis caudalis and oralis, respectively.

Scheibel, 1958; Valverde, 1961). Neuronal circuits of this kind might be involved in the effects exerted by stimulation of one labyrinth on the contralateral vestibular nuclei as indeed appears from the study of Shimazu and Precht (1966). Following midline transections which abolish the inhibitory commissural responses of type-I neurons, these were replaced by excitatory responses on vestibular nerve stimulation strong enough to produce reticular evoked potentials.

A convergence of impulses from the two labyrinths finally occurs in the spinal cord as well as in the oculomotor nuclei and the small nuclei in the mesencephalon adjacent to the latter (nucleus of Darkschewitsch and interstitial nucleus of Cajal). Ascending fibres from the vestibular nuclei are distributed bilaterally to the mesencephalic nuclei mentioned (see Tarlov, 1969; 1970). As to the spinal cord, the medial vestibulospinal tract, arising in the medial vestibular nucleus, gives off crossed as well as uncrossed fibres (Nyberg-Hansen, 1964). This tract, however, does not descend much below the cervical cord. A secondary collaboration of vestibular impulses from the two labyrinths may occur by commissural connections in the spinal cord, since commissural cells appear to be especially abundant in lamina VIII of Rexed (1952) which is the main site of termination of the medial vestibulospinal tract. In this way impulses descending in the two uncrossed lateral vestibulospinal tracts may also collaborate, since this tract as well has most of its terminations in lamina VIII (Nyberg-Hansen and Mascitti, 1964).

While there are thus several routes by which impulses from the two labyrinths may interact within the central nervous system, the most direct collaboration is by means of commissural connections between the vestibular nuclei. It is obvious from the anatomical data that the vestibular nuclei differ considerably with regard to their commissural connections, and the physiological observations indicate that the anatomical basis for the various commissural effects are probably not identical.

SUMMARY

The labyrinths of the two sides may be imagined to cooperate within the central nervous system by means of several anatomical connections. These are not sufficiently known to permit complete correlations with physiological observations.

There is no convincing evidence for primary vestibular fibres passing to the contralateral vestibular nuclei.

Commissural connections between the vestibular nuclei are well known to exist. In recent experimental anatomical studies (Ladpli and Brodal, 1968) these connections turned out to be more specifically organized than previously known. The main features are shown in the diagram of Fig. 4. The lateral nucleus gives off only few commissural fibres, mainly to the contralateral lateral nucleus. The superior and descending nuclei are amply interconnected with their partners on the opposite side, but in addition send some commissural fibres to all the other main nuclei. The distribution of the commissural fibres from the medial nucleus could not be precisely defined, except for the fact that they are distributed within the sites of termination of the commissural fibres from the descending nucleus. All commissural connections terminate mainly in the ventral parts of the contralateral nuclei, except those which interconnect the two superior nuclei.

There is no clear evidence that impulses entering in the few primary vestibular fibres which have been traced to the reticular formation can be transmitted to the vestibular nuclei.

Many efferent fibres from the vestibular nuclei terminate in fairly well circumscribed regions of the reticular formation, contralaterally and ipsilaterally. Cells in these regions give off axons or collaterals to the vestibular nuclei, but the detailed course and distribution of these connections are not known in detail.

A collaboration between the two labyrinths may finally occur in more peripheral regions (spinal cord and oculomotor nuclei), since fibres from certain of the vestibular nuclei of the two sides meet here. With regard to the spinal cord a collaboration may further be mediated by commissural cells, especially abundant in Rexed's lamina VIII, which receives most of the vestibulospinal fibres.

REFERENCES

BRODAL, A. (1972a) Anatomy of the vestibuloreticular connections and possible 'ascending' vestibular pathways from the reticular formation. In A. BRODAL AND O. POMPEIANO (Eds.), *Progress in Brain Research. Vol. 37. Basic aspects of central vestibular mechanisms.* Elsevier, Amsterdam, pp. 553–565.

BRODAL, A. (1972b) Anatomy of the vestibular nuclei and their connections. In H. H. KORNHUBER (Ed.), *Handbook of Sensory Physiology. Vol. VI. Vestibular System.* Springer Verlag, Berlin, Heidelberg, New York, in press.

BRODAL, A., POMPEIANO, O. AND WALBERG, F. (1962) *The Vestibular Nuclei and their Connections, Anatomy and Functional Correlations.* Oliver and Boyd, Edinburgh, London, pp. VIII-193.

CAJAL, S. R. Y (1909–1911) *Histologie du Système Nerveux de l'Homme et des Vertébrés.* Maloine, Paris.

CARPENTER, M. B. (1960a) Fiber projections from the descending and lateral vestibular nuclei in the cat. *Amer. J. Anat.,* 107, 1–22.

CARPENTER, M. B. (1960b) Experimental anatomical-physiological studies of the vestibular nerve and cerebellar connections. In G. L. RASMUSSEN AND W. WINDLE (Eds.), *Neural Mechanisms of the Auditory and Vestibular Systems.* C. C. Thomas, Springfield, Illinois, pp. 297–323.

FERRARO, A., PACELLA, B. L. AND BARRERA, S. E. (1940) Effects of lesions of the medial vestibular nucleus. An anatomical and physiological study in Macacus Rhesus monkeys. *J. comp. Neurol.,* 73, 7–36.

GRAY, L. P., (1926) Some experimental evidence on the connections of the vestibular mechanism in the cat. *J. comp. Neurol.,* 41, 319–364.

HAUGLIE–HANSSEN, E. (1968) Intrinsic neuronal organization of the vestibular nuclear complex in the cat. A Golgi study. *Ergebn. Anat. Entwickl.-Gesch.,* 40/5, 1–105.

INGVAR, S. (1918) Zur Phylo- und Ontogenese des Kleinhirns nebst einem Versuche zu einheitlicher Erklärung der zerebellaren Funktion und Lokalisation. *Folia neuro-biol. (Lpz.),* 11, 205–495.

KASAHARA, M., MANO, N., OSHIMA, T., OZAWA, S. AND SHIMAZU, H. (1968) Contralateral short latency inhibition of central vestibular neurons in the horizontal canal system. *Brain Res.,* 8, 376–378.

LADPLI, R. AND BRODAL, A. (1968) Experimental studies of commissural and reticular formation projections from the vestibular nuclei in the cat. *Brain Res.,* 8, 65–96.

LEIDLER, R. (1914) Experimentelle Untersuchungen über das Endigungsgebiet des Nervus vestibularis. *Arb. neurol. Inst. Univ. Wien,* 21, 151–212.

LORENTE DE NÓ, R. (1933) Vestibulo-ocular reflex arc. *Arch. Neurol. Psychiat. (Chicago),* 30, 245–291.

McMASTERS, R. E., WEISS A. H. AND CARPENTER M. B. (1966) Vestibular projections to the nuclei of the extraocular muscles. Degeneration resulting from discrete partial lesions of the vestibular nuclei in the monkey. *Amer. J. Anat.*, **118**, 163–194.

MANO, N., OSHIMA, T. AND SHIMAZU, H. (1968) Inhibitory commissural fibers interconnecting the bilateral vestibular nuclei. *Brain Res.*, **8**, 378–382.

MARKHAM, C. H. (1968) Midbrain and contralateral labyrinth influences on brain stem vestibular neurons in the cat. *Brain Res.*, **9**, 312–333.

NYBERG-HANSEN, R. (1964) Origin and termination of fibers from the vestibular nuclei descending in the medial longitudinal fasciculus. An experimental study with silver impregnation methods in the cat. *J. comp. Neurol.*, **122**, 355–367.

NYBERG-HANSEN, R. AND MASCITTI, T. A. (1964) Sites and mode of termination of fibers of the vestibulospinal tract in the cat. An experimental study with silver impregnation methods. *J. comp. Neurol.*, **122**, 369–387.

RASMUSSEN, A. T. (1932) Secondary vestibular tracts in the cat. *J. comp. Neurol.*, **54**, 143–171.

REXED, B. (1952) The cytoarchitectonic organization of the spinal cord in the cat. *J. comp. Neurol.*, **96**, 415–496.

SCHEIBEL, M. E. AND SCHEIBEL, A. B. (1958) Structural substrates for integrative patterns in the brain stem reticular core. In H. H. JASPER, L. D. PROCTOR, R. S. KNIGHTON, W. C. NOSHAY AND R. T. COSTELLO (Eds.), *Reticular Formation of the Brain*. Henry Ford Hospital Symposium, Little, Brown and Co., Boston, Mass., pp. 31–55.

SHIMAZU, H. AND PRECHT, W. (1966) Inhibition of central vestibular neurons from the contralateral labyrinth and its mediating pathway. *J. Neurophysiol.*, **29**, 467–492.

TARLOV, E. (1969) The rostral projections of the primate vestibular nuclei. An experimental study in macaque, baboon and chimpanzee. *J. comp. Neurol.*, **135**, 27–56.

TARLOV, E. (1970) Organization of vestibulo-oculomotor projections in the cat. *Brain Res.*, **20**, 159–179.

VALVERDE, F. (1961) Reticular formation of the pons and medulla oblongata. A Golgi study. *J. comp. Neurol.*, **116**, 71–100.

WALBERG, F., BOWSHER, D. AND BRODAL, A. (1958) The termination of primary vestibular fibers in the vestibular nuclei in the cat. An experimental study with silver methods. *J. comp. Neurol.*, **110**, 391–419.

WILSON, V. J., WYLIE, R. M. AND MARCO, L. A. (1968) Synaptic inputs to cells in the medial vestibular nucleus. *J. Neurophysiol.*, **31**, 176–185.

Organization of the Commissural Connections: Physiology

H. SHIMAZU

Department of Neurophysiology, Institute of Brain Research, School of Medicine, University of Tokyo, Hongo, Bunkyo-ku, Tokyo, Japan

Histological studies have shown that neurons in the vestibular nuclei send commissural fibers to the contralateral vestibular nuclei (Gray, 1926; Rasmussen, 1932; Ferraro *et al.*, 1940). Recently Ladpli and Brodal (1968) have made an extensive study on the commissural connections between the bilateral vestibular nuclei in the cat (Brodal, 1972).

With respect to physiological studies on crossed labyrinthine effects, de Vito *et al.* (1956) and Pompeiano and Cotti (1959) described that polarization of the unilateral labyrinth caused activation or depression of unit activities in the contra-lateral Deiters' nucleus. Multisynaptic pathways were presumed to mediate these crossed effects. A different approach to this problem was made by Moruzzi and Pompeiano (1957) and Batini, Moruzzi and Pompeiano (1957) who observed the postural changes caused by interruption of the vestibular nerves in the decerebrate and decerebellate animal and suggested that the vestibular nuclei receive an inhibitory influence from the contralateral labyrinth. In those days, however, no substantial evoked potentials were found in the vestibular nuclei after single shocks to the contralateral vestibular nerve (Mickle and Ades, 1954; Gernandt *et al.*, 1959). Thus, these negative results cast doubt upon any contribution of the commissural fibers to significant physiological function (Gernandt, 1960).

FUNCTIONAL CONNECTION OF THE COMMISSURAL FIBERS

The existence of contralaterally induced electric activities in the vestibular nuclei was found by Shimazu and Precht (1966). As shown in Fig. 1A, the field potentials in the vestibular nuclei induced after contralateral vestibular nerve stimulation consisted of an initial positive, or positive-negative, deflection and a later slow negative wave. The intensity of stimulation was less than two times threshold for evoking the N_1 potential ($2 \times N_1 T$) in the vestibular nuclei on the stimulated side, thus no evoked potentials being found in the pontobulbar reticular formation (Precht and Shimazu, 1965; Shimazu and Precht, 1966). The field potentials were induced in a fairly localized region in the ventral part of the medial nucleus and ventromedial part of the superior and lateral nuclei. The initial positive deflection was attributed to nerve impulses propagated along commissural fibers running beneath the fourth ventricle. The later slow negative wave was explained by activation of type-II vestibular neurons (see

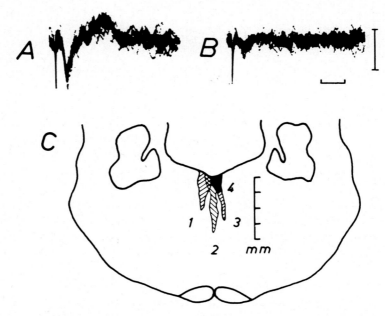

Fig. 1. Effects of incision of the dorsal brain stem along the midline on the contralaterally evoked field potentials in the vestibular nuclei. A: control response. B: after incision indicated by hatched area, 1. Each record is composed of 15 superimposed traces. Time: 5 msec, calibration: 100 μV. Upward deflection indicates negative. C: line drawing of histological section of the brain stem showing the depth of incision. Contralateral vestibular field potentials were almost completely abolished by the incision, 1–3, and only slightly decreased, 4. From Shimazu and Precht (1966).

below). These neurons were excited by weak stimulation of the contralateral vestibular nerve, and most of them were located in the ventral part of the medial nucleus and in the ventromedial part of the superior nucleus in agreement with the location of the later slow negative field potential.

After incising the dorsal brain stem beneath the fourth ventricle along the midline from the inferior colliculus to obex, both the initial positive and later slow negative waves were remarkably decreased or completely abolished (Fig. 1B). Fig. 1C shows examples of histological examination indicating the depth of incision necessary to abolish the contralateral field potentials. It was concluded that the midline incision should be about 2 mm deep and should extend just ventral to the medial longitudinal fasciculus in order to abolish them. These findings appear to be in good agreement with anatomical studies on the course and termination of the commissural fibers (Ladpli and Brodal, 1968).

The effects of commissural pathway on the contralateral vestibular neurons were analyzed in the horizontal canal system (Shimazu and Precht, 1966). Unit activities of type-I neurons were recorded extracellularly in the vestibular nuclei and were identified by their responses to horizontal rotation of the head. Type-I denotes their responses to horizontal angular acceleration in parallel with receptor activities in the ipsilateral horizontal canal (Gernandt, 1949; Duensing and Schaefer, 1958), thus indicating that these neurons are the secondary vestibular neurons in the horizontal canal system (Shimazu and Precht, 1965). Spontaneous discharges of tonic type-I neurons defined by their characteristic responses to rotation (Shimazu and Precht, 1965) were found to be distinctly suppressed by weak repetitive stimulation of the contralateral vestibular nerve (Fig. 2A). The intensity of stimulation was less than that for producing field potentials in the pontobulbar reticular formation. The discharges of kinetic neurons (Shimazu and Precht, 1965) induced by ipsilateral vestibular nerve stimulation (Fig. 2Da) were also suppressed by contralateral vestibular nerve stimulation (Fig. 2Db). No excitation was observed in any type-I neuron with stimulus intensity less than that for evoking reticular potentials.

Type-II neurons were consistently excited by weak stimulation of the contralateral vestibular nerve in marked contrast to the inhibitory responses of type-I neurons to identical stimulation. Type-II denotes their responses to horizontal angular acceleration in parallel with receptor activities in the contralateral horizontal canal (Duensing and Schaefer, 1958).

The effects of incision of the dorsal brain stem along the midline were examined on the crossed inhibitory influences on type-I neurons and the crossed excitatory influences on type-II neurons. On all type-I neurons tested after interrupting the commissural fibers (Fig. 2C), the crossed inhibitory effects were completely abolished. No type-II neurons were found to be excited by contralateral vestibular nerve stimulation after

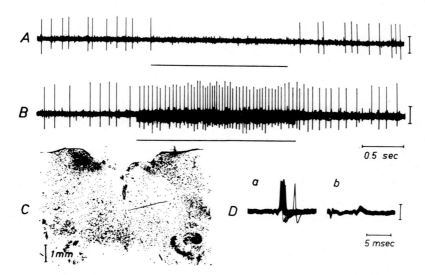

Fig. 2. Effects of contralateral vestibular nerve stimulation on type-I neurons before (A) and after (B) incising the midline of the dorsal brain stem. A: control response of tonic type-I neuron. B: after incision, about 2 mm deep, indicated in the microphotograh (C). A horizontal line below each record indicates 100/sec repetitive stimulation. Intensities of stimulation are 1.5 (A) and 3.0 (B) xN₁T. D: effect of contralateral vestibular nerve stimulation on kinetic type-I neuron; a, spikes were evoked by 50/sec electric stimulation of the ipsilateral vestibular nerve; b, additional 50/sec stimulation was applied to the contralateral vestibular nerve. Each record in D is composed of about 30 superimposed traces. Calibration: 500 µV for all records. From Shimazu and Precht (1966).

cutting the commissural fibers, when stimulus intensity was less than that for evoking reticular responses. The depth of the incision necessary to abolish the contralateral inhibition of type-I neurons was 1.5–2.0 mm, which was almost the same as the depth required to abolish the contralateral field potentials as mentioned above. When stimulus intensity was increased to induce reticular potentials after cutting the commissural fibers, the inhibitory response of type-I neurons was invariably replaced by an excitation (Fig. 2B). From these results it was concluded that type-I neurons are inhibited and type-II neurons are excited through the commissural pathway from the contralateral vestibular nuclei and that the reticulo-vestibular connections may be overall excitatory.

The impulses producing inhibition of type-I neurons and excitation of type-II neurons presumably originate from the contralateral horizontal canal, because in the chronically hemilabyrinthectomized animal type-I and type-II responses of vestibular neurons to horizontal rotatory stimulation were still found on the affected side (Precht et al., 1966). The studies on vestibular neurons of the horizontal canal were extended to those of the anterior canal (Markham, 1968). Commissural effects on type-I and type-II neurons of the anterior canal were found to be quite similar to those of the horizontal canal, though the strength of inhibition of type-I neurons was weaker in the anterior canal system than that in the horizontal canal system according to Markham. The origin of the inhibitory influence on type-I neurons of the anterior canal was presumed to be the contralateral posterior canal.

With respect to the functional significance of the commissural inhibition of type-I neurons it was inferred that during ipsilateral angular acceleration discharge frequencies of type-I neurons are increased not only by activation of the ipsilateral horizontal canal but also by a decrease of commissural inhibition (disinhibition) resulting from decreased activities of the contralateral horizontal canal. During contralateral angular acceleration, the commissural inhibition acts on type-I neurons in addition to a decrease in excitation (disfacilitation) from the ipsilateral horizontal canal. These functionally additive influences from the ipsi- and contralateral horizontal canal will elevate the sensitivity of secondary relay neurons to natural, rotatory stimulation (Shimazu and Precht, 1966).

NEURONAL ORGANIZATION OF THE COMMISSURAL PATHWAY

In the study of Shimazu and Precht (1966) inhibition of spontaneous activities of tonic type-I neurons had a relatively long latency (4 msec on the average) after contralateral vestibular nerve stimulation. Activation of type-II neurons occurred slightly earlier than the onset of the inhibition. It was thus postulated that the commissural inhibition of tonic type-I neurons is mediated through a multisynaptic pathway and that some of type-II neurons are intercalated inhibitory neurons acting on the homolateral type-I neurons.

Synaptic nature of the commissural inhibition and the neuronal organization of the related pathway mediating the inhibitory action on kinetic and tonic type-I neurons have been further studied by correlating the intracellular records of the postsynaptic

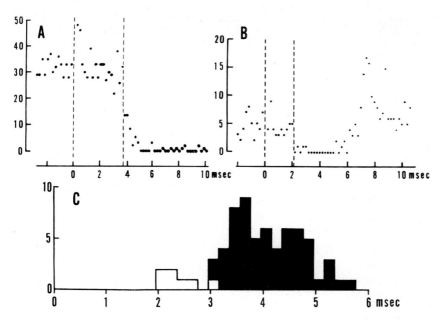

Fig. 3. A: spike distribution constructed with 6000 sweeps for a tonic type-I unit. B: that for a kinetic type-I unit with 10000 sweeps. Ordinates: number of spikes counted at each bin. Bin width, 0.2 msec. Left and right vertical broken lines in each of A and B indicate time of contralateral vestibular nerve stimulation and onset of inhibition, respectively. In B background discharges were induced by ipsilateral labyrinthine cathodal polarization of less than 100 μA (modified from Kasahara *et al.*, 1968). C: frequency distribution histogram of the latency of contralateral inhibition in 7 kinetic (open) and in 62 tonic (filled) type-I units. Class width, 0.2 msec.

potentials in the vestibular nucleus neurons with the extracellular records of functionally identified type-I neurons (Kasahara *et al.*, 1968; Mano *et al.*, 1968; Kasahara, Mano, Oshima, Ozawa and Shimazu, in preparation). These studies have been carried out with the unanesthetized, decerebrate cat in order to keep the presumed multisynaptic chains of the commissural pathway intact.

Repetitive discharges of tonic type-I neurons were depressed for a certain period following a single shock to the contralateral vestibular nerve. Since kinetic type-I neurons were spontaneously silent (Shimazu and Precht, 1965), their repetitive discharges were induced by cathodal polarization of the ipsilateral labyrinth. The latter were also highly sensitive to the inhibitory influence from the contralateral vestibular nerve. The frequencies of occurrence of these spikes at successive intervals of 0.2–0.4 msec before and after each shock (applied at 3–5/sec to the contralateral vestibular nerve) were counted over 3000–10000 sweeps by means of an electronic computer in order to yield the histogram of spike distribution. Fig. 3A exemplifies the histogram obtained from a tonic neuron, in which the inhibition started at the 19th bin. The bin width was 0.2 msec and therefore the latency was determined to be 3.8 msec in this case. Fig. 3B illustrates an example of the histogram for a kinetic type-I neuron, in which the latency of inhibition was 2.2 msec. The onset of the inhibition was usually abrupt enough to minimize a possible error of latency determination by superposition of a large number of sweeps.

In 62 tonic type-I neurons the latencies of the commissural inhibition after contralateral vestibular nerve stimulation ranged from 3.0 to 5.6 msec, the mean latency being 4.1 msec (Fig. 3C, filled histogram). This value was in good agreement with the mean value, 4 msec, obtained in a previous study on tonic type-I neurons (Shimazu and Precht, 1966). The mean value of the latencies for 7 kinetic neurons was 2.3 msec (range: 2.0–3.0 msec) (Fig. 3C, open histogram). Thus, the commissural inhibition of kinetic type-I neurons was found to start definitely earlier than that of tonic type-I neurons. These results suggest that the neuronal organization of the commissural pathway acting on kinetic neurons differs from that on tonic neurons.

In the next stage of experiments intracellular recording was made from the secondary vestibular neurons in the medial or superior nucleus where many type-I neurons were located (Shimazu and Precht, 1965). Since the type-I unit spikes identified by horizontal rotation were consistently activated ipsilaterally and inhibited contralaterally by vestibular nerve stimulation, only neurons that received these effects from each labyrinth were sampled. Fig. 4A–D illustrates the excitatory postsynaptic potenti-

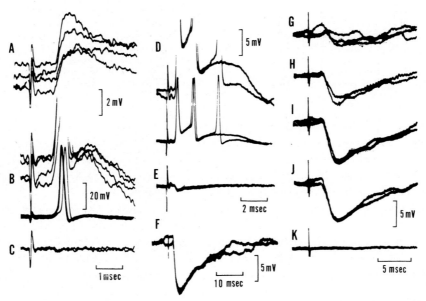

Fig. 4. Intracellular recording from a medial vestibular nucleus neuron. A–E: effects of ipsilateral vestibular nerve stimulation with intensities of 1.2 (A), 1.4 (B, C) and 3.8 (D, E) xN₁T. C and E: extracellular control recorded after withdrawal of microelectrode with same amplifications as upper traces in B and D, respectively. F–K: effects of contralateral vestibular nerve stimulation with intensities of 2.9 (F), 1.6 (G), 1.9 (H), 2.3 (I) and 2.6 (J, K) xN₁T. K: extracellular field potentials. Oscillographic records are taken by superimposing 2–10 traces at a repetition rate of 1–5/sec. Voltage calibration (upward positive): 2 mV for A, C and upper traces in B; 20 mV for lower traces of B and D; 5 mV for others. Time scale: 1 msec applies to A–C; 2 msec to D and E; 10 msec to F; 5 msec to G–K.

als (EPSPs) and action potentials elicited in a medial vestibular nucleus neuron with varied intensity of ipsilateral vestibular nerve stimulation. When a single shock was applied to the contralateral vestibular nerve, a membrane hyperpolarization was produced in the same neuron as in Fig. 4A–D with an amplitude amounting to 10 mV and a duration of 10–40 msec (Fig. 4F). This hyperpolarization was concluded to be the inhibitory postsynaptic potential (IPSP) in view of its inhibitory action on spontaneous discharges and of its reversal to a depolarization by passing hyperpolarizing currents through the recording microelectrode or by electrophoretic injection of Cl⁻ ions into the cell (Mano *et al.*, 1968).

Fig. 4G–J shows the IPSPs produced at varied intensity of contralateral vestibular nerve stimulation. The amplitude of the IPSP attained its maximum at stimulus intensity of 2.5–3.0 xN_1T. The threshold of contralateral vestibular nerve stimulation for inducing the IPSP ranged from 1.2 to 2.0 xN_1T. This range of stimulus intensity was within the range for producing the commissural inhibition of type-I neurons (1.2–2.8 xN_1T), and much less than the stimulus intensity for activating the crossed pathway through the deeper bulbopontine structures (2.3–5.9 xN_1T) (Shimazu and Precht, 1966). The course of development of the crossed IPSP amplitude in relation to stimulus intensity (Fig. 4F–J) was similar to that of the commissural-induced field potentials. On the basis of these correspondences it is most likely that the IPSPs are induced through the commissural pathway.

Latencies of the commissural IPSP ranged widely in different neurons, *i.e.*, 1.7–4.6 msec after stimulation of the contralateral vestibular nerve. The open histogram in Fig. 5G shows the frequency distribution of latencies of the commissural IPSPs in 127 vestibular neurons. These values may be divided into three groups; 1.7–2.9 msec for the first group (mean: 2.3 msec), 3.0–4.1 msec for the second group (mean: 3.5 msec), and 4.2–4.6 msec for the third group (mean: 4.5 msec). When latencies of the commissural IPSPs in Fig. 5G are compared with those of the commissural inhibition of functionally identified type-I neurons (Fig. 3C), the first group of IPSP corresponds to the inhibition of kinetic type-I neurons, and the second and third groups of IPSP to the inhibition of tonic type-I neurons.

Fig. 5A shows the commissural IPSP (bottom trace) in response to contralateral vestibular nerve stimulation and its reversal to a depolarization by Cl⁻ ions injection (top trace). When the shock stimuli were applied directly to the contralateral medial vestibular nucleus (see Fig. 5E), similar IPSPs were produced with an appreciably shorter latency (Fig. 5B). (Compare the diverging point, arrow, of superimposed traces of the original and the inverted IPSPs in Fig. 5D with that in Fig. 5C.) The filled histogram in Fig. 5G shows the frequency distribution of latencies of the IPSPs induced by stimulation of the contralateral medial vestibular nucleus. The latencies are clearly divided into two groups and the mean latency of each group is approximately 1 msec shorter than each of the first and second group of IPSP induced from the contralateral nerve, respectively (open histogram in Fig. 5G).

Fig. 6 represents the latency of the contralateral nucleus-induced IPSP plotted against the latency of the contralateral nerve-induced IPSP measured on each neuron. It is clear that three groups of the contralateral nerve-induced IPSP in Fig. 5G (open

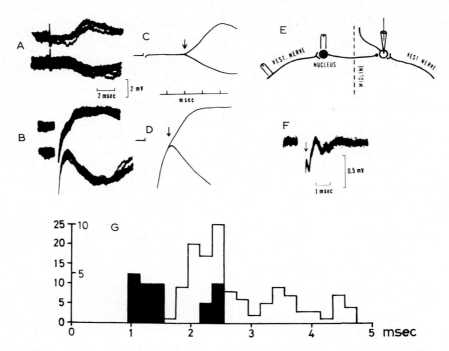

Fig. 5. A and B: intracellular recording from a medial nucleus neuron. A: IPSP induced by contralateral vestibular nerve stimulation (bottom) and its reversal to depolarizing potential by Cl⁻ ions
(top). B: same arrangement as in A but record made in response to stimulation of the contralateral
medial vestibular nucleus. C and D: superimposed traces of the top and bottom records in A and B,
respectively, with an expanded time scale. Arrow indicates the diverging point of these two potential
curves. E: schematic drawing of neuronal connections for the shortest latency inhibition of kinetic
type-I neurons from the contralateral labyrinth. Filled neuron indicates inhibitory commissural
neuron. F: field potentials recorded from the ventral part of the medial vestibular nucleus in response
to single shocks to the contralateral medial vestibular nucleus. In all records upward deflection
represents positivity (modified from Mano, Oshima and Shimazu, 1968). G: frequency distribution
histogram of latencies of the commissural IPSPs after stimulation of the contralateral vestibular nerve
(open) and the contralateral medial vestibular nucleus (filled). Left and right scales (number of
neurons) in ordinate apply to open and filled histograms, respectively.

histogram) correspond to the clusters a, b and c in Fig. 6, respectively, and that two
groups of the contralateral nucleus-induced IPSP in Fig. 5G (filled histogram)
correspond to the cluster a and the clusters b and c, respectively.

   In the cluster a in Fig. 6, the shortest latency of the contralateral nucleus-induced
IPSP was 1.0 msec. Stimulation of the contralateral medial nucleus produced field
potentials composed of an early sharp negative deflection (arrow in Fig. 5F) followed
by a slow negativity. The former may indicate the action potentials of directly excited
commissural fibers together with those of antidromically excited commissural neurons,
while the latter would represent the activities of transsynaptically excited vestibular
neurons. The latency of onset of the initial negative deflection was 0.55 msec, which
may be the conduction time of impulses along the commissural fibers. When this value

of 0.55 msec is subtracted from the 1.0 msec which is the shortest latency of the contra-lateral nucleus-induced IPSP, the remaining delay, 0.45 msec, is of the order of a single synaptic delay time as determined in the spinal cord (Eccles, 1964) and the brain stem (Ito and Yoshida, 1966). It can thus be postulated that the stimulation of the contralateral medial nucleus induces IPSPs monosynaptically through the commissural fibers which by themselves have an inhibitory nature (Fig. 5E).

The latency difference between the IPSPs evoked from the contralateral vestibular nerve and medial nucleus was 1.05 msec on the average in the cluster a in Fig. 6. This difference would be the time required for monosynaptic activation of the inhibitory commissural neurons (Fig. 5E, filled neuron) by the primary vestibular nerve volley. Actually, as seen above (Fig. 4A–D), the monosynaptic EPSPs were induced in the medial nucleus neurons during ipsilateral vestibular nerve stimulation with latencies of 0.6–0.9 msec. The contralateral nucleus-induced IPSP was facilitated by a preceding weak shock to the contralateral vestibular nerve, the optimal interval between the conditioning and test stimuli being around 1.0 msec. It is therefore concluded for the IPSPs in the cluster a in Fig. 6 that impulses along the primary afferent fibers excite monosynaptically the inhibitory commissural neurons, impulses from which in turn cross the midline, eventually producing the IPSPs monosynaptically in the contralateral vestibular neurons (Fig. 5E). In view of the good agreement between the latencies of the IPSPs and those of inhibition of functionally identified type-I neurons as mentioned above, the vestibular neurons which receive the IPSP through the fastest commissural pathway (disynaptic from the contralateral vestibular nerve) are presumably the kinetic type-I neurons.

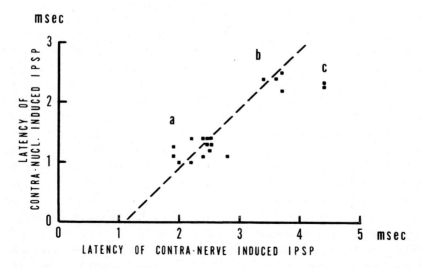

Fig. 6. Relation between latency of the contralateral nucleus-induced IPSP (ordinate) and that of the contralateral nerve-induced IPSP (abscissa) measured on each vestibular neuron. Broken line is drawn with gradient of 45° crossing the mean value of the cluster a.

Regarding the cluster b in Fig. 6, both the latencies of the contralateral nerve-induced and nucleus-induced IPSPs were 1.0–1.2 msec longer than those of the respective IPSPs in the cluster a. Therefore this additional delay time should be spent either along the commissural pathway or at the internuncial relay after crossing the midline. The latter possibility is more likely than the possibility of slowly conducting impulses along the inhibitory commissural fibers producing the monosynaptic IPSP, because threshold stimulation of the contralateral vestibular nuclei for inducing the commissural IPSP showed a clear temporal summation with double or triple shocks. Furthermore, while the IPSP in the cluster a could follow high frequency (*e.g.* 100/sec) stimulation, the IPSP in the cluster b could not even lower frequency of stimulation. It is thus inferred that the primary afferent fibers excite monosynaptically the excitatory commissural neurons, impulses from which in turn cross the midline and produce disynaptically the IPSP in the contralateral vestibular neurons through activation of the inhibitory interneurons (probably type-II neurons).

The IPSPs in the cluster c in Fig. 6 were induced from the contralateral vestibular nucleus with the latencies similar to those of the IPSPs in the cluster b (disynaptic), but from the contralateral vestibular nerve the latencies were about 1 msec longer than those of the cluster b. This suggests intercalation of one synapse in the contralateral vestibular nuclei. This slowest commissural pathway is similar to that suggested by Shimazu and Precht (1966). The IPSPs in the cluster b and c in Fig. 6 have similar latencies to those of commissural inhibition of tonic type-I neurons as mentioned above. Thus, the vestibular neurons receiving the commissural inhibition from the contralateral vestibular nerve through three or four synapses are presumably the tonic type-I neurons.

It has been suggested that the commissural inhibition of type-I neurons of the horizontal canal originates from the contralateral horizontal canal (Shimazu and Precht, 1966; Precht *et al.*, 1966), and that of the anterior canal originates from the contralateral posterior canal (Markham, 1968). Direct evidence has been provided for the selective mode of commissural inhibition related to activation of each specific end organ (Kasahara and Uchino, 1971). Using the techniques of electric stimulation of individual semicircular canal nerves developed by Suzuki *et al.* (1969), it was found that the secondary neuron excited from the ipsilateral anterior (A), horizontal (H) or posterior (P) canal receives the IPSP on separate stimulation of the contralateral posterior (p), horizontal (h) or anterior (a) canal nerve, respectively. Thus, the fundamental design of the commissural function may be p → A, h → H and a → P inhibitory action. Wilson *et al.* (1968) also studied on the crossed inhibition of medial nucleus neurons and found latencies of crossed inhibition ranging from 1.6 to 3.7 msec after stimulation of the contralateral vestibular nerve. Comparing these values with the mean latency of inhibition of tonic type-I neurons of the horizontal canal (4 msec) (Shimazu and Precht, 1966), they suggested that receptors other than those of the horizontal canal could activate faster pathways. After the end organs were identified, however, a number of the latencies of the horizontal canal-induced IPSPs were found to fall into the range of the fastest group. Thus, evidence has now been provided that the latency differences of the commissural inhibition depend neither on the different test systems nor on the different receptors concerned (Wilson, Wylie and Marco, 1968), but on the functionally different kinds of recipient vestibular neurons. It is conceivable that the properties of the commissural inhibition described above are common in all the canal systems.

With respect to the origin of commissural fibers, Ladpli and Brodal (1968) stated that the superior and descending nuclei send commissural fibers. The findings concerning the medial nucleus have not been conclusive. A physiological study has been attempted to find whether stimulation of the contralateral medial nucleus excites the commissural neurons located in the medial nucleus or excites commissural fibers coming from the more laterally located descending nucleus. In about two thirds of the vestibular neurons which received the disynaptic IPSP from the contralateral vestibular nerve, stimulation of the contralateral medial nucleus produced the IPSP monosynaptically, while stimulation of the contralateral descending nucleus induced the disynaptic IPSP. The latter effect may be explained by activation of primary afferents within the descending nucleus, which in turn excite the commissural neurons located in the medial nucleus. In the remaining one third, both the IPSPs induced from the contralateral medial and descending nuclei had a similar monosynaptic latency. In these cases the possibility of medial nucleus stimulation exciting the commissural fibers coming from the descending nucleus is not excluded.

EXTRA-COMMISSURAL CROSSED EFFECTS

Crossed labyrinthine influences mediated through the extra-commissural connections will be briefly described. These effects were particularly found on the Deiters neurons which responded to lateral tilt of the head under unanesthetized, decerebrate condition (Shimazu and Smith, 1971). These neurons were consistently excited by stimulation of the contralateral vestibular nerve (Fig. 7F) and were never inhibited. The minimal intensities of vestibular nerve stimulation (50/sec repetition) required for producing excitation of contralateral Deiters neurons ranged from 2.4 to 3.8 xN_1T (mean: 3.27). These values were significantly higher than those for excitation of contralateral type-II neurons through the commissural pathway (mean: 1.52 xN_1T), and were strong enough to induce reticular responses (Shimazu and Precht, 1966).

When spikes of Deiters neurons were evoked by single shocks to the contralateral vestibular nerve, the latency was about 7–8 msec or more (Fig. 7A). After cutting the commissural fibers along the midline of the dorsal brain stem from the inferior colliculus to obex (Fig. 7E), the Deiters neurons responding to tilt were still activated by contralateral vestibular nerve stimulation (Fig. 7G). The thresholds of contralateral vestibular nerve stimulation for exciting Deiters neurons were not significantly changed after cutting the commissural fibers as compared with the control value. In these experiments the animal was decerebrated and the medial part of the cerebellum was removed. It may thus be concluded that the crossed excitation of Deiters neurons responding to tilt is mediated through multineuronal chains in the underlying structures including the reticular formation.

References pp. 189–190

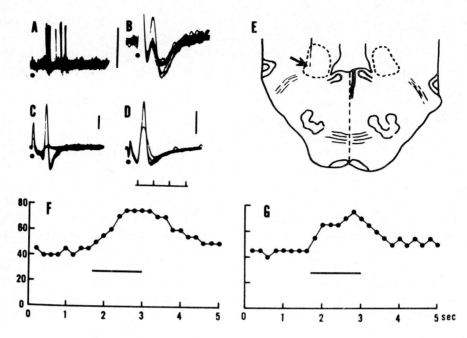

Fig. 7. Influences of the contralateral vestibular nerve activity on Deiters neurons. A: excitation of a Deiters neuron in response to single shocks to the contralateral vestibular nerve. B: antidromic activation of the same neuron as in A by threshold stimulation of the cervical cord. C and D: antidromic activation of other Deiters neurons by threshold stimulation of the cervical cord. Time: 10 msec for A; 1 msec for B, C and D. Calibration: 300 μV. E: line drawing of histological section of the brain stem indicating the longitudinal incision (black area) which was made between recordings of spikes shown in C and D. The arrow indicates the location of the electrode tip with which the spikes in D were recorded. F: frequency responses of the neuron shown in C to repetitive stimulation of the contralateral vestibular nerve. G: responses of the neuron shown in D to the same stimulation as in F after cutting the commissural fibers indicated in E. In each of F and G, the ordinate represents spikes per second measured in each 0.2 sec, and a horizontal line indicates the period of stimulation. Each neuron responded sensitively to lateral tilt of the head. From Shimazu and Smith (1971).

SUMMARY

Synaptic nature of the commissural inhibition and the neuronal organization of the related pathway mediating the inhibitory action on kinetic and tonic type-I neurons of the horizontal canal have been studied with the unanesthetized, decerebrate cat. These studies were carried out by correlating the intracellular records of the postsynaptic potentials in the vestibular nucleus neurons with the extracellular records of functionally identified type-I neurons. The commissural inhibition is caused by a production of the IPSP in the recipient vestibular neuron. The commissural pathway acting on the kinetic type-I neurons is composed of two neuron chains from the vestibular nerve; impulses along the primary afferent fibers excite monosynaptically the inhibitory commissural neurons, impulses from which in turn cross the midline, eventually producing the IPSP monosynaptically in the contralateral kinetic neurons. The commissural pathway for tonic type-I neurons has one or two more synapses along its path from the primary vestibular nerve, and the inhibitory neuron (probably type-II neuron) is located on the same side as the type-I neuron that receives the commissural inhibition. Extra-commissural crossed effects on Deiters neurons responding to lateral tilt of the head are briefly described; they are consistently excitatory.

REFERENCES

BATINI, C., MORUZZI, G. AND POMPEIANO, O. (1957) Cerebellar release phenomena. *Arch. ital. Biol.*, **95**, 71–95.

BRODAL, A. (1972) Organization of the commissural connections: anatomy. In A. BRODAL AND O. POMPEIANO (Eds.), *Progress in Brain Research. Vol. 37. Basic aspects of central vestibular mechanisms.* Elsevier, Amsterdam, pp. 167–176.

DUENSING, F. AND SCHAEFER, K. P. (1958) Die Aktivität einzelner Neurone im Bereich der Vestibulariskerne bei Horizontalbeschleunigungen unter besonderer Berücksichtigung des vestibulären Nystagmus. *Arch. Psychiat. Nervenkr.*, **198**, 225–252.

ECCLES, J. C. (1964) *The Physiology of Synapses.* Springer, Berlin, pp. 316.

FERRARO, A., PACELLA, B. L. AND BARRERA, S. E. (1940) Effects of lesions of the medial vestibular nucleus. An anatomical and physiological study in *Macacus rhesus* monkeys. *J. comp. Neurol.*, **73**, 7–36.

GERNANDT, B. E. (1949) Response of mammalian vestibular neurons to horizontal rotation and caloric stimulation. *J. Neurophysiol.*, **12**, 173–184.

GERNANDT, B. E. (1960) Generation of labyrinthine impulses, descending vestibular pathway, and modulation of vestibular activity by proprioceptive, cerebellar, and reticular influences. In G. L. RASMUSSEN AND W. F. WINDLE (Eds.), *Neural Mechanisms of the Auditory and Vestibular Systems.* C. C. Thomas, Springfield, Ill., pp. 324–348.

GERNANDT, B. E., IRANYI, M. AND LIVINGSTON, R. B. (1959) Vestibular influences on spinal mechanisms. *Exp. Neurol.*, **1**, 248–273.

GRAY, L. P. (1926) Some experimental evidence on the connections of the vestibular mechanism in the cat. *J. comp. Neurol.*, **41**, 319–364.

ITO, M. AND YOSHIDA, M. (1966) The origin of cerebellar-induced inhibition of Deiters neurons. I. Monosynaptic initiation of the inhibitory postsynaptic potentials. *Exp. Brain Res.*, **2**, 330–349.

KASAHARA, M., MANO, N., OSHIMA, T., OZAWA, S. AND SHIMAZU, H. (1968) Contralateral short latency inhibition of central vestibular neurons in the horizontal canal system. *Brain Res.*, **8**, 376–378.

KASAHARA, M. AND UCHINO, Y. (1971) Selective mode of commissural inhibition induced by semicircular canal afferents on secondary vestibular neurons in the cat. *Brain Res.*, **34**, 366–369.

LADPLI, R. AND BRODAL, A. (1968) Experimental studies of commissural and reticular formation projections from the vestibular nuclei in the cat. *Brain Res.*, **8**, 65–96.

MANO, N., OSHIMA, T. AND SHIMAZU, H. (1968) Inhibitory commissural fibers interconnecting the bilateral vestibular nuclei. *Brain Res.*, **8**, 378–382.

MARKHAM, C. H. (1968) Midbrain and contralateral labyrinth influences on brain stem vestibular neurons in the cat. *Brain Res.*, **9**, 312–333.

MICKLE, W. A. AND ADES, H. W. (1954) Rostral projection pathway of the vestibular system. *Amer. J. Physiol.*, **176**, 243–252.

MORUZZI, G. AND POMPEIANO, O. (1957) Inhibitory mechanisms underlying the collapse of decerebrate rigidity after unilateral fastigial lesions. *J. comp. Neurol.*, **107**, 1–26.

POMPEIANO, O. AND COTTI, E. (1959) Analisi microelettrodica delle proiezioni cerebello-deitersiane. *Arch. Sci. biol. (Bologna)*, **43**: 57–101.

PRECHT, W. AND SHIMAZU, H. (1965) Functional connections of tonic and kinetic vestibular neurons with primary vestibular afferents. *J. Neurophysiol.*, **28**, 1014–1028.

PRECHT, W., SHIMAZU, H. AND MARKHAM, C. H. (1966) A mechanism of central compensation of vestibular function following hemilabyrinthectomy. *J. Neurophysiol.*, **29**, 996–1010.

RASMUSSEN, A. T. (1932) Secondary vestibular tracts in the cat. *J. comp. Neurol.*, **54**, 143–171.

Shimazu, H. and Precht, W. (1965) Tonic and kinetic responses of cat's vestibular neurons to horizontal angular acceleration. *J. Neurophysiol.*, **28**, 991–1013.

Shimazu, H. and Precht, W. (1966) Inhibition of central vestibular neurons from the contralateral labyrinth and its mediating pathway. *J. Neurophysiol.*, **29**, 467–492.

Shimazu, H. and Smith, C. M. (1971) Cerebellar and labyrinthine influences on single vestibular neurons identified by natural stimuli. *J. Neurophysiol.*, **34**, 493–508.

Suzuki, J., Goto, K., Tokumasu, K. and Cohen, B. (1969) Implantation of electrodes near individual vestibular nerve branches in mammals. *Ann. Otol. (St. Louis)*, **78**, 815–826.

Vito, R. V. de, Brusa, A. and Arduini, A. (1956) Cerebellar and vestibular influences on Deitersian units. *J. Neurophysiol.*, **19**, 241–253.

Wilson, V. J., Wylie, R. M. and Marco, L. A. (1968) Synaptic inputs to cells in the medial vestibular nucleus. *J. Neurophysiol.*, **31**, 176–185.

COMMENTS TO CHAPTER III

Input to Type-II Neuron from the Labyrinths

G. MELVILL JONES

Canadian Defence Research Board, Aviation Medical Research Unit, Department of Physiology, McGill University, Montreal, Quebec, Canada

H. SHIMAZU

Department of Neurophysiology, Institute of Brain Research, School of Medicine, University of Tokyo, Hongo, Bunkyo-ku, Tokyo, Japan

C. H. MARKHAM

Department of Neurology, School of Medicine, University of California, Los Angeles, California, U.S.A.

G. MELVILL JONES: It was rather surprising to hear that, despite section of commissural vestibular fibres, Markham and Curthoys (1972) found no change in the ratio of type-I and II cells, since there is good evidence that a group of type-II cells receives excitatory influence only from the contralateral labyrinth (Shimazu and Precht, 1966). Perhaps Dr. Shimazu and Dr. Markham would care to comment on this apparent anomaly.

H. SHIMAZU: As described previously in detail (Shimazu and Precht, 1966), a group of type-II neuron receives an excitatory influence only from the contralateral labyrinth and no excitatory influence from the ipsilateral side. These neurons respond very sensitively to horizontal rotation. The thresholds of electric stimulation of the contralateral vestibular nerve for exciting these type-II neurons are within the range of intensities for activating the commissural pathway and are much lower than those for reticular activation. No type-II neurons are excited with such a low intensity of stimulation of the contralateral vestibular nerve after interrupting the commissural pathway. The excitation was induced only with stimulation strong enough to produce reticular responses. Most of the type-II neurons excited only from the contralateral labyrinth are located in the ventral part of the medial nucleus and in the ventromedial part of the superior nucleus. These type-II neurons were presumed to be inhibitory neurons mediating the commissural inhibition of type-I neurons.

The other group of type-II neurons, however, is excited not only from the contralateral but also from the ipsilateral vestibular nerve. The ipsilateral excitation seems to originate from end organs other than the horizontal canal. The thresholds of contralateral vestibular nerve stimulation for exciting these neurons are higher than those for activation of the above mentioned type-II neurons. Some of the contralateral effects on this group of type-II neuron appear to be mediated through the reticular formation, but not related to the commissural pathway. Type-II neurons are still found even after destruction of the contralateral labyrinth, suggesting that the type-II response is caused by inhibitory influences from the ipsilateral horizontal canal. The location of these type-II neurons is not restricted to the ventral part of the vestibular nuclei, but is scattered in various parts of the nuclei. Some type-II neurons are found in the Deiters nucleus and are antidromically excited from the spinal cord. These neurons may not be inhibitory neurons intercalated in the commissural pathway.

It would be expected that the thresholds of rotation for activating the above mentioned first group of type-II neurons will be considerably elevated after interrupting the commissural connections. Judging from amplitudes of extracellularly recorded spikes, the type-II neurons which are presumed to be inhibitory neurons in the commissural pathway appear to be much smaller in size than the ipsilaterally excited type-II neurons. This suggests that, with random sampling which is necessary for statistical analysis, the latter might be more frequently recorded than the former. If type-II neurons tested were mainly those activated from both labyrinths, it would not be unreasonable that the probability of picking up these neurons is not much reduced after interrupting the commissural pathway. I would stress that the identification of type-II neurons not only by horizontal rotation but also by stimulation of various sources as well as their anatomical location is highly important.

C. H. MARKHAM: The point which my old colleague, Dr. Shimazu, refers to, our finding no percentage change in type-I: type-II on sectioning the vestibular commissural fibers, was also a surprise to us. Since it was not the main purpose of our experiment, we did not do tests to better characterize the type-II neurons. However, it is unlikely in this experiment we selectively avoid a certain group of type-II neurons since we used searching and identification procedures which were the same as past experiments including some with Shimazu and Precht (1966).

I would hypothesize that those type-II's responding to labyrinthine influence only from the contralateral side may have more powerful pathways through the reticular formation than heretofore considered. The contralateral labyrinth might act on some type-II's solely by a reticular path; on a few others solely by the commissural path; and the majority by both paths. Differences in latency and threshold of these connections might not be apparent with natural stimulation at $4°/\text{sec}^2$.

I hope to have data shortly to prove (or reject) these considerations.

REFERENCES

MARKHAM, C. H. AND CURTHOYS, I. S. (1972) Labyrinthine convergence on vestibular nuclear neurons using natural and electrical stimulation. In A. BRODAL AND O. POMPEIANO (Eds.), *Progress in Brain Research. Vol. 37. Basic aspects of central vestibular mechanisms.* Elsevier, Amsterdam, pp. 121–137.
SHIMAZU, H. AND PRECHT, W. (1966) Inhibition of central vestibular neurons from the contralateral labyrinth and its mediating pathway. *J. Neurophysiol.*, **29**, 467–492.

IV. RELATIONS BETWEEN THE VESTIBULAR NUCLEI AND THE SPINAL CORD

Vestibulospinal Relations: Vestibular Influences on Gamma Motoneurons and Primary Afferents

O. POMPEIANO

Institute of Physiology II, University of Pisa, Pisa, Italy

A detailed study of the anatomo-functional organization of the vestibulospinal pathways is required in order to understand the mechanisms through which the vestibular system affects the spinal cord activities. It should be noticed, however, that the vestibular nuclei project also to reticulospinal and propriospinal neurons, which actually contribute together with the vestibulospinal projections to the vestibular control of different spinal mechanisms.

VESTIBULOSPINAL RELATIONS: ANATOMICAL AND PHYSIOLOGICAL ASPECTS

There are two main fiber systems which project from the vestibular nuclei to the spinal cord: the lateral vestibulospinal tract, originating from Deiters' nucleus and the medial vestibulospinal tract, originating mainly, but not exclusively, from the medial vestibular nucleus (Brodal *et al.*, 1962).

(*i*) *The lateral vestibulospinal tract.* Using the modified Gudden method (Brodal, 1940), Pompeiano and Brodal (1957) have shown that the lateral vestibulospinal tract originates from the lateral vestibular nucleus of Deiters (Fig. 1). Not only the large, giant cells but also the medium-sized and the small neurons on this nucleus project to the spinal cord. This was later confirmed by physiologists who found that the conduction velocity of the fibers of the lateral vestibulospinal tract varies between 24 and 140 m/sec (Ito *et al.*, 1964a, b; Wilson *et al.*, 1965, 1966b, 1967a) with an average conduction velocity at 90–100 m/sec (Ito *et al.*, 1964a; Lund and Pompeiano, 1968; Wilson and Yoshida, 1969c). If Hursh's (1939) proportion factor between the conduction velocity and the fiber diameter holds for the vestibulospinal tract, its fiber spectrum would cover a wide range from 4 to 23 μm with the peak at 16 μm.

In their experimental anatomical study, Pompeiano and Brodal (1957) demonstrated that the lateral vestibulospinal tract was somatotopically organized. Following lesions of the tract at various levels of the cord, the retrograde cellular changes in the nucleus have a different location. On the basis of these findings the pattern shown in Fig. 1 was established. In particular the rostroventral part of the lateral vestibular nucleus projects to the cervical cord, while the dorsocaudal part projects to the lumbosacral cord. Fibers to the thoracic cord come from intermediate regions. It is of interest that

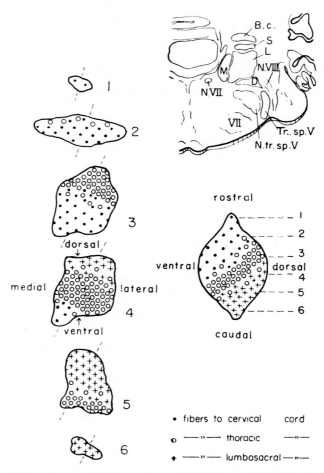

Fig. 1. Diagram showing the somatotopical pattern within the lateral vestibulospinal projection in the cat as demonstrated with experimental anatomical method by Pompeiano and Brodal. To the left a series of transverse sections through the lateral vestibular nucleus, to the right a longitudinal reconstruction of the nucleus. Key below shows that the rostroventral part of the nucleus may be considered as the forelimb region, the dorsocaudal part as the hindlimb region. Abbreviations for all figures. B.c., brachium conjunctivum; D., descending vestibular nucleus; L., lateral vestibular nucleus of Deiters; M., medial vestibular nucleus; N.tr.sp.V., nucleus of spinal trigeminal tract; N.VII, N.VIII, VII and VIII cranial nerve; S., superior vestibular nucleus; Tr.sp.V, spinal trigeminal tract; VII, motor nucleus of the VII nerve. From Pompeiano and Brodal (1957).

in the rostroventral part of Deiters' nucleus smaller cells are more abundant than large and giant cells, while in the dorsocaudal region giant cells are more numerous.

The same cytoarchitectonic differences observed between the rostroventral and the dorsocaudal part of Deiters' nucleus in the cat have been found between the medial and the lateral part of Deiters' nucleus in man (Sadjadpour and Brodal, 1968). It appears that there is also in man a somatotopical pattern in the vestibulospinal projection (Løken and Brodal, 1970; cf. Foerster and Gagel, 1932).

The somatotopic organization of the lateral vestibulospinal tract has been confirmed in cat both anatomically with silver impregnation methods, following localized lesions of Deiters' nucleus (Nyberg–Hansen and Mascitti, 1964: Nyberg–Hansen, 1966, 1970) and physiologically (Pompeiano, 1960; Ito et al., 1964a, b; Wilson et al., 1965, 1966a, b, 1967a; Wilson, 1970). It should be noted that diagrams like those of Fig. 1 can give no more than the main principles of organization. Pompeiano and Brodal (1957) have pointed out that there are no clear cut borders between nuclear regions supplying different levels of the cord but a fair degree of overlapping. This is shown by the fact that while the dorsocaudal region of the nucleus consists pre-dominantly of lumbar cells, scattered cells projecting to the lumbar cord have been identified by antidromic stimulation as being situated within the forelimb region of the nucleus (Precht et al., 1967; Wilson et al., 1967a).

The intramedullary course of the lateral vestibulospinal tract has been followed both anatomically (Rasmussen, 1932; Busch, 1961) and physiologically (Cook et al., 1969a). In the medulla this tract courses dorsolaterally to the inferior olive. From this part of the tract a short latency monosynaptic (followed by a disynaptic) potential can be recorded on single shock stimulation of the ipsilateral vestibular nerve (Cook et al., 1969a). The lateral vestibulospinal tract descends purely ipsilaterally along the periphery of the ventrolateral funiculus in the cervical cord; during its descent in the thoracic cord the tract is gradually displaced in a dorsomedial direction and in the lumbar enlargement it is medially located in the ventral funiculus along the anterior median fissure (cf. Pompeiano and Brodal, 1957; Nyberg–Hansen and Mascitti, 1964; Nyberg–Hansen, 1966, 1970).

The lateral vestibulospinal fibers enter the spinal grey matter of the ventral horn at the level of the ventromedial aspect of laminae VIII and VII (Nyberg–Hansen and Mascitti, 1964). They then spread dorsolaterally to terminate on the soma and particularly the dendrites of neurons localized in the entire lamina VIII and the neighbouring medial and central parts of lamina VII (Fig. 2A). Occasional fibers are seen in the ventral part of lamina VI and in lamina IX, but they are never seen in

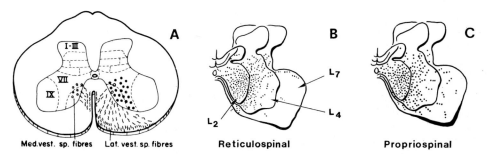

Fig. 2. Diagram comparing the distribution of the vestibulospinal, the reticulospinal and the long propriospinal fibers in the grey matter of the lumbosacral cord of the cat. A, Sites of termination of the lateral and medial vestibulospinal tract. Both tracts terminate in laminae VII and VIII. From Nyberg–Hansen (1970). B, C, Note the similarities in the distribution of the reticulospinal and the long propriospinal fibers. From Giovannelli Barilari and Kuypers (1969).

contact with nerve cells in these laminae. Moreover no fibers terminate in the inter-mediolateral cell column or in the column of Clarke (Nyberg–Hansen and Mascitti, 1964).

It should be mentioned here that according to some anatomical (Kuypers, 1966; Sterling and Kuypers, 1968) as well as physiological findings (Lloyd, 1941; Bernhard and Rexed, 1945; Appelberg, 1962) the interneurons located primarily in the ventro-medial part of the internuncial zone are leading to proximal motoneurons, while those located primarily in the dorsolateral parts of the internuncial zone lead to distal moto-neurons. This anatomical finding should be kept in mind in evaluating the action of the lateral vestibulospinal tract on spinal motoneurons.

The statement by Schimert (1938) that the vestibulospinal fibers terminate almost exclusively on medial motoneurons is not confirmed, since the majority of vestibulo-spinal fibers seem to end on the interneurons of lamina VIII (Nyberg–Hansen, 1970). The almost complete lack of terminations on motoneurons is in agreement with previous and more recent findings (Rasdolsky, 1923; Carpenter, 1960; Staal, 1961; Kuypers et al., 1962; Petras, 1967; Nyberg–Hansen, 1969).

It does not necessarily follow from these anatomical studies that the lateral vestibulo-spinal tract does not make monosynaptic contact with the motoneurons. It was shown by several authors that stimulation of the ventral funiculus and the ventral part of the lateral funiculus excited monosynaptically the lumbar motoneurons (Lloyd, 1941; Eide et al., 1961; Lund and Pompeiano, 1965, 1958; Willis et al., 1967; Skinner et al., 1970). Recent experiments have demonstrated that the vestibulospinal projection from Deiters' nucleus makes monosynaptic excitatory contact with hindlimb extensor motoneurons (Lund and Pompeiano, 1965, 1968; Pompeiano, 1966a) or with moto-neurons not classified as to function (Shapovalov, 1966; Shapovalov et al., 1966). As discussed by Grillner and Hongo (1972) vestibulospinal monosynaptic EPSPs occur particularly in ankle (GS) (Lund and Pompeiano, 1965, 1968; Grillner et al., 1966a, 1968, 1970; Wilson and Yoshida, 1968a, 1969c) and knee (quadriceps) extensor moto-neurons (Grillner et al., 1968, 1970), while there is little evidence of a monosynaptic vestibulospinal input to hip (ABSm) and toe (FDL) extensors (Grillner et al., 1968, 1970; Grillner and Lund, 1968; Wilson and Yoshida, 1969c; cf. also Lund and Pompe-iano, 1968). Stimulation of Deiters' nucleus also produced disynaptic and polysynaptic EPSPs in all extensor α motoneurons (Lund and Pompeiano, 1968; Grillner et al., 1968, 1970; Shapovalov, 1969; Wilson and Yoshida, 1969c; cf. Sasaki et al., 1962; Sasaki and Tanaka, 1964) as well as in a large number of pretibial flexor (DP) moto-neurons, but not in more proximal flexors (PBST, Sart, Grac) (Grillner et al., 1970). Contrary to extensor motoneurons, the vestibulospinal projection from Deiters' nucleus exerts disynaptic (Lund and Pompeiano, 1968; Grillner et al., 1968, 1970) or polysynaptic IPSP (Wilson and Yoshida, 1969c) in knee and ankle flexor motoneu-rons, as well as in some hip extensor (ABSm) motoneurons (Grillner et al., 1970).*

---

* Monosynaptic activation of ankle and knee flexors as well as of some hip (ABSm) and toe (FDL) extensor motoneurons occurs by stimulation of the medial brain stem reticular formation (Grillner et al., 1966a, 1968, 1970; Grillner and Lund, 1966, 1968; Wilson and Yoshida, 1968a, 1969c).

Since the dendrites of spinal motoneurons extend for considerable distances from the perikarya in lamina IX into laminae VIII and VII (Lenhossek, 1895; Cajal, 1909–11; Lorente de Nó, 1938; Aitken and Bridger, 1961; Sprague and Ha, 1964; Scheibel and Scheibel, 1966) it has been suggested that some of the vestibulospinal fibers terminating on these laminae may end on dendrites of motoneurons (Lund and Pompeiano, 1968). Physiological observations seem to support this conclusion (Shapovalov, 1966, 1969; Shapovalov et al., 1966; Grillner and Lund, 1968; Shapovalov and Safyants, 1968; Wilson and Yoshida, 1969c; Grillner et al., 1970, 1971). There is little doubt, however, that the late polysynaptic EPSPs in extensor motoneurons and the disynaptic IPSP on flexor motoneurons elicited by stimulation of Deiters' nucleus are due to activation of interneurons located in laminae VII and VIII (Lund and Pompeiano, 1968). These interneurons are known to send axon collaterals into the lateral motor nuclei (Matsushita, 1969). It should be anticipated here that the disynaptic IPSPs on flexor motoneurons (Lund and Pompeiano, 1968) elicited by Deiters' stimulation are due to monosynaptic activation of interneurons mediating the antagonistic extensor Ia inhibition to flexor motoneurons (Grillner et al., 1966c; Lundberg, 1970). It is of interest that these interneurons have been localized to the ventral part of lamina VII, just medial to lamina IX (Hultborn et al., 1968).*

There is no anatomical evidence that lateral vestibulospinal fibers cross within the spinal cord. However stimulation of the spinal cord in the L1 segment produces monosynaptic EPSPs on hindlimb α and γ motoneurons which could be mediated by fibers in both the ipsilateral and contralateral ventral quadrant (Willis et al., 1967; Grillner et al., 1969). Crossed effects from Deiters' nucleus may be mediated either by collaterals of the lateral vestibulospinal tract to reticulospinal or propriospinal neurons, or else by commissural fibers originating from neurons in laminae VII and VIII which cross the midline in the anterior commissure (Szentágothai, 1951, 1964, 1967; Rexed, 1952; Nyberg–Hansen and Mascitti, 1964; Scheibel and Scheibel, 1966; Willis and Willis, 1966; Sterling and Kuypers, 1968; Matsushita, 1969).

(ii) *The medial vestibulospinal tract.* The early anatomical observations on the medial vestibulospinal tract have been reviewed by Pompeiano and Brodal (1957). Although retrograde changes affect only the lateral vestibular nucleus, it was concluded at that time on the basis of the available evidence that fibers descending in the medial longitudinal fascicle (MLF) most probably originate from the medial vestibular nucleus. This is consistent with the fact that axons originating in the medial vestibular nucleus descend to the spinal cord in the MLF, as shown in anatomical (Busch, 1961; Nyberg–Hansen, 1964, 1966, 1970; McMaster et al., 1966) as well as physiological studies (Gernandt et al., 1959; Gernandt, 1968, 1970; Cook et al., 1969a). Following selective lesions of the medial vestibular nucleus, degenerating fibers course in the dorsal part of the ventral funiculus along the anterior median fissure (Nyberg–Hansen,

---

* There is also evidence suggesting that the lateral vestibulospinal tract excites the last order interneurons of the crossed extensor reflex pathway (Bruggencate et al., 1969; Hongo et al., 1971). It likely therefore that even these interneurons are located within laminae VII and VIII.

1964). These fibers do not extend as far ventrolaterally as the lateral vestibulospinal fibers. The medial vestibulospinal projection is bilateral and only few if any fibers have been traced below the cervical enlargement in cat (Petras, 1967) or monkey (McMaster et al., 1966). According to Nyberg–Hansen (1966) and Gernandt (1970) however descending fibers from the medial vestibular nucleus can be traced to midthoracic levels and it has been maintained by some anatomists (Matano et al., 1964; McMaster et al., 1966) and physiologists (Precht et al., 1967) that some of these fibers reach the lumbar cord on each side. Moreover, the fibers on the ipsilateral side outnumber those of the contralateral side (Nyberg–Hansen, 1964, 1966; Wilson et al., 1968; cf. however Matano et al., 1964).

The number of medial vestibulospinal fibers is very modest when compared with those in the lateral vestibulospinal tract (Nyberg–Hansen, 1964, 1966; cf. also Wilson et al., 1968); moreover the fibers of the medial tract are of medium to fine caliber (Busch, 1961; Nyberg–Hansen, 1964, 1966; Petras, 1967), i.e., smaller in size than those in the lateral tract. Conduction velocity of the fibers in the MLF ranges from 47–75 m/sec (Gernandt, 1968), while fibers descending from the medial vestibular nucleus conduct at 13–76 m/sec, with a mode of 36 m/sec (Wilson et al., 1968).

While a large fraction of Deiters' cells in all regions of the nucleus send axons to the spinal cord (Wilson et al., 1966b, 1967a), only 17% of medial cells seem to have long descending axons: these cells are apparently chiefly found at rostral levels in the medial vestibular nucleus (Wilson et al., 1968; Wilson, 1970).

It is generally assumed that most of the axons of medial nucleus cells that descend to the spinal cord are branches of dichotomizing axons, with another long branch ascending in a rostral direction (Brodal and Pompeiano, 1957). According to Wilson et al. (1968) however, only 24% of the medial nucleus projecting to the spinal cord could also be activated antidromically from the ascending MLF. The conclusion that a large fraction of descending medial vestibular neurons do not have long ascending axons is, however, weakened by the fact that the ascending MLF was antidromically activated by an electrode inserted into the midline of the floor of the IV ventricle about two mm rostral to the tip of Deiters nucleus. Unfortunately, at this level the nucleus raphe dorsalis displaces the ascending MLF in a lateral direction. This may explain that no monosynaptic response can be recorded in the MLF at this level on single shock stimulation of the vestibular nerve (Cook et al., 1969a). It seems reasonable, therefore, to assume that some of the non-driven cells in the experiments mentioned above consisted of rostrally projecting units whose axons escaped stimulation.

Contrary to the opinion of Matano et al. (1964) it is generally assumed on the basis of anatomical findings that the superior, lateral (Nyberg–Hansen, 1964) and the descending vestibular nucleus (Carpenter, 1960; Carpenter et al., 1960; Nyberg–Hansen, 1964) do not contribute to the medial vestibulospinal tract. Physiological observations however indicate that a modest contribution to this tract originate from the descending nucleus (Wilson et al., 1967b; Kawai et al., 1969; Peterson, 1970). This discrepancy may be only apparent (see Brodal, 1972).

The fibers of the medial vestibulospinal tract terminate in the medial part of the ventral horn (Nyberg–Hansen, 1964; McMasters et al., 1966; Petras, 1967). In particular they enter the grey matter of the ventral horn corresponding to the dorsomedial aspect of lamina VIII and terminate in the dorsal half of this lamina and the neighbouring medial part of lamina VII (Nyberg–Hansen, 1964, 1966, 1970). According to this author no fibers terminate among the soma of the motoneurons in lamina IX, neither in the intermedio-lateral cell column, nor in the column of Clarke. Fig. 2A shows that the area of termination is much less extensive than is that of the lateral vestibulospinal tract. Physiological observations made recently (Wilson and Yoshida, 1968b, 1969a–c) indicate that axons originating in the medial vestibular nucleus: (i) make monosynaptic connection with motoneurons in the upper cervical cord and (ii) they are inhibitory in function, thus exerting monosynaptic IPSPs on cervical motoneurons. Here again we have physiological evidence that supraspinal descending fibers terminate monosynaptically on spinal motoneurons, although they do not invade lamina IX.

Since stimulation of the medial (and descending) vestibular nucleus may influence the lumbar segments of the spinal cord of both sides, there are two main pathways through which the vestibular impulses may reach the lumbar cord: (i) one via vestibuloreticular fibers from the medial and descending vestibular nuclei (Ladpli and Brodal, 1968) and further relayed to the cord by way of the bilateral reticulospinal projection, which reaches not only the upper (Torvik and Brodal, 1957) but also the lower segments of the spinal cord (Nyberg–Hansen, 1965b, 1966; cf. Gernandt and Thulin, 1952; Gernandt et al., 1959; Diete–Spiff et al., 1967b); (ii) via descending propriospinal fibers interconnecting the spinal enlargements. Recent observations indicate that these descending propriospinal fibers (Giovannelli Barilari and Kuypers 1969) similarly to the reticulospinal fibers (Nyberg–Hansen, 1965b, 1966), are distributed bilaterally to the ventromedial parts of the grey substance, corresponding to lamina VIII and the medial parts of lamina VII (Fig. 2B, C).

There is evidence that the interneurons responding to both ipsilateral and contralateral vestibular nerve stimulation are concentrated in lamina VIII, with some neurons scattered in the medial part of laminae IV–VI (Erulkar et al., 1966).

VESTIBULAR INFLUENCES ON γ MOTONEURONS

Fusimotor activity induced by labyrinthine volleys

Fusimotor activity leading to muscle spindle afferent discharge can be elicited by natural labyrinthine stimulation (Eldred et al., 1953; Granit et al., 1955; Poppele, 1964, 1967; Van der Meulen and Gilman, 1965; Gilman and Van der Meulen, 1966) or by electrical stimulation of the vestibular nerve (Andersson and Gernandt, 1956; Gernandt et al., 1959; Diete–Spiff et al., 1966, 1967a, b; Gernandt, 1967).

Eldred et al. (1953) and Granit et al. (1955) gave the first demonstration that stimulation of vestibular and neck receptors produced a reflex activation of the γ system. The frequency of discharge of the spindle receptors could be either increased or decreased, according to the position of the head. After deafferentation the spindle retained its previous pattern of response but the accompanying reflex contraction was absent. This indicated that in these reflexes the α motoneurons were actively influenced through the loop via the muscle spindles. Since these experiments were carried out in animals with intact cervical roots it is not possible to decide how much of the reflex activation of the γ system is due to stimulation of vestibular receptors, how much to receptors in the neck.

That the muscle spindle afferent discharge can be modified by natural labyrinthine stimulation has been documented in several studies (Van der Meulen and Gilman 1965; Gilman and Van der Meulen 1966). In the experiments made by Poppele (1964, 1967; cf. Ajala and Poppele, 1967) vestibular stimulation was produced by rotating the head about the antero–posterior axis: in this way the vertical semicircular canals and the macular receptors were preferentially stimulated. The observations were performed by recording the spindle discharge from the gastrocnemius muscle after contralateral labyrinthectomy. Both phasic and tonic components of the spindle responses appeared; while the phasic response consisted of a transient increase in impulse frequency coincident with the head rotation in either direction, the tonic response consisted of a sustained increase in spindle discharge frequency particularly caused by contralateral rotation. The magnitude of the phasic response to rotation was found to be a function of the velocity of rotation thus being attributed to ampullar receptors. On the other hand the magnitude of the tonic changes was dependent on the angle of rotation, thus being attributed to stimulation of macular receptors.

Electrical stimulation of certain peripheral branches of the vestibular nerve also influence the activity of the γ fibers isolated from ventral root filaments of L7–S1 (Andersson and Gernandt, 1956). It appears from this study that the small γ efferents are activated at lower strengths of stimuli than the α fibers and show a higher frequency of discharge during vestibular stimulation than the α fibers. These findings have been confirmed by Diete–Spiff et al., (1967b) who found that the spindles from the gastrocnemius muscle were excited by repetitive stimulation of the ipsilateral VIII cranial nerve at lower threshold frequencies (at optimum voltage) than that needed to produce extrafusal contraction also.

After the demonstration that the muscle spindles are innervated by static and dynamic fusimotor neurons (Matthews, 1962; Crowe and Matthews, 1964a, b; Appelberg et al., 1965, 1966; Brown et al., 1965; Bessou et al., 1966, 1968), the problem arises whether orthodromic labyrinthine volleys are able to affect the two population of fusimotor neurons and whether there is a relative segregation of the static and dynamic fusimotor effects in the lateral and medial vestibular nuclei. The observation by Diete–Spiff et al. (1967b), i.e., that stimulation of the VIII nerve produced acceleration not only of primary but also of secondary endings suggests that static fusimotor neurons are influenced by the labyrinthine volleys. It is likely, although not definitely proved, that this effect is mediated by Deiters' nucleus, since stimulation of this structure is able to activate static fusimotor neurons to extensor muscles (see page 213). In addition to these events, however, there is also evidence that stimulation of the labyrinth by direct current produces large dynamic responses to stretch (Jansen and Matthews, 1962). Further experiments are required to find out whether the static effects induced by vestibular nerve stimulation are abolished by selective lesion of

Deiters' nucleus and whether the dynamic effects still persist after this lesion. It would then be possible to decide which type of fusimotor neurons is influenced by the medial vestibular nucleus.

Fusimotor activity induced by Deiters' nucleus

Two pathways have been defined by which a supraspinal center may induce muscle's motor units to contract (Merton, 1953). One, a fast direct pathway (α route), is a straight-through connection from supraspinal structures to the anterior horn cells and hence to the muscle fibers by the large α motor fibers. It was suggested that this pathway is used only for rapid movements. The other pathway, referred to as the γ route, is the one supposedly concerned with the postural type of contraction. In this, supraspinal structures act on the small γ motoneurons, which activate the intrafusal muscle fibers of the spindle and thus excite the spindle receptors. The resultant impulses are then conveyed through the monosynaptic reflex path to the α anterior horn cells and contraction of the main muscle follows the contraction of the spindle (Merton, 1951; 1953; Eldred et al., 1953; Granit, 1955; Hammond et al., 1956; Granit et al., 1959a). What is implied and in fact specifically stated is that the motor units are not activated directly by impulses impinging on their motoneurons from supraspinal structures but only by those impulses which utilize the γ loop. Electrical stimulation of fusimotor axons can indeed excite the α motoneurons of the gastrocnemius–soleus muscle of the cat over the γ loop (Granit, 1966; Granit et al., 1966).

It is well known that decerebrate rigidity depends mainly upon the activity of Deiters' nucleus (cf. Brodal et al., 1962). Electrical stimulation of Deiters' nucleus enhances the activity in extensor muscles (Sprague et al., 1948; Pompeiano, 1960) and increases the excitability of extensor motoneurons as indicated by the effect on monosynaptic test reflexes (Gernandt and Thulin, 1955; Sasaki et al., 1962). On the other hand a lesion of Deiters' nucleus greatly reduces or abolishes the decerebrate rigidity in the ipsilateral limbs (cf. Brodal et al., 1962). Since the decerebrate rigidity is abolished by deafferentation, one could suggest that this postural type of contraction is exclusively mediated through the γ-loop and that Deiters' nucleus is responsible for the tonic discharge of the spindle receptors from extensor muscles.

The demonstration by Lund and Pompeiano (1965, 1968) that Deiters' nucleus exerts a monosynaptic (followed by a polysynaptic) excitation of ipsilateral extensor motoneurons raised some questions. First of all it would be of interest to know the extent and the nature of the linkage between this vestibular structure and the γ motoneurons supplying the muscle spindles of the extensor muscles. It would further be of interest to look for changes in afferent signalling without changes in muscle tension, for increasing signalling during the development of tension, for maintenance of signalling during shortening of the muscle, and finally whether there is a preponderance of direct control over servo-control in this output system.

Stimulation of Deiters' nucleus was originally made by Granit et al. (1959b) who found that single shock stimulation of this structure elicited both extrafusal contraction and spindle discharge. More recently two groups of experiments were performed.

The first was made by Carli *et al.* (1966a–c, 1967a–d) and Pompeiano *et al.* (1967a, b) who studied the effects of repetitive stimulation of Deiters' nucleus on spindle discharge and extrafusal contraction of the gastrocnemius muscle in cats either anesthetized or decerebrated at precollicular level. The second group of experiments was made by Grillner *et al.* (1966b, 1969) and Grillner (1969a) who studied the effects of stimulation of Deiters' nucleus on γ motoneurons recorded with both extracellular and intracellular recording.

Effects of stimulation of Deiters' nucleus on muscle spindle discharge in anesthetized

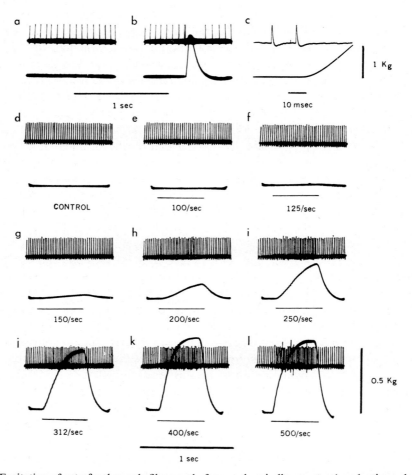

Fig. 3. Excitation of extrafusal muscle fibers and of a muscle spindle receptor (conduction velocity of fiber: 64 m/sec) on stimulation of Deiters' nucleus. Gastrocnemius muscle, de-afferented. Initial muscle extension, 10 mm. Pentobarbitone anesthesia. a, Spontaneous discharge; b, the 'pause' during a maximal twitch; c, expanded sweep for determination of conduction time. In d–l, Deiters' nucleus was stimulated with 0.5 msec pulses, at 7V and at the different frequencies indicated below each of the appropriate records. Stimulation period indicated by a bar. The upper trace in each frame is the spindle receptor discharge recorded from a dorsal root filament, the lower trace shows the tension developed in the muscle. Note the different time scales: for a and b, for c, and for the other frames. From Carli, Diete–Spiff and Pompeiano (1967a).

cats. Selective stimulation of Deiters' nucleus performed in cats anesthetized with pentobarbitone sodium (Nembutal) produced both spindle activation and extrafusal contraction of the ipsilateral gastrocnemius muscle (Carli *et al.*, 1966a–c, 1967a; Diete–Spiff *et al.*, 1967b). Both these events occurred at about the same latency and had a parallel time course. Although in some cases spindle receptor activation occurred at lower stimulus strength than induced extrafusal contraction, spindle discharge acceleration and tension development increased *pari passu* with increase in stimulus strength. The spindle receptors were on the whole excited at about the same frequency of stimulation (100–125/sec) as that which resulted in extrafusal contraction. Fig. 3 shows the responses of a muscle spindle receptor (conduction velocity of fiber: 64 m/sec) and of the extrafusal muscle fibers of the gastrocnemius muscle to stimulation of the ipsilateral Deiters' nucleus in a preparation with the ipsilateral dorsal root cut. The muscle contracted isometrically. Extrafusal contraction and spindle receptor acceleration occurred in this experiment when the stimulus frequency was 125/sec. Both responses increased with increasing frequency of stimulation but extrafusal contractile tension reached its peak at a stimulus frequency of 400/sec, whereas spindle receptor acceleration continued to increase up to stimulus frequency of 500/sec.

The spindle receptors in the gastrocnemius muscle were seen to be excited in slack muscle, *i.e.*, in a muscle contracting isotonically with minimal external load. Both in

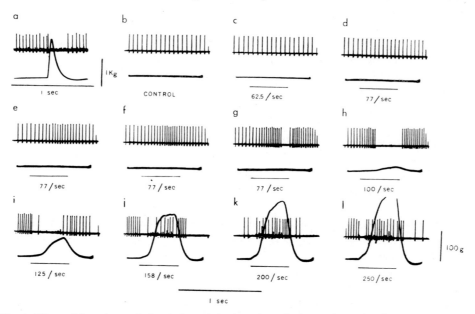

Fig. 4. Effect of frequency of stimulation of the lateral vestibular nucleus of Deiters on the tension developed by the ipsilateral gastrocnemius muscle and on the discharge of one of its spindle receptors. Decerebrate cat, dorsal roots intact. Conduction velocity of receptor fiber: 87 m/sec. Initial muscle extension: 4 mm. a, The 'pause' during a maximal twitch; b, control, no stimulus; c–l; stimulation of the ipsilateral Deiters' nucleus with 0.5 msec pulses, 1.8V, at the frequencies indicated beneath each record. Note acceleration in the second stimulation period at 77/sec, followed in records g–i by a definite 'pause'. Note also the filling up of the 'pause' in j–l, with higher frequencies of stimulation. From Diete–Spiff, Carli and Pompeiano (1967b).

slack muscle and in muscle contracting isometrically spindle receptor activation following stimulation of Deiters' nucleus barely outlasted the stimulus or the extra-fusal contraction induced by the stimulus.

It is of interest to notice that most of the extrafusal contraction elicited by stimula-tion of Deiters' nucleus was due to direct vestibulospinal influence in α motoneurons since only a slight reduction in the extrafusal contraction occurred after ipsilateral deafferentation.

Effects of stimulation of Deiters' nucleus on muscle spindle discharge in decerebrate cats. Spindle receptors of the gastrocnemius muscle were investigated in decerebrate preparations (Carli *et al.*, 1966a–c, 1967a). Even in this group of experiments spindle activation and extrafusal contraction tended both to occur at the same voltage when Deiters' nucleus was stimulated repetitively. An outstanding feature of the spindle response was its long-lasting duration. This contrasted markedly with the characteris-tic spindle response to stimulation of Deiters' nucleus seen in cats under pentobarbi-tone anesthesia. The responses outlasted the stimulus and the induced contraction by a period of some seconds.

There was usually no unloading of the spindle receptor whose discharge was acceler-ated even when the extrafusal muscle fibers developed a tension of over 500 g. In one experiment, however, the phenomenon of unloading of the spindle by extrafusal con-traction was observed (Fig. 4). The dorsal roots were virtually intact in this case. It is of interest that in this experiment the quantity of fusimotor activity induced by low frequencies of stimulation was too small to offset the mechanical effect of unloading. However, when the frequency of stimulation increased there was no silencing by un-loading and possibly a small increase in the spindle discharge. In other words a larger extrafusal contraction unloaded the spindle only slightly, presumably because the effect of unloading was partially compensated by a large fusimotor activity persisting throughout the period of stimulation.

Experiments of dorsal root section performed in decerebrate animals produced a slight decrease in the tension developed in response to stimulation of Deiters' nucleus.

Conduction velocity of spindle receptor afferents excited from Deiters' nucleus. Using the generally accepted criterion for the subdivision of their fibers, those above 72 m/ sec being primary and those below 72 m/sec secondary, both types of spindle receptor endings were found to have been excited from Deiters' nucleus (Carli *et al.*, 1967a).

Dissociation of extrafusal from fusimotor effects by gallamine. The time relations between the extrafusal contractions and the spindle receptor activation obtained from stimulating Deiters' nucleus suggested that some of the spindle excitation might have arisen as a consequence of the extrafusal contraction. Stimulation of Deiters' nucleus after injection of 0.7–1.4 mg/kg of gallamine tri-ethiodide, which blocks extra-fusal endplates before intrafusal neuromuscular junctions, produces spindle accelera-tion even in the absence of extrafusal contraction (Fig. 5) (Carli *et al.*, 1967a). If larger doses of gallamine were injected as to paralyze both intrafusal and extrafusal neuromuscular junctions, a stage was observed during the recovery of the extrafusal junctions in which the intrafusal junctions were selectively blocked (Carli *et al.*, 1967b–d). During this stage of selective intrafusal neuromuscular block by gallamine,

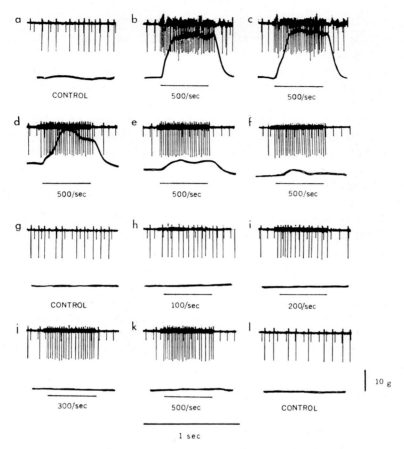

Fig. 5. Differential paralysis by gallamine of extrafusal muscle fibers, leaving excitation of a muscle spindle receptor in response to stimulation of Deiters' nucleus. Gastrocnemius muscle, dorsal roots intact. Initial extension: 6 mm. Pentobarbitone anesthesia. Conduction velocity of receptor fiber: 89 m/sec. After a control record (a), Deiters' nucleus was stimulated at 500/sec (0.5 msec pulses, 4 V). After b, 1.4 mg/kg body weight gallamine tri-ethiodide was injected intravenously with the animal on artificial respiration. c–f form part of a consecutive series of records taken at 5 sec intervals after the injection, stimulating Deiters' nucleus for the period indicated by the bar beneath each record during each sweep of the oscilloscope. g, l, Controls, and h–k, responses of the spindle receptor to different frequencies of stimulation of Deiters' nucleus after the ext.afusal endplates had been blocked by gallamine. From Carli, Diete–Spiff and Pompeiano (1967a).

tension changes from Deiters' stimulation, comparable in magnitude to those obtained before administration of the drug, failed to excite muscle spindle receptors. Spindle activation in response to supraspinal stimulation reappeared only after there had been a spontaneous recovery from the intrafusal neuromuscular block. At all times and in all stages of differential block the spindle receptor response to passive stretch remained unimpaired. It appears therefore that the contracting extrafusal muscle fibers are incapable of exciting the spindle receptors by pull, by re-extension, by other forms of distortion or ephaptically.

References pp. 224–232

In summary, all these experiments indicate that both primary and secondary spindle receptors of the gastrocnemius muscle are activated by repetitive stimulation of the ipsilateral nucleus of Deiters. Evidence was presented indicating that the unloading effect due to submaximal contraction of the gastrocnemius muscle (Hammond *et al.*, 1956) was clearly offset by coactivation of fusimotor neurons. It is also of interest that this activation was observed not only when the muscle constrained by the isometric myograph was not allowed to shorten freely, but also when the muscle contracted isotonically. This spindle activation then persisted throughout the period of stimulation in spite of the unloading effect due to shortening of the contracting extrafusal muscle fibers.

Indeed the works presented above gave very little evidence for an independent projection from Deiters' nucleus to the fusimotor neurons and to the α motoneurons. On the whole the responses of the spindle receptors and of extrafusal muscle fibers appeared at about the same threshold. The threshold frequencies for the skeletomotor and the fusimotor effect were also comparable. These findings indicate that the vestibulospinal action on muscle spindles and on motor units are functionally linked to a certain extent. The possibility that spindle acceleration during Deiters' stimulation was due to mechanical stimulation of the spindles resulting from extrafusal contraction was excluded by experiments showing that the excitation of spindle receptors was still obtained after the extrafusal contraction had been completely blocked by gallamine. It appears therefore that the spindle discharge due to Deiters' stimulation is a truly fusimotor effect due to activation of γ motoneurons.

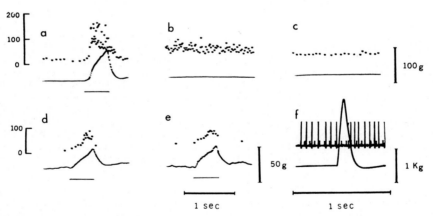

Fig. 6. Effect of barbiturate anesthesia on the responses of a gastrocnemius muscle spindle receptor (primary ending; conduction velocity of fiber: 94 m/sec) to stimulation of the medial vestibular nucleus close to Deiters' nucleus. Gastrocnemius muscle, de-afferented. Initial extension: 4 mm. Precollicular decerebrate cat. Stimulus indicated by a bar beneath each appropriate record (7 V, 0.5 msec pulses, 159/sec). a, 'Vestibular' stimulation; b, c, successive frames without stimulation; d, e, consecutive responses to 'vestibular' stimulation following the i.v. injection of 1 ml of a 5% solution (w/v in distilled water) of sodium methyl-thioethyl-2 pentyl-thiobarbiturate. In a, b, c and in d, e, the repetition rate of the sweep is 1 every 4 sec. f, The 'pause' of the receptor discharge during a maximum twitch. From Carli, Diete–Spiff and Pompeiano (1967a).

Dissociation of long-lasting from short-lasting fusimotor effects by anesthesia. It has already been mentioned that repetitive stimulation of Deiters' nucleus produces two types of spindle responses in the decerebrate preparation: an early acceleration closely correlated in time with the extrafusal contraction (Fig. 6a) and a late long-lasting response which outlasted the stimulus for several seconds (Fig. 6b, c).

After i.v. injection of 1 ml of a 5 mg/ml solution of sodium methyl-thioethyl-2 pentyl-thiobarbiturate, both the resting discharge as well as the brisk initial high frequency spindle response were only reduced, while the long-lasting component was abolished (Fig. 6d, e). The excitation of the spindle receptor ran a parallel time course with that of the muscle tension and lasted only for the duration of the stimulus (Pompeiano *et al.*, 1967a, b; Carli *et al.*, 1967a).

It may be assumed that this long-lasting excitatory response of the spindle receptors is due to excitation of interneurons interposed in the vestibulospinal projection to the γ motoneurons. Since spinal interneurons discharge repetitively (McIntyre *et al.*, 1956; Hunt and Kuno, 1959; Wall, 1959), the fusimotor neurons concerned apparently follow the repetitive discharges thus leading to sustained contraction of the intrafusal muscle fibers (Smith 1966; *cf.* Corvaja *et al.*, 1969), with a resultant long-lasting excitation of the spindle receptor endings.

The effects seen in short-term barbiturate anesthesia support this interpretation since the long-lasting portion of the spindle response to stimulation of Deiters' nucleus is abolished by the anesthesia. Anesthetics are known to affect interneurons quickly and profoundly; this was also shown by the fact that intravenous injection of small doses (5 mg/kg) of Nembutal greatly decreased or even abolished the polysynaptic EPSP in α motoneurons on stimulation of the vestibulospinal pathway, while the monosynaptic EPSP was apparently unmodified or only slightly reduced (Lund and Pompeiano, 1968).

If such an organization of vestibulospinal connections is valid also for the γ motoneurons, then the excitation of the spindle receptors which persists during barbiturate anesthesia and whose time-course runs parallel with the muscle tension record could be attributed to activity of a more direct pathway, such as the vestibulospinal fibers making monosynaptic connection with the γ motoneurons. This hypothesis, put forward by Pompeiano *et al.* (1967a, b) and Carli *et al.* (1967a) has been verified by later investigators who have followed a more direct approach to the problem, as will be discussed presently.

Effects of stimulation of Deiters' nucleus on γ motoneurons. Grillner *et al.* (1966b, 1969) and Grillner (1969a) have studied the response of γ motoneurons to stimulation of Deiters' nucleus and the medial reticular formation in the MLF region. The control of γ motoneurons from these supraspinal structures has been studied with both extracellular and intracellular recording from lumbosacral γ motoneurons in cat. Preliminary observations indicated that stimulation of the ipsilateral ventral quadrant at the lower thoracic level produced monosynaptic EPSPs in γ motoneurons belonging to flexor and extensor motor nuclei. However not all γ motoneurons were excited with short latencies from descending fibers.

It is of interest that in most extensor motor nuclei monosynaptic EPSPs are evoked exclusively from Deiters' nucleus, in a few from MLF and in flexor motor nuclei from the latter region (Grillner *et al.*, 1968). An important question is whether there are parallel effects on α and γ motoneurons of the same muscle from the two brain stem regions. Although their material is small the observations by Grillner *et al.* (1969) suggest that this is the case. In particular stimulation of Deiters' nucleus produced monosynaptic EPSP in extensor γ motoneurons. In one instance a GS γ motoneuron received monosynaptic EPSP on single shock stimulation of Deiters' nucleus and IPSP from the MLF originating in the pontine reticular formation. This reciprocal pattern from the two regions resembles that evoked by the same regions in α motoneurons to extensors (Grillner *et al.*, 1968). These findings suggest parallel effect to α and part of the γ motoneuron population supplying one muscle. Quite recently it has been shown that stimulation of Deiters' nucleus facilitated extensor γ motoneurons and inhibited flexor γ motoneurons (Kato and Tanji, 1971).

The descending monosynaptic effects to γ motoneurons originating in Deiters' nucleus are mediated by fast conducting fibers located in the ipsilateral ventral quadrant of the cord. It should be mentioned that the α motoneurons supplying a particular muscle are located within the group of α motoneurons innervating the same muscle (Eccles *et al.*, 1960; Nyberg–Hansen, 1965a). It is likely, although not definitely proved, that the lateral vestibulospinal fibers terminate on the dendrites rather than on the soma of these motoneurons, as postulated for the α motoneurons.

It is of interest that the descending monosynaptic EPSP is larger in γ than in α motoneurons. In α motoneurons with resting potentials of 60–70 mV the average value of the descending monosynaptic EPSP was 0.8 mV, while the average value in 8 γ motoneurons with descending monosynaptic EPSPs was 3.1 mV (Grillner *et al.*, 1969). This large value does not imply a difference in synaptic organization of descending effects to α and γ motoneurons, but may be attributed to the fact that γ motoneurons having smaller cell size than α motoneurons, have a higher input resistance. The same quantal release, giving rise to the same synaptic current, will yield a larger PSP in a cell with high input resistance as compared to one with a low input resistance (Katz and Thesleff, 1957; Henneman *et al.*, 1965; Burke, 1968).

It has already been mentioned that the γ-efferents are of two kinds (Jansen and Matthews, 1962; Matthews, 1962, 1964), one type controlling mainly the dynamic sensitivity of primary endings (Ia afferents) and the other the discharge rate and presumably also the static sensitivity of the primary endings and in addition the activity in secondary endings (group II afferents) (*cf.* Appelberg *et al.*, 1966).

Since not all γ motoneurons receive the descending monosynaptic EPSP, the question was raised whether the monosynaptic control was exerted only on one type of γ motoneuron. The demonstration by Carli *et al.* (1967a) that stimulation of Deiters' nucleus produced acceleration not only of primary but also of secondary endings from extensors, already suggested that this vestibular structure affected the static γ motoneurons, since it is known that the secondary endings of muscle spindles are influenced only by static γ motoneurons (Appelberg *et al.*, 1966; Brown *et al.*, 1967). To test this hypothesis the static and dynamic γ efferents were tested for descending effects by stimulation of the ipsilateral ventrolateral funicle (Bergmans and Grillner, 1968;

Grillner, 1969b); and indeed monosynaptic effects were revealed in static but never in dynamic γ motoneurons.

The demonstration that Deiters' nucleus affects the static fusimotor neurons opens the question as to whether this structure is responsible for the γ activity which occurs in the decerebrate cat. It is generally assumed that γ activity leading to intrafusal contraction is an important feature of the extensor rigidity (Hunt, 1951; Granit and Kaada, 1952; Kobayashi et al., 1952; Eldred et al., 1953; Granit, 1955; cf. however Barrios et al., 1968). A great reduction of fusimotor activity to extensor muscles occurs, however, in the decerebrate preparation following a transverse section of the spinal cord (Kobayashi et al., 1952; Diete–Spiff et al., 1962; Voorhoeve and van Kanten, 1962; Barrios et al., 1968). It is of interest that while in the decerebrate cat there is a background activity in both static and dynamic fusimotor efferents to extensor muscle spindles (Jansen and Matthews, 1962; Jansen, 1966), spinalization results in a severe decrease in the activity of static fusimotor efferents without a corresponding loss of function of dynamic fusimotor efferents (Alnaes et al., 1965; Jansen, 1966; cf. however Barrios et al., 1968). This finding leads to the conclusion that activity in the static fusimotor efferents depends mainly upon descending suprasegmental activation, whereas the dynamic fusimotor neurons are mainly influenced by dorsal root inflow (cf. Hunt, 1951). The demonstration that Deiters' nucleus exerts a monosynaptic effect on static γ motoneurons to extensor muscles (Bergmans and Grillner, 1968; cf. also Pompeiano et al., 1967a, b; Carli et al., 1967a) suggests that this nucleus represents the tonogenic structure of the brain stem which is responsible for the tonic discharge of the static γ motoneurons to extensor muscles, leading to the decerebrate rigidity.

In summary, all the experiments reported in this chapter clearly indicate that there is a linkage in the descending effects from Deiters' nucleus on α and static γ motoneurons of the same motor nuclei. Merton (1953) in his follow-up length-servo hypothesis postulated that the γ loop constituted an independent route for motor control. The author clearly pointed out that the direct activation of α motoneurons would be a disturbing factor for this kind of servo, since during muscle contraction the unloading mechanisms provide a negative feedback, which counteracts any shortening. Subsequent work of Granit et al. (1955, 1959b) has shown that in most cases α and γ motoneurons are coactivated. The results presented on Deiters' stimulation provide further evidence for an α–γ linkage. The tonic contraction of the extensor muscle induced by Deiters' stimulation can be mediated and sustained by primary activation of α motoneurons associated with sufficient fusimotor activity to prevent any decrease in spindle discharge occurring during the contraction. It is particularly the coactivation of static γ motoneurons produced by Deiters' stimulation which prevents the unloading effect of the primary endings. In this case the γ loop does have servo properties (Matthews, 1964), thus contributing with the accelerated spindle discharge to support the direct influence of Deiters' nucleus on α motoneurons. The vestibulospinal tract would then increase the excitability of α motoneurons not only directly with EPSPs of descending origin, but also indirectly through increased activity in the γ loop, the latter part being dependent on muscle length.* It has already been mentioned that deafferentation slightly reduces the contractile tension of the gastrocnemius muscle in response to stimulation of Deiters' nucleus (Carli et al., 1967a). However, when the γ fusimotor fibers are blocked by local application of procaine on the gastrocnemius nerve, the tension in the homonymous muscle due to stimulation of Deiters' nucleus is clearly reduced (Carli et al., 1966b,c). This indicates the importance of the spindle discharge in potentiating the response of the α motoneurons to Deiters' stimulation.

VESTIBULAR INFLUENCES ON PRIMARY AFFERENTS

Presynaptic depolarization of the primary afferents induced by labyrinthine volleys. The problem of the vestibular influence on γ motoneurons is closely related to that of the vestibular effects on primary afferents. Indeed there is evidence indicating that vestibular nerve stimulation evokes depolarization in spinal afferents. Erulkar et al. (1966) reported that current pulses delivered to the labyrinth of the anesthetized cat provoke centrifugal dorsal root discharges. This study, however, did not reveal what types of somatosensory fibers, cutaneous or muscular, were engaged in centrifugal activity. Similar results were also obtained by Megirian (1971) who found that in unanesthetized, decerebrate-decerebellate phalangers, vestibular nerve stimulation evoked bilateral centrifugal discharges in cutaneous fibers supplying the posterior extremities. The computed conduction velocity for vestibular evoked centrifugal cutaneous nerve discharges (19–24 m/sec) indicates that the reflex discharges occur in fine myelinated cutaneous fibers.

In precollicular decerebrate cats Cook et al. (1968a, b; 1969b) have shown that repetitive electrical stimulation of the VIII cranial nerve or of the vestibular component of the VIII nerve evoked negative dorsal root potentials (DRPs) in both the ipsilateral and the contralateral lumbar dorsal roots. A close relationship existed between the amplitude of the DRPs and that of the monosynaptic vestibular response elicited from the ascending MLF at different stimulus intensities (Fig. 7). The finding that the DRPs elicited by VIII nerve stimulation persisted after deafferentation or following immobilization with gallamine tri-ethiodide indicates that these potentials are not due to proprioceptive reverberation, but rather to a central mechanism triggered by supraspinal descending volleys.

Repetitive stimulation of the VIII cranial nerve produced not only DRPs in the lumbar spinal cord but also contraction of ipsilateral extensor hindlimb muscles (Fig. 8A). With the stimulating voltage held constant to 2–6 times the threshold (T) for the monosynaptic vestibular response recorded from the ascending MLF, both tension and DRP appeared at the threshold frequency of about 100/sec and increased to a maximum with increasing frequency of stimulation up to 500/sec.

---

* The increased activity in Ia afferents also causes 'direct' inhibition of antagonist motor nuclei and it is of considerable interest that these inhibitory effects on at least knee flexor motoneurons are strongly facilitated from the vestibulospinal tract by its monosynaptic action (Grillner et al., 1966c; Lundberg, 1970).

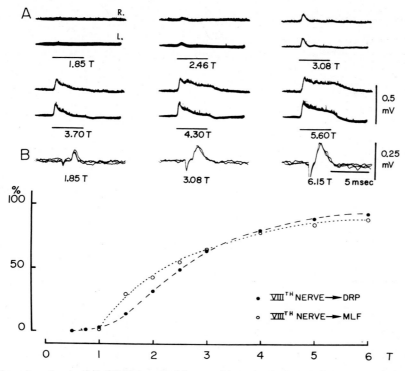

Fig. 7. Dorsal root potentials (DRPs) evoked by repetitive stimulation of the VIII cranial nerve at different stimulus intensities. Precollicular decerebrate cat. A, Development of the DRPs evoked from the right (R) and left (L) sides of lower L6 by a 400 msec tetanus applied to the left VIII nerve at 500/sec and at the indicated stimulus intensities. These are expressed in multiples of the threshold (T) for the monosynaptic evoked potential recorded from the ascending medial longitudinal fasciculus (MLF). B, Superimposed traces of the monosynaptic evoked potential recorded from the ascending MLF following single shock stimulation of the ipsilateral VIII nerve. The diagram summarizes the results obtained from 5 experiments. The percentage increases in amplitude of the initial peak of the DRPs and of the monosynaptic ascending MLF potential elicited from the ipsilateral VIII nerve are plotted as a function of the intensities of stimulation. From Cook, Cangiano and Pompeiano (1969b).

Experiments were also performed to study the effects of repetitive stimulation of the VIII nerve: (i) on the excitability of the central terminals of muscular and cutaneous afferents and (ii) on transmission in monosynaptic and polysynaptic reflex pathways (Cook et al., 1968a, b; 1969c).

Stimulation of the ipsilateral VIII nerve evoked primary afferent depolarization (PAD) in group I afferents from both extensor and flexor muscles, as well as in cutaneous afferents. Fig. 9A shows the time course of the excitability changes of the presynaptic terminals of the group I afferents from GS muscle elicited by repetitive stimulation of the VIII nerve. With near maximal stimulation of the VIII nerve the threshold frequency responsible for PAD in group I afferents from both extensor and flexor muscles was 100/sec, i.e., the same threshold frequency responsible for the DRPs. This effect increased progressively with increasing frequencies of stimulation up to

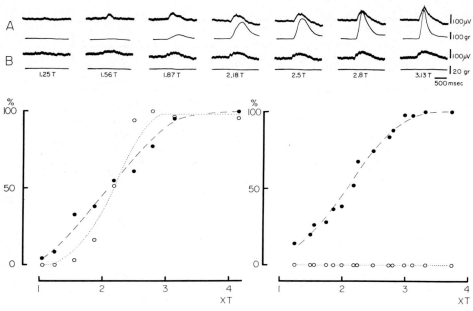

Fig. 8. Selective abolition of the muscle tension and persistence of the DRPs evoked by repetitive stimulation of the VIII cranial nerve following lesion of the ipsilateral Deiters nucleus. Precollicular decerebrate cat. The records illustrate the DRPs elicited from lower L6 on the left side (upper traces) and the contractile tension of the left GS muscle recorded isometrically at an initial extension of 6 mm (lower records). A, Effects of repetitive stimulation of the left VIII nerve with a 200 msec tetanus at 312/sec, 0.2 msec pulse duration and at different intensities expressed in multiples of the threshold (T) for the monosynaptic vestibular response recorded from the ascending MLF (same values as in B). The diagram on the left illustrates the amplitude of the evoked tension (circles) and DRPs (dots) plotted as a function of the stimulus intensity applied to the VIII nerve. B, Effects of repetitive stimulation of the left VIII nerve after electrolytic lesion of the hindlimb region of Deiters' nucleus. Stimulation at 312/sec, 0.2 msec pulse duration, and at the intensities indicated below each record. Note the reduction in amplitude of the DRPs and the complete suppression of the evoked contraction of the GS muscle. The diagram on the right illustrates the changes in amplitude of the tension (circles) and of the DRPs (dots) induced by Deiters' lesion. The responses are plotted as a function of the intensity of stimulation applied to the VIII nerve. Each diagram represents the average of 3 consecutive series of responses in which the intensity of stimulation was progressively increased. Each symbol corresponds to the mean value of 12–15 responses. From Barnes and Pompeiano (1970c).

500/sec. The results of collision experiments provide evidence that the increase in excitability of the group I volley involved the Ia pathway (Fig. 10). PAD in the group I muscular afferents from extensor muscles was also elicited by stimulation of the contralateral VIII nerve.

If we study now the changes in the spinal reflex evoked from the VIII nerve stimulation it appears that stimulation of the VIII nerve facilitated the extensor monosynaptic reflex evoked by single shock stimulation of the ipsilateral GS nerve. Fig. 9B shows the time course of this facilitation (left diagram) as well as the relative increase in amplitude of the monosynaptic reflex as a function of the frequency of stimulation of the ipsilateral VIII nerve (right diagram). The two diagrams also show the increased excitability of the terminal arborization of the group I afferents which parallels

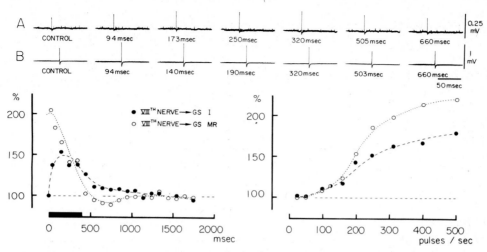

Fig. 9. Facilitation of the gastrocnemius-soleus (GS) monosynaptic reflex and primary afferent depolarization (PAD) in its group I afferents evoked from the ipsilateral VIII cranial nerve. Precollicular decerebrate cat. The left VIII nerve was stimulated in A and B with a 400 msec tetanus (500/sec, 0.2 msec pulse duration, 3.4 T). The effect of VIII nerve stimulation on the excitability of group I afferent terminals from GS muscle and on monosynaptic reflex transmission through the GS motoneuronal pool of the ipsilateral side are shown respectively in A and B. Intervals between onset of conditioning volleys and test volley are indicated in msec. The amplitudes of the antidromic volleys (dots) and monosynaptic reflexes (circles) from 10 experiments made in 8 animals are summarized in the left diagram (500/sec and 2–5 T). In the right diagram the amplitude of the extensor monosynaptic reflex and the group I antidromic volley from GS nerve are plotted as a function of the frequency of stimulation of the ipsilateral VIII nerve (8 animals, 2.8–6 T, intervals of 24–315 msec). From Cook, Cangiano and Pompeiano (1969c).

the facilitation of the monosynaptic reflex. Contrary to the monosynaptic extensor reflex which was facilitated, the monosynaptic and the polysynaptic flexor reflexes were generally depressed by conditioning stimulation of the ipsilateral VIII nerve. Stimulation of the VIII nerve also produced a depression of the contralateral GS monosynaptic reflex whose time course paralleled the time course of the increased excitability in the group I afferents.

In summary, the main results of these experiments indicate that orthodromic vestibular volleys exert a depolarizing influence on both extensor motoneurons and central endings of the group I afferents from ipsilateral extensor muscles. It is generally assumed that transmission in reflex pathways to motoneurons can be presynaptically inhibited at a primary afferent level (Eccles, 1964). One might expect, therefore, that the extensor motoneurons would be uncoupled from the primary afferents due to descending vestibular volleys. Contrary to this assumption it was found that the monosynaptic extensor reflex was facilitated by conditioning impulses in the ipsilateral VIII nerve which also produced PAD in the corresponding group I extensor pathway. One may suggest that the reduced postsynaptic efficacy of the orthodromic volley due to presynaptic depolarization was compensated for by the simultaneous excitation of the ipsilateral extensor motoneurons exerted by the descending vestibular volleys. In support of this hypothesis is the finding that repetitive stimulation of the VIII

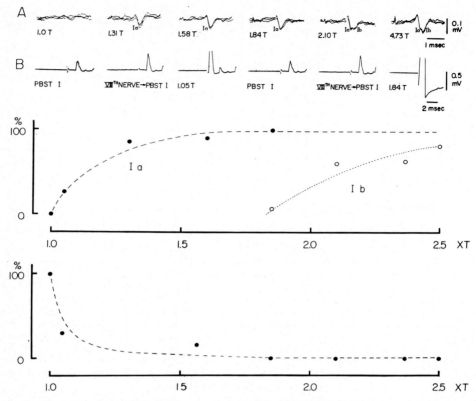

Fig. 10. The composition of the antidromic group I volley facilitated by stimulation of the ipsilateral VIII cranial nerve. Precollicular decerebrate cat. A, The ingoing volleys were recorded from the dorsal root entry zone of lower L7 following single shock stimulation of the ipsilateral posterior biceps-semitendinous (PBST) nerve (0.05 msec pulses). The stimulus intensities are expressed in terms of times threshold (T) for the group Ia volley. In this series of responses negativity is recorded as a downward deflection and the development of the response with increasing stimulus strengths into its two component parts is labelled. The amplitudes of the two responses (Ia and Ib) are plotted as a function of the stimulating voltage in the upper graph. B, the responses should be read left to right. Stimulation of the motor nucleus to the PBST nerve with 0.1 msec pulses. The antidromic test response (PBST I) was recorded from the PBST nerve and conditioning stimulation of the ipsilateral VIII nerve at 500/sec 0.3 msec pulse duration, 3.0 T (VIIIth Nerve → PBST I) resulted in marked facilitation. The facilitated antidromic volley was then preceded by an orthodromic volley in the PBST nerve at 1.05 T and the nearly complete depression of the facilitated antidromic response is shown in the third record. The last 3 records are identical except that the size of the orthodromic volley was increased to 1.84 T which resulted in total collision of the facilitated antidromic response. The experiment is plotted in the lower graph, where 100% equals the amplitude of the facilitated antidromic response. The stimulus strengths for the orthodromic colliding volley are indicated on the abscissa and should be compared with the upper graph. From Cook, Cangiano and Pompeiano (1969c).

nerve elicited a depression of the monosynaptic extensor reflex of the contralateral side, as well as of the monosynaptic and the polysynaptic flexor reflexes of the ipsilateral side. Additional studies, however, are required to find out whether this reflex depression is due not only to presynaptic but also to postsynaptic inhibition.

Presynaptic depolarization of the primary afferents induced by the vestibular nuclei.

It may be asked now whether there is a segregation within the vestibular nuclear complex of those neurons which depolarize the extensor motoneurons and those which depolarize the primary afferents.

Stimulation of the medial (Carpenter *et al.*, 1966; Cook *et al.*, 1969b, c), the descending and the lateral vestibular nuclei (Cook *et al.*, 1969b, c) performed in precollicular decerebrate cats, elicits ipsilateral DRPs due to PAD in different groups of primary afferents, including the group Ia and the Ib muscle afferents and the cutaneous fibers. Furthermore stimulation of the same structures is also able to elicit contraction of the GS muscle (Cook *et al.*, 1969b, c).

Since stimulation within the vestibular complex of primary vestibular and fastigio-vestibular afferents may lead through axo-axonic reflex to activation of vestibular nuclei different from those which are directly stimulated, experiments were performed several days after complete bilateral lesion of the fastigial nuclei and section of the ipsilateral VIII nerve (Barnes and Pompeiano, 1970c). It appears that stimulation of both the lateral and medial vestibular nucleus produced negative DRPs as well as contraction of ipsilateral extensor muscles. However for the same parameters of stimulation, the largest contraction of the ipsilateral GS muscle was elicited by stimulation

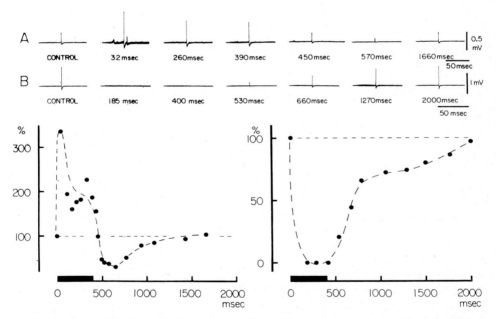

Fig. 11. Effects of stimulation of the lateral and medial vestibular nucleus on the ipsilateral GS monosynaptic reflex in two separate experiments. Precollicular decerebrate cats. A, Facilitation of the GS monosynaptic reflex elicited at the indicated times after the onset of a 400 msec tetanus to the lateral vestibular nucleus at 500/sec, 0.2 msec pulse duration, 2.0 times the threshold for the monosynaptic response from the ipsilateral ascending MLF. The responses partially shown in A are plotted in the left diagram. B, inhibition of the GS monosynaptic reflex elicited at the indicated times after the onset of a 400 msec tetanus to the medial vestibular nucleus at 500/sec, 0.5 msec pulse duration, 2.0 times the threshold for the monosynaptic response from the ipsilateral ascending MLF. The responses partially shown in B are plotted in the right diagram. From Barnes and Pompeiano (1970c).

of the lateral vestibular nucleus, while the largest DRP was evoked by stimulation of the medial vestibular nucleus. Moreover while stimulation of the lateral vestibular nucleus elicits a large facilitation of the ipsilateral extensor monosynaptic reflex followed by a late depression, stimulation of the medial vestibular nucleus elicited a great and prolonged depression of that reflex, which outlasted the duration of the conditioning stimulus by several hundred msec (Fig. 11). On the basis of these experiments one may suggest that the medial and lateral vestibular nuclei are basically responsible for PAD in the group I afferents, and contraction of the ipsilateral extensor muscle respectively.

The conclusion of these experiments, namely that the medial vestibular nucleus is critically responsible for the effects on the primary afferents, is supported by the studies of the pathway responsible for PAD in the Ia afferents, indicating that this effect is due to activation of the descending efferent vestibular projection coursing along the MLF (Carpenter *et al.*, 1966; Cook *et al.*, 1969c). Since the medial vestibular

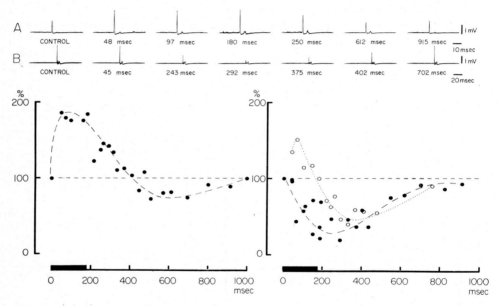

Fig. 12. Inhibition of the GS monosynaptic reflex evoked from the ipsilateral VIII cranial nerve following lesion of Deiters' nucleus. Same experiment as in Fig. 8. A, Control records showing facilitation of the GS monosynaptic extensor reflex elicited by single shock stimulation of the GS nerve (0.1 msec pulses at 2.0 times the threshold for the monosynaptic reflex) at the indicated times following the onset of a 180 msec tetanus applied to the ipsilateral VIII nerve (at 312 /sec, 0.2 msec pulse duration and 2.5 T). These data are plotted in the diagram on the left side. B, same experiment as in A, 20 min after electrolytic lesion of the hindlimb region of the ipsilateral Deiters' nucleus. Note the inhibition of the GS monosynaptic reflex for the same parameters of conditioning stimulation of the left VIII nerve which elicited a large facilitation of the reflex in the intact preparation (A). The data partially shown here are plotted in the right diagram (dots). In this figure the circles indicate the changes in amplitude of the GS monosynaptic reflex for the same parameters of stimulation of the VIII nerve applied only 5 min after electrolytic lesion of Deiters' nucleus. Note the persistence of some early facilitation of the monosynaptic reflex soon after the lesion. From Barnes and Pompeiano (1970c).

nucleus mainly contributes to the descending MLF and stimulation of this pathway at brain stem level evokes group Ia PAD, this structure would appear to be relevant to the study of the involved pathways. A problem however is presented by the fact that most of the medial vestibulospinal fibers do not extend in the cat to the lumbar cord (see page 202). As a matter of fact the propriospinal or the reticulospinal systems would seem to be implicated by exclusion since bilateral destruction of the medial part of the ventral funiculi at cervical level, *i.e.*, where the medial vestibulospinal tract courses, did not alter the bilateral DRPs evoked by VIII nerve stimulation (Cook *et al.*, 1969b). Control experiments have actually shown that after chronic degeneration of all descending fibers obtained by a complete hemisection of the left cord at T10, stimulation of the ventral and lateral funiculi of the lumbar cord was unable to produce PAD in the group I afferents from the ipsilateral GS muscle. One may conclude that all the descending propriospinal pathways originating below T10 are unable to produce PAD in the Ia afferents. The effects from the vestibular system on the group Ia afferents may then be mediated by supraspinal structures probably located in the reticular formation which are activated by the vestibular volleys.

The hypothesis that different vestibular nuclei subserve entirely different functions is supported by experiments of stimulation of primary vestibular afferents. It has been mentioned that repetitive electrical stimulation of the VIII cranial nerve evokes both DRP in the lumbar cord and contraction of the ipsilateral extensor muscles (Fig. 8A). Both these effects are abolished by complete destruction of the medial and lateral vestibular nuclei (Cook *et al.*, 1969b; Barnes and Pompeiano, 1970a–c). However after electrolytic lesion limited to the hindlimb region of Deiters' nucleus, the contraction of the ipsilateral extensor muscles elicited by repetitive stimulation of primary vestibular afferents is selectively abolished, while the induced DRP is not greatly impaired by the lesion (Fig. 8B). Excitability measurements of the central terminals of primary afferents indicate that in this condition PAD of the group I afferents from the GS muscle still contributes to the induced DRP. A striking finding in these experiments is that conditioning stimulation of the VIII nerve with the same parameters which in the intact preparation facilitated the monosynaptic extensor reflex is now able to depress the response (Fig. 12).*

The presynaptic depolarization of the group I primary afferents, which persists after electrolytic lesion of Deiters' nucleus, appears thus to be critically responsible for the blockage of the orthodromic transmission of the group Ia volley from the GS muscle. In the absence of excitation of the extensor motoneurons the monosynaptic extensor reflex is completely depressed due to the induced PAD. The dissociation of PAD from the muscle tension eliminates the possibility that the depolarization of the primary afferents resulted from the motoneuronal activity (*e.g.*, field effects, or extra-

---

* By studying the effects of stimulation of the peripheral branches of the vestibular nerve in an animal in which all the descending pathways but the MLF had been interrupted at medullary level, Gernandt (1970) was unable to find any motor outflow through the ventral lumbosacral roots which could be mediated through the medial vestibulospinal pathway. However no visible effects upon the local segmental reflexes were obtained in these preparations.

References pp. 224–232

cellular accumulation of potassium: Frankenhaeuser and Hodgkin, 1956; Kuffler and Nicholls, 1966; Orkand et al., 1966).

The demonstration that a segregation exists within the vestibular nuclei of those neurons which depolarize the extensor motoneurons and those which depolarize the primary afferents is supported by earlier observations made on the hypnic depression of spinal reflexes during sleep. It was shown that during the outbursts of rapid eye movements (REM) typical of the desynchronized phase of sleep there is a short-lasting depression of all the spinal reflexes including the monosynaptic extensor reflex (Gassel et al., 1964), which is due to presynaptic depolarization of the group I afferents (Morrison and Pompeiano, 1965). Furthermore bilateral electrolytic lesions limited to the medial and descending vestibular nuclei, but sparing Deiters' nucleus, abolished not only the bursts of rapid eye movements (Pompeiano and Morrison, 1965) but also the related phasic inhibition of the monosynaptic reflexes (Pompeiano and Morrison, 1966). Since the firing of units located particularly in the medial vestibular nuclei but not in Deiters' is strikingly enhanced during the bursts of REM (Bizzi et al., 1964a, b), the conclusion has been drawn that the phasic outbursts of activity occurring within the vestibular nuclei synchronously with the REM give rise to descending volleys which are in turn responsible for the phasic presynaptic inhibition of the monosynaptic reflexes (Pompeiano, 1966b, 1967).

CONCLUSION

The conclusion that different vestibular structures influence different spinal cord mechanisms will gain further support from studies where natural stimulation of different receptor organs is performed. Since there is both anatomical (Lorente de Nó, 1926, 1933; Stein and Carpenter, 1967; Gacek, 1969) and physiological evidence (Adrian, 1943; Gernandt and Thulin, 1952; Eckel, 1954; Duensing and Schaefer, 1959; Hiebert and Fernandez, 1965; Precht and Shimazu, 1965; Shimazu and Precht, 1965, 1966; Markham et al., 1966; Peterson, 1967, 1970; Precht et al., 1967; Fujita et al., 1968) indicating that the primary vestibular afferents originating from different receptor organs are distributed to particular subdivisions of the vestibular complex, one may suggest that differential effects on the spinal cord can be elicited by impulses originating selectively from the maculae and the cristae.

It is known in particular that fibers associated with the otolith receptors, which sense orientation of the head with respect to gravity, terminate in the ventral part of Deiters' nucleus, as well as in the descending nucleus, with a few fibers also reaching the medial nucleus (Lorente de Nó, 1926, 1933; Stein and Carpenter, 1967; Gacek 1969). Moreover, responses to tilting have been recorded from neurons in Deiters' nucleus (Adrian, 1943; Duensing and Schaefer, 1959; Hiebert and Fernandez, 1965; Fujita et al., 1968), particularly in the ventral Deiters' nucleus and in the descending and medial vestibular nuclei (Peterson, 1967, 1970). It is likely that among these vestibular structures Deiters' nucleus contributes to the static vestibular reflexes involving not only the skeletomotor but also the static fusimotor system to extensor hindlimb muscles (Poppele, 1964, 1967; Roberts, 1967; Ehrhardt and Wagner, 1970).

As to the fibers associated with semicircular canal receptors, which sense angular acceleration, it is known that they impinge mainly upon the superior and the rostral part of the medial nucleus, with a few semicircular canal fibers also reaching the ventral part of Deiters' nucleus (Lorente de Nó, 1926, 1933; Stein and Carpenter, 1967; Gacek, 1969). Moreover units responding to horizontal angular acceleration are located particularly although not exclusively in the medial vestibular nucleus (Adrian, 1943; Gernandt and Thulin, 1952; Eckel, 1954; Duensing and Schaefer, 1958; Precht and Shimazu, 1965; Shimazu and Precht, 1965, 1966; Markham *et al.*, 1966; Precht *et al.*, 1967). The possible activation of Deiters' neurons during horizontal angular acceleration should be kept in mind to explain in part at least the responses of the α (Ehrhardt and Wagner, 1970) and the γ motoneurons (Poppele, 1964, 1967) during dynamic vestibular reflexes. One may suggest, however, that the depression of some monosynaptic hindlimb reflexes during or after stimulation of the horizontal semicircular canals (Gernandt and Thulin, 1953; Ehrhardt and Wagner, 1970; Ghez *et al.*, 1970) is due to presynaptic inhibitory events in the group Ia pathway to spinal motoneurons induced by descending vestibular volleys originating from the medial vestibular nucleus. The occurrence of PAD during dynamic labyrinthine stimulation may explain why a pronounced γ activation can be elicited without any recordable change in muscle tension, and why in those instances in which tension responses occur, they are little affected by ipsilateral deafferentation (Poppele, 1964, 1967; Ajala and Poppele, 1967). If future experiments will prove that transmission of the proprioceptive group Ia volleys to spinal ascending pathways is unaffected by dynamic labyrinthine stimulation (contrary to that in the corresponding Ia pathway to spinal motoneurons), it would then be possible to attribute to the fusimotor discharge the function of signalling to the supraspinal structures, namely to the cerebral and the cerebellar cortices, the changes in muscle spindle length induced by labyrinthine volleys.

SUMMARY

There are two main fiber systems which project from the vestibular nuclei to the spinal cord: the lateral vestibulospinal tract originating from the lateral vestibular nucleus of Deiters and the medial vestibulospinal tract, originating from the medial and to some extent the descending vestibular nuclei. The vestibulospinal fibers from the lateral vestibular nucleus show a somatotopical arrangement, those to the cervical cord coming mainly from the rostroventral regions, those to the lumbosacral cord from the dorsocaudal regions, while the fibers to the thoracic cord are derived from areas intermediate between the two others. The lateral vestibulospinal fibers terminate ipsilaterally in laminae VII and VIII, but not in lamina IX where the soma of the motoneurons are located. The medial vestibulospinal projection is not somatotopically organized. Their descending fibers can be traced bilaterally to midthoracic levels where they terminate in laminae VII and VIII.

The lateral vestibular nucleus exerts a monosynaptic as well as a polysynaptic excitatory influence on some extensor motoneurons to ipsilateral hindlimb muscles and this effect involves not only α motoneurons but also static γ motoneurons. The possibility that the monosynaptic excitation of these extensor motoneurons is due to activation of axo-dendritic rather than axo-somatic synapses may explain why the lateral vestibulospinal fibers have not been found to terminate anatomically in lamina IX. The fusimotor activation of static γ motoneurons from Deiters' nucleus is responsible for the γ rigidity which occurs in the decerebrate preparation.

Contrary to Deiters' nucleus, however, the medial vestibular nucleus is apparently unable to excite the α motoneurons to ipsilateral extensor hindlimb muscles. Fusimotor effects can also be elicited by this structure, but it is still open to question whether static and/or dynamic fusimotor influences are elicited by this vestibular nucleus.

An additional phenomenon induced by selective stimulation of the medial vestibular nucleus is the appearance of a depolarization in primary afferents, including the group Ia afferents from both extensor and flexor hindlimb motoneurons, which leads to presynaptic inhibition in the monosynaptic reflex pathway to spinal motoneurons.

The conclusion that different vestibular structures influence different spinal cord mechanisms must be expected to receive further support from studies where natural stimulation of different receptor organs is performed.

ACKNOWLEDGEMENTS

This work was supported by P.H.S. Research Grant NB 07685-03 from the National Institute of Neurological Diseases and Blindness, N.I.H., Public Health Service, U.S.A. and by a research grant from the Consiglio Nazionale delle Ricerche, Italia.

REFERENCES

ADRIAN, E. D. (1943) Discharges from vestibular receptors in the cat. *J. Physiol. (Lond.)*, **101**, 389–407.

AITKEN, J. T. AND BRIDGER, J. E. (1961) Neuron size and neuron population density in the lumbosacral region of the cat's spinal cord. *J. Anat. (Lond.)*, **95**, 38–53.

AJALA, G. F. AND POPPELE, R. E. (1967) Some problems in the central actions of vestibular inputs. In M. D. YAHR AND D. P. PURPURA (Eds.), *Neurophysiological Basis of Normal and Abnormal Motor Activities*. Raven Press, Hewlett, N.Y., pp. 141–154.

ALNAES, E., JANSEN, J. K. S. AND RUDJORD, T. (1965) Fusimotor activity in the spinal cat. *Acta physiol. scand.*, **63**, 197–212.

ANDERSSON, S. AND GERNANDT, B. E. (1956) Ventral root discharge in response to vestibular and proprioceptive stimulation. *J. Neurophysiol.*, **19**, 524–543.

APPELBERG, B. (1962) The effect of electrical stimulation of nucleus ruber on the gamma motor system. *Acta physiol. scand.*, **55**, 150–159.

APPELBERG, B., BESSOU, P. AND LAPORTE, Y. (1965) Effects of dynamic and static fusimotor γ-fibres on the responses of primary and secondary endings belonging to the same spindle. *J. Physiol. (Lond.)*, **177**, 29–30P.

APPELBERG, B., BESSOU, P. AND LAPORTE, Y. (1966) Action of static and dynamic fusimotor fibres on secondary endings of cat's spindles. *J. Physiol. (Lond.)*, **185**, 160–171.

BARNES, C. D. E POMPEIANO, O. (1970a) Dissociazione delle risposte presinaptiche e postsinaptiche prodotte nel midollo lombare da stimoli vestibolari. *Boll. Soc. ital. Biol. sper.*, **46**, 203–205.

BARNES, C. D. AND POMPEIANO, O. (1970b) The contribution of the medial and lateral vestibular nuclei to presynaptic and postsynaptic effects produced in the lumbar cord by vestibular volleys. *Pflügers Arch. ges. Physiol.*, **317**, 1–9.

BARNES, C. D. AND POMPEIANO, O. (1970c) Dissociation of presynaptic and postsynaptic effects produced in the lumbar cord by vestibular volleys. *Arch. ital. Biol.*, **108**, 295–324.

BARRIOS, P., HAASE, J., NASSR–ESFAHANI, H., NOTH, J. UND ROPTE, H. (1968) Statische und dynamische Aktivitätsänderungen primärer Spindelafferenzen aus den Fussextensoren und prätibialen Flexoren der anaesthesierten und deafferenzierten Katze nach intercolliculärer Dezerebrierung, tiefer Spinalisierung und Deefferentierung. *Pflügers Arch. ges. Physiol.*, **299**, 128–148.

BERGMANS, J. AND GRILLNER, S. (1968) Monosynaptic control of static γ-motoneurones from the lower brain stem. *Experientia (Basel)*, **24**, 146–147.

BERNHARD, C. G. AND REXED, B. (1945) The localization of the premotor interneurons discharging through the peroneal nerve. *J. Neurophysiol.*, **8**, 387–392.

BESSOU, P., LAPORTE, Y. ET PAGÈS, B. (1966) Similitude des effets (statiques ou dynamiques) exercés par des fibres fusimotrices uniques sur les terminaisons primaires de plusieurs fuseaux chez le chat. *J. Physiol. (Paris)*, **58**, 31–39.

BESSOU, P., LAPORTE, Y. AND PAGÈS, B. (1968) Frequencygrams of spindle primary endings elicited by stimulation of static and dynamic fusimotor fibres. *J. Physiol. (Lond.)*, **196**, 47–63.

BIZZI, E., POMPEIANO, O. AND SOMOGYI, I. (1964a) Vestibular nuclei: activity of single neurons during natural sleep and wakefulness. *Science*, **145**, 414–415.

BIZZI, E., POMPEIANO, O. AND SOMOGYI, I. (1964b) Spontaneous activity of single vestibular neurons of unrestrained cats during sleep and wakefulness. *Arch. ital. Biol.*, **102**, 308–330.

BRODAL, A. (1940) Modification of Gudden method for study of cerebral localization. *Arch. Neurol. (Chicago)*, **43**, 46–58.

BRODAL, A. (1972) Some features in the anatomical organization of the vestibular nuclear complex in the cat. In A. BRODAL AND O. POMPEIANO (Eds.), *Progress in Brain Research. Vol. 37. Basic aspects of central vestibular mechanisms*. Elsevier, Amsterdam, pp. 31–53.

BRODAL, A. AND POMPEIANO, O. (1957) The origin of ascending fibres of the medial longitudinal fasciculus from the vestibular nuclei. An experimental study in the cat. *Acta morph. neerl.-scand.*, **1**, 306–328.

BRODAL, A., POMPEIANO, O. AND WALBERG, F. (1962) *The Vestibular Nuclei and Their Connections. Anatomy and Functional Correlations*. Oliver and Boyd, Edinburgh, London, pp. VIII–193.

BROWN, M. C., CROWE, A. AND MATTHEWS, P. B. C. (1965) Observations on the fusimotor fibres of the tibialis posterior muscle of the cat. *J. Physiol. (Lond.)*, **177**, 140–159.

BROWN, M. C., ENGBERG, I. AND MATTHEWS, P. B. C. (1967) Fusimotor stimulation and the dynamic sensitivity of the secondary ending of the muscle spindles. *J. Physiol. (Lond.)*, **189**, 545–550.

BRUGGENCATE, G. TEN, BURKE, R. E., LUNDBERG, A. AND UDO, M. (1969) Interaction between the vestibulospinal tract and contralateral flexor reflex afferents. *Brain Res.*, **14**, 529–532.

BURKE, R. (1968) Group Ia synaptic input to fast and slow twitch motor units of cat triceps surae. *J. Physiol. (Lond.)*, **196**, 605–630.

BUSCH, H. F. M. (1961) *An Anatomical Analysis of the White Matter in the Brain Stem of the Cat*. Van Gorcum, Leiden, pp. 116.

CAJAL, S., RAMÓN Y (1909–1911) *Histologie du Système Nerveux de l'Homme et des Vertébrés*. Maloine, Paris.

CARLI, G., DIETE–SPIFF, K. E POMPEIANO, O. (1966a) Effetti della stimolazione elettrica del nucleo di Deiters sulla scarica afferente fusale e sulla tensione muscolare nel gastrocnemio di gatto. *Boll. Soc. ital. Biol. sper.*, **42**, 999–1001.

CARLI, G., DIETE-SPIFF, K. E POMPEIANO, O. (1966b) Persistenza della risposta di recettori fusali alla stimolazione del nucleo di Deiters dopo blocco periferico dei γ-motoneuroni. *Boll. Soc. ital. Biol. sper.*, **42**, 1001–1003.

CARLI, G., DIETE–SPIFF, K. AND POMPEIANO, O. (1966c) Skeletomotor and fusimotor control of gastrocnemius muscle from Deiters' nucleus. *Experientia (Basel)*, **22**, 583–584.

CARLI, G., DIETE-SPIFF, K. AND POMPEIANO, O. (1967a) Responses of the muscle spindles and of the extrafusal fibres in an extensor muscle to stimulation of the lateral vestibular nucleus in the cat. *Arch. ital. Biol.*, **105**, 209–242.

CARLI, G., DIETE–SPIFF, K. E POMPEIANO, O. (1967b) Meccanismi attivi e passivi responsabili dell'eccitazione dei recettori fusali. *Boll. Soc. ital. Biol. sper.*, **43**, 275–277.

CARLI, G., DIETE–SPIFF, K. AND POMPEIANO, O. (1967c) Active and passive factors in muscle spindle excitation. *Nature (Lond.)*, **214**, 838–839.

CARLI, G., DIETE–SPIFF, K. AND POMPEIANO, O. (1967d) Mechanisms of muscle spindle excitation. *Arch. ital. Biol.*, **105**, 273–289.

CARPENTER, D., ENGBERG, I. AND LUNDBERG, A. (1966) Primary afferent depolarization evoked from the brain stem and the cerebellum. *Arch. ital. Biol.*, **104**, 73–85.

CARPENTER, M. B. (1960) Fiber projections from the descending and lateral vestibular nuclei in the cat. *Amer. J. Anat.*, **107**, 1–22.

CARPENTER, M. B., ALLING, F. A. AND BARD, D. S. (1960) Lesions of the descending vestibular nucleus in the cat. *J. comp. Neurol.*, **114**, 39–50.

COOK, W. A., JR., CANGIANO, A. AND POMPEIANO, O. (1968a) Vestibular evoked primary afferent depolarization in the lumbar spinal cord. *Proc. XXIV int. Congr. physiol. Sci.*, Washington, D.C., VII, n. 272, 91.

COOK, W. A., JR., CANGIANO, A. AND POMPEIANO, O. (1968b) Vestibular influences on primary afferents in the spinal cord. *Pflügers Arch. ges. Physiol.*, **299**, 334–338.

COOK, W. A., JR., CANGIANO, A. AND POMPEIANO, O. (1969a) An electrical investigation of the efferent pathways from the vestibular nuclei. *Arch. ital. Biol.*, **107**, 235–274.

COOK, W. A., JR., CANGIANO, A. AND POMPEIANO, O. (1969b) Dorsal root potentials in the lumbar cord evoked from the vestibular system. *Arch. ital. Biol.*, **107**, 275–295.

COOK, W. A., JR., CANGIANO, A. AND POMPEIANO, O. (1969c) Vestibular control of transmission in primary afferents to the lumbar spinal cord. *Arch. ital. Biol.*, **107**, 296–320.

CORVAJA, N., MARINOZZI, V. AND POMPEIANO, O. (1969) Muscle spindles in the lumbrical muscle of the adult cat. Electron microscopic observations and functional considerations. *Arch. ital. Biol.*, **107**, 365–543.

CROWE, A. AND MATTHEWS, P. B. C. (1964a) The effects of stimulation of static and dynamic fusimotor fibres on the response to stretching of the primary endings of muscle spindles. *J. Physiol. (Lond.)*, **174**, 109–131.

CROWE, A. AND MATTHEWS, P. B. C. (1964b) Further studies of static and dynamic fusimotor fibres. *J. Physiol. (Lond.)*, **174**, 132–151.

DIETE–SPIFF, K., CARLI, G. E POMPEIANO, O. (1966) Analisi delle risposte motorie extra- ed intrafusali prodotte della stimolazione elettrica del nervo ottavo e dei nuclei vestibolari nel gastrocnemio di gatto. *Boll. Soc. ital. Biol. sper.*, **42**, fasc. 20 bis, n. 1.

DIETE–SPIFF, K., CARLI, G. AND POMPEIANO, O. (1967a) Spindle responses and extrafusal contraction on stimulation of the VIIIth cranial nerve or the vestibular nuclei in the cat. *Pflügers Arch. ges. Physiol.*, **293**, 276–280.

DIETE–SPIFF, K., CARLI, G. AND POMPEIANO, O. (1967b) Comparison of the effects of stimulation of the VIIIth cranial nerve, the vestibular nuclei or the reticular formation on the gastrocnemius muscle and its spindles. *Arch. ital. Biol.*, **105**, 243–272.

DIETE–SPIFF, K., DODSWORTH, H. AND PASCOE, J. E. (1962) An analysis of the effect of ether and ethyl chloride on the discharge frequency of gastrocnemius fusimotor neurones in the rabbit. In D. BARKER (Ed.), *Symposium on Muscle Receptors*. Hong Kong Univ. Press, Hong Kong, pp. 43–47.

DUENSING, F. UND SCHAEFER, K. P. (1958) Die Aktivität einzelner Neurone im Bereich der Vestibulariskerne bei Horizontalbeschleunigungen unter besonderer Berücksichtigung der vestibulären Nystagmus. *Arch. Psychiat. Nervenkr.*, **198**, 225–252.

DUENSING, F. UND SCHAEFER, K. P. (1959) Über die Konvergenz verschiedener labyrinthärer Afferenzen auf einzelne Neurone des Vestibulariskerngebietes. *Arch. Psychiat. Nervenkr.*, **199**, 345–371.

ECCLES, J. C. (1964) *The Physiology of Synapses*. Springer, Berlin, pp. 316.

ECCLES, J. C., ECCLES, R. M., IGGO, A. AND LUNDBERG, A. (1960) Electrophysiological studies on gamma motoneurones. *Acta physiol. scand.*, **50**, 32–40.

ECKEL, W. (1954) Elektrophysiologische und histologische Untersuchungen im Vestibulariskerngebiet bei Drehreizen. *Arch. Ohr.-, Nas.- u. Kehlk.-Heilk.*, **164**, 487–513.

EHRHARDT, K. J. AND WAGNER, A. (1970) Labyrinthine and neck reflexes recorded from spinal single motoneurons in the cat. *Brain Res.*, **19**, 87–104.

EIDE, E., LUNDBERG, A. AND VOORHOEVE, P. (1961) Monosynaptically evoked inhibitory post-synaptic potentials in motoneurones. *Acta physiol. scand.*, **53**, 185–195.

ELDRED, E., GRANIT, R. AND MERTON, P. A. (1953) Supraspinal control of the muscle spindles and its significance. *J. Physiol. (Lond.)*, **122**, 498–523.

ERULKAR, S. D., SPRAGUE, J. M., WHITSEL, B. L., DOGAN, S. AND JANNETTA, P. J. (1966) Organization of the vestibular projection to the spinal cord of the cat. *J. Neurophysiol.*, **29**, 626–664.

FOERSTER, O. UND GAGEL, O. (1932) Die Vorderseitenstrangdurchschneidung beim Menschen: Eine klinisch-patho-physiologisch-anatomische Studie. *Z. ges. Neurol. Psychiat.*, **138**, 1–92.

FRANKENHAEUSER, B. AND HODGKIN, A. L. (1956) The after-effects of impulses in the giant nerve fibres of Loligo. *J. Physiol. (Lond.)*, **131**, 341–376.

FUJITA, Y., ROSENBERG, J. AND SEGUNDO, J. P. (1968) Activity of cells in the lateral vestibular nucleus as a function of head position. *J. Physiol. (Lond.)*, **196**, 1–18.

GACEK, R. (1969) The course and central termination of first order neurons supplying vestibular endorgans in the cat. *Acta oto-laryng. (Stockh.)*, Suppl. 254, 1–66.

GASSEL, M. M., MARCHIAFAVA, P. L. AND POMPEIANO, O. (1964) Tonic and phasic inhibition of spinal reflexes during deep, desynchronized sleep in unrestrained cats. *Arch. ital. Biol.*, **102**, 471–499.

GERNANDT, B. E. (1967) Vestibular influence upon spinal reflex activity. In A. V. S. DE REUCK AND J. KNIGHT (Eds.), *Myotatic, Kinesthetic and Vestibular Mechanisms*. Churchill Ltd., London, pp. 170–183.

GERNANDT, B. E. (1968) Functional properties of the descending medial longitudinal fasciculus. *Exp. Neurol.*, **22**, 326–342.

GERNANDT, B. E. (1970) Vestibular activity in the descending medial longitudinal fasciculus. In *Fourth Symposium on the Role of the Vestibular Organs in Space Exploration. NASA SP-*187, 237–241.

GERNANDT, B. E., IRANYI, M. AND LIVINGSTON, R. B. (1959) Vestibular influences on spinal mechanisms. *Exp. Neurol.*, **1**, 248–273.

GERNANDT, B. E. AND THULIN, C.-A. (1952) Vestibular connections of the brain stem. *Amer. J. Physiol.*, **71**, 121–127.

GERNANDT, B. E. AND THULIN, C.-A. (1953) Vestibular mechanisms of facilitation and inhibition of cord reflexes. *Amer. J. Physiol.*, **172**, 653–660.

GERNANDT, B. E. AND THULIN, C.-A. (1955) Reciprocal effects upon spinal motoneurons from stimulation of bulbar reticular formation. *J. Neurophysiol.*, **18**, 113–129.

GHEZ, C., LENZI, G. L. E POMPEIANO, O. (1970) Inibizione dei reflessi spinali prodotta dalla stimolazione naturale dei canali semicircolari orizzontali nel gatto decerebrato. *Arch. Fisiol.*, **68**, 68–69.

GILMAN, S. AND VAN DER MEULEN, J. P. (1966) Muscle spindle activity in dystonic and spastic monkeys. *Arch. Neurol. (Chicago)*, **14**, 553–563.

GIOVANELLI BARILARI, M. AND KUYPERS, H. G. J. M. (1969) Propriospinal fibers interconnecting the spinal enlargements in the cat. *Brain Res.*, **14**, 321–330.

GRANIT, R. (1955) *Receptors and Sensory Perception*. Yale Univ. Press, New Haven, pp. 237–276.

GRANIT, R. (1966) Effects of stretch and contraction on the membrane of motoneurones. In R. GRANIT (Ed.), *Nobel Symposium I. Muscular Afferents and Motor Control*. Almqvist and Wiksell, Stockholm, pp. 37–50.

GRANIT, R., HOLMGREN, B. AND MERTON, P. A. (1955) The two routes for excitation of muscle and their subservience to the cerebellum. *J. Physiol. (Lond.)*, **130**, 213–224.

GRANIT, R., HOMMA, S. AND MATTHEWS, P. B. C. (1959a) Prolonged changes in the discharge of mammalian muscle spindles following tendon taps or muscle twitches. *Acta physiol. scand.*, **46**, 185–193.

GRANIT, R. AND KAADA, B. (1952) Influence of stimulation of central nervous structures on muscle spindles in cat. *Acta physiol. scand.*, **27**, 130–160.

GRANIT, R., KELLERTH, J.-O. AND SZUMSKI, A. J. (1966) Intracellular recording from extensor motoneurons activated across the gamma loop. *J. Neurophysiol.*, **29**, 530–544.

GRANIT, R., POMPEIANO, O. AND WALTMAN, B. (1959b) Fast supraspinal control of mammalian muscle spindles: extra- and intrafusal co-activation. *J. Physiol. (Lond.)*, **147**, 385–398.

GRILLNER, S. (1969a) Supraspinal and segmental control of static and dynamic γ-motoneurons in the cat. *Acta physiol. scand.*, Suppl. 327, 1–34.

GRILLNER, S. (1969b) The influence of DOPA on the static and dynamic fusimotor activity to the triceps surae of the spinal cat. *Acta physiol. scand.*, **77**, 490–509.

GRILLNER, S. AND HONGO, T. (1972) Vestibulospinal effects on motoneurones and interneurones in the lumbosacral cord. In A. BRODAL AND O. POMPEIANO (Eds.), *Progress in Brain Research. Vol. 37. Basic aspects of central vestibular mechanisms*, Elsevier, Amsterdam, pp. 243–262.

GRILLNER, S., HONGO, T. AND LUND, S. (1966a) Descending pathways with monosynaptic action on motoneurones. *Acta physiol. scand.*, **68**, Suppl. 277, 60.

GRILLNER, S., HONGO, T. AND LUND, S. (1966b) Monosynaptic excitation of spinal γ-motoneurones from the brain stem. *Experientia (Basel)*, **22**, 691.

GRILLNER, S., HONGO, T. AND LUND, S. (1966c) Interaction between the inhibitory pathways from the Deiters' nucleus and Ia afferents to flexor motoneurones. *Acta physiol. scand.*, **68**, Suppl. 277, 61.

GRILLNER, S., HONGO, T. AND LUND, S. (1968) Reciprocal effects between two descending bulbospinal systems with monosynaptic connections to spinal motoneurones. *Brain Res.*, **10**, 477–480.

GRILLNER, S., HONGO T. AND LUND, S. (1969) Descending monosynaptic and reflex control of γ-motoneurones. *Acta physiol. scand.*, **75**, 592–613.

GRILLNER, S., HONGO, T. AND LUND, S. (1970) The vestibulospinal tract. Effects on alpha-motoneurones in the lumbosacral spinal cord in the cat. *Exp. Brain Res.*, **10**, 94–120.

GRILLNER, S., HONGO, T. AND LUND, S. (1971) Convergent effects on alpha motoneurones from the vestibulospinal tract and a pathway descending in the medial longitudinal fasciculus. *Exp. Brain Res.*, **12**, 457–479.

GRILLNER, S. AND LUND, S. (1966) A descending pathway with monosynaptic action on flexor motoneurones. *Experientia (Basel)*, **22**, 390.

GRILLNER, S. AND LUND, S. (1968) The origin of a descending pathway with monosynaptic action on flexor motoneurones. *Acta physiol. scand.*, **74**, 274–284.

HAMMOND, P. H., MERTON, P. A. AND SUTTON, C. G. (1956) Nervous gradation of muscular contraction. *Brit. med. Bull.*, **12**, 214–218.

HENNEMAN, E., SOMJEN, G. AND CARPENTER, D. O. (1965) Functional significance of cell size in spinal motoneurones. *J. Neurophysiol.*, **28**, 560–580.

HIEBERT, T. G. AND FERNANDEZ, C. (1965) Deitersian response to tilt. *Acta oto-laryng. (Stockh.)*, **60**, 180–190.

HONGO, T., KUDO, N. AND TANAKA, R. (1971) Effects from the vestibulospinal tract on the contralateral hindlimb motoneurones in the cat. *Brain Res.*, **31**, 220–223.

HULTBORN, H., JANKOWSKA, E. AND LINDSTRØM, S. (1968) Recurrent inhibition from motor axon collaterals in interneurones monosynaptically activated from Ia afferents. *Brain Res.*, **9**, 367–369.

HUNT, C. C. (1951) The reflex activity of mammalian small-nerve fibres. *J. Physiol. (Lond.)*, **115**, 456–469.

HUNT, C. C. AND KUNO, M. (1959) Properties of spinal interneurones. *J. Physiol. (Lond.)*, **147**, 346–363.

HURSCH, J. B. (1939) Conduction velocity and diameter of nerve fibers. *Amer. J. Physiol.*, **127**, 131–139.

ITO, M., HONGO, T., YOSHIDA, M., OKADA, Y. AND OBATA, K. (1964a) Antidromic and trans-synaptic activation of Deiters' neurones induced from the spinal cord. *Jap. J. Physiol.*, **14**, 638–658.

ITO, M., HONGO, T., YOSHIDA, M., OKADA, Y. AND OBATA, K. (1964b) Intracellularly recorded antidromic responses of Deiters' neurones. *Experientia (Basel)*, **20**, 295–296.

JANSEN, J. K. S. (1966) On fusimotor reflex activity. In R. GRANIT (Ed.), *Nobel Symposium I. Muscular Afferents and Motor Control*. Almqvist and Wiksell, Stockholm, pp. 91–105.

JANSEN, J. K. S. AND MATTHEWS, P. B. C. (1962) The central control of the dynamic response of muscle spindle receptors. *J. Physiol. (Lond.)*, **161**, 357–378.

KATO, M. AND TANJI, J. (1971) The effects of electrical stimulation of Deiters' nucleus upon hindlimb γ-motoneurons in the cat. *Brain Res.*, **30**, 385–395.

KATZ, B. AND THESLEFF, S. (1957) On the factors which determine the amplitude of the miniature endplate potentials. *J. Physiol. (Lond.)*, **137**, 267–278.

KAWAI, N., ITO, M. AND NOZUE, M. (1969) Postsynaptic influences on the vestibular non-Deiters nuclei from primary vestibular nerve. *Exp. Brain Res.*, **8**, 190–200.

KOBAYASHI, Y., OSHIMA, K. AND TASAKI, I. (1952) Analysis of afferent and efferent systems in the muscle nerve of the toad and cat. *J. Physiol. (Lond.)*, **117**, 152–171.

KUFFLER, S. W. AND NICHOLLS, J. G. (1966) The physiology of neuroglial cells. *Ergebn. Physiol.*, **57**, 1–90.

KUYPERS, H. G. J. M. (1966) The descending pathways to the spinal cord. Second Symposium on Parkinson's Disease. *J. Neurosurg.*, Suppl., part II, 200–202.

KUYPERS, H. G. J. M., FLEMING, W. R. AND FARINHOLT, J. W. (1962) Subcortical projections in the rhesus monkey. *J. comp. Neurol.*, **118**, 107–137.

LADPLI, R. AND BRODAL, A. (1968) Experimental studies of commissural and reticular formation projections from the vestibular nuclei in the cat. *Brain Res.*, **8**, 65–96.

LENHOSSEK, M. VON, (1895) *Feinere Bau des Nervensystems im Lichte neuerster Forschungen*. Fischers Medicinische Buchhandlung H. Kornfeld, Berlin.

LLOYD, D. P. C. (1941) Activity in neurons of the bulbospinal correlation system. *J. Neurophysiol.*, **4**, 115–134.

LORENTE DE NÓ, R. (1926) Études sur l'anatomie et la physiologie du labyrinthe de l'oreille et du VIIIe nerf. II. Quelques données au sujet de l'anatomie des organes sensoriels du labyrinthe. *Trav. Lab. Rech. Biol. Univ. Madr.*, **24**, 53–153.

LORENTE DE NÓ, R. (1933) Anatomy of the eighth nerve. The central projection of the nerve endings of the internal ear. *Laryngoscope (St. Louis)*, **43**, 1–38.

LORENTE DE NÓ, R. (1938) Synaptic stimulation of motoneurons as a local process. *J. Neurophysiol.*, **1**, 195–206.

LUND, S. AND POMPEIANO, O. (1965) Descending pathways with monosynaptic action on motoneurones. *Experientia (Basel)*, **21**, 602–603.

LUND, S. AND POMPEIANO, O. (1968) Monosynaptic excitation of alpha motoneurones from supraspinal structures in the cat. *Acta physiol. scand.*, **73**, 1–21.

LUNDBERG, A. (1970) The excitatory control of the Ia inhibitory pathway. In P. ANDERSEN AND J. K. S. JANSEN (Eds.), *Excitatory Synaptic Mechanisms*. Universitetsforlaget, Oslo, pp. 333–340.

LØKEN, A. C. AND BRODAL, A. (1970) A somatotopical pattern in the human lateral vestibular nucleus. *Arch. Neurol. (Chicago)*, **23**, 350–357.

MARKHAM, C. H., PRECHT, W. AND SHIMAZU, H. (1966) Effect of stimulation of interstitial nucleus of Cajal on vestibular unit activity in the cat. *J. Neurophysiol.*, **29**, 493–507.

MATANO, S., ZYO, K. AND BAN, T. (1964) Experimental studies on the medial longitudinal fasciculus in the rabbit. I. Fibers originating in the vestibular nuclei. *Med. J. Osaka Univ.*, **14**, 339–370.

MATSUSHITA, M. (1969) Some aspects of the interneuronal connections in cat's spinal gray matter. *J. comp. Neurol.*, **136**, 57–80.

MATTHEWS, P. B. C. (1962) The differentiation of two types of fusimotor fibres by their effects on dynamic response of muscle spindle primary endings. *Quart. J. exp. Physiol.*, **47**, 324–333.

MATTHEWS, P. B. C. (1964) Muscle spindles and their motor control. *Physiol. Rev.*, **44**, 219–288.

McINTYRE, A. K., MARK, R. F. AND STEINER, J. (1956) Multiple firing at central synapses. *Nature (Lond.)*, **178**, 302–304.

McMASTER, R. E., WEISS, A. H. AND CARPENTER, M. B. (1966) Vestibular projections to the nuclei of the extraocular muscles. Degeneration resulting from discrete partial lesions of the vestibular nuclei in the monkey. *Amer. J. Anat.*, **118**, 163–194.

MEGIRIAN, D. (1971) Vestibular and somatosensory evoked centrifugal cutaneous nerve discharges in the decerebrate-decerebellate phalanger, *Tricosurus vulpecula*. *Arch. ital. Biol.*, **109**, 152–165.

MERTON, P. A. (1951) The silent period in a muscle of the human hand. *J. Physiol. (Lond.)*, **114**, 183–198.

MERTON, P. A. (1953) Speculation on the servo-control of movement. In G. E. W. WOLSTENHOLME (Ed.), *The Spinal Cord*. Churchill, London, pp. 247–255.

MORRISON, A. R. AND POMPEIANO, O. (1965) Central depolarization of group Ia afferent fibers during desynchronized sleep. *Arch. ital. Biol.*, **103**, 517–537.

NYBERG–HANSEN, R. (1964) Origin and termination of fibers from the vestibular nuclei descending in the medial longitudinal fasciculus. An experimental study with silver impregnation methods in the cat. *J. comp. Neurol.*, **122**, 355–367.

NYBERG–HANSEN, R. (1965a) Anatomical demonstration of gamma motoneurones in the cat's spinal cord. *Exp. Neurol.*, **13**, 71–81.

NYBERG–HANSEN, R. (1965b) Sites and mode of termination of reticulo-spinal fibers in the cat. An experimental study with silver impregnation methods. *J. comp. Neurol.*, **124**, 71–100.

NYBERG–HANSEN, R. (1966) Functional organization of descending supraspinal fibre systems to the spinal cord. Anatomical observations and physiological correlations. *Ergebn. Anat. Entwickl.-Gesch.*, **39**, 1–48.

NYBERG–HANSEN, R. (1969) Do cat spinal motoneurones receive direct supraspinal fibre connections? A supplementary silver study. *Arch. ital. Biol.*, **107**, 67–78.

NYBERG–HANSEN, R. (1970) Anatomical aspects on the functional organization of the vestibulospinal projection, with special reference to the sites of termination. In *Fourth Symposium on the Role of the Vestibular Organs in Space Exploration. NASA SP*-187, 167–181.

NYBERG–HANSEN, R. AND MASCITTI, T. A. (1964) Sites and mode of termination of fibers of the vestibulospinal tract in the cat. An experimental study with silver impregnation methods. *J. comp. Neurol.*, **122**, 369–387.

ORKAND, R. K., NICHOLLS, J. G. AND KUFFLER, S. W. (1966) Effect of nerve impulses on the membrane potential of glial cells in the central nervous system of amphibia. *J. Neurophysiol.*, **29**, 788–806.

PETERSON, B. W. (1967) Effect of tilting on the activity of neurons in the vestibular nuclei of the cat. *Brain Res.*, **6**, 606–609.

PETERSON, B. W. (1970) Distribution of neural responses to tilting within vestibular nuclei of the cat. *J. Neurophysiol.*, **33**, 750–767.

PETRAS, J. M. (1967) Cortical, tectal and tegmental fiber connections in the spinal cord of the cat. *Brain Res.*, **6**, 275–324.

POMPEIANO, O. (1960) Organizzazione somatotopica delle risposte posturali alla stimolazione elettrica del nucleo di Deiters nel gatto decerebrato. *Arch. Sci. biol. (Bologna)*, **44**, 497–511.

POMPEIANO, O. (1966a) Discussion of Dr. Shapovalov's paper. In R. GRANIT (Ed.), *Nobel Symposium I. Muscular Afferents and Motor Control*. Almqvist and Wiksell, Stockholm, p. 348.

POMPEIANO, O. (1966b) Muscular afferents and motor control during sleep. In R. GRANIT (Ed.), *Nobel Symposium I. Muscular Afferents and Motor Control*. Almqvist and Wiksell, Stockholm, pp. 415–436.

POMPEIANO, O. (1967) The neurophysiological mechanisms of the postural and motor events during desynchronized sleep. *Res. Publ. Ass. nerv. ment. Dis.*, **45**, 351–423.

POMPEIANO, O. AND BRODAL, A. (1957) The origin of vestibulospinal fibres in the cat. An experimental-anatomical study, with comments on the descending medial longitudinal fasciculus. *Arch. ital. Biol.*, **95**, 166–195.

POMPEIANO, O., DIETE–SPIFF, K. E CARLI, G. (1967a) Componenti precoci e tardive nella risposta dei recettori fusali alla stimolazione del nucleo di Deiters. *Boll. Soc. ital. Biol. sper.*, **43**, 273–275.

POMPEIANO, O., DIETE–SPIFF, K. AND CARLI, G. (1967b) Two pathways transmitting vestibulospinal influences from the lateral vestibular nucleus of Deiters to extensor fusimotor neurones. *Pflügers Arch. ges. Physiol.*, **293**, 272–275.

POMPEIANO, O. AND MORRISON, A. R. (1965) Vestibular influences during sleep. I. Abolition of the rapid eye movements during desynchronized sleep following vestibular lesions. *Arch. ital. Biol.*, **103**, 569–595.

POMPEIANO, O. AND MORRISON, A. R. (1966) Vestibular influences during sleep. III. Dissociation of the tonic and phasic inhibition of spinal reflexes during desynchronized sleep following vestibular lesions. *Arch. ital. Biol.*, **104**, 231–246.

POPPELE, R. E. (1964) Response of lumbar motoneurons to natural vestibular stimulation. *Physiologist*, **7**, 226.

POPPELE, R. E. (1967) Response of gamma and alpha motor systems to phasic and tonic vestibular inputs. *Brain Res.*, **6**, 535–547.

PRECHT, W., GRIPPO, J. AND WAGNER, A. (1967) Contribution of different types of central vestibular neurons to the vestibulospinal system. *Brain Res.*, **4**, 119–123.

PRECHT, W. AND SHIMAZU, H. (1965) Functional connections of tonic and kinetic vestibular neurons with primary vestibular afferents. *J. Neurophysiol.*, **28**, 1014–1028.

RASDOLSKY, J. (1923) Über die Endigung der extraspinalen Bewegungssysteme im Rüchenmark. *Z. ges. Neurol. Psychiat.*, **86**, 360–374.

RASMUSSEN, A. T. (1932) Secondary vestibular tracts in the cat. *J. comp. Neurol.*, **54**, 143–171.

REXED, B. (1952) The cytoarchitectonic organization of the spinal cord in the cat. *J. comp. Neurol.*, **96**, 415–496.

ROBERTS, T. D. M. (1967) Labyrinthine control of the postural muscles. In *Third Symposium on the Role of the Vestibular Organs in Space Exploration*. NASA SP-152, 149–168.

SADJADPOUR, K. AND BRODAL, A. (1968) The vestibular nuclei in man. A morphological study in the light of experimental findings in the cat. *J. Hirnforsch.*, **10**, 299–323.

SASAKI, K. AND TANAKA, T. (1964) Phasic and tonic innervation of spinal alpha motoneurons from upper brain centers. *Jap. J. Physiol.*, **14**, 56–66.

SASAKI, K., TANAKA, T. AND MORI, K. (1962) Effects of stimulation of pontine and bulbar reticular formation upon spinal motoneurons of the cat. *Jap. J. Physiol.*, **12**, 45–62.

SCHEIBEL, M. E. AND SCHEIBEL, A. B. (1966) Spinal motoneurons, interneurons and Renshaw cells. A Golgi study. *Arch. ital. Biol.*, **104**, 328–353.

SCHIMERT, J. S. (1938) Die Endigungsweise des Tractus vestibulospinalis. *Z. Anat. Entwickl.-Gesch.*, **108**, 761–767.

SHAPOVALOV, A. I. (1966) Excitation and inhibition of spinal neurones during supraspinal stimulation. In R. GRANIT (Ed.), *Nobel Symposium I. Muscular Afferents and Motor Control*. Almqvist and Wiksell, Stockholm, pp. 331–348.

SHAPOVALOV, A. I. (1969) Posttetanic potentiation of monosynaptic and disynaptic actions from supraspinal structures on lumbar motoneurons. *J. Neurophysiol.*, **32**, 948–959.

SHAPOVALOV, A. I., KURCHAVYI, G. G. AND STROGONOVA, M. P. (1966) Synaptic mechanisms of vestibulo-spinal influences on alpha-motoneurons. *Sechenov J. Physiol., U.S.S.R.*, **52**, 1401–1409. *Neurosci. Transl.*, **1**, (1967–68) 91–100.

SHAPOVALOV, A. I. AND SAFYANTS, V. I. (1968) Potentiation of suprasegmentary synaptic influences on α-motoneurons. *Sechenov J. Physiol., U.S.S.R.*, **54**, 1261–1270.

SHIMAZU, H. AND PRECHT, W. (1965) Tonic and kinetic responses of cat's vestibular neurons to horizontal angular acceleration. *J. Neurophysiol.*, **28**, 991–1013.

SHIMAZU, H. AND PRECHT, W. (1966) Inhibiton of central vestibular neurones from the contralateral labyrinth and its mediating pathway. *J. Neurophysiol.*, **29**, 467–492.

SKINNER, R. D., WILLIS, W. D. AND HANCOCK, M. B. (1970) Actions of ventral cord pathways on spinal neurons. *Exp. Neurol.*, **27**, 318–333.

SMITH, R. S. (1966) Properties of intrafusal muscle fibres. In R. GRANIT (Ed.), *Nobel Symposium I. Muscular Afferents and Motor Control.* Almqvist and Wiksell, Stockholm. pp. 69–80.

SPRAGUE, J. M. AND HA, H. (1964) The terminal fields of dorsal root fibers in the lumbosacral spinal cord of the cat, and the dendritic organization of the motor nuclei. In J. C. ECCLES AND J. P. SCHADÉ (Eds.), *Progress in Brain Research. Vol. 11. Organization of the spinal cord.* Elsevier, Amsterdam, pp. 120–152.

SPRAGUE, J. M., SCHREINER, L. H., LINDSLEY, D. B. AND MAGOUN, H. W. (1948) Reticulo-spinal influences on stretch reflexes. *J. Neurophysiol.*, **11**, 501–507.

STAAL, A. (1961) *Subcortical Projections on the Spinal Grey Matter of the Cat.* Thesis, Koninklijke Drukkerijen Lankhout, Immig N.V., 's-Gravenhage, Leiden, pp. 164.

STEIN, B. M. AND CARPENTER, M. B. (1967) Central projections of portions of the vestibular ganglia innervating specific parts of the labyrinth in the rhesus monkey. *Amer. J. Anat.*, **120**, 281–317.

STERLING, P. AND KUYPERS, H. G. J. M. (1968) Anatomical organization of the brachial spinal cord of the cat. III. The propriospinal connections. *Brain Res.*, **7**, 419–443.

SZENTÁGOTHAI, J. (1951) Short propriospinal neurons and intrinsic connections of the spinal grey matter. *Acta morph. Acad. Sci. hung.*, **1**, 81–94.

SZENTÁGOTHAI, J. (1964) Propriospinal pathways and their synapses. In J. C. ECCLES AND J. P. SCHADÉ (Eds.), *Progress in Brain Research. Vol. 11. Organization of the spinal cord.* Elsevier, Amsterdam, pp. 155–177.

SZENTÁGOTHAI, J. (1967) Synaptic architecture of the spinal motoneuron pool. *Electroenceph. clin. Neurophysiol.*, **25**, Suppl., 4–19.

TARLOV, E. (1970) Organization of vestibulo-oculomotor projections in the cat. *Brain Res.*, **20**, 159–179.

TORVIK, A. AND BRODAL, A. (1957) The origin of reticulospinal fibers in the cat. An experimental study. *Anat. Rec.*, **128**, 113–138.

VAN DER MEULEN, J. P. AND GILMAN, S. (1965) Recovery of muscle spindle activity in cats after cerebellar ablation. *J. Neurophysiol.*, **28**, 943–957.

VOORHOEVE, P. E. AND KANTEN, R. W. VAN (1962) Reflex behaviour of fusimotor neurones of the cat upon electrical stimulation of various afferent fibres. *Acta physiol. pharmacol. neerl.*, **10**, 391–407.

WALL, P. D. (1959) Repetitive discharge of neurones. *J. Neurophysiol.*, **22**, 305–319.

WILLIS, W. D. AND WILLIS, J. C. (1966) Properties of interneurons in the ventral spinal cord. *Arch. ital. Biol.*, **104**, 354–386.

WILLIS, W. D., WILLIS, J. C. AND THOMSON, W. M. (1967) Synaptic action of fibres in the ventral spinal cord upon lumbosacral motoneurones. *J. Neurophysiol.*, **30**, 382–397.

WILSON, V. J. (1970) Vestibular and somatic inputs to cells of the lateral and medial vestibular nuclei of the cat. In *Fourth Symposium on the Role of the Vestibular Organs in Space Exploration. NASA SP*-187, 145–158.

WILSON, V. J., KATO, M. AND PETERSON, B. W. (1966a) Convergence of inputs on Deiters' neurones. *Nature (Lond.)*, **211**, 1409–1411.

WILSON, V. J., KATO, M., PETERSON, B. W. AND WYLIE, R. M. (1967a) A single-unit analysis of the organization of Deiters' nucleus. *J. Neurophysiol.*, **30**, 603–619.

WILSON, V. J., KATO, M. AND THOMAS, R. C. (1965) Excitation of lateral vestibular neurones. *Nature (Lond.)*, **206**, 96–97.

WILSON, V. J., KATO, M., THOMAS, R. C. AND PETERSON, B. W. (1966b) Excitation of lateral vestibular neurons by peripheral afferent fibers. *J. Neurophysiol.*, **29**, 508–529.

WILSON, V. J., WYLIE, R. M. AND MARCO, L. A. (1967b) Projection to the spinal cord from the medial and descending nuclei of the cat. *Nature (Lond.)*, **215**, 429–430.

WILSON, V. J., WYLIE, R. M. AND MARCO, L. A. (1968) Organization of the medial vestibular nucleus. *J. Neurophysiol.*, **31**, 166–175.

WILSON, V. J. AND YOSHIDA, M. (1968a) Vestibulospinal and reticulospinal effects on hindlimb, fore-limb, and neck alpha motoneurons of the cat. *Proc. nat. Acad. Sci. (Wash.)*, **60**, 836–840.

WILSON, V. J. AND YOSHIDA, M. (1968b) Monosynaptic inhibition of neck motoneurons by fibers originating in the brain stem. *Brain Res.*, **11**, 691–694.

WILSON, V. J. AND YOSHIDA, M. (1969a) Bilateral connections between labyrinths and neck moto-neurons. *Brain Res.*, **13**, 603–607.

WILSON, V. J. AND YOSHIDA, M. (1969b) Monosynaptic inhibition of neck motoneurons by the medial
   vestibular nucleus. *Exp. Brain Res.*, **9**, 365–380.
WILSON, V. J. AND YOSHIDA, M. (1969c) Comparison of effects of stimulation of Deiters' nucleus and
   medial longitudinal fasciculus on neck, forelimb, and hindlimb motoneurons. *J. Neurophysiol*
   32, 743–758.

Vestibular Influences on Alpha Motoneurons in the Cervical and Thoracic Cord

V. J. WILSON

The Rockefeller University, New York, N.Y., U.S.A.

The vestibular nuclei, acting as a relay for inputs from the labyrinth and from various regions of the central nervous system, notably the cerebellum, exert an important influence on spinal motoneurons (see Brodal *et al.*, 1962; Wilson, 1972). This influence is conveyed principally by two groups of fibers, the lateral and medial vestibulospinal tracts (VST and MVST); the former originates in Deiters' nucleus, the latter mainly in the medial (Nyberg–Hansen, 1966). Whereas it is well known that impulses in VST fibers increase the excitability of ipsilateral extensor motoneurons, the function of the MVST has remained obscure until recently. This brief review will describe current views on monosynaptic and simple polysynaptic actions of the two tracts upon cervical and thoracic alpha motoneurons in the cat, without touching on the actions descending fibers may exert on segmental reflex arcs (see Grillner *et al.*, 1970, for examples in hindlimb segments). It is appropriate to discuss axial and limb motoneurons separately and they will be dealt with sequentially, with emphasis on axial motoneurons.

EXCITATORY AND INHIBITORY ACTIONS ON AXIAL MOTONEURONS

Neck motoneurons

Because the labyrinth is closely linked functionally to the neck musculature (Magnus, 1926; Batini *et al.*, 1957), Wilson and Yoshida (1969a, b) investigated, in cats anesthetized with pentobarbital, the effect of electrical stimulation of the vestibular nuclei on a population of extensor motoneurons in the C2 and C3 segments. The cells were identified by antidromic stimulation of the splenius nerve or of the remainder of the dorsal rami (DR) of the spinal nerves, and all may be classified as extensors of the head. Stimulation of the vestibular nuclei evokes excitatory and inhibitory postsynaptic potentials (EPSPs and IPSPs) in many of these motoneurons. In addition to potentials that are obviously at least disynaptic, there is a group of early EPSPs and IPSPs with a latency range of 0.9–1.5 msec. As the earliest descending volleys arrive in the corresponding segments at 0.4–0.7 msec, and the mean delay between the positive peak of this volley and the start of the PSP is 0.6–0.7 msec, the early EPSPs and IPSPs are monosynaptic (Wilson and Yoshida, 1969a, b). This is particularly interesting in the case of IPSPs, since it has generally been held that inhibition of supraspinal origin is mediated by descending excitatory fibers that activate segmental inhibitory interneurons.

Excitation

Stimulation of the vestibular nuclei produces monosynaptic EPSPs with a mean amplitude of 0.8 mV (range 0.3–2.0, n = 46), such as those shown in Fig. 1, in more than 50% of extensor motoneurons in C2 and C3 (Wilson and Yoshida, 1969a). In order to identify the source of these potentials stimulating arrays consisting of several metal electrodes were used. This procedure permits comparison of the effectiveness of stimulation of various loci within and outside the vestibular nuclei. Results show that monosynaptic EPSPs are evoked at low threshold by electrodes that are located in Deiters' nucleus and presumably activate cells giving rise to VST fibers. Monosynaptic EPSPs are also produced in many motoneurons by a stimulating electrode placed in the medial longitudinal fasciculus (MLF) or nearby reticular formation in the medulla or lower pons (Fig. 1). By analogy with potentials evoked in hindlimb and other motoneurons by a similarly placed electrode (Grillner and Lund, 1968; Wilson and Yoshida, 1969a; Wilson *et al.*, 1970), it may be assumed that these EPSPs are mainly produced by stimulation of rapidly conducting reticulospinal fibers. In many

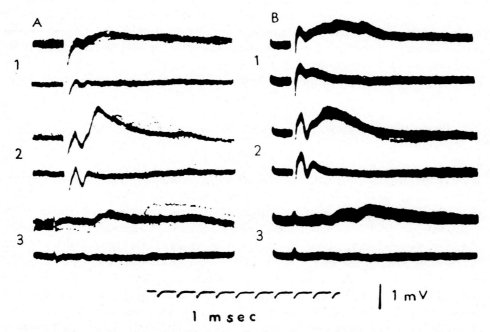

Fig. 1. EPSPs evoked in neck extensor motoneurons by stimulation of Deiters' nucleus, the MLF, and the labyrinth. A, C3 splenius motoneuron. Stimulus to Deiters' nucleus (1) and MLF (2) of 0.33 mA. EPSP in (3) evoked by stimulation of ipsilateral labyrinth at 3.1 times N_1 threshold. B, C3 DR motoneurons. Stimulus of 0.28 mA to Deiters' (1) and MLF (2). Labyrinthine stimulus (3) at 1.5 times N_1 threshold. Lower records of each pair show field potentials recorded juxtacellularly.
Upward deflection positive in this and other figures. From Wilson and Yoshida (1969a).

cells EPSPs result from stimulation of Deiters' nucleus and the MLF, simultaneous stimulation of the two structures leading to summation of the potentials. The lack of occlusion shows that the vestibulospinal and reticulospinal inputs are separate, and not due either to stimulus spread from one region to the other or to stimulation of branches of the same fibers. Both descending systems also evoke polysynaptic potentials in neck motoneurons, but these have not been studied in any detail.

In many neck motoneurons stimulation of the ipsilateral, and contralateral (Wilson and Yoshida, 1969c) labyrinth with single shocks of the strength required for monosynaptic activation of vestibular nucleus neurons evokes di- or polysynaptic EPSPs (Fig. 1). These EPSPs resemble those produced by stimulation of Deiters' nucleus, which is assumed to be the principal relay in the excitatory pathway. The distribution of the labyrinthine input within the nucleus, in relation to the location of neurons projecting to different levels of the spinal cord, supports this assumption (Brodal et al., 1962; Wilson et al., 1967). There are other possible relays for labyrinthine excitation. One is the MVST, coming from the medial and descending nuclei. The role of the MVST is considered below. Another is the reticular formation, acting on motoneurons by means of reticulospinal fibers. It is hardly likely that any disynaptic actions originating in the labyrinth are due to activity of reticulospinal neurons: (i) there is no anatomical evidence for termination of vestibular afferents on reticular neurons, and (ii) in response to labyrinthine stimulation neurons in the medial bulbar reticular formation fire multisynaptically if at all (Peterson and Felpel, 1971) and the earliest EPSPs recorded from the cells are disynaptic (Peterson, Filion and Wilson, unpublished observations).

Inhibition

Localized stimulation of the vestibular nuclei, followed by systematic mapping of low-threshold points in the horizontal and transverse planes, demonstrates that inhibitory fibers to the neck segments originate in the medial vestibular nucleus. (Wilson and Yoshida, 1969b). Therefore the MVST contains an inhibitory component. This does not mean the tract is of necessity entirely inhibitory, or that the medial nucleus contains only inhibitory neurons.

Monosynaptic inhibition is found in many (40/61) neck motoneurons, and a longer-latency inhibition is frequently produced by stimulation of the labyrinth with weak shocks (Fig. 2). The labyrinth-evoked IPSP resembles that produced by medial nucleus stimulation and in many instances the latency difference between the two potentials is that of one synaptic delay. It is therefore postulated that the inhibitory pathway linking the labyrinth to neck extensor motoneurons relays in the medial vestibular nucleus. Previous experiments support this assumption, having shown that 80% of the medial nucleus neurons projecting to the spinal cord are driven monosynaptically by stimulation of the labyrinth (Wilson et al., 1968). Ito et al. (1970b) have proposed the existence of inhibitory reticulospinal neurons; anatomical evidence and the work of Peterson and his colleagues (1971), described above, argues against the involvement of any such reticulospinal neurons in the disynaptic inhibitory pathway.

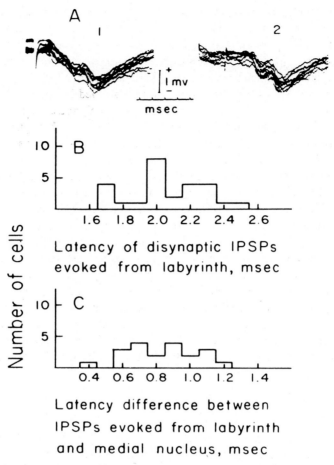

Fig. 2. Medial nucleus and labyrinthine IPSP in neck motoneurons. A, Typical IPSP evoked in a motoneuron by stimulation of the medial nucleus (1) and labyrinth (2). Stimulus to medial nucleus 6 V, threshold 2.4 V (0.14 mA). Threshold of labyrinthine IPSP 1.4 times N_1 threshold. B, Distribution of latencies of those labyrinthine IPSPs considered disynaptic; results from C2 and C3 pooled in the histogram. C, Latency differences between IPSPs evoked in the same cell by stimulation of medial nucleus and labyrinth. From Wilson and Yoshida (1969b).

The pharmacology of the inhibitory pathway has recently been studied (Felpel, 1972). Disynaptic IPSPs evoked by labyrinthine stimulation are blocked by intravenously applied strychnine, unaffected by bicuculline or picrotoxin. While such results do not identify the inhibitory transmitter, they do suggest that glycine, rather than GABA, is a likely candidate (Curtis *et al.*, 1969; Curtis *et al.*, 1970).

Back motoneurons

Like neck motoneurons, the cells innervating thoracic back muscles are axial motoneurons, and it could be expected that the pattern of connections between labyrinth, vestibular nuclei and these motoneurons resembles that found in the upper cervical segments. This expectation has been confirmed (Wilson *et al.*, 1970).

Motoneurons innervating several different muscles, all acting as extensors of the vertebral column and located in the Th 1-Th 10 segments, were studied. In some, particularly in longissimus dorsi motoneurons, monosynaptic EPSPs were evoked by stimulation of Deiters' nucleus and disynaptic EPSPs by stimulation of the labyrinth. The VST apparently synapses with some of these cells. The presence of such synapses was suggested by earlier anatomical findings that VST fibers terminate in the vicinity of thoracic motoneurons, medially in the ventral horn (Nyberg–Hansen and Mascitti, 1964).

Whereas monosynaptic excitation originating in Deiters' nucleus is seen in *some* types of back motoneurons, MLF stimulation produces monosynaptic EPSPs in the great majority of *all* types of cells. This excitation is presumably reticular in origin. Linear regression analysis, to which this population of cells lends itself particularly

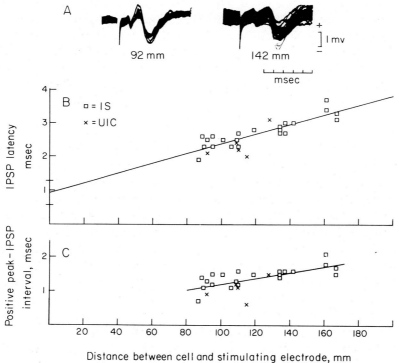

Fig. 3. Relation between latency of IPSP evoked by MLF stimulation and distance between stimulating electrode and motoneuron. A, IPSPs recorded in two interspinales motoneurons located 92 and 142 mm from the stimulating electrode. B, Regression line of latency versus distance. Marks denoting 90% confidence bounds are on each side of the y-intercept. C, Regression line of interval between positive peak of descending volley and IPSP onset versus distance. Each point in B and C represents a measurement on one cell. IS, interspinales; UIC, unidentified motoneuron. From Wilson, Yoshida and Schor (1970).

well (see below), shows that in the spinal cord the average conduction velocity of the descending fibers producing the foot of the EPSP is 127 m/sec.

Of greater interest is that MLF stimulation with single shocks evokes IPSPs in many cells, especially in motoneurons innervating interspinales muscles. The apparent segmental delay between the arrival of the visible, fast, descending volley and the start of the IPSP ranges from 0.6–2.1 msec. On this basis most IPSPs appear at least disynaptic. It cannot be assumed *a priori*, however, that the rapidly conducted tract potential reflects the activity of fibers in the inhibitory pathway. It is possible to take advantage of the long distance over which the motoneurons are scattered, plot IPSP latency against distance between stimulating and recording electrodes, and apply linear regression analysis to the data (Fig. 3). This procedure reveals that the tract potential produced by rapidly conducting fibers is not causally related to the IPSP: the time interval between the positive peak of this potential and the IPSP increases with distance. Instead, the IPSP is produced monosynaptically by fibers with an average conduction velocity of 69 m/sec: inhibitory fibers of supraspinal origin reach at least as far as the lower thoracic cord. The precise origin of these inhibitory fibers is not known, but it is not the ipsilateral medial vestibular nucleus. Stimulation of the contra-lateral labyrinth may evoke disynaptic IPSPs in interspinales motoneurons, and we therefore suggest that inhibitory fibers arise from the contralateral vestibular nuclei, perhaps from the medial nucleus. This is consistent with the fact that the MVST is bilateral, and has been traced as far caudally as midthoracic levels by Nyberg–Hansen (1964); physiological evidence suggests it may descend even lower (Precht *et al.*, 1967).

DISCUSSION

As pointed out by Sherrington (1910), 'labyrinthine proprioceptors are largely the equilibrators of the head', and it is therefore not surprising that there is a close rela-tion between labyrinth and neck (and other axial) motoneurons. Deiters' nucleus and the medial vestibular nucleus are the main relays, excitatory and inhibitory, linking the labyrinth to neck segments. As far as their relation with the most rostral cord seg-ments is concerned, the two nuclei seem to act mainly as labyrinthine relays. The vesti-bular input is the dominant one to neurons giving rise to MVST fibers, and an impor-tant one to Deiters' cells projecting to the upper cervical cord, although the activity of both cell groups is modulated by other inputs (Wilson, 1972).

The pathways described above provide discrete excitatory and inhibitory inputs to neck motoneurons, and can subserve the variety of neck reflex responses to labyrin-thine stimulation described by Szentágothai (1952). As the neck is a bilateral structure, there must be close coordination between the corresponding motor nuclei on the two sides in the execution of these reflexes: sometimes the muscles must contract together (for example the splenii during dorsiflexion), sometimes reciprocally (splenii during lateral flexion). In another bilateral structure, the tail, such coordination is aided by the presence in motoneurons of crossed inhibitory, and to a lesser extent excitatory, actions originating in low-threshold, presumably group Ia, fibers (Curtis *et al.*, 1958; Lloyd and Wilson, 1959). Even though head extensor muscles perform tasks that require elaborate spindle control, and contain large numbers of spindles (Granit, 1970, p. 54), no such crossed effects are present in the neck segments (M. E. Anderson, personal communication). Bilateral coordination in reflex activity is apparently due to descending pathways, for example vestibulospinal, and tecto-reticulo-spinal (Anderson *et al.*, 1971).

Some important questions concerning vestibulospinal pathways remain. (*i*) Which receptors have access to the pathways, particularly the inhibitory one? During position change, do impulses arising in the utricle activate inhibitory MVST neurons, or is control of the extensor motoneurons governed by facilitation and disfacilitation through the Deiters'–neck motoneuron pathway? It is possible that inhibition relayed via the medial nucleus is reserved for faster reactions that follow canal activation: many more canal than utricular afferents terminate in the nucleus (Stein and Carpenter, 1967). (*ii*) The relation between the inhibitory fibers to neck motoneurons and those to extraocular motoneurons needs clarification. Recent work suggests that some inhibitory fibers to extraocular (trochlear) motoneurons originate in the superior vestibular nucleus (Baker *et al.*, 1971; Precht and Baker, personal communication). A dual origin of inhibitory fibers is suggested by the fact that whereas labyrinthine disynaptic inhibition of neck motoneurons is blocked by strychnine (Felpel, 1972), inhibition of rabbit oculomotor neurons is blocked by picrotoxin (Ito, Highstein and Tsuchiya, 1970a). Pharmacological investigation of labyrinthine inhibition of abducens motoneurons, believed to relay in the rostral medial nucleus (Baker *et al.*, 1969), is called for. (*iii*) As previously suggested (Wilson and Yoshida, 1969b), there are also excitatory cells in the medial nucleus (Baker *et al.*, 1971; Precht and Baker, personal communication). Are then the dichotomizing fibers known to arise in the nucleus excitatory or inhibitory? (*iv*) Finally, what is the origin of inhibitory fibers to back motoneurons? Answers to these and similar questions, hopefully soon forthcoming, will greatly increase our understanding of the functional organization of the vestibular nuclei and their spinal projection.

VESTIBULOSPINAL ACTIONS ON FORELIMB MOTONEURONS

There has been some recording from forelimb motoneurons, as part of a series of experiments in which hindlimb and neck cells were also studied and Deiters' nucleus was stimulated as described above (Wilson and Yoshida, 1969a). Motoneurons studied included some with axons in the elbow extensors long and lateral heads of triceps; the elbow flexor musculocutaneous; and the mixed extensor and flexor wrist and digit nerves median, ulnar and dorsal interosseus. The results differ from those obtained with neck and back extensor motoneurons in two respects. (1) Stimulation of Deiters' nucleus did not produce monosynaptic excitation of forelimb motoneurons. Polysynaptic EPSPs were often evoked in extensor, and sometimes in flexor, motoneurons by multiple shocks to Deiters', which also evoked polysynaptic IPSPs in flexor motoneurons, and sometimes in extensors. This pattern of effects resembles that found in hindlimb motoneurons by ourselves and others and described elsewhere in this volume, with one exception: the vestibulospinal tract does excite some hindlimb extensors monosynaptically, specifically those of the knee and ankle extensors quadriceps and gastrocnemius (Lund and Pompeiano, 1968; Wilson and Yoshida, 1969a; Grillner et al., 1970). (2) Stimulation of the labyrinth did not evoke synaptic potentials in any cells in response to either single or multiple shocks. Apparently in the case of forelimb motoneurons, as with hindlimb motoneurons (Wilson and Yoshida, 1969a), Deiters' nucleus is not *primarily* a labyrinthine relay, although pathways linking the labyrinth to motoneurons at both levels and including Deiters' nucleus exist (Szentágothai, 1952; Gernandt and Gilman, 1959; Diete–Spiff et al., 1967; Yamauchi and Kato, 1969; Barnes and Pompeiano, 1970).

Our results involve a reasonably small sample of cells (54) and muscle nerves (6). They suggest that monosynaptic connection is not an important feature of the linkage between Deiters' nucleus and forelimb extensor motoneurons but do not rule out its presence, particularly in view of the presence of a quite specific monosynaptic input to some hindlimb extensor motoneurons. Further, more detailed study of Deiters'–forelimb relations is worthwhile, perhaps as part of a more general investigation of the relative importance of mono- and polysynaptic connections between Deiters' nucleus and motoneurons in different animal species.

It should be noted that the MVST apparently has no inhibitory action on motoneurons in forelimb or hindlimb (Wilson and Yoshida, 1969b). Inhibition seems to be produced disynaptically by the VST, acting through segmental inhibitory neurons. While this matter should also be investigated more closely, results so far suggest another difference between vestibular inputs to neck and limb motoneurons: in the former population precise control is present because of the presence of specific excitatory and inhibitory fibers; in the latter one set of descending fibers carries out both functions, and control is less direct and therefore less precise.

SUMMARY

Deiters' nucleus and the medial vestibular nucleus influence cervical and thoracic motoneurons by means of the lateral and medial vestibulospinal tracts. The former consists of excitatory, the latter, at least in part, of inhibitory fibers. The two tracts act as labyrinthine relays to the cells innervating the neck and back muscles, but the activity of the cells of origin is also modulated by other inputs. Excitatory and inhibitory connections between VST and MVST fibers on the one hand, and neck motoneurons on the other, are monosynaptic, permitting direct and precise vestibular control of the neck musculature.

By means of pathways, at least disynaptic, excitatory VST fibers originating in Deiters' nucleus facilitate and inhibit extensor and flexor forelimb motoneurons respectively. In its actions on these neurons the VST does not act primarily as a labyrinthine relay. No MVST action has been observed in forelimb neurons. This pattern of connections resembles that observed in hindlimb motoneurons, with the exception that the VST makes some monosynaptic connections with the latter.

ACKNOWLEDGEMENT

Supported in part by Grants NS 02619 and NS 05463 from the U.S. Public Health Service.

REFERENCES

ANDERSON, M. E., YOSHIDA, M. AND WILSON, V. J., (1971) Influence of the superior colliculus on cat neck motoneurons. *J. Neurophysiol.*, **34**, 898–907.
BAKER, R. G., MANO, N. AND SHIMAZU, H. (1969) Postsynaptic potentials in abducens motoneurons induced by vestibular stimulation. *Brain Res.*, **15**, 577–580.
BAKER, R. G., PRECHT, W. AND LLINÁS, R. (1971) Intracellular potentials evoked in trochlear motoneurons by vestibular nerve activation. *Fed. Proc.*, **30**, 213 (Abstr.).
BARNES, C. D. AND POMPEIANO, O. (1970) Dissociation of presynaptic and postsynaptic effects produced in the lumbar cord by vestibular volleys. *Arch. ital. Biol.*, **108**, 295–324.
BATINI, C., MORUZZI, G. AND POMPEIANO, O. (1957) Cerebellar release phenomena. *Arch. ital. Biol.*, **95**, 71–95.
BRODAL, A., POMPEIANO, O. AND WALBERG, F. (1962) *The Vestibular Nuclei and their Connections. Anatomy and Functional Correlations*. Oliver and Boyd, London, pp. VIII–193.
CURTIS, D. R., DUGGAN, A. W., FELIX, D. AND JOHNSTON, G. A. R. (1970) GABA, bicuculline and central inhibition. *Nature (Lond.)*, **226**, 1222–1224.
CURTIS, D. R., DUGGAN, A. W. AND JOHNSTON, G. A. R. (1969) Glycine, strychnine, picrotoxin and spinal inhibition. *Brain Res.*, **14**, 759–762.
CURTIS, D. R., KRNJEVIC, K. AND MILEDI, R. (1958) Crossed inhibition of sacral motoneurones. *J. Neurophysiol.*, **21**, 319–326.
DIETE–SPIFF, K., CARLI, G. AND POMPEIANO, O. (1967) Comparison of the effects of stimulation of the VIIIth cranial nerve, the vestibular nuclei or the reticular formation on the gastrocnemius muscle and its spindles. *Arch. ital. Biol.*, **105**, 243–272.
FELPEL, L. P. (1972) Effect of strychnine, bicuculline and picrotoxin on labyrinthine-evoked inhibition in neck motoneurons of the cat. *Exp. Brain Res.*, **14**, 494–502.
GERNANDT, B. E. AND GILMAN, S. (1959) Descending vestibular activity and its modulation by proprioceptive, cerebellar and reticular influences. *Exp. Neurol.*, **1**, 274–304.
GRANIT, R. (1970) *The Basis of Motor Control*. Academic Press, London, New York, pp. VI–346.
GRILLNER, S., HONGO, T. AND LUND, S. (1970) The vestibulospinal tract. Effects on alpha motoneurones in the lumbosacral spinal cord in the cat. *Exp. Brain Res.*, **10**, 94–120.
GRILLNER, S. AND LUND, S. (1968) The origin of a descending pathway with monosynaptic action on flexor motoneurones. *Acta physiol. scand.*, **74**, 274–284.
ITO, M., HIGHSTEIN, S. M. AND TSUCHIYA, T. (1970a) The postsynaptic inhibition of rabbit oculomotor neurones by secondary vestibular impulses and its blockage by picrotoxin. *Brain Res.*, **17**, 520–523.
ITO, M., UDO, M. AND MANO, N. (1970b) Long inhibitory and excitatory pathways converging onto cat reticular and Deiters' neurons and their relevance to reticulofugal axons. *J. Neurophysiol.*, **33**, 210–226.
LLOYD, D. P. C. AND WILSON, V. J. (1959) Functional organization in the terminal segments of the spinal cord with a consideration of central excitatory and inhibitory latencies in monosynaptic reflex systems. *J. gen. Physiol.*, **42**, 1219–1232.
LUND, S. AND POMPEIANO, O. (1968) Monosynaptic excitation of alpha motoneurones from supraspinal structures in the cat. *Acta physiol. scand.*, **73**, 1–21.
MAGNUS, R. (1926) Some results of studies in the physiology of posture. *Lancet*, **211**, 531–536, 585–588.
NYBERG-HANSEN, R. (1966) Functional organization of descending supraspinal fibre systems to the spinal cord. Anatomical observations and physiological correlations. *Ergebn. Anat. Entwickl.-Gesch.*, **39**, 1–48.
NYBERG-HANSEN, R. AND MASCITTI, T. A. (1964) Sites and mode of termination of fibers of the vestibulospinal tract in the cat. An experimental study with silver impregnation methods. *J. comp. Neurol.*, **122**, 369–388.

PETERSON, B. W. AND FELPEL, L. P. (1971) Excitation and inhibition of reticulospinal neurons by vestibular, cortical and cutaneous stimulation. *Brain Res.*, **27**, 373–376.

PRECHT, W., GRIPPO, J. AND WAGNER, A. (1967) Contribution of different types of central vestibular neurons to the vestibulospinal system. *Brain Res.*, **4**, 119–123.

SHERRINGTON, C. S. (1910) *The Integrative Action of the Nervous System.* A. Constable, London, pp. XVI–393.

STEIN, B. M. AND CARPENTER, M. B. (1967) Central projections of portions of the vestibular ganglia innervating specific parts of the labyrinth in the Rhesus monkey. *Amer. J. Anat.*, **120**, 281–318.

SZENTÁGOTHAI, J. (1952) *Die Rolle der einzelnen Labyrinthrezeptoren bei der Orientation von Augen und Kopf im Raume.* Akadémiai Kiadó, Budapest, pp. 129.

WILSON, V. J. (1972) Physiological pathways through the vestibular nuclei. *Int. Rev. Neurobiol.*, in press.

WILSON, V. J., KATO, M., PETERSON, B. W. AND WYLIE, R. M. (1967) A single-unit analysis of the organization of Deiters' nucleus. *J. Neurophysiol.*, **30**, 603–619.

WILSON, V. J., WYLIE, R. M. AND MARCO, L. A. (1968) Synaptic inputs to cells in the medial vestibular nucleus. *J. Neurophysiol.*, **31**, 176–185.

WILSON, V. J. AND YOSHIDA, M. (1969a) Comparison of effects of stimulation of Deiters' nucleus and medial longitudinal fasciculus on neck, forelimb and hindlimb motoneurons. *J. Neurophysiol.*, **32**, 743–758.

WILSON, V. J. AND YOSHIDA, M. (1969b) Monosynaptic inhibition of neck motoneurons by the medial vestibular nucleus. *Exp. Brain Res.*, **9**, 365–380.

WILSON, V. J. AND YOSHIDA, M. (1969c) Bilateral connections between labyrinths and neck motoneurons. *Brain Res.*, **13**, 603–607.

WILSON, V. J., YOSHIDA, M. AND SCHOR, R. H. (1970) Supraspinal monosynaptic excitation and inhibition of thoracic back motoneurons. *Exp. Brain Res.*, **11**, 282–295.

YAMAUCHI, T. AND KATO, M. (1969) The effects of electrical stimulation of vestibular nerve from lateral semicircular canal upon spinal cord. *Brain Res.*, **14**, 227–230.

TABLE I

DISTRIBUTION OF PREDOMINANT SYNAPTIC EFFECTS EVOKED FROM THE IPSI- AND CONTRA-
LATERAL VESTIBULOSPINAL TRACTS AND THE MEDIAL LONGITUDINAL FASCICULUS
(MLF, IPSILATERAL) AMONG HINDLIMB MOTONEURONES FUNCTIONING AT DIFFERENT
JOINTS

MS, monosynaptic; DS, disynaptic; TS, trisynaptic; exc., excitation; inh., inhibition. Only the monosynaptic effects from the MLF have been included since other effects have not definitely been proved to originate from the same system. For the effects labelled with * Bruggencate, Lundberg and Udo (unpublished) have shown that among hip extensors adductor femoris and semimembranosus but not the anterior biceps receive disynaptic excitation from the vestibulospinal tract. For the DP motoneurones which can receive either excitation or inhibition (Grillner, Hongo and Lund, 1970), they also found that the ankle flexor, anterior tibial (part of DP), received mainly inhibition but the toe flexor EDL (also part of DP) mainly excitation. Toe and ankle flexor motoneurones were not differentiated in the experiments of contralateral vestibulospinal effects. From Grillner, Hongo and Lund (1971) and Hongo, Kudo and Tanaka (1971).

	Ipsilateral				Contralateral	
	Vestibulospinal			MLF	Vestibulospinal	
	MS exc.	DS exc.	DS inh.	MS exc.	DS exc.	TS inh.
Extensors						
Toe		+		+	+	
Ankle	+	+			+	
Knee	+	+			+	
Hip		+*	(+)	+	+	
Flexors						
Toe		+*		+	} +	
Ankle			+*	+	}	} +
Knee			+	+		+

252 and Hongo *et al.*, 1971). It is hence inferred that the relays are in the lumbosacral spinal cord and that the EPSPs are evoked disynaptically and the IPSPs trisynaptically on the basis of the segmental latencies. The vestibulospinal fibres responsible are descending ipsilaterally (to Deiters' nucleus) in the ventral quadrant to a level below the lower thoracic segments, and it is most likely that the fibres terminate ipsilaterally (*cf.* Nyberg–Hansen and Mascitti, 1964) on interneurones which either cross to the contralateral side directly or influence neurones crossing to the other side.

The disynaptic EPSP can be evoked in hip, knee, ankle and toe extensors, as well as in a group of pretibial flexor cells (Table I). On the other hand the trisynaptic IPSP occurs predominantly in knee and a population of pretibial flexor cells. It is noteworthy that these patterns of distribution of excitatory and inhibitory effects resemble markedly those of polysynaptic excitation and inhibition onto ipsilateral motor nuclei (*cf.* Table I). In fact, the effects from the ipsi- and the contralateral vestibulospinal tract were similar in terms of excitation or inhibition in most of the motoneurones in which effects from both sides were examined. In some motoneurones to thigh muscles (anterior biceps-semimembranosus, gracilis), however, reciprocal effects from the two sides were also observed. It should be noted that the effects exerted on the contralateral side is weaker than the ipsilateral effects, but since they are polysynaptic they might easily be facilitated by other systems.

The monosynaptic effects to motoneurones are direct signals that can be interacted with from other sources only on the motoneuronal level or via presynaptic mechanisms. Concerning the latter possibility, Eide *et al.* (1968) failed to observe inhibition of the descending monosynaptic EPSP after peripheral stimulation that caused presynaptic inhibition of Ia EPSPs in motoneurones. The di- or trisynaptic pathways, on the other hand, have their relay on the segmental level or at least below the lower thoracic level (Grillner *et al.*, 1970), and hence there should be ample opportunities for interaction with other systems in the relay cells. In order to evaluate the possible interaction at the interneuronal level, the effect of conditioning vestibulospinal volleys on test PSPs elicited through segmental reflex arcs has been studied and the reversed conditioning-test situation has also been used. Also the convergence from peripheral nerves on individual interneurones monosynaptically excited from the Deiters' nucleus has been investigated in order to obtain a more general knowledge of the vestibulospinal action on the spinal cord.

Interaction with segmental pathways to motoneurones

Fig. 3 shows recordings from a knee flexor motoneurone (PBSt, *cf.* A) in which a stimulation of Deiters' nucleus with single shock gives no IPSP (B) but stimulation of group I fibres from the knee extensor quadriceps at 1.18 times threshold gives a reciprocal disynaptic Ia IPSP (C). In D–F they are stimulated together at different time intervals; the IPSP is markedly facilitated. The time course of this facilitatory process is shown in the graph below (G, *cf.* legend) which shows that the vestibulospinal tract activates monosynaptically the inhibitory interneurone of the disynaptic Ia inhibitory pathway from extensor to flexor. The corresponding pathway from flexor to extensor was never facilitated. This effect is very constant and occurred in 46 out of 48 tested knee flexor motoneurones but corresponding effects were not found for the motoneurones of the ankle joint. Note that the vestibulospinal tract itself is inhibitory to flexors. IPSPs in extensors, being the excitatory target of the vestibulospinal tract, were never influenced.

The Ia interneurones responsible for the above effects receive recurrent inhibition from the ventral roots (Hultborn and Udo, 1972) as shown in Fig. 4 in which a PBSt motoneurone receives only a very small IPSP from Deiters' nucleus (A) and from the nerve to quadriceps at 1.1 times threshold (B). The facilitation of the interneuronal transmission is very marked (Fig. 4C) when both inputs are activated at a suitable interval. This disynaptic IPSP is completely suppressed in D, when these two volleys are preceded by a stimulation of L5 and L6 ventral roots. From these data it can be concluded that the common interneurones of the Ia inhibitory pathway and the vestibulospinal disynaptic pathway to motoneurones receive recurrent inhibition

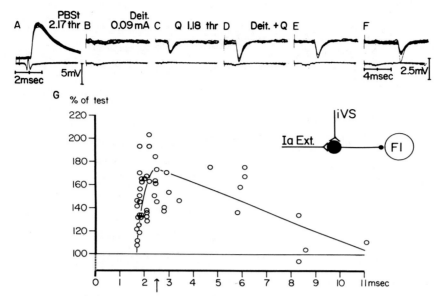

Fig. 3. Vestibulospinal monosynaptic facilitation of the Ia inhibitory pathway to knee flexors. The upper traces in A–F show intracellular records from a PBSt cell and the lower traces the cord dorsum potential recorded at the segmental level. In D–F quadriceps group I fibres are stimulated at different intervals of time after a conditioning stimulus to the Deiters' nucleus, and a marked facilitation occurs of the disynaptic Ia IPSP. The time course of the facilitation is shown in the graph. Ordinate: amplitude of Ia IPSP in relation to control (C). Abscissa: at 0 the Deiters' nucleus is stimulated with single shock, and the time delay (msec) between this stimulation and the incoming nerve volley from quadriceps is plotted. The arrow indicates the arrival of the descending volley to the segment of L7. The line connecting the different points is fitted by eye. Note that the facilitation is maximal when the descending (vestibulospinal) and the incoming (nerve) volley arrive simultaneously to the segment. Since the Ia inhibitory pathway is disynaptic, this implies that there is a monosynaptic activation of the Ia inhibitory interneurones as outlined in the diagram to the right in the figure.

From Grillner, Hongo and Lund (unpublished).

from the ventral roots. This recurrent inhibition of the Ia interneurones is mainly responsible (Hultborn *et al.*, 1971) for the 'recurrent disinhibition' (Wilson and Burgess, 1962) of motoneurones and is organized so that the recurrent inhibition from the knee extensors inhibits the transmission in the Ia inhibitory pathway to flexors and consequently disinhibits these motoneurones.

Fig. 5 shows that the Ia IPSP from quadriceps in a knee flexor motoneurone is markedly facilitated if it is preceded by a volley from the Deiters' nucleus contralateral to the recorded motoneurone (*cf.* legend). The time course of this facilitation is shown in the graph of Fig. 5 (*cf.* Fig. 3 for the facilitation of ipsilateral effects, also legend) from which it is evident that the Ia inhibitory interneurone is not impinged upon monosynaptically as for the ipsilateral effects, but at least one extra interneurone should be interposed between the vestibulospinal fibres and the inhibitory last order interneurone.

The extensive convergence found on this 'Ia inhibitory interneurone' is summarized in Fig. 6, which includes also an input from contralateral cutaneous and high threshold

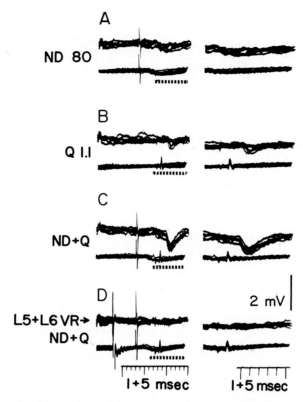

Fig. 4. Recurrent inhibition from the ventral roots of the common inhibitory path to knee flexor motoneurones from the Ia afferents and the vestibulospinal tract. The upper traces show intracellular records from a flexor motoneuıone and the lower traces were recorded on the cord dorsum. Records in the right column show the same events as in the left but at a faster time base. In A and B the Deiters' nucleus (80 μA) and the nerve to quadriceps (1.1 × threshold) were stimulated separately with no marked postsynaptic effects. When both were stimulated together at appropriate intervals a marked spatial facilitation occurs (C), indicating that the resulting IPSP is due to interneurones common for the two inputs. If this IPSP is preceded by an antidromic single volley in L5 and L6 ventral roots, it is entirely abolished (D). Hence these inhibitory interneurones receive recurrent inhibition from the ventral roots. From Hultborn and Udo (1972).

muscle afferents (coFRA) found by Bruggencate *et al.* (1969). Also other descending pathways impinge upon this type of interneurone (*cf.* Lundberg, 1970). In view of this wide convergence pattern it may be asked if it is misleading to call them 'Ia inhibitory interneurones'.

Reflex effects from other ipsilateral afferents (Ib, II, III muscle, cutaneous) were not facilitated from the ipsilateral Deiters' nucleus when the short-latency segmental reflex pattern was investigated (Grillner *et al.*, 1966b). However, the disynaptic EPSPs (Fig. 7) and IPSPs evoked from the ipsilateral Deiters' nucleus could readily be facilitated by volleys in contralateral high threshold (group II and III) muscle and cutaneous afferents, which evoke the crossed extension reflex (Bruggencate *et al.*, 1969). This indicates that the facilitatory convergence occurs at the last order inter-

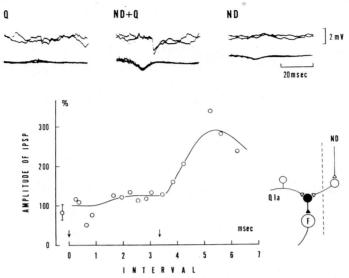

Fig. 5. Convergence between the contralateral vestibulospinal tract and the Ia inhibitory pathway to knee flexors. The upper traces were recorded intracellularly from a knee flexor motoneurone (PBSt) and the lower show the cord dorsum potentials. Stimulation of the nerve to quadriceps (Q, 1.2 × threshold) gave rise to a small IPSP, whereas the Deiters' nucleus (ND) gave virtually no postsynaptic effects. If the stimulation of Q was preceded by a stimulation of Deiters' nucleus (4 shocks at 50 μA) a disynaptic Ia IPSP was strongly facilitated (ND + Q). The time course of this facilitation is illustrated in the graph below (another PBSt cell). The ordinate shows the amplitude of the conditioned IPSP in relation to the control (S.D. indicated by a vertical bar on the left) and the abscissa the interval between the arrival of the descending volley of the first pulse to Deiters' nucleus and the arrival of the Ia afferent volley to the segment. The arrows indicate the arrival of the first (left) and the second descending volley. Note that the peak of facilitation occurs when the incoming nerve volley arrives later (by 1.5–2.0 msec) than the descending volley (*cf.* right arrow) and that the facilitation appears to start with about 1.0–1.4 msec longer latencies compared with ipsilateral effects (note the difference from the ipsilateral effects, *cf.* Fig. 3). This would indicate that one additional interneurone is intercalated between the vestibulospinal fiber and the Ia inhibitory interneurone as outlined in the diagram to the right. From Hongo, Kudo and Tanaka (unpublished).

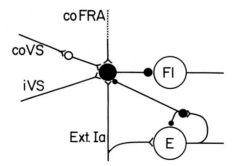

Fig. 6. Convergence on the interneuronal level in the Ia inhibitory pathway to knee flexor motoneurones. The different inputs to the Ia inhibitory interneurone are summarized. Large and small filled circles indicate inhibitory neurones and synapses respectively; open circles and dichotomizing lines indicate excitatory neurones and synapses respectively. The abbreviations stand for Fl, flexor; E, extensor; coFRA, contralateral flexor reflex afferents, *i.e.*, cutaneous and high threshold muscle afferents; iVS and coVS, ipsi- and contralateral vestibulospinal tract.

References pp. 260–262

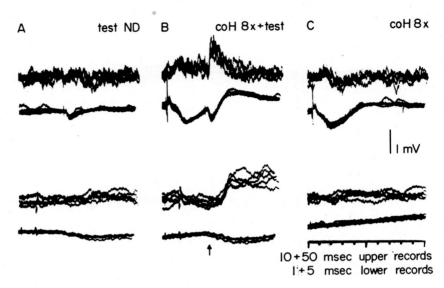

Fig. 7. Facilitation of the disynaptic vestibulospinal EPSP in extensors by a volley from the contralateral hamstring nerve. The upper beams show intracellular records from an ankle extensor motoneurone and the lower beam the cord dorsum potentials. Each column shows the same event at a slow (upper pair) and a fast timebase (lower pair). Single shock to Deiters' nucleus gives virtually no effect (A), whereas a volley in the contralateral hamstring including group II afferents (no effects by a group I volley) gives small mixed effects (C). When both inputs are stimulated together a large EPSP occurs as a response to the stimulation of Deiters' nucleus with a segmental latency of 1.1 msec (cf. lower records in B, arrow indicates arrival of first peak of initial descending volley) which only allows a disynaptic linkage. Hence convergence occurs on the last order excitatory interneurone. From Bruggencate et al. (1969).

TABLE II

EFFECTS FROM THE VESTIBULOSPINAL TRACT ON SPINAL REFLEX PATHWAYS

Abbreviations are Ext, extensor; Flex, flexor; i, ipsilateral, i.e., cutaneous and high threshold muscle and joint afferents; Inh., inhibition; Exc., excitation; di, disynaptic; poly, polysynaptic. 'ipsilateral' or 'contralateral' is in reference to the side of motoneuronal recording. Where marked with asterisk, some effects could be observed on rare occasions.

Kinds of reflexes examined		Effects from ipsilateral tract	Effects from contralateral tract
Ia	Inh. (di) Ext → Flex (knee)	facilitation	facilitation
	Flex → Ext	none	none
Ib	Exc. (di)	none	none
	Inh. (di)	none	none
iFRA	Exc. (poly)	none*	none*
	Inh. (poly)	none*	none*
coFRA	Exc. (poly) to Ext	facilitation	facilitation
	Inh. (poly) to Flex	facilitation	facilitation

neurones of the reflex pathway. Corresponding findings have been made for the crossed vestibulospinal effects (Hongo et al., 1971), i.e., disynaptic EPSPs and trisynaptic IPSPs from the contralateral Deiters' nucleus are facilitated at an interneuronal level by volleys from the contralateral FRA to the recording side.

Table II summarizes which reflex paths are influenced from the Deiters' nucleus, the exact correspondence between the ipsi- and the contralateral side is striking. *To summarize, a surprisingly simple pattern has emerged, the vestibulospinal tract facilitates generally reflex arcs which give the same effect to α-motoneurones as it gives itself, i.e., excitation to extensors and inhibition to flexors. The effects are exerted bilaterally and the convergence with the reflex pathways is on the last order interneurone.* *

Facilitatory interaction between the ipsi- and the contralateral vestibulospinal tract at the spinal level

Similarities in effects of the ipsilateral and the contralateral vestibulospinal tract on

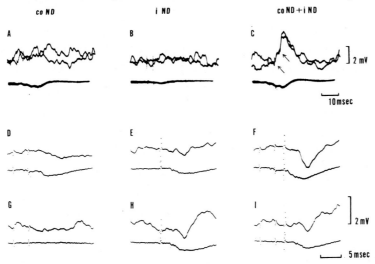

Fig. 8. Facilitation of ipsilateral vestibulospinal effects by volleys in the contralateral vestibulospinal tract. Upper beams are intracellularly recorded in a flexor digitorum-hallucis longus motoneurone (A–C) and a knee flexor motoneurone (PBSt) (D–I) and the lower on the cord dorsum. The left and the middle columns respectively show effects of stimulation of the contralateral Deiters' nucleus (200 μA in A and 80 μA in D and G) and of the ipsilateral Deiters' nucleus (90 μA in B and 85 μA in E and H), and in the right column the contralateral side was stimulated prior to the ipsilateral side. Note the marked facilitation of disynaptic EPSPs and IPSPs respectively in C and F. In G–I the contralateral ventral quadrant (the dorsal quadrant had been cut before the start of experiments) was cut at lower thoracic level. The IPSP in H was then not influenced when conditioned by a contralateral Deiters' volley (I), which shows that the effects seen in F are due to descending impulses on the contralateral side. After the partial spinal transection the test volley from the ipsilateral Deiters' nucleus evoked EPSPs following the disynaptic IPSP (H). From Aoyama, Hongo, Kudo and Tanaka (1971).

---

* This is, however, uncertain for the facilitatory interaction of inhibition between the tract and the FRA, both contralateral to the recording side.

many motoneurones and on reflex pathways as described above would suggest the existence of common interneuronal paths shared by both vestibulospinal tracts, which has been verified by Aoyama *et al.* (1971). Fig. 8D–F shows that the disynaptic IPSP evoked from the ipsilateral vestibulospinal tract in a knee flexor cell (E) is markedly facilitated after conditioning stimuli to the contralateral Deiters' nucleus (F), the effect of the latter being negligible by itself (D). Similarly, ipsilateral excitation, di- or polysynaptic, to extensor motoneurones may be facilitated by contralateral stimulation (Fig. 8A–C). In these experiments the commissural fibres between the vestibular nuclei of both sides were transected by a vertical incision in the midline from obex to the inferior colliculi (depths 3–4 mm). The following results support the notion that the main site of the facilitation is not in the Deiters' nucleus used as a test (ipsilateral) but in the lumbar segments: (*i*) ipsilateral effects evoked from the axonal region of the Deiters' nucleus are also facilitated by stimulation of the contralateral Deiters' nucleus; (*ii*) the facilitation evoked from the contralateral Deiters' nucleus is abolished by transection of the contralateral spinal half at the lowest thoracic level (Fig. 8G–I, compare with D–F).

The latency for the facilitation as indicated by the time interval between the first conditioning and the test shocks can be in the order of 3–4 msec for the inhibitory effects. These data do not allow a conclusion on whether the contralateral vestibulo-spinal tract impinges disynaptically on the inhibitory interneurone which is excited monosynaptically from the ipsilateral side or if a more complex relay is responsible. Usually, longer latencies (9–15 msec from the first conditioning volley) are required to facilitate excitatory effects to extensor motoneurones, indicating a rather complex pathway for interaction. However, recent experiments under different anaesthetic conditions showed that the excitatory effects can interact with as short latencies as the inhibitory ones.

Effects on interneurones

The data above give indirect information regarding what kind of interneurones can be influenced by vestibulospinal volleys. Interneurones (L5–L7, *cf.* legend) monosynapti-cally activated from the vestibulospinal tract are located in the ventromedial part of the gray matter, largely in Rexed's lamina VII–VIII, which coincides with the region where the vestibulospinal tract gives a large and sharp negative field potential (Grill-ner, Hongo and Lund, unpublished paper). Many of these interneurones were readily activated by descending volleys and could follow very high frequencies (600 Hz) of stimulation as shown in Fig. 9A–J. This is a necessary property for the interneurones mediating, for example, the disynaptic PSPs to motoneurones, which require at an average only 0.6 msec longer latency than the monosynaptic EPSPs (Grillner *et al.*, 1970). The majority of the interneurones monosynaptically excited from Deiters' nucleus also received convergence of polysynaptic excitatory effects from the ipsilateral FRA but not from group I muscular afferents. This was in cats in which the reflex effects from FRA to α-motoneurones were mainly excitatory to flexors and inhibitory to extensors, and it is therefore difficult to believe that these interneurones should be

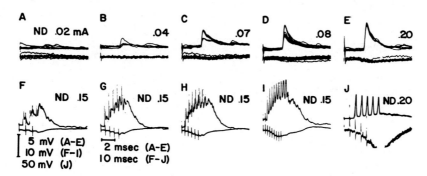

Fig. 9. Monosynaptic activation of an interneurone in Rexed's layer VIII (L6). The upper traces show intracellular records in response to single shock stimulation of Deiters' nucleus at progressively increasing strength (A–E) and to repetitive stimulation at different frequencies (F–I). The lower beams show recordings from the cord dorsum. In A–E the cell was hyperpolarized by a constant current (5 nA) in order to block the generation of action potentials. Note in F–J that the spike is generated directly during the rise of the monosynaptic EPSP and hence this type of interneurone is very effectively activated. From Grillner, Hongo and Lund (unpublished).

intercalated in a pathway to ipsilateral α-motoneurones or at least not in a short latency pathway that can be revealed under the present experimental conditions with an anaesthetized cat 'at rest'.

The vestibulospinal tract gives, however, disynaptic excitation and trisynaptic inhibition to contralateral α-motoneurones and it is thus possible that these recorded interneurones send their axons to the contralateral side of the spinal cord, particularly since these effects can be facilitated from cutaneous and high threshold muscle afferents ipsilateral to the stimulated Deiters' nucleus. Also a few interneurones with convergence both from quadriceps Ia afferents and from the vestibulospinal tract were found in a region which coincides with that found for the Ia interneurones transmitting Ia inhibition to α-motoneurones (Hultborn et al., 1971; Jankowska and Roberts, 1971). These interneurones are very likely responsible for transmitting the ipsilateral disynaptic and the contralateral trisynaptic inhibitory effects where the Ia afferents interact with the vestibulospinal tract volleys.

Aoyama et al. (1971) hence found the same type of interneurones which in addition receive polysynaptic excitation from Deiters' nucleus of the contralateral side. This would be expected from the results obtained in motoneurones regarding facilitation of reflex paths and also between descending effects from Deiters' nuclei of both sides. The interneurone of Fig. 10 receives monosynaptic excitation from the ipsilateral Deiters' nucleus (A, B) and polysynaptic effects from the contralateral side (C).

An additional group of cells deserve some comments. They constitute a substantial part of the whole sample of cells recorded from the medial part of the ventral horn. By contrast to the previously described cells, they receive reciprocal effects from the two sides of the Deiters' nuclei, excitation from the ipsilateral (Fig. 10D) and inhibition from the contralateral side (Fig. 10E). The shortest linkage is monosynaptic for the excitation and disynaptic for the inhibition. The evidence for a disynaptic linkage of the contralateral inhibition was derived from comparison of latencies of the IPSPs

256   S. GRILLNER, T. HONGO

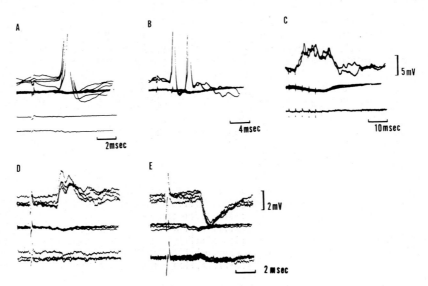

Fig. 10. Two lumbar interneurones receiving convergent excitatory (A–C) and reciprocal (D–E) synaptic effects from ipsi- and contralateral Deiters' nucleus. The uppermost traces are intracellular records, the second traces cord dorsum potentials, the third traces extracellular field potentials just outside the cells and the fourth trace (only in A) the cord dorsum potentials. The ipsilateral Deiters' nucleus was stimulated in A and B (150 μA) and in D (200 μA), and the contralateral Deiters' nucleus was stimulated in C (150 μA) and E (200 μA). From Aoyama, Hongo, Kudo and Tanaka (unpublished).

evoked from two levels, Deiters' nucleus and the lowest thoracic cord, in the same interneurone. Similar reciprocal effects were found also in some ascending cells in the ventral horn with their axons on the contralateral side (Aoyama, Hongo, Kudo and Tanaka, unpublished paper).

Although some of the patterns of convergence between the vestibulospinal pathway and the periphery are easy to correlate to the findings in α-motoneurones described above, some interneuronal convergence patterns are difficult to understand. It must be realized that the vestibulospinal tract might well influence reflex pathways that are concealed under ordinary experimental conditions (Holmqvist and Lundberg, 1961; Lundberg, 1966) and moreover many of these interneurones might terminate on ascending cells, particularly those situated in the ventral horn (Grillner, Hongo and Lund, unpublished paper). The vestibulospinal tract terminates not only on moto-neurones and interneurones of the spinal cord but also on ascending cells as spino-reticulo-cerebellar neurones (Grillner et al., 1968b) and ventral spinocerebellar tract neurones (Baldissera and Weight, 1969; Baldissera and Bruggencate, 1969). The former neurones receive a very strong monosynaptic activation, and single volleys in the vestibulospinal tract regularly discharge the spinoreticular neurones which are part of a cerebello-vestibulo-spino-reticulo-cerebellar loop (see diagram in Fig. 11). It is interesting to note that the ipsilateral vestibulospinal tract can influence the ipsilateral lateral reticular nucleus directly (Ladpli and Brodal, 1968) as well as the contralateral lateral reticular nucleus via the spinoreticular neurones (Grillner et al., 1968b;

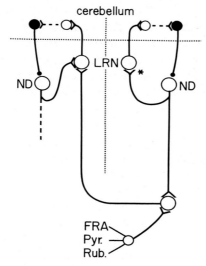

Fig. 11. The vestibulospinal control of the spinoreticulo-cerebellar pathway and the relation to cerebellum. Large and small filled circles indicate inhibitory neurones and synapses respectively; open circles and dichotomizing lines indicate excitatory neurones and synapses respectively. Abbreviations used are ND, Deiters' nucleus; LRN, lateral reticular nucleus; FRA, flexor reflex afferents, *i.e.*, cutaneous and high threshold muscle and joint afferents; Pyr, pyramidal tract; Rub, rubrospinal tract. The direct connexions from Deiters' nucleus to the lateral reticular nucleus, indicated by an asterisk, is established anatomically but not physiologically (Ladpli and Brodal, 1968). The vertical interrupted line indicates the midline, and the horizontal the limit to the cerebellum. The possible cerebellar circuitry is drawn in a simplified and tentative fashion.

Grant *et al.*, 1966). The latter are strongly influenced from interneurones activated from cutaneous and high threshold muscular afferents (Lundberg and Oscarsson, 1962; Oscarsson, 1967) and from the pyramidal and the rubrospinal tracts (Lundberg *et al.*, 1963; Magni and Oscarsson, 1961; Baldissera, Hultborn, Lundberg and Weight, unpublished paper). It is thought that this ascending tract signals the ongoing interneuronal activity rather than any particular peripheral events (Lundberg, 1959, 1964).

FUNCTIONAL CONSIDERATIONS

In a discussion of the physiological role in motor control of this system it is necessary to consider the descending effects not only to α- but also to γ-motoneurones. With regard to the direct effects to α- and γ-motoneurones, the vestibulospinal tract provides the most striking example of α-γ-linkage (Fig. 12) with monosynaptic as well as disynaptic excitatory connexions to both kinds of motoneurones (Grillner *et al.*, 1966a, c; 1969, 1970). Grillner (1969a) found indirect evidence suggesting that only static but not dynamic γ-motoneurones are influenced from the vestibulospinal tract. It is important to note that during a muscle contraction (with shortening) the spindle afferents can increase their discharge rate only if they are under bias from static γ-motoneurones, and hence a linkage between α- and static γ-motoneurones would be particularly purposeful (Grillner, 1969b). In addition Fig. 12 demonstrates that the reciprocal Ia inhibition exerted through the 'extensor γ-loop' is facilitated by direct vestibulospinal effects on the Ia inhibitory interneurones (*cf.* above) as well as a reciprocal inhibition of the γ-motoneurones indicated tentatively (*cf.* Kato and Tanji, 1971). Some caution must of course be taken in the interpretation of the finding that α- and γ-motoneurones belonging to the same motor nucleus receive monosynaptic excitation from vestibulospinal fibres with the same conduction velocity, since this does not necessarily mean that the same fibres are responsible, although this possibility seems to us more likely.

Except for the findings of Fulton *et al.* (1930) suggesting that the vestibulospinal tract should be one of the pathways responsible for the maintenance of decerebrate rigidity (assuming a relation to postural mechanisms) very little has been known about this pathway from the functional point of view. However, Orlovski (1972) has recently shown that 67% of antidromically identified vestibulospinal neurones were modulated in phase with the locomotor cycle during walk or trot. Fifty-five per cent of the total number had their maximal activity at the end of the swing or at the beginning of the stance phase. Note that the EMG-activity of extensors commences in the end of the swing phase (*e.g.*, Engberg and Lundberg, 1969). The activity of these vestibulospinal neurones thus coincides with the activity of the extensor muscles. Twelve per cent of the recorded neurones were also modulated in the locomotor rhythm but in a somewhat different phase relation to the locomotor cycle. These data were obtained on mesencephalic cats, which can perform good locomotion on a tread-mill if the 'locomotor region' beneath the inferior colliculi is stimulated continuously (Shik *et al.*, 1966). Cerebellectomized mesencephalic cats can also perform locomotion,

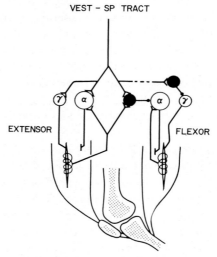

Fig. 12. Vestibulospinal connexions to α- and γ-motoneurones controlling the knee joint muscles. Large and small filled circles indicate inhibitory neurones and synapses respectively; open circles and dichotomizing lines indicate excitatory neurones and synapses respectively. For simplicity the disynaptic excitatory connexions to α- and γ-motoneurones from the vestibulospinal tract has been excluded from the diagram. Note that the γ-motoneurones probably are of the static type (*cf.* text).

which, however, is somewhat less well coordinated. Thus it is interesting that cerebellectomy invariably causes a complete disappearance of modulation of vestibulospinal neurones in the locomotor rhythm. It can be concluded that the phasic modulation itself of the neurones in Deiters' nucleus is not responsible for the phasic extensor activity during locomotion. The fact that locomotion can remain also after destruction of the Deiters' nucleus (even if the locomotion is weak) shows that the vestibulospinal tract itself is not responsible for the basic neuronal mechanism of locomotion. *It seems likely that the function of the vestibulospinal tract during locomotion is to coordinate and adjust the extensor activity to an optimal level during each cycle, presumably through the influence of cerebellum or its nuclei.*

In relation to locomotion, the vestibulospinal effects on the ipsilateral side are easy to understand. But the fact that the vestibulospinal tract exerts identical effects also on the contralateral lumbosacral enlargement (Hongo *et al.*, 1971) is somewhat difficult to understand, since during trot and walk the two hindlimbs have a different phase relation to each other. However, during the gallop in cats they are activated simultaneously (Roberts, 1967). The contra- and the ipsilateral effects might be exerted by different vestibulospinal fibres. If this is not the case, it is possible that the effects to the contralateral side can be blocked at an interneuronal level when not needed (*e.g.*, during trot or walk) but can be opened when bilateral extensor activity is required as in gallop, jumping or other postural conditions. The reciprocal effects on interneurones from the two sides of Deiters' nuclei (Fig. 10 D, E) might be interpreted along this line assuming that such interneurones are relays to the contralateral side.

Finally it must be recognized that the Deiters' nucleus is derived ontogenetically from the same structures as the reticular formation (Ariens Kappers *et al.*, 1960; *cf.* also Vraa–Jensen, 1956) and it is probably not correct to look at this system as primarily a vestibular system. There is a fast reticulospinal pathway descending in MLF (Grillner and Lund, 1966, 1968) that has striking similarities with the vestibulospinal system, the difference being that they often act reciprocally at the same joints. It has been suggested that these two descending systems might constitute parts of one control system for control of flexors and extensors particularly related to cerebellum (Grillner *et al.*, 1971). Whether this is so remains to be shown.

SUMMARY

The report deals with effects from the vestibulospinal tract on neurones in the lumbosacral spinal cord.

1. Effects of the vestibulospinal tract on α- and γ-motoneurones: (a) monosynaptic and disynaptic effects exerted ipsilaterally: (b) di- and trisynaptic effects exerted contralaterally.

2. Effects on the segmental interneuronal apparatus: (a) vestibulospinal effects on transmission in segmental reflex arcs to motoneurones; (b) interaction between the ipsi- and the contralateral vestibulospinal tract on interneurones influencing α-motoneurones; (c) convergence pattern on interneurones and ascending lumbosacral neurones with monosynaptic excitation from Deiters' nucleus.

3. Functional considerations: (a) α-γ-linkage; (b) the vestibulospinal tract during locomotion; (c) relations with a reticulospinal system descending in MLF.

ACKNOWLEDGEMENTS

The authors are greatly indebted to Drs. Aoyama, Baldissera, Hultborn, Kudo, Lundberg, Orlovski, Tanaka, Udo and Weight for permission to reproduce and discuss their unpublished data.

REFERENCES

AOYAMA, M., HONGO, T., KUDO, N. AND TANAKA, R. (1971) Convergent effects from the bilateral vestibulospinal tracts on spinal interneurons. *Brain Res.*, **35**, 250–253.
ARIENS KAPPERS, C. U., HUBER, G. C. AND CROSBY, E. C. (1960) *The Comparative Anatomy of the Nervous System of Vertebrates, Including Man.* Hafner, New York, pp. 645–689.
BALDISSERA, F. AND BRUGGENCATE, G. TEN (1969) Rubrospinal effects on spinal border cells. *Acta physiol. scand.*, **77**, Suppl. 330, 119.
BALDISSERA, F. AND WEIGHT, F. (1969) Descending monosynaptic connexions to spinal border cells. *Acta physiol. scand.*, **76**, 28–29A.
BRUGGENCATE, G. TEN, BURKE, R., LUNDBERG, A. AND UDO, M. (1969) Interaction between the vestibulospinal tract, contralateral flexor reflex afferents and Ia afferents. *Brain Res.*, **14**, 529–532.
CARLI, G., DIETE–SPIFF, K. AND POMPEIANO, O. (1966) Skeletomotor and fusimotor control of gastrocnemius muscle from Deiters' nucleus. *Experientia (Basel)*, **22**, 583–584.
CARLI, G., DIETE–SPIFF, K. AND POMPEIANO, O. (1967) Responses of the muscle spindles and of extrafusal fibres in an extensor muscle to stimulation of the lateral vestibular nucleus in the cat. *Arch. ital. Biol.*, **105**, 209–242.
EIDE, E., JURNA, I. AND LUNDBERG, A. (1968) Conductance measurements from motoneurons during presynaptic inhibition. In C. VON EULER, S. SKOGLUND AND U. SÖDERBERG (Eds.), *Structure and Functions of Inhibitory Neuronal Mechanisms*, Pergamon Press, Oxford, pp. 215–219.
ENGBERG, I. AND LUNDBERG, A. (1969) An electromyographic analysis of muscular activity in the hindlimb of the cat during unrestrained locomotion. *Acta physiol. scand.*, **75**, 614–630.
FULTON, J. F., LIDDELL, E. G. T. AND RIOCH, D. MCK. (1930) The influence of unilateral destruction of the vestibular nuclei upon posture and the knee-jerk. *Brain*, **53**, 327–343.
GACEK, R. R. (1969) The course and central termination of first order neurons supplying vestibular endorgans in the cat. *Acta oto-laryng. (Stockh.)*, Supp. 254, 1–66.
GRANT, G., OSCARSSON, O. AND ROSÉN, I. (1966) Functional organization of the spino-reticulo-cerebellar path with identification of its spinal component. *Exp. Brain Res.*, **1**, 306–319.
GRILLNER, S. (1969a) The influence of DOPA on the static and the dynamic fusimotor activity to the triceps surae of the spinal cat. *Acta physiol. scand.*, **77**, 490–509.
GRILLNER, S. (1969b) Supraspinal and segmental control of static and dynamic γ-motoneurones in the cat. *Acta physiol. scand.*, **77**, Suppl. 327, 1–34.
GRILLNER, S., HONGO, T. AND LUND, S. (1966a) Descending pathways with monosynaptic action on motoneurones. *Acta physiol. scand.*, **68**, Suppl. 277, 60.
GRILLNER, S., HONGO, T. AND LUND, S. (1966b) Interaction between the inhibitory pathways from the Deiters' nucleus and Ia afferents to flexor motoneurones. *Acta physiol. scand.*, **68**, Suppl. 277, 61.
GRILLNER, S., HONGO, T. AND LUND, S. (1966c) Monosynaptic excitation of spinal γ-motoneurones from the brain stem. *Experientia (Basel)*, **22**, 691.
GRILLNER, S., HONGO, T. AND LUND, S., (1968a) Reciprocal effects between two descending bulbospinal systems with monosynaptic connections to spinal motoneurones. *Brain Res.*, **10**, 477–480.
GRILLNER, S., HONGO, T. AND LUND, S. (1968b) The origin of descending fibres monosynaptically activating spinoreticular neurones, *Brain Res.*, **10**, 259–262.
GRILLNER, S., HONGO, T. AND LUND, S. (1969) Descending monosynaptic and reflex control of γ-motoneurones. *Acta physiol. scand.*, **75**, 592–613.

GRILLNER, S., HONGO, T. AND LUND, S. (1970) The vestibulospinal tract. Effects on alpha-moto-neurones in the lumbosacral spinal cord in the cat. *Exp. Brain Res.*, **10**, 94–120.

GRILLNER, S., HONGO, T. AND LUND, S. (1971) Convergent effects on alpha motoneurones from the vestibulospinal tract and a pathway descending in the medial longitudinal fasciculus. *Exp. Brain Res.*, **12**, 457–479.

GRILLNER, S. AND LUND, S. (1966) A descending pathway with monosynaptic action on flexor motoneurones. *Experientia (Basel)*, **22**, 390.

GRILLNER, S. AND LUND, S. (1968) The origin of a descending pathway with monosynaptic action on flexor motoneurones. *Acta physiol. scand.*, **74**, 274–284.

HOLMQVIST, B. AND LUNDBERG, A. (1961) Differential supraspinal control of synaptic actions evoked by volleys in the flexion reflex afferents in alpha motoneurones. *Acta physiol. scand.*, **54**, Suppl. 186, 1–51.

HONGO, T., KUDO, N. AND TANAKA, R. (1971) Effects from the vestibulospinal tract on the contralateral hindlimb motoneurones in the cat. *Brain Res.*, **31**, 220–223.

HULTBORN, H., JANKOWSKA, E. AND LINDSTRÖM, S. (1971) Recurrent inhibition of interneurones monosynaptically activated from group Ia afferents. *J. Physiol (Lond.)*, **215**, 613–636.

HULTBORN, H. AND UDO, M., (1971) Convergence in the reciprocal Ia inhibitory pathway of excitation from descending pathways and inhibition from motor axon collaterals. *Acta physiol. scand.*, **84**, 95–108.

ITO, M., HONGO, T., YOSHIDA, M., OKADA, Y. AND OBATA, K. (1964) Antidromic and trans-synaptic activation of Deiters' neurones induced from the spinal cord. *Jap. J. Physiol.*, **14**, 638–658.

JANKOWSKA, E. AND ROBERTS, W. (1971) Function of single interneurones established by their mono-synaptic inhibitory effects on motoneurones. *Acta physiol. scand.*, **82**, 24–25A.

KATO, M. AND TANJI, J. (1971) Effects of Deiters' nucleus stimulation on hindlimb fusimotor neurons in cats. *Proc. XXV int. Congr. physiol. Sci.*, Munich, IX, n. 866, 293.

LADPLI, R. AND BRODAL, A. (1968) Experimental studies of commissural and reticular formation projections from the vestibular nuclei in the cat. *Brain Res.*, **8**, 65–96.

LORENTE DE NÓ, R. (1933) Anatomy of the eighth nerve. The central projection of the nerve endings of the internal ear. *Laryngoscope (St. Louis)*, **43**, 1–38.

LUND, S. AND POMPEIANO, O. (1965) Descending pathways with monosynaptic action on moto-neurones. *Experientia (Basel)*, **21**, 602–603.

LUND, S. AND POMPEIANO, O. (1968) Monosynaptic excitation of alpha motoneurones from supra-spinal structures in the cat. *Acta physiol. scand.*, **73**, 1–21.

LUNDBERG, A. (1959) Integrative significance of patterns of connections made by muscle afferents in the spinal cord. *Proc. XXI int. Congr. physiol. Sci.*, Buenos Aires, 1–5.

LUNDBERG, A. (1964) Ascending spinal hindlimb pathways in the cat. In J. C. ECCLES AND J. P. SCHADÉ (Eds.), *Progress in Brain Research. Vol. 12. Physiology of spinal neurons*. Elsevier, Amsterdam, pp. 135–163.

LUNDBERG, A. (1966) Integration in the reflex pathway. In R. GRANIT (Ed.), *Muscular Afferents and Motor Control. Nobel Symposium I*. Almqvist and Wiksell, Stockholm, pp. 275–305.

LUNDBERG, A. (1970) The excitatory control of the Ia inhibitory pathway. In P. ANDERSEN AND J. K. S. JANSEN (Eds.), *Excitatory Synaptic Mechanisms*. Universitetsforlaget, Oslo, pp. 333–340.

LUNDBERG, A., NORRSELL, U. AND VOORHOEVE, P. (1963) Effects from the sensorimotor cortex on ascending spinal pathways. *Acta physiol. scand.*, **59**, 462–473.

LUNDBERG, A. AND OSCARSSON, O. (1962) Two ascending spinal pathways in the ventral part of the cord. *Acta physiol. scand.*, **54**, 270–286.

MAGNI, F. AND OSCARSSON, O. (1961) Cerebral control of transmission to the ventral spinocerebellar tract. *Arch. ital. Biol.*, **99**, 369–396.

NYBERG-HANSEN, R. (1964) Origin and termination of fibers from the vestibular nuclei descending in the medial longitudinal fasciculus. An experimental study with silver impregnation methods in the cat. *J. comp. Neurol.*, **122**, 355–367.

NYBERG-HANSEN, R. (1969) Do cat spinal motoneurones receive direct supraspinal fibre connections? A supplementary silver study. *Arch. ital. Biol.*, **107**, 67–78.

NYBERG-HANSEN, R. AND MASCITTI, T. A. (1964) Sites and mode of termination of fibers of the vestibulospinal tract in the cat. An experimental study with silver impregnation methods. *J. comp. Neurol.*, **122**, 369–387.

ORLOVSKII, G. N. (1972) The activity of vestibulospinal neurones to the lumbosacral cord during locomotion, *Brain Res.*, in press.

Oscarsson, O. (1967) Functional significance of information channels from the spinal cord to the cerebellum. In D. P. Purpura and M. D. Yahr (Eds.), *Neurophysiological Basis of Normal and Abnormal Motor Activities*, Raven Press, Hewlett, N.Y., pp. 93–117.

Pompeiano, O., Diete–Spiff, K. and Carli, G. (1967) Two pathways transmitting vestibulospinal influences from the lateral vestibular nucleus of Deiters' to extensor fusimotor neurones. *Pflügers Arch. ges. Physiol.*, **293**, 272–275.

Rexed, B. (1954) A cytoarchitectonic atlas of the spinal cord in the cat. *J. comp. Neurol.*, **100**, 297–379.

Roberts, T. D. M. (1967) *Neurophysiology of Postural Mechanisms*. Butterworths, London, pp. XVII–354.

Sasaki, K., Tanaka, T. and Mori, K. (1962) Effects of stimulation of pontine and bulbar reticular formation upon spinal motoneurons of the cat. *Jap. J. Physiol.*, **12**, 45–62.

Shapovalov, A. I. (1966) Excitation and inhibition of spinal neurones during supraspinal stimulation. In R. Granit (Ed.), *Muscular Afferents and Motor Control. Nobel Symposium I*. Almqvist and Wiksell, Stockholm, pp. 331–348.

Shapovalov, A. I. (1969) Posttetanic potentiation of monosynaptic and disynaptic actions from supraspinal structures on lumbar motoneurones. *J. Neurophysiol.*, **32**, 948–959.

Shik, M. L., Orlovskii, G. N. and Severin, F. V. (1966) Organization of locomotor synergism. *Biophysics*, **11**, 1011–1019.

Shimazu, H. and Smith, C. M. (1971) Cerebellar and labyrinthine influences on single vestibular neurons identified by natural stimuli. *J. Neurophysiol.*, **34**, 493–508.

Vraa–Jensen, G. (1956) On the correlation between the function and structure of nerve cells. *Acta psychiat. scand.*, **31**, Suppl. 109, 1–88.

Wilson, V. J. and Burgess, P. R. (1962) Disinhibition in the cat spinal cord. *J. Neurophysiol.*, **25**, 392–404.

Wilson, V. J., Kato, M., Peterson, B. W. and Wylie, R. M. (1967) A single-unit analysis of the organization of Deiters' nucleus. *J. Neurophysiol.*, **30**, 603–619.

Wilson, V. J. and Yoshida, M., (1968) Vestibulospinal and reticulospinal effects on hindlimb, fore-limb and neck alpha motoneurones of the cat. *Proc. N.Y. Acad. Sci.*, **60**, 836–840.

Wilson, V. J. and Yoshida, M. (1969) Comparison of effects of stimulation of Deiters' nucleus and medial longitudinal fasciculus on neck, forelimb and hindlimb motoneurones. *J. Neurophysiol.*, **32**, 743–758.

Spinovestibular Relations: Anatomical and Physiological Aspects

O. POMPEIANO

Institute of Physiology II, University of Pisa, Pisa, Italy

INTRODUCTION

The main function of the vestibular apparatus is to record information about static and dynamic changes in head position. As a result of labyrinthine stimulations, rapid reflex adjustments occur which involve the oculomotor and the spinal motoneurons.

Classic neurophysiological investigations (Sherrington, 1898; Magnus and De Kleijn, 1912; Magnus, 1924; McNally and Tait, 1925) had already demonstrated the need for integration of vestibular and deep somatosensory afferents in postural regulation.

The problem of the interaction between vestibular and proprioceptive activity has been investigated by several authors, who found that vestibular impulses converge with somatic afferent volleys at spinal cord level, thus contributing to control the posture and locomotion (Gernandt and Thulin, 1953; Andersson and Gernandt, 1956; Koella *et al.*, 1956; Gernandt *et al.*, 1957, 1959; Gernandt and Gilman, 1959, 1960a, b; Gernandt, 1959, 1962, 1964, 1967; Gernandt and Proler, 1965; Kim and Partridge, 1969). The experimental evidence presented here indicates that an interaction between labyrinthine and somatic impulses may also occur within the vestibular nuclei, as shown by the fact that somatosensory volleys influence the activity of neurons localized in different vestibular nuclei. Somatic afferent impulses may reach the vestibular complex through a direct spinovestibular pathway. In addition to this pathway, however, it will be shown that ascending spinal impulses may influence the vestibular nuclei indirectly, via the reticular formation or the cerebellum.

ANATOMY OF THE SPINOVESTIBULAR PROJECTION

There are several reports in the literature of the termination of spinal afferents in the vestibular nuclei. Most authors used the Marchi method on human or animal material and found that the fibers end in Deiters' nucleus or in the descending vestibular nucleus (Brodal, Pompeiano and Walberg, 1962). In Golgi studies of the mouse, Lorente de Nó (1924) describes collaterals of the dorsal spinocerebellar tract which pass to the vestibular nuclei and assumes that the great majority of these enter the ventrocaudal part of the descending vestibular nucleus, with only a few ending in the

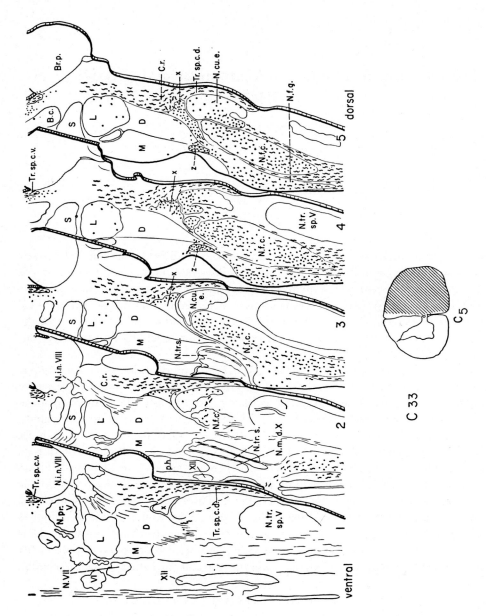

Fig. 1. Diagrammatic representation of the termination of spinovestibular fibers in an adult cat following hemisection of the spinal cord at C5 10 days before sacrifice. Degenerating coarser fibers (shown as wavy lines) and terminal degenerating fibers and boutons (shown as dots) are shown in a series of horizontal sections through the brain stem at approximately equal intervals. Degenerating fibers are seen to ascend in the area of the dorsal spinocerebellar tract and to enter the inferior cerebellar peduncle. Unequivocal terminal degeneration is found in the caudodorsal part of the lateral nucleus, in the caudalmost regions of the medial and descending vestibular nuclei and, more abundantly, in the groups x and z. Terminal degeneration in the gracile, cuneate and accessory cuneate nuclei is shown, but has not been mapped in detail. From Pompeiano and Brodal (1957b).

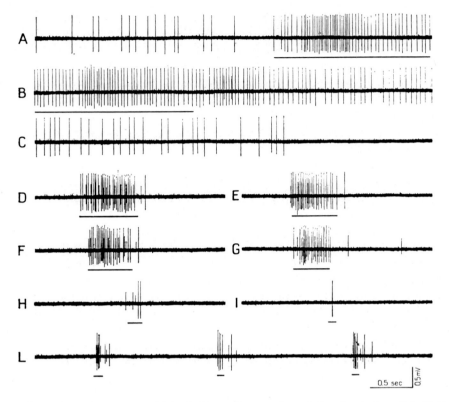

Fig. 2. Effects of somatosensory and labyrinthine volleys on the activity of a single unit in Deiters' nucleus. Precollicular decerebrate cat, with the cerebellum intact. A, B, C: increase in the frequency of discharge produced by cathodal polarization of the ipsilateral labyrinth with 0.3 mA. D, E: tappings applied to the tendon of the left triceps (forelimb) and quadriceps (hindlimb) muscles, respectively. F, G: tappings applied to the right triceps and quadriceps muscles, respectively. H: slight compression of the tail. I: quick displacement of hairs in the tail; L: slight repetitive tappings on the muzzle. From Pompeiano and Cotti (1959).

ventrolateral part of the medial nucleus. These collaterals have also been found with the Golgi method in kittens (Hauglie-Hanssen, 1968). Observations made with silver impregnation methods confirm the existence of spinovestibular fibers. In particular Johnson (1954) using the Nauta method in the cat, describes such fibers ending in Deiters' nucleus. It thus appears from the data in the literature that the terminal region of the spinovestibular fibers may be restricted to certain parts of the vestibular nuclei. The fibers are almost exclusively homolateral. Although some authors had stated that the majority of spinovestibular fibers are derived from the lumbar spinal cord, there was no general agreement.

Pompeiano and Brodal (1957b), using the silver impregnation method of Glees, studied this projection in order to obtain detailed information of the levels of origin of the spinovestibular fibers and to map their terminal distribution within the vestibular complex. From a comparison of cases with various lesions of the spinal cord it was concluded that the spinovestibular fibers ascend with those of the dorsal spino-cerebellar tract. The fibers to the vestibular nuclei may well be collaterals of dorsal spinocerebellar fibers, as observed by Lorente de Nó (1924) in Golgi preparations, but probably there are also direct spinovestibular fibers as shown by the fact that some of them are derived from levels of the spinal cord below the caudal end of the column of Clarke (L4 in the cat according to Rexed, 1954). A considerable number of spino-vestibular fibers originate from the lumbosacral levels of the spinal cord. However, the extent to which the cervical and thoracic segments give off spinovestibular fibers cannot be decided.

Fig. 1 shows that following hemisection of the spinal cord at C5 terminal degenera-tion is found ipsilaterally in the medial, descending and lateral vestibular nuclei as well as in the nuclei *x* and *z* originally described by Brodal and Pompeiano (1957) as subnuclei of the vestibular complex of the cat. In particular very few spinovestibular fibers terminate in the caudalmost regions of the medial and descending vestibular nuclei. Very slight degeneration is also found in the dorsal and caudal part of the lateral vestibular nucleus. In the nuclei *x* and *z* degeneration is much more abundant than in any of the vestibular nuclei proper. It is of interest to notice that in Fig. 1 the most medial ventral region of the nucleus *x* contains no degenerating fibers. In cases with lesions at successively lower levels of the cord, the degeneration is limited more and more to the dorsolateral regions of the group, thus indicating a somatotopical arrangement within the termination of its spinal afferents. The distribution of degene-rating spinovestibular fibers in cats studied recently with the Nauta method (Brodal and Angaut, 1967) corresponds closely to that found with the Glees method (Pompei-ano and Brodal, 1957b). It is of interest that the spinovestibular fibers in rat (Mehler, 1968), monkey (Mehler, Feferman and Nauta, 1960) and man (Bowsher, 1962) appear to be organized in the same way as in the cat. As to the mode of termination of the fibers it may tentatively be suggested that most of them establish synaptic contact with thin dendrites. However, definite conclusions concerning synaptic relationship can be made only with experimental electron microscopical studies*.

It is of interest that the spinal afferents like the vestibulospinal afferents are homo-lateral. However, while the lateral vestibulospinal tract is fairly large and is distributed to all segments of the spinal cord, the direct spinal afferents to Deiters' nucleus are scanty and end in its most dorsocaudal part only, *i.e.*, in that region which is not supplied by primary vestibular fibers (Walberg *et al.*, 1958). In view of the somato-

---

* In addition to the spinal afferents treated here, there are a few dorsal root fibers of the upper cer-vical roots which may terminate in the vestibular nuclei, particularly in the caudal ventrolateral part of the descending nucleus, of different animal species such as cat, rabbit and monkey (Corbin and Hinsey 1935; Corbin, Lhamon and Petit, 1937; Yee and Corbin, 1939; Escolar 1948). The number of these fibers appears to be scanty as shown by the fact that they have been missed in Nauta study applied on squirrel monkey (Igarashi *et al.*, 1969). Our study (Pompeiano and Brodal 1957b) supports the conclusion that such fibers do exist and they pass particularly in the first cervical dorsal root. Some fibers appear to be distributed to the small group *z*. These fibers may have been observed by Gehuchten (1900), Ranson *et al.* (1932) and perhaps by Escolar (1948). Dorsal root fibers L6 and S1 also terminate in very scanty numbers in the most caudolateral region of the ipsilateral nucleus *z* (Hand, 1966).

topical pattern in the vestibulospinal projection (Pompeiano and Brodal, 1957a), it appears that the terminal region of the spinal afferents is restricted to the "hindlimb" region of Deiters' nucleus, *i.e.*, the part of the nucleus which sends its fibers to the lower parts of the spinal cord. Since a considerable proportion of the spinovestibular fibers are derived from the lower segments of the spinal cord, it appears that the dorsocaudal part of the nucleus of Deiters is particularly related to the lower part of the spinal cord.

Further, it is noteworthy that in the descending and medial vestibular nuclei the spinal afferents likewise end in regions which do not receive primary vestibular afferents. It is also of interest that group *x* and *z*, which receive abundant spinal afferents, are not supplied by primary vestibular fibers (Walberg *et al.*, 1958). In particular the ample termination of spinal afferents in the group *x* points to a supplementary, usually neglected spinocerebellar pathway; since this group projects onto the flocculonodular lobe (Brodal and Torvik, 1957), it appears to produce a fairly direct pathway for spinal impulses to the vestibular part of the cerebellum. The group *z* in the cat does not receive primary vestibular afferents (Walberg *et al.*, 1958), while it receives some spinal afferents as does the group *x* (Pompeiano and Brodal, 1957b). Unlike the latter it does not send fibers to the cerebellum (Brodal and Torvik, 1957), but it projects to the rostral end of the lateral subdivision of nucleus ventralis posterolateralis and to the nucleus ventralis lateralis of the thalamus (Boivie *et al.*, 1970).

It has been mentioned in the introduction that spinal impulses can reach the vestibular nuclei not only directly but also indirectly, through the reticular formation (Brodal *et al.*, 1962) or the cerebellum. Ito, Obata and Ochi (1966) maintain that impulses from the spinal cord entering the inferior olive are propagated directly via collaterals of olivocerebellar fibers to Deiters' nucleus. Although collaterals of the olivocerebellar fibers to the vestibular nuclei have been postulated (Lorente de Nó, 1924), no clearcut anatomical evidence for these collaterals has been brought forward recently (Hauglie–Hanssen, 1968). However, restricted small parts of the medial accessory olive have been found to project onto the vestibular nuclei (Brodal, 1940).

SOMATIC INFLUENCES ON NEURONS IN THE LATERAL VESTIBULAR NUCLEUS

Pompeiano and Cotti (1959a–c) recorded the responses of single units of Deiters' nucleus to peripheral stimulation in precollicular decerebrate cats with the cerebellum intact. The units were influenced by proprioceptive and exteroceptive stimuli applied to the limbs of the animal, such as passive movements of the limbs, tapping of the tendons of extensor muscles and displacement of the hairs of the legs. The same units were also influenced by natural stimuli applied to the muzzle and to the tail. Fig. 2 shows the convergence on the same Deiters' unit of impulses originating from natural stimulation of the four limbs, the tail and the muzzle. The effect of stimulation was an increased frequency of the unit discharge. Deiters' units could also be influenced by single rectangular pulses applied to the radial and sciatic nerves of both sides. Most of these units were excited, while only a few were inhibited by peripheral nerve stimulation. In all instances these responses followed the large positive potential evoked in the vermal cortex of the anterior lobe by peripheral stimuli.

Unit responses similar to those described above were also elicited from unspecified structures of the vestibular nuclear complex with nociceptive stimulations or by stimulating the forelimb nerves with arousing stimuli in different types of preparations with the cerebellum intact (Dumont, 1960; Dumont-Tyč, 1964, 1966). In most instances units responsive to peripheral nerve stimulation were also influenced by labyrinthine volleys (Fig. 2) (Pompeiano and Cotti, 1959c; Dumont 1960; Dumont-Tyč, 1964).

The responses of Deiters' neurons to stimulation of forelimb (superficial and deep radial) nerves and hindlimb (hamstring) nerve of both sides were also recorded by Giaquinto, Pompeiano and Santini (1963) in precollicular decerebrate cat with the cerebellum intact. The responses of Deiters' units to stimulation of cutaneous and muscular nerves were generally excitatory (Fig. 3), rarely inhibitory (Fig. 4). An increase in intensity of stimulation generally potentiated the response without altering the sign of it. In addition to these neurons, units were found which responded to low

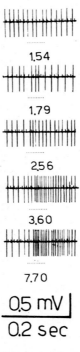

Fig. 3. Facilitatory response of a single unit in Deiters' nucleus elicited by stimulation of a muscular nerve. Precollicular decerebrate cat, with the cerebellum intact. Unit recorded from the left Deiters' nucleus. In this and the following two figures the nerves were stimulated at 200/sec, 0.1 msec pulse duration. The train duration was always 50 msec. The stimulus strengths are expressed in multiples of the threshold for the most excitable afferent fibers (T). The figure illustrates the effects of stimulation of the ipsilateral deep radial nerve at progressively increasing stimulus strengths. The threshold for the response was 1.79 T. The same unit was also facilitated by threshold stimulation of the contralateral deep radial nerve at 3.42 T as well as by stimulation of both the ipsilateral and contralateral superficial radial nerves at the threshold values of 1.88 T and 1.43 T respectively. From Giaquinto, Pompeiano and Santini (unpublished.)

intensity stimulation of cutaneous or muscular nerves with a train of spikes. However this early facilitatory response was followed for high intensity stimulation by a late response, characterized by a silent period followed by a rebound (Fig. 5). This silent period was due to some inhibitory process since it increased in duration and overwhelmed the early facilitatory response with progressively increasing stimulus intensities.

It is of interest that similar complex patterns of discharge had previously been recorded from reticular neurons in unanesthetized, decerebrate cats with the cerebellum intact (Pompeiano and Swett, 1963b), but not in cerebellectomized preparations, where the reticular neurons generally responded with an increased discharge to the somatic sensory volleys (Pompeiano and Swett, 1963a). In these studies the early acceleration was attributed to a direct influence of spinal afferents on the reticular neurons, while the anatomical and functional integrity of the cerebellum was considered to be responsible for the delayed components of the responses. Similarly one may assume that the early acceleration is due to some extracerebellar influence of spinal

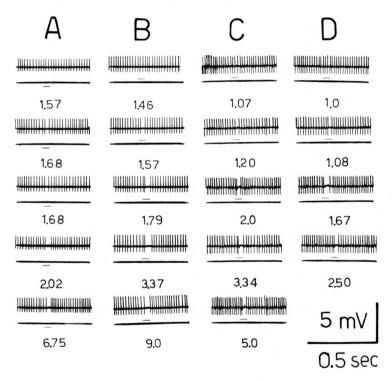

Fig. 4. Inhibitory responses of a single unit in Deiters' nucleus by stimulation of muscular and cutaneous nerves. Precollicular decerebrate cat, with the cerebellum intact. Unit recorded from the left Deiters' nucleus. A: effects of stimulating the left deep radial nerve. The threshold for the inhibitory response was 1.68 T. B: stimulation of the right deep radial nerve. The threshold for inhibition corresponded to 1.57 T. C: stimulation of the left superficial radial nerve. The threshold for the inhibitory response was 1.20 T. D: stimulation of the right superficial radial nerve. The threshold for inhibition corresponded to 1.08 T. From Giaquinto, Pompeiano and Santini (unpublished).

afferents on Deiters' neurons, while the late inhibition followed by rebound may be attributed to excitation followed by inhibition of those Purkinje neurons projecting directly to Deiters' nucleus. The first assumption has been demonstrated to be correct by Wilson *et al.* (1966b, 1967; *cf.* Wilson, 1970), who recorded extracellularly the responses of Deiters' neurons to somatosensory volleys in cerebellectomized preparations. The second assumption is supported by the experiments made by Wylie and Felpel (1971), who compared the extracellularly recorded activity of Deiters' cells in decerebellate cats and in those with an intact cerebellum, and by the observations made by Bruggencate *et al.* (1971), who recorded intracellularly the responses of Deiters' neurons to peripheral volleys.

Somatic input to lateral vestibular neurons via the reticular formation

The possibility that the spinal influences on the vestibular nuclei are diffusely mediated through the bulbar reticular formation is suggested by Feldman, Wagman and Bender (1961), who found that unilateral stimulation of the sciatic nerve evoked a bilateral response in unidentified regions of the vestibular nuclei, which was greatly depressed or even abolished by small doses of pentobarbital. The usual response was a negative wave of 10–20 msec latency. On some occasions the negativity was preceded by a short latency (5 to 8 msec) positive wave.

Wilson, Kato and Thomas (1965), Wilson, Kato and Peterson (1966a) and Wilson, Kato, Thomas and Peterson (1966b), Wilson, Kato, Peterson and Wylie (1967) (*cf.* Wilson, 1970) have recently studied the activity of single lateral vestibular neurons in cerebellectomized cats, anesthetized with choloralose-urethane. Stimulation of various fore- and hindlimb nerves produced a relatively long-lasting facilitation of the firing in most of the single units in Deiters' nucleus. Occasionally the leg nerve stimulus caused inhibition of spontaneous discharge. The peripheral activation of Deiters' cells had the following characteristics; (*i*) it has quite a long latency (usually 10–35 msec on stimulation of hindlimb nerves) compared to the latency of the antidromic firing (2.2–5.5 msec); (*ii*) the pathway that produces the response has a spinal conduction velocity ranging from 11 to 80 m/sec, usually 40 m/sec or less, *i.e.*, slower than that of the vestibulospinal fibers (from 31 to 140 m/sec); (*iii*) the facilitation lasts 100–200 msec; (*iv*) while single shocks to cutaneous or mixed nerves are effective in producing facilitation, multiple shocks to muscle nerves are usually required. The facilitation is not organized somatotopically (Wilson *et al.*, 1967) in that cells projecting to the forelimb or hindlimb regions of the spinal cord could be facilitated by activity of both forelimb and hindlimb afferents. Moreover, stimulation of both ipsilateral and contralateral nerves are effective*. The facilitatory effect described above cannot be attributed to

---

* Stimulation of neck receptors induced by joint movements may influence Deiters' neurons (Fredrickson *et al.*, 1966). Since the recorded units appear to be located in the caudal part of Deiters' nucleus, further experiments are required to find out whether there is convergence of this somatic input on those Deiters' neurons which project to the cervical motoneurons (Pompeiano and Brodal, 1957a) and which are particularly influenced by labyrinthine volleys (Batini, Moruzzi and Pompeiano, 1957).

passage of spinal impulses through the cerebellum since the experiments were performed in decerebellate animals. Experiments with chronic lesions of the spinal cord indicate that the facilitation is due in part to fibers that ascend in the ventral or ventrolateral white matter. This finding as well as the bilateral nature of the effect exclude that this effect is due to activation by spinovestibular fibers which are ipsilateral and course along the dorsolateral quadrant of the cord. The nature of the ascending pathway is apparently quite complex and it may include pathways through the reticular formation, as well as collaterals to Deiters' neurons of reticulocerebellar (Brodal *et al.*, 1962), olivocerebellar (Lorente de Nó, 1924) and spinocerebellar fibers (*cf.* Eccles *et al.*, 1967). This possibility is supported by the observation that Deiters' neurons may receive excitation through collaterals of some cerebellar afferents (Ito and Kawai, 1964; Ito and Yoshida, 1964, 1966; Ito *et al.*, 1965, 1966, 1969, 1970b, c; Ito, 1968, 1970, 1972; *cf.* also Allen *et al.*, 1971; Bruggencate *et al.*, 1971).

Since any localized spinovestibular action may be masked by the generalized effect of somatic afferent volleys on Deiters' neurons, experiments with intracellular recording were performed. Short latency monosynaptic EPSPs have been recorded from Deiters' cells following stimulation of the ventral and lateral funiculi of the cervical spinal cord (Ito *et al.*, 1964, 1969; *cf.* also Bruggencate *et al.*, 1971). This effect was attributed to stimulation of the ascending spinal tract which makes direct contact on Deiters' neurons (Ito *et al.*, 1964). Unfortunately it is not clear in these experiments whether the responsive neurons were located in the caudal part of Deiters' nucleus. Moreover the observation that supramaximal stimulation at the C_3 segment produced monosynaptic EPSP in 50% of the Deiters' neurons contrasts with the fact that the direct spinovestibular fibers to these neurons are rather scanty. It is likely that the induced effect is due in part at least to antidromic activation of descending reticulospinal axons and monosynaptic excitation of Deiters' neurons through axo-axonic reflex (Ito *et al.*, 1970a; Udo and Mano, 1970).

Somatic input to lateral vestibular neurons via the cerebellum

Wylie and Felpel (1971) found that in the decerebellate cat, stimulation of either ipsi- or contralateral limb nerves facilitates many Deiters' cells, whereas in the presence of the cerebellum, peripheral stimulation evokes facilitation followed by inhibition (*cf.* also Giaquinto *et al.*, 1963). The inhibition was ascribed to activation by peripheral stimulation of Purkinje cells projecting to Deiters' nucleus from the cerebellum. Activity in segmental primary afferents can ascend to the cerebellum via direct spinocerebellar tracts (Oscarsson, 1965) and via indirect paths relayed in the reticular formation (Grant, Oscarsson and Rosén, 1966) and the inferior olive (Miller and Oscarsson, 1969). The spino-olivocerebellar paths probably terminate as climbing fibers, the other paths as mossy fibers (Eccles, Ito and Szentágothai, 1967). Activation of the climbing fibers evokes excitation of the Purkinje neurons. On the other hand activation of the mossy fiber-granule cell path should evoke excitation of the Purkinje neurons leading to monosynaptic inhibition of Deiters' neurons (Ito and Yoshida, 1966), succeeded by inhibition of Purkinje cells through cerebellar inhibitory interneurons

References pp. 290–296

(Eccles, Ito and Szentágothai, 1967) which would lead to disinhibition of Deiters' neurons (Ito, 1968, 1970, 1972; Ito *et al.*, 1968b). Recently, attempts have been made, to identify the cerebellar components of the spinal evoked responses of Deiters' neurons mediated by mossy fibers and climbing fibers. In particular the activity of Deiters' neurons was recorded intracellularly in cats anesthetized with chloralose-Nembutal (Bruggencate *et al.*, 1971). Two typical responses were found. In some instances stimulation of the spinal cord evoked in Deiters' neurons a sharp IPSP (*cf.* also Ito *et al.*, 1964, 1969; Ito, Obata and Ochi, 1966). The second type of response appeared with stimulation of the peripheral nerves or the lumbar cord. It consisted of a more slowly developing hyperpolarization, which then turned into a prolonged depolarization.

The experimental evidence indicates that the sharp hyperpolarization is due to excitation of Purkinje cells induced via climbing fibers, leading to inhibition of Deiters' neurons. On the other hand, the prolonged hyperpolarization-depolarization sequence has been attributed to activation of the mossy fiber-granule cell path. This path should evoke excitation of Purkinje cells (leading to inhibition of Deiters' neurons), succeeded by inhibition of Purkinje cells through cerebellar inhibitory interneurones (leading to disinhibition of Deiters' neurons). Both IPSPs and disinhibition did not survive after anemic decerebration leading to ischemia of the cerebellar anterior lobe.

Experiments were also performed (Bruggencate *et al.*, 1971) to study the type of synaptic pattern evoked from different peripheral nerves in many Deiters' units. Stimulation of both fore- and hindlimb nerves elicits a slowly developing hyperpolarization (latency of 8–12 msec from forelimb, 10–14 msec from hindlimb nerves), as well as a sharp IPSP (latency 17–20 msec from forelimb, 22–25 msec from hindlimb) which rides on the initial phase of the slow hyperpolarization. However, when recording was made from lumbar Deiters' units, the sharp IPSP occurred only when hindlimb nerves were stimulated (see also Allen *et al.*, 1971a, b). It appears, therefore, that the sharp IPSPs are evoked mainly from nerves to the segmental level of which the Deiters' neurons project. The somatotopic pattern shown in this study with sharp IPSPs evoked mainly in lumbar units from the hindlimb, and prolonged events evoked from the nerves of both fore- and hindlimb, fits with the longitudinal-transversal organization of climbing fiber and mossy fiber inputs to the cerebellum (Miller and Oscarsson, 1969), if one takes into account the longitudinal organization of Purkinje cells projecting onto Deiters' neurons (Ito, Kawai and Udo, 1968a).

Types of afferent volleys influencing the lateral vestibular neurons

Since Deiters' nucleus influences the activity of the γ motoneurons (*cf.* Pompeiano, 1972), it would be of interest to know whether in their turn the Ia afferent volleys originating from the primary endings of muscle spindles are able to influence Deiters' neurons.

Giaquinto *et al.* (1963) recorded the responses of Deiters' neurons to graded stimulation of forelimb (superficial and deep radial) nerves and hindlimb (hamstring) nerves of both sides. The experiments were performed in precollicular decerebrate cats with the cerebellum intact. The nerves were stimulated with trains of impulses at 200/sec and all the stimulus intensities were expressed in terms of multiples of the threshold (T) for the most excitable afferent fibers.

The Deiters' units responded to threshold stimulation of the ipsilateral deep radial nerve with intensities of current ranging from 1.52 to 2.10 T (mean 1.75 T). The same neurons also responded to threshold stimulation of the contralateral deep radial nerve with intensities ranging from 1.57 to 3.42 T (mean 2.12 T) (Figs. 3–5). Considering the thresholds of activation of group II and III afferents which occur at approximately two and five times the threshold of the largest fibers respectively (Eccles and Lundberg, 1959), it appears that most of the Deiters' units were influenced by threshold or slightly suprathreshold stimulation of group II afferents. However a more limited

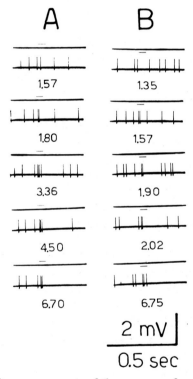

Fig. 5. Facilitatory and inhibitory components of the response of a single unit in Deiters' nucleus following stimulation of a muscular nerve. Same experiment as in Fig. 4. Unit recorded from the left Deiters' nucleus. A: stimulation of the left deep radial nerve. The threshold for the facilitatory response was 1.57 T. By increasing progressively the stimulus strength the number of spikes which characterizes the early response first increases and then decreases; contemporaneously one observes a progressive increase in duration of the silent period following the burst. B: stimulation of the right deep radial nerve. The threshold for the facilitatory response was 1.57 T. For higher stimulus intensities the pattern of response is modified as in A. The same unit was also influenced by cutaneous nerve stimulation. However, the thresholds for the early facilitatory response elicited by stimulation of the left and right superficial radial nerve corresponded respectively to 1.1 T and 1.18 T. From Giaquinto, Pompeiano and Santini (unpublished.)

number of Deiters' units was influenced by higher threshold group I afferents. It is of interest that in most instances it was necessary to activate at least 50% of the group I muscle fibers in order to elicit these responses. Additional stimulation of group II and III muscle afferents greatly potentiated the responses. The same Deiters' units which were influenced by stimulation of the deep radial nerves were also influenced by the two hamstring nerves with intensities of stimulation which were generally higher than 2 T. Some units however responded to threshold stimulation of these nerves corresponding to 1.70–1.80 T. For these intensities of stimulation 70–90% of the group I fibers were stimulated.

The same lateral vestibular units which responded to stimulation of muscular nerves with the intensities mentioned above were also submitted to graded stimulation of the superficial radial nerves of both sides. The threshold values responsible for the unitary responses ranged from 1.10 to 1.62 T (mean 1.32 T) for the ipsilateral superficial radial nerve and from 1.08 to 1.45 T (mean 1.28 T) for the contralateral superficial radial nerve. With these stimulus intensities only the low threshold group II cutaneous afferents are stimulated. It is of interest that the lowest threshold values capable of eliciting the unit responses, activated only 5% of the group II cutaneous afferents. There is therefore a striking difference between the threshold of responses of Deiters' units to cutaneous and muscular nerve stimulation as expressed in terms of multiples of T.

It seems surprising that the impulses coursing along the low threshold group I muscle afferents are apparently unable to influence the Deiters' units in spite of the anatomical and functional integrity of the cerebellum. It is known, however, that stimulation of group I muscle afferents elicits small potentials from the cerebellar cortex which contrast with the large potentials evoked by stimulation of cutaneous afferents (McIntyre, 1951; Mountcastle et al., 1952; Laporte et al., 1956; Oscarsson, 1956, 1965; Lundberg and Oscarsson, 1960; Pompeiano and Swett, 1963b; Körlin and Larson, 1970).

Preliminary observations by Eccles et al. (1968a, b), based on the analysis of field potentials elicited by stimulation of hindlimb nerves, indicate that the group I muscle afferent volleys are relatively uneffective in inducing mossy fiber and climbing fiber responses. The arrival of the group I volleys to the granular layer of the cerebellum, however, has been clearly documented with unit analysis (Eccles et al., 1971a). Responses of Purkinje cells to a mossy fiber and climbing fiber input from muscle afferents have also been recorded. Although high threshold (group II and III) muscle afferents were generally recruited in order to elicit such unit responses, mossy fiber responses of Purkinje cells could be evoked by stimulus intensities below 2 T (Eccles et al., 1969, 1970, 1971b, c). Since the threshold stimuli generally ranged between 1.5 and 2.0 T, it seems very likely that the action depended in part at least on Ib impulses (see Fig. 5F in Eccles et al., 1971b). It should be mentioned that because of the overlapping thresholds to nerve stimulation and the weakness of the effects observed, it is difficult to discriminate the effects of group Ia and Ib impulses in this group of experiments.

A recently devised method allows stimulation of primary endings of muscle spindles ₗMaṭṭhews, 1966; Morelli *et al.*, 1970). It was reported that muscle vibration provides a powerful stimulus for the primary endings of the muscle spindles while it has less effect in exciting secondary endings of the spindles (Bianconi and Van der Meulen, 1963; Brown *et al.*, 1967). This method has been used recently by Faber *et al.* (1971) who studied the effects of vibration of the anterior tibial muscle group of the hindlimb in 130 Purkinje cells which responded to electrical stimulation of the common peroneal nerve at strengths no greater than 5 times the group I threshold. Of these 52 (40%) were responsive to vibration with climbing fiber responses only, with purely mossy fiber induced effects or with both. The threshold of the responsive units extended from 15 up to 600 μm, but only 50% of the responsive units were affected at amplitudes less than 200 μm. The opinion of the authors, *i.e.*, that all the effects induced by these amplitudes of vibration are due to group Ia afferents and not to group II afferents is contradicted by the fact that a vibration of 60 μm amplitude or less which activated 95% of the Ia fibers activated also 41% of the group II fibers (Stuart *et al.*, 1970). Experiments are in progress to determine the relative contribution of the Ia, Ib and group II inputs to the climbing fiber and the mossy fiber responses of Purkinje neurons to vibration (Iosif *et al.*, 1972).

The observation that low threshold muscle afferents are apparently unable to produce any changes of the spontaneous activity of Deiters' units, does not exclude that intracellular recording might reveal a sign of weak group Ia input so far undetected. The experimental evidence, however, does not support this hypothesis. It has already been reported that stimulation of hindlimb nerves evoked in lumbar Deiters' units a slowly developing hyperpolarization which has been attributed to activation of Purkinje cells via the mossy fiber-granule cell path. In addition a sharp IPSP attributed to synchronous activity in Purkinje cells induced via climbing fibers, rides on the initial phase of the slow hyperpolarization (Bruggencate *et al.*, 1971). While the slowly developing hyperpolarization showed up with a stimulation strength slightly above threshold (T) for cutaneous nerves, from muscle nerves the responses could be evoked at about 1.5 T, but higher strengths were often needed. The sharp IPSP was evokable at 2–6 T from both cutaneous and muscle nerves (Bruggencate *et al.*, 1971). It seems therefore that even in these experiments there is no clear evidence indicating that the low threshold group I muscle afferents are able to influence postsynaptically the activity of Deiters' neurons. The same neurons, however, can be modified, particularly when the cutaneous and the high threshold (group II and III) muscle afferents are stimulated.

The observations made by Giaquinto *et al.* (1963) in preparations with the cerebellum intact have been confirmed also in decerebellate animals (Wilson *et al.*, 1966 b 1967). Activation of lateral vestibular cells by stimuli to cutaneous or mixed hindlimb nerves has been obtained with shocks as weak as 1.3–1.4 times the threshold for the largest fibers in the nerve. On the other hand the threshold of the effect from muscle hindlimb nerves corresponded to 6–9 T. When bursts of 3 shocks (at 300/sec) were applied to muscle nerves, intensities greater than 2.5–3 T were required to produce facilitation by forelimb muscle nerves, while shocks only 4–5 T to hindlimb muscle nerves produced a definite facilitating action. The threshold values responsible for the

responses of lateral vestibular neurons induced by stimulation of muscular and cutaneous nerves in decerebellate preparations closely correspond to those recorded in the
same experimental condition from the brain stem reticular neurons (Pompeiano and
Swett, 1963a). This finding further supports the hypothesis that the responses of
Deiters' neurons to peripheral nerve stimulation after ablation of the cerebellum are
mainly, if not exclusively, mediated via the reticular formation.

In conclusion, it appears that the Deiters' nucleus, which is involved in the regulation of posture and muscle tone, is little affected by stimulation of the low threshold
group I muscle afferents, which originate from the primary endings of muscle spindles.
This finding, obtained in preparations with the cerebellum intact, contrasts with the
responses recorded in the same preparation from several Deiters' units by stimulating
the high threshold group I muscle afferents, which originate from Golgi tendon
organs. In most instances, however, a response of Deiters' units occurs only when the
cutaneous and the high threshold (group II and III) muscular afferents are stimulated.
It should be mentioned here that these afferent impulses which are responsible for the
ipsilateral flexion reflex at segmental level are also able to activate the neurons of the
ascending spinoreticular pathway (Lundberg, 1964). Recent experiments have shown
that the vestibulospinal tract originating from Deiters' nucleus produces monosynaptic excitation on these spinoreticular neurons (Grillner et al., 1968). A close loop therefore exists between the ascending spinoreticular pathway which excites the Deiters'
neurons and the descending vestibulospinal tract which exerts a monosynaptic effect
on the spinoreticular neurons. The importance of this loop in the motor control should
be kept in mind.

SOMATIC INFLUENCES ON NEURONS IN THE MEDIAL AND DESCENDING VESTIBULAR NUCLEI

The effects of somatic afferent volleys on medial and descending vestibular neurons
have been investigated in experiments of electrical stimulation of peripheral nerves
and natural stimulation of different receptors.

Electrical stimulation of peripheral nerves

This approach was followed by Wilson et al. (1968; cf. Wilson, 1970) who studied the
responses of medial vestibular neurons to spinal cord or peripheral nerve stimulation
in cats anesthetized with chloralose–urethane and cerebellectomized. It was found that
38 cells in the medial vestibular nucleus were activated synaptically by single shock
stimulation of the descending medial longitudinal fasciculus at cervical level. The
latency of the response ranged from 2–5 msec up to, and even longer than, 15 msec.
The cells were scattered throughout the rostrocaudal extent of the nucleus and most of
them were located ventrally. These responses cannot be attributed exclusively to
activation of ascending spinal pathways since reticulospinal excitatory neurons may
send their axon to the spinal cord along the midline and may excite neighbouring
neurons through their collaterals (Udo and Mano, 1970). Stimulation of peripheral
nerves, principally hindlimb mixed nerves (peroneal and tibial), was tried with a

number of cells; 17 of 52 neurons recorded from the medial vestibular nucleus were facilitated by strong shocks above group III threshold. Latency of synaptic activation from leg nerves ranged from 12 to 30 msec.

Natural stimulation of somatosensory receptors

Two separate groups of investigators have recently studied the responses of the medial and descending vestibular neurons to stimulation of different groups of receptors, namely (i) the joint receptors (Fredrickson *et al.*, 1964, 1966; *cf.* Fredrickson and Schwarz, 1970) and (ii) the muscle receptors (Barnes and Pompeiano, 1971a; Pompeiano and Barnes, 1971 a, b).

(1) Deep neck proprioceptors, localized in the neck joints (McCouch *et al.*, 1951; Gernandt, Iranyi and Livingston, 1959; *cf.* Ehrhardt and Wagner, 1970), play an important role in the control of body equilibrium (Magnus and Storm van Leeuwen, 1914; Cohen, 1961; Hinoki and Kurosawa, 1965; Igarashi *et al.*, 1969) as well as in the regulation of eye movements (De Kleijn, 1921; Koella, 1947; Trincker, 1961; Philipszoon, 1962; Bos and Philipszoon, 1963; Philipszoon and Bos, 1963; Jongkees and Philipszoon, 1964; Hinoki and Terayama, 1966; Igarashi *et al.*, 1969). These observations suggest that a good deal of the neck-vestibular integration takes place in the vestibular nuclei. In addition to these findings there is evidence indicating that manipulation of the joints of the foot has a facilitatory effect on vestibular ventral root responses (Gernandt, Katsuki and Livingston, 1957; Gernandt, Iranyi and Livingston, 1959; Gernandt, 1967).

Fredrickson, Schwarz and Kornhuber (1964, 1966; *cf.* Fredrickson and Schwarz, 1970) have studied the responses of vestibular units to somatic inputs particularly originating from joint receptors. The experiments were performed either in cats paralyzed with Flaxedil, with or without cerebellum, or in anesthetized preparations. Somatic stimuli included blowing on the fur, gently touching the skin, deep muscle pressure and joint movements. Of the 149 vestibular neurons obtained only 18 were located in the lateral vestibular nucleus, while 78 were located in the descending and 53 in the medial vestibular nucleus. 106 of the 128 neurons analyzed for the labyrinthine influence responded to somatic stimulation. Of the 106 responsive neurons, 103 reacted to joint movement and only 3 to exteroceptive somatic stimulation; on the other hand there were no responses to deep muscle pressure. Ipsilateral joint responses exceeded contralateral responses by 2 to 1, and proximal joint responses exceeded peripheral responses by 5 to 1.

Approximately 45% of the total number of joint-responsive units responded to neck movement. The great majority of the responses were excitatory in nature, while only a few neurons appeared to be inhibited by reciprocal joint movement. This was especially true for units influenced by neck movement. All units affected by joint movement responded almost immediately. Moreover the maximum rate of neuronal discharge appeared to correspond with the maximum joint displacement.

The observation that these unit responses persisted in barbiturate preparations as well as after cerebellectomy has lead the authors to suggest that somatic influence has a direct effect upon some units in the vestibular nuclei, rather than being mediated through the reticular formation and the cerebellum. It seems unlikely, however, that the few direct spinovestibular fibers may account for the extensive effect of joint stimulation on a large population of vestibular neurons. The possibility therefore exists that this effect is mediated, in part at least, through the reticular formation.

It would appear from these observations that proximal limb and neck joints play a prominent role in supplying postural information to the vestibular nuclei. The discharge patterns and frequencies of the units studied in the vestibular nuclei responding to joint movement provide information concerning the direction, rate of movement and the steady position of the limbs. It is of interest that units located in the descend-

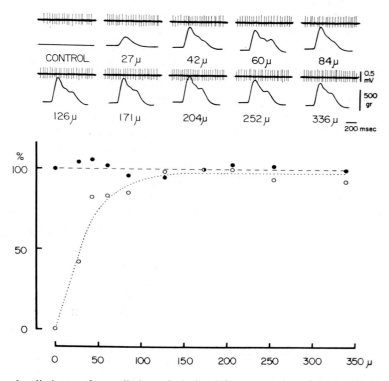

Fig. 6. Regular discharge of a vestibular unit during reflex contraction of the gastrocnemius-soleus (GS) muscle elicited by a series of vibrations of increasing amplitudes applied to the Achilles tendon. Precollicular decerebrate cat with the cerebellum intact. GS muscle at 6 mm of initial extension. In each group of records the upper traces represent the discharge recorded from a neuron localized in the descending vestibular nucleus of the left side, while the lower traces represent the reflex contraction of the left GS muscle elicited by vibration applied to the Achilles tendon. Vibrations applied for 350 msec, at 200/sec and increasing peak-to-peak amplitudes, as indicated at the bottom of the records. The responses partially shown above have been plotted diagrammatically. The changes in frequency of unit discharge relative to the control values (dots), as well as the changes in amplitude of the induced tension (circles), are plotted as a function of the amplitude of vibration. The mean frequency of the unit discharge in the absence of vibration (control) corresponded to 25.6/sec. The maximum tension (580 g) was obtained at 126 μm amplitude of vibration. In this figure 10 controls and 10 responses for each value of vibration were recorded and averaged. From Pompeiano and Barnes (1971b).

ing vestibular nucleus may respond not only to stimulation of proprioceptive afferents such as movements of a joint, but also to adequate stimulation of pressure and tactile receptors (Yamamoto and Miyajima, 1961).

(2) The main aim of the experiments performed by Barnes and Pompeiano (1971a) and Pompeiano and Barnes (1971a, b) was to determine if the proprioceptive group Ia volleys could affect the spontaneous activity of brain stem vestibular and reticular units. This question is relevant in view of the fact that stimulation of the medial and descending vestibular nuclei as well as of the medullary reticular formation produces primary afferent depolarization of different systems of spinal afferents, including the group Ia pathway from extensor muscles (Carpenter, Engberg and Lundberg, 1966; Cook *et al.*, 1969a, b; Barnes and Pompeiano, 1970c, d). Transmission in the monosynaptic reflex path to extensor motoneurons can thus be presynaptically inhibited at primary afferent level by supraspinal descending volleys (Barnes and Pompeiano, 1970c, d; *cf.* Pompeiano, 1972).

It has been reported that vibration of a muscle provides a powerful stimulus for the primary endings of the muscle spindles, while it has less effect in exciting secondary endings of the spindles (Bianconi and Van der Meulen, 1963; Brown *et al.*, 1967; Stuart *et al.*, 1970). By applying a small-amplitude longitudinal vibration to the isolated muscle (Matthews, 1966; Morelli *et al.*, 1970), a contraction of the vibrated muscle occurs which is due to monosynaptic reflex excitation of the corresponding motoneurons (Matthews, 1966; Barnes and Pompeiano, 1970a, b). By using this method it was possible to study the effects of spindle receptors on the unit discharge recorded from vestibular and reticular neurons in precollicular decerebrate cats (Barnes and Pompeiano, 1971a; Pompeiano and Barnes, 1971a, b). In particular the vestibular units were located in the medial and descending vestibular nuclei ipsilateral to the side of vibration, while the reticular units were located in the nucleus reticularis pontis caudalis, gigantocellularis, parvicellularis, reticularis centralis and reticularis lateralis of both sides.

In decerebrate cats with intact afferent pathways, vibration of the gastrocnemius-soleus (GS) muscle at 200/sec for about 200–400 msec produced a reflex contraction of the muscle, with a threshold amplitude of 15–30 μm. The response increased progressively up to an approximate plateau for amplitudes of 100–150 μm (Fig. 6). Further increases in vibration amplitude to 400 μm did not produce any significant change in the reflex contraction. In spite of the complete activation of the primary endings of muscle spindles, demonstrated by the reflex contraction of the GS muscle, neither the frequency, nor the pattern of discharge of the vestibular and reticular units were altered. Increases in reflex muscle contraction produced by increasing either the frequency of vibration in the range 10–300/sec or the initial muscle extension from 0 up to 10 mm were also unable to affect the unit discharge.

Of the 40 vestibular and 83 reticular units recorded, 35 and 61, respectively, were not affected by muscle vibration applied to the GS muscle. In all these units negative results were obtained even when the amplitude of vibration was increased up to 400–450 μm. The 5 vestibular and the 22 reticular units which were affected by muscle vibration were either facilitated or inhibited by vibration amplitudes less than those which produced a maximum reflex muscle contraction (100–150 μm). In 11 units the injection of Flaxedil abolished both muscle contraction and brain stem unit responses indicating that these units were being influenced by the activation of Golgi tendon organs as a result of the tension induced by reflex. In the remaining 16 units which still responded to muscle vibration after Flaxedil, the threshold of vibration amplitude was greater than 100–150 μm. The responses of these units could be attributed to stimulation of the secondary endings of the GS muscle spindles or to receptor organs outside the muscle.

The activity of 71 reticular and 13 vestibular units was recorded in deefferented preparations. Vibrations of the GS muscle for about 200–400 msec at 200–300/sec and amplitudes of vibration up to 400 μm were without effect on 65 reticular and in all vestibular units. These negative effects were obtained even when the initial muscle extension was increased up to 10 mm. Many of these units could be excited by isometric contraction resulting from electrical stimulation of the distal cut ventral roots L7 or S1. The remaining 6 reticular units were influenced (either excited or inhibited) by muscle vibration. Only in one of these units could the responses be attributed to group Ia afferent volleys since the threshold for activation corresponded to 52 μm and the unit discharge was not greatly potentiated by increasing the amplitude of vibration from 100 μm up to 400 μm. On the contrary the remaining 5 units were influenced only by amplitudes of vibration larger than 100 μm, which is required to produce maximal activation of the primary endings of muscle spindles. The secondary endings of muscle spindles or costimulation of receptors other than the spindles was probably responsible for these effects.

The effectiveness of vibration in activating group Ia muscle afferents in the deefferented preparations was shown by the fact that amplitudes of vibration as low as 5–10 μm applied to the ankle extensor muscles elicited a series of monosynaptic reflex discharges from the ventral roots which increased in amplitude until vibration amplitudes reached about 60 μm. In the same preparation conditioning vibration of the lateral gastrocnemius-soleus (LGS) muscle at 200/sec facilitated the heteronymous monosynaptic reflex of the medial gastrocnemius (MG) nerve at a threshold amplitude of vibration of 5–10 μm, while the maximum facilitation was reached at about 70 μm* (cf. Barnes and Pompeiano, 1970a, b).

It is concluded that the primary endings of muscle spindles from the GS muscle are unable to influence most of the brain stem vestibular and reticular units. While the vestibular and the reticular systems can inhibit presynaptically the orthodromic transmission of the group Ia volleys to the extensor motoneurons (Carpenter, Engberg and Lundberg, 1966; Cook, Cangiano and Pompeiano, 1969a, b; Barnes and Pompeiano, 1970c, d; cf. Pompeiano, 1972), the proprioceptive volleys coursing along the Ia pathway are apparently unable to influence the discharge of most the reticular and the vestibular neurons.

---

* The maximum monosynaptic reflex facilitation was generally achieved at a threshold amplitude (70 μm) lower than that responsible for maximum reflex tension (100–150 μm) in the preparation with ventral roots intact. The sensitivity of primary endings to vibration is in fact reduced by muscle contraction (Brown, Engberg and Matthews, 1967).

EFFECTS OF CUTANEOUS AND MUSCULAR AFFERENT VOLLEYS ON SUPRA-
SPINAL DESCENDING INHIBITORY MECHANISMS INVOLVING THE VESTIBULAR
NUCLEI AND THE CEREBELLUM

Stimulation of a spinal dorsal root in decerebrate cats results in the well known
segmental reflexes in the corresponding ventral root which are followed, after a period
of little or no ventral root activity, by an additional delayed reflex response indicated
as spino–bulbo–spinal (SBS) reflex (Gernandt and Shimamura, 1961; Shimamura
and Livingston, 1963; Shimamura et al., 1964, 1967a). This delayed response which
affects flexor but not extensor motoneurons (Shimamura et al., 1964) has been
attributed to reflex activation of a bulbospinal reticular mechanism. These late
reflex discharges can be elicited particularly by stimulation of low threshold cutaneous
afferents. On the other hand stimulation of a muscle nerve produces weak and inconstant late reflex discharges, which may be observed only when high threshold
muscle afferents are involved (Shimamura and Akert, 1965). In addition to these
findings, the descending volleys induced by stimulation of ipsilateral cutaneous afferents are also able to inhibit the monosynaptic extensor and flexor hindlimb reflexes
through a presynaptic inhibitory mechanism (Shimamura, Mori and Yamauchi,
1967b; Shimamura and Aoki, 1969; cf. Giaquinto and Pompeiano, 1964).

The presynaptic inhibition of the monosynaptic extensor reflex elicited by the
descending volleys of the SBS reflex implies the existence of a medullary "center"
exerting primary afferent depolarization in the terminal arborization of the group Ia
afferents. Experiments of stimulation of either the medulla or the vestibular nerve
indicate that this "center" include the medial vestibular nucleus and the bulbar reticular formation (Carpenter, Engberg and Lundberg, 1966; Cook, Cangiano and Pompeiano, 1969a, b; Barnes and Pompeiano, 1970c, d).

Thoden, Magherini and Pompeiano (1971a, b) have made experiments to find out
whether proprioceptive volleys originating from muscle spindles are able to trigger
this supraspinal inhibitory mechanism. The experiments were performed on precollicular, decerebrate cats with the cerebellum intact. Sinusoidal muscle stretch of short
duration (two cycles at 250–300 cycles/sec) and variable amplitude was applied to the
deefferented soleus (S) or GS muscle pulled at 6–8 mm of initial extension. Conditioning mechanical stimulation of the S muscle elicited an early facilitation of the MG
monosynaptic reflex which reached a peak amplitude at the latency of 10–12 msec
(Fig. 7). A similar effect was also obtained by conditioning stimulation of the whole
GS muscle on the test plantaris–flexor digitorum and hallucis longus (Pl–FDHL)
monosynaptic reflex (Fig. 8B). In all instances this early facilitation, referred to heteronymous monosynaptic excitation, was followed by a small amplitude prolonged inhibition, which lasted up to 100–150 msec after the application of the conditioning
stimulus. This late inhibition is segmental in origin since it persists after complete
transection of the spinal cord at postbrachial level and is generally associated with
presynaptic depolarization in the heteronymous group Ia pathway (Barnes and Pompeiano, 1970a, b). Maximum facilitation and inhibition occurred at the peak–to–peak

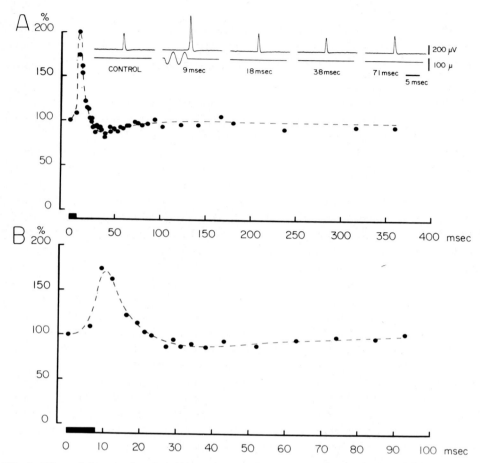

Fig. 7. Effect of short-lasting sinusoidal stretch of the left soleus muscle on the ipsilateral medial gastrocnemius (MG) monosynaptic reflex. Precollicular decerebrate cat, with the cerebellum intact. Conditioning vibration of the left soleus muscle pulled at 6 mm of initial extension with two cycles at 250/sec, 100 μm peak-to-peak amplitude. Testing stimulation applied to the left MG nerve with double shock of 0.05 msec in duration, at very short interval. The diagrams illustrate the percentage changes in amplitude of the monosynaptic reflex occurring at various intervals after the beginning of the conditioning stretch. Each dot represents the average of 10 conditioned responses matched with 10 controls. A: the results obtained from two successive series in which the interval between conditioning vibration and testing shock was increased progressively from 0 up to 358 msec have been plotted. Note an early facilitation at an optimal interval of 10 msec followed by a late inhibition, which reaches the maximum at the optimal interval of 38 msec. B: another series taken on a more expanded baseline to show in detail the time course of the facilitatory and inhibitory interactions.
From Thoden, Magherini and Pompeiano (unpublished).

amplitudes of 70–100 μm. It is assumed that at such amplitudes all the group Ia afferents are stimulated.

Contrary to these findings, a conditioning volley applied in the same preparation to the ipsilateral dorsal root L6 or the sural nerve produced first a marked decrease in amplitude of the extensor monosynaptic reflexes at an average interval of 10 msec

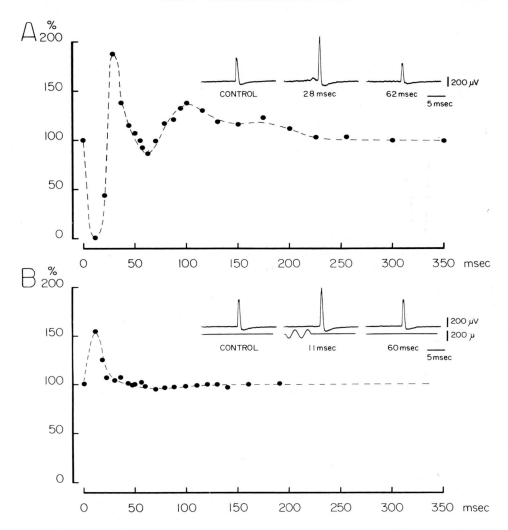

Fig. 8. Effects of conditioning stimulation of a lumbar dorsal root or sinusoidal stretch of the GS muscle on ipsilateral monosynaptic extensor reflex before intravenous injection of eserine. Precollicular decerebrate cat, with the cerebellum intact. A: conditioning stimulation of the left dorsal root L6 with two 0.05 msec rectangular pulses delivered at the interval of 1.4 msec, 10 times the threshold for the segmental polysynaptic reflex recorded from ipsilateral ventral root L7. Testing stimulation applied to the left plantaris-flexor digitorum and hallucis longus (Pl-FDHL) nerves with single pulses of 0.1 msec in duration, 2.0 times the threshold for the monosynaptic reflex. B: conditioning stimulation with two cycles at 280 cycles/sec, 178 μm peak-to-peak amplitude, applied to the Achilles tendon. Testing stimulation as in A. From Thoden, Magherini and Pompeiano (1971a).

(early inhibition) followed by another decrease in amplitude, which reached a maximum at the interval of 55–60 msec (late inhibition) (Fig. 8A). The maximum amount of inhibition was generally achieved by low intensities of conditioning stimulation, indicating that the group II cutaneous afferents were mainly responsible for the late inhibitory effect (Magherini et al., 1971). It is of interest that this late inhibition of the test

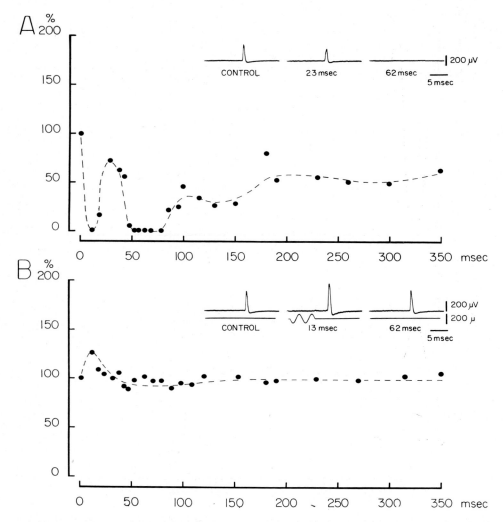

Fig. 9. Effects of conditioning stimulation of a lumbar dorsal root or sinusoidal stretch of the GS muscle on ipsilateral monosynaptic extensor reflex after intravenous injection of eserine. Same experiment as in Fig. 8. A: same experimental condition as in Fig. 8A, 5 min after i.v. injection of eserine sulphate (0.1 mg/kg). B: same as in Fig. 8B, 17 min after injection of the drug. From Thoden, Magherini and Pompeiano (1971a).

reflexes was generally superimposed on a wave of facilitation which reached its peak at a latency of about 25–30 msec and slowly decayed (Fig. 8A).

Both the delayed inhibition and the delayed facilitation of the test reflex were abolished by a postbrachial transection of the spinal cord, while the early inhibition persisted after this lesion. This implies that the late interactions on the monosynaptic reflexes are concerned with long reflex activities which probably engage supraspinal descending mechanisms.

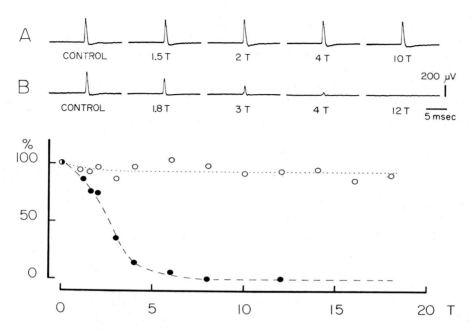

Fig. 10. Comparison of the delayed inhibitory effects on ipsilateral monosynaptic extensor reflexes elicited by conditioning electrical stimulation of the dorsal root L6 or of the GS nerve following intravenous injection of eserine. Precollicular decerebrate cat, with the cerebellum intact. Records taken 15–20 min after i.v. injection of eserine sulphate (0.1 mg/kg). The *dots* indicate the percentage depression of the Pl-FDHL monosynaptic reflex of the left side (0.1 msec rectangular pulses, 2.0 times the threshold for the monosynaptic reflex) as a function of the intensity of conditioning stimulation applied to the left DR L6 (two 0.05 msec pulses delivered at very short interval). The intensities of stimulation are expressed in multiples of the threshold (T) for the polysynaptic reflex recorded from the ipsilateral ventral root L7. Some of the records measured are illustrated in B. The *circles* indicate the percentage changes in amplitude of the same Pl-FDHL monosynaptic reflex as a function of the intensity of conditioning stimulation applied to the ipsilateral GS nerve (two 0.05 msec pulses delivered at very short interval). The intensities of stimulation are expressed in multiples of the threshold (T) for the GS monosynaptic reflex recorded from the ipsilateral ventral root L7. Some of the records measured are illustrated in A. Most of these responses are only slightly depressed. In both the experimental series the interval between conditioning stimulation and testing shock corresponded to the appropriate interval for the SBS inhibition (66 msec). From Thoden, Magherini and Pompeiano (1971b).

Recent observations (Barnes, 1970; Barnes and Pompeiano, 1971b) have shown that the inhibitory phase of the SBS reflex involves a cholinergic mechanism in the brain stem. Intravenous injection of eserine sulphate, a cholinesterase inhibitor, at the dosis of 0.1 mg/kg, abolished the late facilitation and greatly potentiated the late inhibition of the monosynaptic extensor reflex elicited by conditioning stimulation of the ipsilateral dorsal root L6 (Fig. 9A) or the sural nerve.

It would be of interest to know whether group I*a* volleys were able to trigger the supraspinal descending inhibitory mechanism which appears to be potentiated by the cholinesterase inhibitor. Administration of eserine (0.1 mg/kg) in preparations with intact spinal cord slightly depressed the heteronymous monosynaptic reflex facilitation elicited by sinusoidal stretch applied to the ipsilateral GS muscle. The same condition-

ing stimulus, however, was unable to bring to light any late interaction which could be
attributed to long-loop reflex inhibition (Fig. 9B). It appears, therefore, that while
somatic afferent volleys originating from cutaneous afferents are able to trigger the
supraspinal descending inhibitory mechanism exerting presynaptic depolarization in
the group Ia pathway (Shimamura *et al.*, 1967b; Shimamura and Aoki, 1969), the
proprioceptive afferent volleys originating from the primary endings of muscle spindles apparently do not have access to this supraspinal descending inhibitory mechanism. This is true even when this supraspinal inhibitory mechanism is greatly potentiated by the cholinesterase inhibitor.

Negative results were also obtained when the conditioning stimulus was made by
electrical shocks applied to the group I muscle afferents from the GS muscle. Costimulation of the group II and low threshold group III muscle afferents add very little inhibition. Fig. 10 shows the marked SBS inhibition of the Pl–FDHL monosynaptic
reflex as a function of the intensity of conditioning stimulation applied to the ipsilateral dorsal root L6. This result contrasts with the very slight depression of the same
test reflex when conditioning stimulation of increasing intensities was applied to the
ipsilateral GS nerve.

The conclusion that group Ia volleys are unable to drive reflex inhibition via SBS
mechanisms can be correlated with the results of previously reported experiments
showing that stimulation of the primary endings of muscle spindles induced by muscle
vibration did not apparently affect either the frequency or the pattern of discharge of
reticular neurons as well as of neurons localized in the medial and descending vestibular nuclei.

A final comment should be devoted to the fact that the proprioceptive afferent
volleys originating from the primary endings of muscle spindles, contrary to the
cutaneous afferent volleys, are unable to produce not only a spino–bulbo–spinal reflex
inhibition but also any delayed facilitation of monosynaptic extensor reflexes. Observations made in humans have shown that an intercurrent facilitation of the H reflex
involving the GS muscle occurs after a conditioning H reflex or a sudden plantar
flexion of ankle (Táboříková *et al.*, 1966; *cf.* Eccles, 1967). This effect has been attributed to group Ia impulses which reach the cerebellum through the dorsal spinocerebellar tract, thus leading to a *powerful* inhibition of the Purkinje cells by the pathway:
mossy fibers, granule cells, parallel fibers, basket cells, inhibitory synapses on Purkinje
cell somata. Since Purkinje neurons in turn inhibit Deiters' nucleus, which is known
to excite monosynaptically the extensor GS motoneurons (Lund and Pompeiano,
1965, 1968), the reduced activity of the Purkinje cells would lead to disinhibition of
Deiters' neurons, which would then be responsible for the intercurrent facilitation.

The observation that selective stimulation of the primary endings of muscle spindles
induced by sinusoidal stretch of the GS muscle is unable to elicit any delayed intercurrent facilitation of the ipsilateral extensor reflex suggests that receptor organs
other than those innervated by the Ia fibers are responsible for this long-loop reflex.
Indeed, there is evidence indicating that the threshold for the monosynaptic H reflex,
due to stimulation of Ia afferents, may be higher than that for the polysynaptic spinal
reflex, which is attributed to stimulation of group II afferents (Pompeiano, 1968;

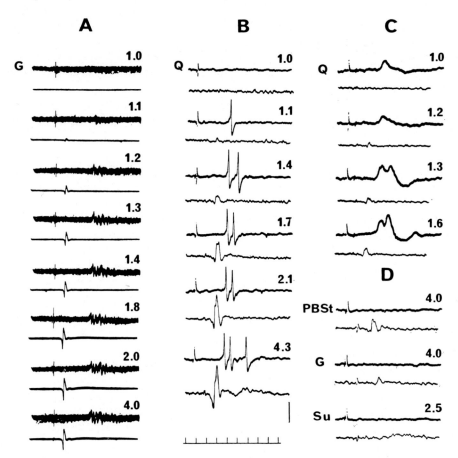

Fig. 11. Records of focal and single unit potentials obtained in nucleus z and evoked by group I hindlimb afferents. Positivity is recorded upwards in all the upper records, and downwards in all the lower records of the afferent volley obtained from the lumbar dorsal roots. A, upper records: focal potential evoked by increasing strength of electrical stimulation of the gastrocnemius nerve (G). Threshold multiples indicated. B, upper records: extracellular single unit responses evoked by electrical stimulation of the quadriceps nerve (Q), at strengths indicated. C, upper records: intra-cellular potentials of the same unit shown in B in response to electrical stimulation of Q. The membrane potential of the cell was not measured. D, upper records: lack of excitatory convergence on the same unit shown in B and C. Intracellular recording. Electrical stimulation of PBST, G and Su nerves were made at strengths indicated. Time: 2 sec. Voltage bar for A–D: 400 μV. From Landgren and Silfvenius (1971).

Lund and Pompeiano, 1970). The negative finding reported above is in line with the observation that repetitive electrical stimulation of low threshold muscle afferents is apparently unable to modify the spontaneous activity of Deiters' neurons.

SOMATIC INFLUENCES ON NEURONS IN THE NUCLEI x AND z

While nothing is known so far about the information transmitted by the spinal afferents to the nucleus x, recent experiments have clarified the nature of the somatic afferent volleys impinging upon nucleus z.

Observations made by Landgren and Silfvenius (1969a) and Landgren (1969) had shown that group I muscle afferents from the cat's hindlimb project to the cerebral cortex. The cortical projections were found in two places, one rostromedial to the postcruciate dimple and another near the cruciate sulcus on the medial surface of the hemisphere. It was also demonstrated that the ascending path travelled in the dorsolateral fasciculus of the spinal cord and that it crossed to the contralateral side above the level of the first cervical segments. The path did not pass via the cerebellum. Since the nucleus z of Brodal and Pompeiano (1957) receives spinal afferents travelling only in the dorsolateral fasciculus and does not send axons to the cerebellum, experiments were performed to investigate whether group I relay cells were located in the region of nucleus z (Landgren, 1969; Landgren and Silfvenius, 1969b, 1971).

The observations made by these authors clearly demonstrate that the medullary relay in the group I muscular path from the hindlimb to the cerebral cortex is located in nucleus z. Focal and unitary responses appeared at threshold strengths of the afferent volleys (Fig. 11). The latencies of the focal potentials varied between 4.5 and 7.0 msec, while those of the unitary ones between 5.1 and 11.0 msec. Group II muscle afferents and low threshold cutaneous afferents also projected to nucleus z. The physiological observations confirm the anatomical finding that the afferents to nucleus z travel in the dorsolateral fascicle, since a superficial transection of the ipsilateral dorsolateral fascicle at the first cervical segment abolished the potentials evoked in nucleus z (cf. also Landgren and Silfvenius, 1969a). Moreover, the spinal course of the group I path seems to be identical with that of the dorsal spinocerebellar tract indicating that the segmental relay of the path is at the level of the Clarke's column.

The group I impulses mediated through group z ascend to the contralateral thalamus (Landgren and Silfvenius, 1970) and are there relayed to the group I projection areas in the posterior sigmoid gyrus of the cerebral cortex (Landgren and Silfvenius, 1969a). Moreover a lesion of nucleus z abolished the response evoked in the contralateral posterior sigmoid gyrus of the cerebral cortex by the group I muscle afferents of the hindlimb (Landgren and Silfvenius, 1971).

It is of interest that the relay cells in the nucleus z in many respects resemble the cuneo-thalamic relay cells in the group I path from the forelimb muscles (Rosén, 1969), in so far as they had a high degree of spatial specificity, they followed high frequency afferent stimulation, and they often discharged at a stimulus strength just threshold for the afferent volley indicating that very little spatial summation is required (Fig. 11).

The discharge of the group I relay cells in nucleus z is probably induced by large muscle spindle afferents because action potentials were recorded at the very threshold of the group Ia component of the dorsal root volley. Additional discharges which appeared with increasing strength of stimulation between 1.3 and 2.0 T can probably be due to activation of afferents from Golgi tendon organs.

Seguin et al. (1972) have recently shown that units localized in the region of nucleus z were responsive to longitudinal vibration of the deefferented gastrocnemius–soleus muscle in decerebrate cats. Their threshold amplitude was very low (10–20 μm at 200/sec), and corresponded to that of the monosynaptic reflex discharges recorded in the same preparation from ventral roots L7–S1. On the other hand the maximum intensity of the unit response was reached at about 80 μm, which corresponded to the value responsible for maximum development of the ventral root discharges. The progressive increase in unit responses as a function of the amplitude of vibration may therefore be related to recruitment of the primary endings of muscle spindles.

SUMMARY

Anatomical observations have shown that the spinovestibular pathway originates mainly, although not exclusively, from the lumbosacral levels of the spinal cord. Their fibers ascend with those of the dorsal spinocerebellar tract along the dorsal part of the lateral funiculus. Direct spinovestibular fibers as well as collaterals of the dorsal spinocerebellar tract terminate in very small numbers in the caudalmost regions of the medial and descending vestibular nuclei, and in the hindlimb region of the lateral vestibular nucleus, while an abundant projection impinges upon the nuclei x and z of Brodal and Pompeiano (1957). All these nuclear regions receiving spinal afferents are not supplied by primary vestibular fibers.

There is no direct evidence so far concerning the functional significance of the spinovestibular pathway, with the exception of the spinal afferents to nucleus z. Recent observations indicate in fact that this nucleus represents the medullary relay in the low threshold group I muscular path from the hindlimb to the cerebral cortex. Somatic afferent impulses, however, may reach the vestibular nuclei indirectly, either via the reticular formation or the cerebellum.

The spinal influence on the vestibular nuclei mediated through the reticular formation is mainly an excitatory one. This response is rather generalized, since it involves the neurons of the vestibular nuclear complex of both sides, including the lateral and medial vestibular nuclei. Cutaneous and high threshold (group II and III) muscular afferents, which are responsible for the ipsilateral flexion reflex at segmental level, are particularly able to modify the spontaneous activity of these vestibular neurons. On the contrary the low threshold group I muscle afferents are apparently uneffective. Experiments of natural stimulation of different types of receptors indicate that skin and deep receptors, particularly the joint receptors, may excite the vestibular neurons. This finding contrasts with the negative results obtained by applying longitudinal vibration to deefferented hindlimb muscles at such amplitudes as to produce a complete activation of the primary endings of muscle spindles. It would appear, therefore, that contrary to the spindle receptors, the joint receptors play a prominent role in supplying postural information to the vestibular nuclei. At the level of both the lateral and medial vestibular nuclei the information can be dealt with and lead to rapid reflex postural adjustments which may involve both the lateral and medial vestibulospinal mechanisms. The cerebellar components of the spinal evoked responses of Deiters' neurons mediated by mossy and climbing fibers have been identified and the response of Purkinje neurons to different groups of muscle afferent volleys recorded.

References pp. 290–296

ACKNOWLEDGEMENTS

This work was supported by P.H.S. Research Grant NB 07685-03 from the National Institute of Neurological Diseases and Blindness, N.I.H., Public Health Service, U.S.A. and by a research grant from the Consiglio Nazionale delle Ricerche, Italia.

REFERENCES

ALLEN, G. I., SABAH, N. H. AND TOYAMA, K. (1971a) Afferent nerve volleys acting on Deiters' neurones via the cerebellum. *Proc. XXV Int. Congr. Physiol. Sci.*, Munich, IX, n. 27, 13.

ALLEN, G. I., SABAH, N. H. AND TOYAMA, K. (1971b) Effect of fore- and hindlimb nerve stimulation on Deiters' neurones. *Brain Res.*, **25**, 645–650.

ANDERSSON, S. AND GERNANDT, B. E. (1956) Ventral root discharge in response to vestibular and proprioceptive stimulation. *J. Neurophysiol.*, **19**, 524–543.

BARNES, C. D. (1970) Cholinergic properties of spino-bulbo-spinal reflex inhibition. *Neuropharmacol.*, **9**, 185–190.

BARNES, C. D. AND POMPEIANO, O. (1970a) Effects of muscle vibration on the pre- and postsynaptic components of the extensor monosynaptic reflex. *Brain Res.*, **18**, 384–388.

BARNES, C. D. AND POMPEIANO, O. (1970b) Presynaptic and postsynaptic effects in the monosynaptic reflex pathway to extensor motoneurons following vibration of synergic muscles. *Arch. ital. Biol.*, **108**, 259–294.

BARNES, C. D. AND POMPEIANO, O. (1970c) The contribution of the medial and lateral vestibular nuclei to presynaptic and postsynaptic effects produced in the lumbar cord by vestibular volleys. *Pflügers Arch. ges. Physiol.*, **317**, 1–9.

BARNES, C. D. AND POMPEIANO, O. (1970d) Dissociation of presynaptic and postsynaptic effects produced in the lumbar cord by vestibular volleys. *Arch. ital. Biol.*, **108**, 295–324.

BARNES, C. D. AND POMPEIANO, O. (1971a) Effects of muscle afferents on brain stem reticular and vestibular units. *Brain Res.*, **25**, 179–183.

BARNES, C. D. AND POMPEIANO, O. (1971b) Vestibular nerve activation of a brain stem cholinergic system influencing the spinal cord. *Neuropharmacol.*, **10**, 425–436.

BATINI, C., MORUZZI, G., AND POMPEIANO, O. (1957) Cerebellar release phenomena. *Arch. ital. Biol.*, **95**, 71–95.

BIANCONI, R. AND VAN DER MEULEN, J. F. (1963) The response to vibration of the end-organs of mammalian muscle spindles. *J. Neurophysiol.*, **26**, 177–190.

BOIVIE, J., GRANT, G. AND SILFVENIUS, H. (1970) A projection from nucleus z to the ventral nuclear complex of the thalamus in the cat. *Acta physiol. scand.*, Suppl. 80, 11A.

BOS, J. H. AND PHILIPSZOON, A. J. (1963) Some forms of nystagmus provoked by stimuli other than accelerations. *Pract. oto-rhino-laryng. (Basel)*, **25**, 108–118.

BOWSHER, D. (1962) The topographical projection of fibres from the anterolateral quadrant of the spinal cord to the subdiencephalic brain stem in man. *Psychiat. Neurol. (Basel)*, **143**, 75–99.

BRODAL, A. (1940) Experimentelle Untersuchungen über die olivocerebellare Lokalisation. *Z. ges. Neurol. Psychiat.*, **169**, 1–153.

BRODAL, A. AND ANGAUT, P. (1967) The termination of spinovestibular fibres in the cat. *Brain Res.*, **5**, 494–500.

BRODAL, A. AND POMPEIANO, O., (1957) The vestibular nuclei in the cat. *J. Anat.*, **91**, 438–454.

BRODAL, A., POMPEIANO, O. AND WALBERG, F. (1962) *The Vestibular Nuclei and Their Connections. Anatomy and Functional Correlations.* Oliver and Boyd, Edinburgh, London, pp. VIII-193.

BRODAL, A. AND TORVIK, A. (1957) Über den Ursprung der sekundären vestibulocerebellaren Fasern bei der Katze. Eine experimentall-anatomische Studie. *Arch. Psychiat. Nervenkr.*, **195**, 550–567.

BROWN, M. C., ENGBERG, I. AND MATTHEWS, P. B. C. (1967) The relative sensitivity to vibration of muscle receptors of the cat. *J. Physiol. (Lond.)*, **192**, 773–780.

BRUGGENCATE, G. TEN, SONNHOF, U., TEICHMANN, R. AND WELLER, E. (1971) A study of the synaptic input to Deiters' neurones evoked by stimulation of peripheral nerves and spinal cord. *Brain Res.*, **25**, 207–211.

CARPENTER, D., ENGBERG, I. AND LUNDBERG, A. (1966) Primary afferent depolarization evoked from the brain stem and the cerebellum. *Arch. ital. Biol.*, **104**, 73–85.

COHEN, L. A. (1961) Role of eye and neck proprioceptive mechanisms in body orientation and motor coordination. *J. Neurophysiol.*, **24**, 1–11.

COOK, W. A. JR., CANGIANO, A. AND POMPEIANO, O. (1969a) Dorsal root potentials in the lumbar cord evoked from the vestibular system. *Arch. ital. Biol.*, **107**, 275–295.

COOK, W. A. JR., CANGIANO, A. AND POMPEIANO, O. (1969b) Vestibular control of transmission in primary afferents to the lumbar spinal cord. *Arch. ital. Biol.*, **107**, 296–320.

CORBIN, K. B. AND HINSEY, J. C. (1935) Intramedullary course of the dorsal root fibers of each of the first four cervical nerves. *J. comp. Neurol.*, **63**, 119–126.

CORBIN, K. B., LHAMON, W. T. AND PETIT, D. W. (1937) Peripheral and central connections of the upper cervical dorsal root ganglia in the rhesus monkey. *J. comp. Neurol.*, **66**, 405–414.

DE KLEIJN, A. (1921) Tonische Labyrinth- und Halsreflexe auf die Augen. *Pflügers Arch. ges. Physiol.*, **186**, 82–97.

DUMONT, S. (1960) Effets extralabyrinthiques sur l'activité des cellules des noyaux vestibulaires. *J. Physiologie*, **52**, 87–88.

DUMONT-TYČ, S. (1964) *Contribution à l'Étude du Contrôle d'Origine Réticulaire des Intégrations Sensorimotrices au Cours de la Vigilance.* Thèse à la Faculté des Sciences de l'Université de Paris, pp. 151.

DUMONT-TYČ, S. (1966) Reticular control of a vestibulo-ocular reflex. In M. D. GONZALES AND E. GUMA (Eds.), *Cortico-subcortical Relationship in Sensory Regulation.* Academy of Sciences, Havana, Cuba, pp. 121–140.

ECCLES, J. C. (1967) The way in which the cerebellum processes sensory information from muscle. In M. D. YAHR AND D. P. PURPURA (Eds.), *Neurophysiological Basis of Normal and Abnormal Motor Activities.* Raven Press, Hewlett, New York, pp. 379–414.

ECCLES, J. C., FABER, D. S., MURPHY, J. T., SABAH, N. H. AND TÁBOŘÍKOVA, H. (1969) Firing patterns of Purkinje cells in responses to volleys from limb nerves. *Brain Res.*, **14**, 222–226.

ECCLES, J. C., FABER, D. S., MURPHY, J. T., SABAH, N. H. AND TÁBOŘÍKOVA, H. (1970) The integrative performance of the cerebellar Purkyně cell. In P. ANDERSEN AND J. K. S. JANSEN (Eds.), *Excitatory Synaptic Mechanisms.* Universitetsforlaget, Oslo, pp. 223–236.

ECCLES, J. C., FABER, D. S., MURPHY, J. T., SABAH, N. H. AND TÁBOŘÍKOVÁ, H. (1971a) Afferent volleys in limb nerves influencing impulse discharges in cerebellar cortex. I. In mossy fibers and granule cells. *Exp. Brain Res.*, **13**, 15–35.

ECCLES, J. C., FABER, D. S., MURPHY, J. T., SABAH, N. H. AND TÁBOŘÍKOVÁ, H. (1971b) Afferent volleys in limb nerves influencing impulse discharges in cerebellar cortex. II. In Purkyně cells. *Exp. Brain Res.*, **13**, 36–53.

ECCLES, J. C., FABER, D. S., MURPHY, J. T., SABAH, N. H. AND TÁBOŘÍKOVÁ, H. (1971c) Investigations on integration of mossy fiber inputs to Purkyně cells in the anterior lobe. *Exp. Brain Res.*, **13**, 54–77.

ECCLES, J. C., ITO, M. AND SZENTÁGOTHAI, J. (1967) *The Cerebellum as a Neuronal Machine.* Springer, Berlin, Heidelberg, New York, pp. 335.

ECCLES, J. C., PROVINI, L., STRATA, P. AND TÁBOŘÍKOVÁ, H. (1968a) Analysis of electrical potentials in the cerebellar anterior lobe by stimulation of hindlimb and forelimb nerves. *Exp. Brain Res.*, **6**, 171–194.

ECCLES, J. C., PROVINI, L., STRATA, P. AND TÁBOŘÍKOVÁ, H. (1968b) Topographical investigations on the climbing fiber inputs from forelimb and hindlimb afferents to the cerebellar anterior lobe. *Exp. Brain Res.*, **6**, 195–215.

ECCLES, R. M. AND LUNDBERG, A. (1959) Synaptic actions in motoneurons by afferents which may evoke the flexion reflex. *Arch. ital. Biol.*, **97**, 199–221.

EHRHARDT, K. J. AND WAGNER, A. (1970) Labyrinthine and neck reflexes recorded from spinal single motoneurons in the cat. *Brain Res.*, **19**, 87–104.

ESCOLAR, J. (1948) The afferent connections of the 1st, 2nd and 3rd cervical nerves in the cat. An analysis by Marchi and Rasdolsky methods. *J. comp. Neurol.*, **89**, 79–92.

FABER, D. S., ISHIKAWA, K. AND ROWE, M. J. (1971) The responses of cerebellar Purkyně cells to muscle vibration. *Brain Res.*, **26**, 184–187.

FELDMAN, S., WAGMAN, I. H. AND BENDER, M. B. (1961) Anterior brainstem and sciatic nerve connections to vestibular nuclei in cat. *J. Neurophysiol.*, **24**, 350–363.

FREDRICKSON, J. M. AND SCHWARZ, D. (1970) Multisensory influence upon single units in the vestibular nucleus. In *Fourth Symposium on the Role of the Vestibular Organs in Space Exploration. NASA SP*-187, 203–208.

FREDRICKSON, J. M., SCHWARZ, D. UND KORNHUBER, H. H. (1964) Konvergenz und Interaktion vestibulären und proprioceptiv-somatosensibler Afferenzen au Neuronen der Vestibulariskerne der Katze. *Pflügers Arch. ges. Physiol.*, **281**, 33.

FREDRICKSON, J. M., SCHWARZ, D. AND KORNHUBER, H. H. (1966) Convergence and interaction of vestibular and deep somatic afferents upon neurons in the vestibular nuclei of the cat. *Acta oto-laryng. (Stockh.)*, **61**, 168–188.

GEHUCHTEN, A. VAN (1900) Recherches sur la termination centrale des nerfs sensibles périphériques. La racine postérieure des deux premiers nerfs cervicaux. *Névraxe*, **2**, 229–256.

GERNANDT, B. E. (1959) Vestibular mechanisms. In J. FIELD, H. W. MAGOUN AND V. E. HALL (Eds.), *Handbook of Physiology. Section 1. Neurophysiology. Vol. 1.* Amer. Physiol. Soc., Washington, D.C., pp. 549–564.

GERNANDT, B. E., (1962) Vestibular influence on spinal mechanisms. *Proc. XXII int. Congr. physiol. Sci., Leiden, I*, part II, 497–499.

GERNANDT, B. E. (1964) Somatic and autonomic motor outflow to vestibular stimulation. In W. S. FIELDS AND B. R. ALFORD (Eds.), *Neurological Aspects of Auditory and Vestibular Disorders.* Thomas, Springfield, Ill., pp. 194–211.

GERNANDT, B. E. (1967) Vestibular influences upon spinal reflex activity. In A. V. S. DE REUCK AND J. KNIGHT (Eds.), *Myotatic, Kinesthetic and Vestibular Mechanisms.* J. and A. Churchill, London, pp. 170–183.

GERNANDT, B. E. AND GILMAN, S. (1959) Descending vestibular activity and its modulation by proprioceptive, cerebellar and reticular influences. *Exp. Neurol.*, **1**, 274–304.

GERNANDT, B. E. AND GILMAN, S. (1960a) Vestibular and propriospinal interactions and protracted spinal inhibition by brain stem activation. *J. Neurophysiol.*, **23**, 269–287.

GERNANDT, B. E. AND GILMAN, S. (1960b) Generation of labyrinthine impulses, descending vestibular pathways, and modulation of vestibular activity by proprioceptive, cerebellar, and reticular influences. In G. L. RASMUSSEN AND W. F. WINDLE (Eds.), *Neural Mechanisms of the Auditory and Vestibular Systems.* C. C. Thomas, Springfield, Ill., pp. 324–348.

GERNANDT, B. E., IRANYI, M. AND LIVINGSTON, R. B. (1959) Vestibular influences on spinal mechanisms. *Exp. Neurol.*, **1**, 248–273.

GERNANDT, B. E., KATSUKI, Y. AND LIVINGSTON, R. B. (1957) Functional organization of descending vestibular influences. *J. Neurophysiol.*, **20**, 453–469.

GERNANDT, B. E. AND PROLER, M. L. (1965) Medullary and spinal nerve responses to vestibular stimulation. *Exp. Neurol.*, **11**, 27–37.

GERNANDT, B. E. AND SHIMAMURA, M. (1961) Mechanisms of interlimb reflexes in cat. *J. Neurophysiol.*, **24**, 665–676.

GERNANDT, B. E. AND THULIN, C.-A. (1953) Vestibular mechanisms of facilitation of cord reflexes. *Amer. J. Physiol.*, **172**, 653–660.

GIAQUINTO, S., AND POMPEIANO, O. (1964) Inhibition of proprioceptive spinal reflexes induced by cutaneous afferent volleys in unrestrained cats. *Arch. ital. Biol.*, **102**, 393–417.

GIAQUINTO, S., POMPEIANO, O. E SANTINI, M. (1963) Risposte di unità deitersiane a stimolazione graduata di nervi cutanei e muscolari in animali decerebrati a cervelletto integro. *Boll. Soc. ital. Biol. sper.*, **39**, 524–527.

GRANT, G., OSCARSSON, O. AND ROSÉN, I. (1966) Functional organization of the spinoreticulocerebellar path with identification of its spinal component. *Exp. Brain Res.*, **1**, 306–319.

GRILLNER, S., HONGO, T. AND LUND, S. (1968) The origin of descending fibres monosynaptically activating spinoreticular neurones. *Brain Res.*, **10**, 259–262.

HAND, P. J. (1966) Lumbosacral dorsal root terminations in the nucleus gracilis of the rat. Some observations on terminal degeneration in other medullary sensory nuclei. *J. comp. Neurol.*, **126**, 137–156.

HAUGLIE-HANSSEN, E. (1968) Intrinsic neuronal organization of the vestibular nuclear complex in the cat. A Golgi study. *Ergebn. Anat. Entwickl.-Gesch.*, **40**, 1–105.

HINOKI, M. AND KUROSAWA, R. (1965) Studies on vertigo provoked by neck and nape muscles. Note on vertigo of cervical origin. Some observations on vertiginous attacks caused by injection of procaine solution into neck and nape muscles in man. *Excerpta med.*, **18**, 176.

HINOKI, M. AND TERAYAMA, K. (1966) Physiological role of neck muscles in the occurrence of optic eye nystagmus. *Acta oto-laryng. (Stockh.)*, **62**, 157–170.

IGARASHI, M., ALFORD, B. R., WATANABE, T. AND MAXIAN, P. M. (1969) Role of neck proprioceptors for the maintenance of dynamic bodily equilibrium in the squirrel monkey. *Laryngoscope*, **79**, 1713–1727.

IOSIF, G., POMPEIANO, O., STRATA, P. AND THODEN, U. In preparation.

ITO, M. (1968) Two extensive inhibitory systems for brain stem nuclei. In C. VON EULER, S. SKOGLUND AND U. SÖDERBERG (Eds.), *Structure and Function of Inhibitory Neuronal Mechanisms.* Pergamon Press, Oxford, pp. 309–322.

ITO, M. (1970) The cerebellovestibular interaction in the cat's vestibular nuclei neurons. In *Fourth Symposium on the Role of the Vestibular Organs in Space Exploration. NASA SP*-187, 183–199.

ITO, M. (1972) Cerebellar control of the vestibular neurones: physiology and pharmacology. In A. BRODAL AND O. POMPEIANO, (Eds.), *Progress in Brain Research. Vol. 37. Basic aspects of central vestibular mechanisms.* Elsevier, Amsterdam, pp. 377–390.

ITO, M., HONGO, T., YOSHIDA, N., OKADA, Y. AND OBATA, K. (1964) Antidromic and trans-synaptic activation in Deiters' neurones induced from the spinal cord. *Jap. J. Physiol.,* **14**, 638–658.

ITO, M. AND KAWAI, N. (1964) IPSP-receptive field in the cerebellum for Deiters neurones. *Proc. Jap. Acad.,* **40**, 762–764.

ITO, M., KAWAI, N. AND UDO, M. (1965) The origin of cerebellar-induced inhibition and facilitation in the neurones of Deiters and intracerebellar nuclei. *Proc. XXIII int. Congr. physiol. Sci., Tokyo,* 997.

ITO, M., KAWAI, N. AND UDO, M. (1968a) The origin of cerebellar-induced inhibition of Deiters' neurones. III. Localization of the inhibitory zone. *Exp. Brain Res.,* **4**, 310–320.

ITO, M., KAWAI, N., UDO, M. AND MANO, N. (1969) Axon reflex activation of Deiters' neurones from the cerebellar cortex through collaterals of the cerebellar afferents. *Exp. Brain Res.,* **8**, 249–268.

ITO, M., KAWAI, N., UDO, M. AND SATO, N. (1968b) Cerebellar-evoked disinhibition in dorsal Deiters' neurones. *Exp. Brain Res.,* **6**, 247–264.

ITO, M., OBATA, K., AND OCHI, R. (1966) The origin of cerebellar-induced inhibition of Deiters' neurones. II. Temporal correlation between the trans-synaptic activation of Purkinje cells and the inhibition of Deiters' neurones. *Exp. Brain Res.,* **2**, 350–364.

ITO, M., UDO, M. AND MANO, N. (1970a) Long inhibitory and excitatory pathways converging onto cat reticular and Deiters' neurons and their relevance to reticulofugal axons. *J. Neurophysiol.,* **33**, 210–226.

ITO, M., UDO, M., MANO, N. AND KAWAI, N. (1970b) Synaptic action of the fastigiobulbar impulses upon neurones in the medullary reticular formation and vestibular nuclei. *Exp. Brain Res.,* **11**, 29–47.

ITO, M. AND YOSHIDA, M. (1964) The cerebellar-evoked monosynaptic inhibition of Deiters neurones. *Experienta (Basel),* **20**, 515–516.

ITO, M. AND YOSHIDA, M. (1966) The origin of cerebellar-induced inhibition of Deiters' neurones. I. Monosynaptic initiation of the inhibitory postsynaptic potentials. *Exp. Brain Res.,* **2**, 330–349.

ITO, M., YOSHIDA, M., OBATA, K., KAWAI, N. AND UDO, M. (1970c) Inhibitory control of intracerebellar nuclei by the Purkinje cell axons. *Exp. Brain Res.,* **10**, 64–80.

JOHNSON, F. H. (1954) Experimental study of spino-reticular connections in the cat. *Anat. Rec.,* **118**, 316.

JONGKEES, L. B. W. AND PHILIPSZOON, A. J. (1964) Electronystagmography. *Acta oto-laryng. (Stockh.),* Suppl. 189, 1–111.

KIM, J. H. AND PARTRIDGE, L. D. (1969) Observations on types of response to combinations of neck, vestibular and muscle stretch signals. *J. Neurophysiol.,* **32**, 239–250.

KOELLA, W. (1947) Die Beeinflussbarkeit des postrotatorischen Augennystagmus durch propriozeptive Halsreflexe beim Kaninchen. *Helv. physiol. Acta,* **5**, 430.

KOELLA, W. P., NAKAO, H., EVANS, R. L. AND WADA, J. (1956) Interaction of vestibular and proprioceptive reflexes in the decerebrate cat. *Amer. J. Physiol.,* **185**, 607–613.

KÖRLIN, D. AND LARSON, B. (1970) Differences in cerebellar potentials evoked by the group I and cutaneous components of the cuneocerebellar tract. In P. ANDERSEN AND J. K. S. JANSEN (Eds.), *Excitatory Synaptic Mechanisms.* Universitetsforlaget, Oslo, pp. 237–241.

LANDGREN, S. (1969) Projection of group I muscle afferents to the cerebral cortex. *Acta physiol. scand.,* **77**, Suppl. 330, n. 40, 35.

LANDGREN, S. AND SILFVENIUS, H. (1969a) Projection to cerebral cortex of Group I muscle afferents from the cat's hind limb. *J. Physiol. (Lond.),* **200**, 353–372.

LANDGREN, S. AND SILFVENIUS, H. (1969b) The medullary relay in the path from hind limb muscle spindles to the cerebral cortex of the cat. *Acta physiol. scand.,* **77**, Suppl. 330, n. 190, 119.

LANDGREN, S. AND SILFVENIUS, H. (1970) The projection of Group I muscle afferents from the hind limb to the contralateral thalamus of the cat. *Acta physiol. scand.,* **80**, 10A.

LANDGREN, S. AND SILFVENIUS, H. (1971) Nucleus z, the medullary relay in the projection path to the cerebral cortex of group I muscle afferents from the cat's hind limb. *J. Physiol. (Lond.)*, **218**, 551–571.

LAPORTE, Y., LUNDBERG, A. AND OSCARSSON, O. (1956) Functional organization of the dorsal spino-cerebellar tract in the cat. I. Recording of mass discharge in dissected Flechsig's fasciculus. *Acta physiol. scand.*, **36**, 175–187.

LORENTE DE NÓ, R. (1924) Études sur le cerveau postérieur. III. Sur les connexions extra-cérébelleuses des fascicules afférents au cerveau, et sur la fonction de cet organe. *Trav. Lab. Rech. Biol. Univ. Madr.*, **22**, 51–65.

LUND, S. AND POMPEIANO, O. (1965) Descending pathways with monosynaptic action on motoneurones. *Experientia (Basel)*, **21**, 602–603.

LUND, S. AND POMPEIANO, O., (1968) Monosynaptic excitation of alpha motoneurones from supraspinal structures in the cat. *Acta physiol. scand.*, **73**, 1–21.

LUND, S. AND POMPEIANO, O. (1970) Electrically induced monosynaptic and polysynaptic reflexes involving the same motoneuronal pool in the unrestrained cat. *Arch. ital. Biol.*, **108**, 130–153.

LUNDBERG, A. (1964) Ascending spinal hindlimb pathways in the cat. In J. C. ECCLES AND J. P. SCHADÉ (Eds.), *Progress in Brain Research. Vol. 12. Physiology of spinal neurons*, Elsevier, Amsterdam, pp. 135–163.

LUNDBERG, A. AND OSCARSSON, O. (1960) Functional organization of the dorsal spino-cerebellar tract in the cat. VII. Identification of units by antidromic activation from the cerebellar cortex with recognition of five functional subdivisions. *Acta physiol. scand.*, **50**, 356–374.

MAGHERINI, P. C., THODEN, U. AND POMPEIANO, O. (1971) Spino-bulbo-spinal reflex inhibition of monosynaptic extensor reflexes of hindlimb in cats. *Arch. ital. Biol.*, **109**, 110–129.

MAGNUS, R. (1924) *Körperstellung*. J. Springer, Berlin, pp. 740.

MAGNUS, R. AND DE KLEIJN, A. (1912) Die Abhängigkeit des Tonus der Extremitätenmuskeln von der Kopfstellung. *Pflügers Arch. ges. Physiol.*, **145**, 455–548.

MAGNUS, R. AND STORM VAN LEEUWEN, W. (1914) Die akuten und die dauernden Folgen des Ausfalles der tonischen Hals- und Labyrinthreflexe. *Pflügers Arch. ges. Physiol.*, **159**, 157–217.

MATTHEWS, P. B. C. (1966) The reflex excitation of the soleus muscle of the decerebrate cat caused by vibration applied to its tendon. *J. Physiol. (Lond.)*, **184**, 450–472.

McCOUCH, G. P., DEERING, I. D. AND LING, T. H. (1951) Location of receptors for tonic neck reflexes. *J. Neurophysiol.*, **14**, 191–195.

McINTYRE, A. K. (1951) Spino-cerebellar pathways in the cat. *Proc. Univ. Otago med. School*, **29**, 16.

McNALLY, W. J. AND TAIT, J. (1925) Ablation experiments on the labyrinth of the frog. *Amer. J. Physiol.*, **75**, 155–179.

MEHLER, W. R. (1968) Reticulovestibular connections compared with spinovestibular connections in the rat. *Anat. Rec.*, **160**, 485.

MEHLER, W. R., FEFERMAN, M. E. AND NAUTA, W. J. H. (1960) Ascending axon degeneration following anterolateral chordotomy. An experimental study in the monkey. *Brain*, **83**, 718–750.

MILLER, S. AND OSCARSSON, O. (1969) Termination and functional organization of spino-olivocerebellar paths. In W. S. FIELD AND W. D. WILLIS, JR. (Eds.), *The Cerebellum in Health and Disease*. Green Publ., St. Louis, pp. 172–200.

MORELLI, M., NICOTRA, L., BARNES, C. D., CANGIANO, A., COOK, W. A. JR. AND POMPEIANO, O. (1970) An apparatus for producing small-amplitude high-frequency sinusoidal stretching of the muscle. *Arch. ital. Biol.*, **108**, 222–232.

MOUNTCASTLE, V. B., COVIAN, M. R. AND HARRISON, C. R. (1952) The central representation of some forms of deep sensibility. *Res. Publ. Ass. nerv. ment. Dis.*, **30**, 339–370.

OSCARSSON, O. (1956) Functional organization of the ventral spino-cerebellar tract in the cat. I. Electrophysiological identification of the tract. *Acta physiol. scand.*, **38**, 145–165.

OSCARSSON, O. (1965) Functional organization of the spino- and cuneocerebellar tracts. *Physiol. Rev.*, **45**, 495–522.

PHILIPSZOON, A. J. (1962) Compensatory eye movements and nystagmus provoked by stimulation of the vestibular organ and the cervical nerve roots. *Pract. oto-rhino-laryng. (Basel)*, **24**, 193–202.

PHILIPSZOON, A. J. AND BOS, J. H. (1963) Neck torsion nystagmus. *Pract. oto-rhino-laryng. (Basel)*, **25**, 339–344.

POMPEIANO, O. (1968) Monosynaptic and polysynaptic reflex excitation of motoneurones to plantar muscles in the unrestrained cat. *Brain Res.*, **10**, 252–256.

POMPEIANO, O. (1972) Vestibulospinal relations: vestibular influences on gamma motoneurons and primary afferents. In A. BRODAL AND O. POMPEIANO (Eds.), *Progress in Brain Research. Vol. 37. Basic aspects of central vestibular mechanisms*, Elsevier, Amsterdam, pp. 197–232.

POMPEIANO, O. AND BARNES, C. D. (1971a) Response of brain stem reticular neurons to muscle vibration in the decerebrate cat. *J. Neurophysiol.*, **34**, 709–724.

POMPEIANO, O. AND BARNES, C. D. (1971b) Effect of sinusoidal muscle stretch on neurons in medial and descending vestibular nuclei. *J. Neurophysiol.*, **34**, 725–734.

POMPEIANO, O. AND BRODAL, A. (1957a) The origin of vestibulospinal fibres in the cat. An experimental-anatomical study, with comments on the descending medial longitudinal fasciculus. *Arch. ital. Biol.*, **95**, 166–195.

POMPEIANO, O. AND BRODAL, A. (1957b) Spino-vestibular fibers in the cat. An experimental study. *J. comp. Neurol.*, **108**, 353–382.

POMPEIANO, O. E COTTI, E. (1959a) Modificazione dell'attività di singole unità deitersiane per stimolazioni della periferia sensitiva. *Boll. Soc. ital. Biol. sper.*, **35**, 1221–1222.

POMPEIANO, O. E COTTI, E. (1959b) Convergenza d'impulsi afferenti su unità deitersiane che rispondono alla stimolazione localizzata del cervelletto. *Rend. Accad. naz. Lincei, Cl. Sci. fis., mat. nat.*, Ser. VIII, **27**, 76–79.

POMPEIANO, O. E COTTI, E. (1959c) Analisi microelettrodica delle proiezioni cerebellodeitersiane. *Arch. Sci. biol. (Bologna)*, **43**, 57–101.

POMPEIANO, O. AND SWETT, J. E. (1963a) Actions of graded cutaneous and muscular afferent volleys on brain units in the decerebrate, cerebellectomized cat. *Arch. ital. Biol.*, **101**, 552–583.

POMPEIANO, O. AND SWETT, J. E. (1963b) Cerebellar potentials and responses of reticular units evoked by muscular afferent volleys in the decerebrate cat. *Arch. ital. Biol.*, **101**, 584–613.

RANSON, S. W., DAVENPORT, H. K. AND DOLES, E. A. (1932) Intramedullary course of the dorsal root fibers of the first three cervical nerves. *J. comp. Neurol.*, **54**, 1–12.

REXED, B. (1954) A cytoarchitectonic atlas of the spinal cord in the cat. *J. comp. Neurol.*, **100**, 297–379.

ROSÉN, I. (1969) Afferent connexions to Group I activated cells in the main cuneate nucleus of the cat. *J. Physiol. (Lond.)*, **205**, 209–236.

SEGUIN, J. J., MAGHERINI, P. C. AND POMPEIANO, O. (1972) The response of neurones in the nucleus z to vibration of cat's hindlimb muscles. *Arch. Fisiol.*, **68**, 341–342.

SHERRINGTON, C. S. (1898) Decerebrate rigidity, and reflex coordination of movements. *J. Physiol. (Lond.)*, **22**, 319–332.

SHIMAMURA, J. AND AKERT, K. (1965) Peripheral nervous relations of propriospinal and spino-bulbo-spinal reflex systems. *Jap. J. Physiol.*, **15**, 638–647.

SHIMAMURA, M. AND AOKI, M. (1969) Effects of spino-bulbo-spinal reflex volleys on flexor motoneurons of hindlimb in the cat. *Brain Res.*, **16**, 333–349.

SHIMAMURA, M. AND LIVINGSTON, R. B. (1963) Longitudinal conduction systems serving spinal and brain-stem coordination. *J. Neurophysiol.*, **26**, 258–272.

SHIMAMURA, M., MORI, S., MATSUSHIMA, S. AND FUJIMORI, B. (1964) On the spino-bulbo-spinal reflex in dogs, monkeys and man. *Jap. J. Physiol.*, **14**, 411–421.

SHIMAMURA, M., MORI, S. AND YAMAUCHI, T. (1967a) Interactions of spino-bulbo-spinal reflexes with cortically evoked pyramidal and extrapyramidal activities. *Brain Res.*, **4**, 93–102.

SHIMAMURA, M., MORI, S. AND YAMAUCHI, T. (1967b) Effects of spino-bulbo-spinal reflex volleys on extensor motoneurons of hindlimb in cats. *J. Neurophysiol.*, **30**, 319–332.

STUART, D. G., MOSHER, C. G., GERLACH, R. L. AND REINKING, R. M. (1970) Selective activation of Ia afferents by transient muscle stretch. *Exp. Brain Res.*, **10**, 477–487.

TÁBOŘÍKOVÁ, H., PROVINI, L. AND DECANDIA, M. (1966) Evidence that muscle stretch evokes long-loop reflexes from higher centres. *Brain Res.*, **2**, 192–194.

THODEN, U., MAGHERINI, P. C. AND POMPEIANO, O. (1971a) Effects of muscle afferents on supraspinal descending inhibitory mechanisms. *Brain Res.*, **29**, 339–342.

THODEN, U., MAGHERINI, P. C. AND POMPEIANO, O. (1971b) Proprioceptive control of supraspinal descending inhibitory mechanisms. *Arch. ital. Biol.*, **109**, 130–151.

TRINCKER, D. (1961) Analysis of the physical and neurophysiological principles, underlying vestibular stimulation. *Confin Neurol.*, **21**, 372–379.

UDO, M. AND MANO, N. (1970) Discrimination of different spinal monosynaptic pathways converging onto reticular neurons. *J. Neurophysiol.*, **33**, 227–238.

WALBERG, F., BOWSHER, D. AND BRODAL, A. (1958) The termination of primary vestibular fibers in the vestibular nuclei in the cat. An experimental study with silver methods. *J. comp. Neurol.*, **110**, 391–419.

WILSON, V. J. (1970) Vestibular and somatic inputs to cells of the lateral and medial vestibular nuclei of the cat. In *Fifth Symposium on the Role of the Vestibular Organs in Space Exploration. NASA SP*-187, 145–158.

WILSON, V. J., KATO, M. AND PETERSON, B. W. (1966a) Convergence of inputs on Deiters neurones. *Nature (Lond.)*, **211**, 1409–1411.

WILSON, V. J., KATO, M., PETERSON, B. W. AND WYLIE, R. M. (1967) A single-unit analysis of the organization of Deiters' nucleus. *J. Neurophysiol.*, **30**, 603–619.

WILSON, V. J., KATO, M. AND THOMAS, R. C. (1965) Excitation of lateral vestibular neurones. *Nature, (Lond.)*, **206**, 96–97.

WILSON, V. J., KATO, M., THOMAS, R. C. AND PETERSON, B. W. (1966b) Excitation of lateral vestibular neurons by peripheral afferent fibers. *J. Neurophysiol.*, **29**, 508–529.

WILSON, V. J., WYLIE, R. M. AND MARCO, L. A. (1968) Synaptic inputs to cells in the medial vestibular nucleus. *J. Neurophysiol.*, **31**, 176–185.

WYLIE, R. M. AND FELPEL, L. P. (1971) The influence of the cerebellum and peripheral somatic nerves on the activity of Deiters' cells in the cat. *Exp. Brain Res.*, **12**, 528–546.

YAMAMOTO, S. AND MIYAJIMA, M. (1961) Unit discharges recorded from dorsal portion of medulla responding to adequate exteroceptive and proprioceptive stimulation in cats. *Jap. J. Physiol.*, **11**, 619–626.

YEE, J. AND CORBIN, K. B. (1939) The intramedullary course of the upper five, cervical, dorsal root fibers in the rabbit. *J. comp. Neurol.*, **70**, 297–314.

Vestibulospinal Projection in the Toad

N. CORVAJA AND I. GROFOVÁ

Institute of Physiology II, University of Pisa, Pisa, Italy and
Anatomical Institute, University of Oslo, Oslo, Norway

Experiments performed in frogs and toads have shown that unilateral section of the VIII cranial nerve, as well as lesions localized to its nuclei of termination, produce changes of postural tonus characterized by a decrease in contraction of the extensor muscles ipsilateral to the lesion and by an increase in postural activity on the contra-lateral side. One also observes an asymmetry in the position of the head which is bent towards the side of the lesion (Barale *et al.*, 1971).

Similar observation had been made in cats following unilateral lesion of the lateral vestibular nucleus of Deiters, which projects to the spinal cord via the lateral vestibulo-spinal tract (see Pompeiano, 1972).

The nuclei of termination of the VIII cranial nerve as well as the structural organization of the gray matter in the spinal cord of amphibians have been described by several anatomists (Gaupp, 1899; Larsell, 1934; Ariëns Kappers *et al.*, 1936; Silver, 1942; Nemec, 1951; Kennard, 1959; Nieuwenhuys, 1964; Kemali and Braitenberg, 1969). However, no experimental anatomical data concerning the vestibulospinal tract descending to the spinal cord in the toad could be found in the literature. It is therefore necessary to furnish an anatomical basis for further experimental and refined morphological investigations. Our attention has been primarily focused on the vestibulospinal projection but some other descending spinal tracts have also been considered.

Experiments were carried out in 30 adult toads (*Bufo bufo L.*), mainly females. In a MS-222 (Sandoz, Basle) anesthesia, the fossa rhombencephali was exposed and the head of the animal was then fixed in a special holding system. Electrolytic lesions (0.5–2.5 mA 15–30 sec) were made with a microelectrode, completely isolated except at the tip, which was inserted 0.5 mm deep into the eminentia acustica at a distance of 1.2–1.5 mm (according to the dimension of the brain) from the midline and immediately posterior to the cerebellum.

After the operation the animals were kept at a constant temperature of 28°, in order to accelerate the speed of degeneration. The changes of postural tonus were observed during the whole survival period. After 8–12 days the toads were killed by intravital perfusion with isotonic physiologic saline followed by 10% neutral formalin. The brains and the spinal cords were removed in toto and further fixed in 10% neutral formalin.

References p. 307

The brain stem containing the lesion was separated from the spinal cord and both parts were embedded in yolk (Ebbesson, 1970) and stored in 10 % neutral formalin in the refrigerator. Brain stems of 6 frogs in which a clear-cut postural asymmetry developed following the operation and of some animals without postural changes were cut transversally and stained with the Nissl method for identification of the lesion. In some animals alternating sections were also impregnated according to Nauta (1957) or Land et al. (1970) in order to follow the course and termination of degenerated fibers within the brain stem.

Spinal cords of selected cases were then cut serially in the transversal or sagittal plane and impregnated according to the silver techniques of Nauta (1957), Fink and Heimer (1967), Ebbesson and Heimer (1970) and Land et al. (1970).

In addition, in two toads, hemisection of the spinal cord was made at a high cervical level and the spinal cord was treated in the same way as described above.

Descending fibers following a hemisection of the spinal cord

Fig. 1A illustrates the results obtained in one representative experiment in which the left half of the spinal cord was completely transected between the first and the second spinal nerves. The lesion involved also the adjacent part of the opposite side.

In the cervical cord degenerated fibers are seen in the left dorsal, lateral and ventral funiculi. Some degenerated fibers occur also in the medial part of the right dorsal and ventral funiculi.

The degenerated fibers observed in the *dorsal* funiculus form a thin layer close to the gray matter. They gradually diminish in number during their course through the spinal cord and finally disappear at the upper lumbar level.

The *lateral* funiculus shows degeneration in both its dorsal and ventral halves. Fibers situated dorsolaterally can be followed until the low lumbar level and enter the intermediate gray matter throughout the whole length of the spinal cord. Fibers in the ventral half of the lateral funiculus course close to the border of the ventral horn and do not descend below the thoracic segments. These fibers enter the gray matter of the ventral horn where the large *lateral* column of motoneurons is located (Fig. 1B). Fine degenerated fragments can also be observed around the cell bodies of these motoneurons (Fig. 1C).

Fig. 1. Degeneration following hemisection of the spinal cord of the toad. A: Diagrammatic representation of the distribution of degenerating fibers as seen in transverse section from five representative levels of the spinal cord. 2–3, cranial and caudal levels of the cervical enlargement; 4, thoracic cord, 5–6, cranial and caudal levels of the lumbar enlargement. In this as well as in the following figures *hatchings* indicate the position and the extent of the lesion, *coarse dots* transversally cut degenerating fibers, *wavy lines* obliquely or longitudinally cut fibers, *small dots* terminal fibers; *triangles* indicate motoneurons. B: Photomicrograph of a section from the cervical enlargement illustrating the position of the medial (MC) and lateral (LC) columns of motoneurons. Nauta method. × 100. C: Detail of the previous picture showing degenerating fibers around the lateral column of motoneurons. Nauta method × 215. D: Degenerating fibers (arrows) crossing the midline ventral to the central canal (CC) in the thoracic cord. Nauta method. × 215.

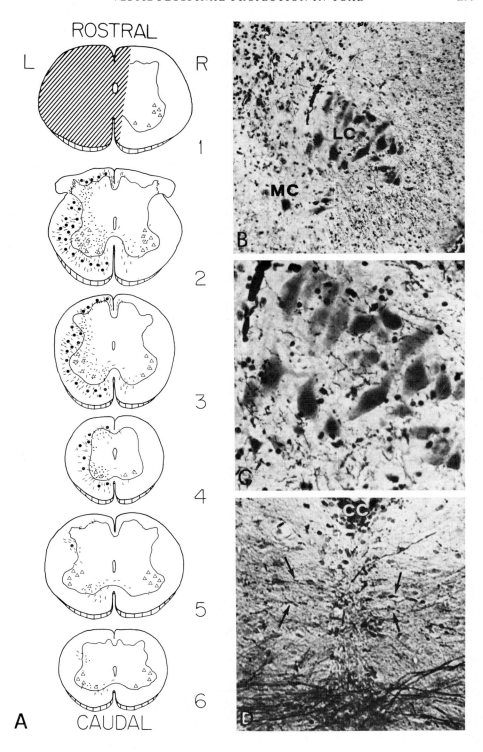

In the *ventral* funiculus degenerated fibers spread in its entire mediolateral extent. During their course through the spinal cord they diminish in number, although they can be followed down to the lowest lumbar level. They enter the medial part of the ventral horn and terminate in this region which includes the *medial* column of moto-neurons (Fig. 1B). Some of the fibers which descend in the ventral funiculus cross the gray matter ventral to the central canal to reach the corresponding region of the opposite side (Fig. 1D).

Descending fibers following lesions of the nuclei of termination of the VIII cranial nerve

In all toads which presented postural asymmetries, lesions involved the ventral nucleus of the VIII cranial nerve. In one case which did not show postural changes, the lesion involved only the upper part of the ventral nucleus. Unfortunately, there was always some injury of the structures adjacent to the nuclei of termination of the VIII nerve which could influence the pattern of degeneration in the spinal cord.

Lesion involving the nuclei of termination of the VIII cranial nerve together with the underlying white matter (Fig. 2). In this experiment the lesion involved both the dorsal and the ventral nuclei of the VIII nerve (Fig. 2, levels 1–3). Caudal to this lesion, degenerating fibers are concentrated in the region of the spinal tract of the V cranial nerve, while some degenerated fragments, probably belonging to the spinal tract of the VIII cranial nerve, appear more dorsally (Fig. 2, levels 4–6).

Degenerating fibers spread in the ventrolateral white matter on the homolateral side and also on the contralateral side. At the level of the nucleus of the XII cranial nerve (Fig. 2, levels 5 and 6) many fibers from the region of the spinal tract of the V cranial nerve descend ventromedially through the gray matter and some of them cross the midline to reach the white matter of the opposite side. They occupy two fields located in the ventral part as well as in the lateral part of the white matter.

In the cervical cord degenerating fibers descend in the dorsal, lateral and ventral funiculi ipsilateral to the side of the lesion and to a smaller extent also in the lateral and ventral funiculi of the contralateral side. Degenerating fibers in the dorsal and ventral funiculi have the same position, course and terminations as following the hemi-section of the spinal cord. Degenerated fields in the lateral funiculi, however, occupy only their dorsal halves and fibers are given off to the intermediate part of the gray matter throughout the whole length of the spinal cord. No degenerated fibers enter the region of the lateral group of motoneurons.

Lesion restricted to the nuclei of termination of the VIII cranial nerve (Fig. 3). In this case the lesion is limited to the dorsal and ventral nuclei of the VIII nerve but it does not involve the surrounding white matter. Crossed degenerated fibers which terminate in part, at least, in the nuclei of termination of the contralateral VIII nerve are observed (Fig. 3, levels 4 and 5). Only the course and the termination of the descending fibers to the spinal cord will be described in detail.

Degenerated fibers descend ventral and ventromedial to the spinal tract of the V cranial nerve which, however, is free of degeneration. At the level of the XII cranial nerve three groups of degenerating fibers can be distinguished.

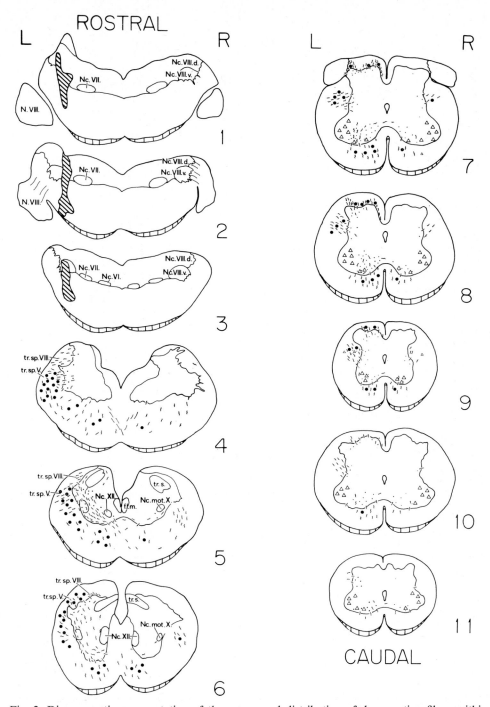

Fig. 2. Diagrammatic representation of the course and distribution of degenerating fibers within the brain stem (4–6) and the spinal cord (7–11) following a lesion involving the dorsal and ventral nuclei of termination of the VIII nerve and extending deep into the white matter of the brain stem. For symbols see legend to Fig. 1. *Abbreviations* for Figs. 2 and 3: f.l.m., fasciculus longitudinalis medialis; N.VIII, VIII cranial nerve; Nc. VI, Nc. VII and Nc XII, nuclei of VI, VII and XII cranial nerves; Nc. VIII d., dorsal nucleus of the VIII nerve; Nc. VIII v., ventral nucleus of the VIII nerve; Nc. mot. X, motor nucleus of the X nerve; tr.s., solitary tract; tr. sp. V., spinal trigeminal tract; tr. sp. VIII, spinal vestibular tract.

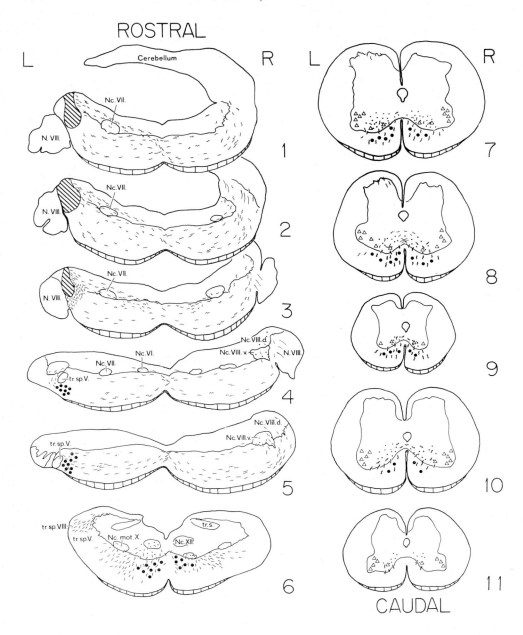

Fig. 3. Diagram illustrating the course and distribution of degenerating fibers following a lesion restricted to the nuclei of termination of the VIII nerve. Symbols and abbreviations as in Figs. 1 and 2.

The first group is relatively small and lies dorsomedial to the spinal tract of the ipsilateral V nerve (Fig. 3, level 6). These fibers descend in the medial part of the dorsal funiculus in the cervical cord and enter the dorsomedial portion of the dorsal horn.

The other two groups are seen in a similar position on both sides of the brain stem. They occupy a rather broad field in the ventrolateral part of the white matter. In the spinal cord they descend in the ventral funiculi and gradually enter the ventromedial portion of the ventral horn. Fine degenerated fragments are seen close to the cell bodies and to the proximal parts of dendrites of the *medial* column of motoneurons especially at high cervical level (Fig. 4A). However, many fibers pass into more dorsal and medial regions of the ventral horn. Moreover, preterminal degeneration is present also at the beginning of the lumbar enlargement where the medial column of motoneurons is absent.

Only scattered degenerated fibers appear to reach the lateral column of motoneurons and pericellular arborizations were never observed in this region (Fig. 4B).

Similar distribution of degeneration was seen in sagittal sections through the spinal cord of another toad in which the lesion involved the nuclei of termination of the VIII nerve and surrounding gray matter, but did not extend into the white matter.

Lesion of the dorsal nucleus of the VIII cranial nerve extending to the upper border of the ventral nucleus. Following this type of lesion degenerated fibers appear within the brain stem, but only very few of them descend into the ipsilateral cervical cord.

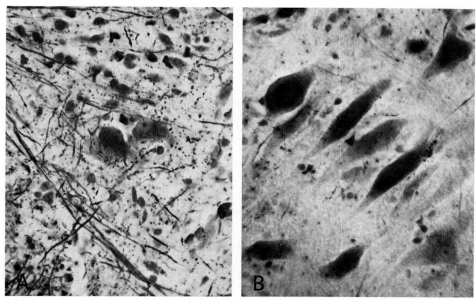

Fig. 4. Photomicrographs from the ventral horn of the cervical enlargement in the case illustrated in Fig. 3. A: preterminal degeneration in the medial region of the ventral horn. Some fine degenerated fragments lie close to the cell bodies of the medial column of motoneurons. Land, Eager and Shepherd method. × 290. B: the lateral column of motoneurons at the same level is free of degenerations. Land, Eager and Shepherd method. × 290.

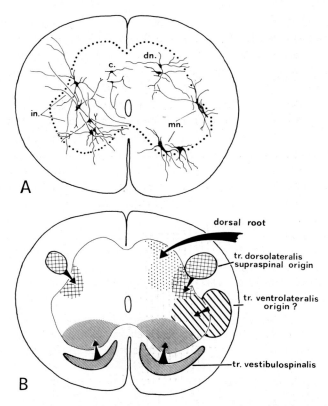

Fig. 5. Diagram summarizing our observations and comparing the areas of termination of different fiber systems within the gray matter of the spinal cord with the cell types and their processes present in these areas. A: Drawing of a transverse Golgi impregnated section of the frog's spinal cord showing the main cell types present. Modified from Silver (1942). c.: commissural cells; dn.: dorsal horn neurons; in.: interneurons; mn.: motoneurons. B: descending fiber tracts and their areas of termination as described in the present study. The region of termination of the dorsal root fibers is depicted according to a drawing of Joseph and Whitlock (1968).

Morphological and functional considerations

The observations reported above give the first experimental anatomical demonstration of the existence of a direct vestibulospinal tract in amphibians. It appears from our material that this tract originates from the ventral nucleus of the VIII cranial nerve and descends in the ipsilateral ventral funiculus throughout the whole length of the spinal cord (Fig. 5B). It thus seems very likely that the ventral nucleus of the VIII nerve of the toad, or at least part of it, is homologous to Deiters' nucleus in mammals.

A striking difference, however, is that in the toad in addition to the ipsilateral there is also a contralateral descending tract, similar in every respect to the ipsilateral one. Fibers crossing the midline could be observed both at the transition between the medulla oblongata and the spinal cord, and in the gray matter of the spinal cord ventral to the central canal. Unfortunately, our material does not allow conclusions as to whether the vestibulospinal tract in the toad is somatotopically organized, as described in cats (Pompeiano and Brodal, 1957) and other mammals (see Pompeiano, 1972). The small size of the ventral nucleus of the VIII nerve in the toad prevents more restricted lesions and only retrograde degeneration studies can probably solve this problem.

In addition to the vestibulospinal tract, other pathways descending in the spinal cord have been observed in our material (Fig. 5B). Their origin could not be ascertained with accuracy. They are:

(*i*) a partially crossed pathway localized in the dorsal part of the lateral funiculus, apparently of supraspinal origin. This tract degenerated following complete hemisection of the spinal cord as well as after lesion of the ventral nucleus of the VIII nerve extending into the white matter. It will here be called the "*tractus dorsolateralis*".

(*ii*) fibers situated in the ventral part of the lateral funiculus, which descend for a distance of 3–4 segments below the hemisection of the spinal cord. They may be propriospinal fibers and/or fibers of supraspinal origin. Because of their position they are here called the "*tractus ventrolateralis*".

(*iii*) fibers descending in the dorsal funiculus corresponding to Wallenberg's spinal roots of the V and VIII cranial nerves (Wallenberg, 1907).

The area and mode of termination of the vestibulospinal tract as well as of the remaining descending pathways are of particular interest especially with regard to a possible monosynaptic contact with the motoneurons.

Physiological observations reported by Brookhart and Kubota (1963) indicate, in fact, that in the frog stimulation of the isolated spinal cord as well as of dorsal root fibers produce monosynaptic EPSPs in lumbosacral motoneurons. There is, however, a striking difference in the time course of the two types of EPSPs which has lead the authors to conclude that the descending fibers coursing in the lateral funiculus terminate monosynaptically on the soma of the lumbosacral motoneurons, while the dorsal root fibers terminate monosynaptically on the distal part of their dendrites. The last finding has also received anatomical support (Liu and Chambers, 1957; Joseph and Whitlock, 1968). Unfortunately it is unknown from the physiological studies reported above, whether the descending pathway producing monosynaptic EPSPs in lumbosacral motoneurons is propriospinal, or whether it originates from the nuclei of termination of the VIII cranial nerve and/or another supraspinal structure. Moreover, it was not stated whether the recorded motoneurons belonged to the medial or to the lateral columns.

Our observations indicate that the vestibulospinal tract terminates in that region of the spinal gray matter which contains the medial column of motoneurons, which is known to innervate the axial musculature (Silver, 1942). The asymmetrical position of the head following lesions of the ventral nucleus of the VIII nerve is likely to be due to disfacilitation of this pool of motoneurons. The presence of fine degenerating fragments close to the cell bodies and the dendrites of the medial motoneurons actually suggests that there may exist a monosynaptic contact of some vestibulospinal fibers with these cells. However, this mode of termination is certainly not the principal one, as many fibers pass more dorsally. Here they can contact either dendrites of the moto-

References p. 307

neurons located in the lateral column or else some interneurons (Fig. 5A). Since the lateral column of motoneurons innervates the muscles of the extremities (Silver, 1942) this may explain that the postural asymmetry following the vestibular lesion involves the limb musculature.

Concerning the distribution of the two others fiber systems descending in the lateral funiculi, the *tractus dorsolateralis* terminates in the intermediate gray matter ventral to the area of termination of the dorsal root fibers as described by previous investigators (Liu and Chambers, 1957; Joseph and Whitlock, 1968). This tract might therefore reach the proximal part of dendrites of lateral motoneurons, but not the cell bodies.

Finally the area of termination of the *tractus ventrolateralis* includes the lateral column of motoneurons. In this instance preterminal arborization, seen around the cell bodies of motoneurons, suggests that this tract may make axosomatic contacts with these motoneurons.

Experimental electron microscopical observations combined with physiological experiments may reveal further details concerning the anatomical and functional organization of these descending projections in the toad.

SUMMARY

The course and distribution of fibers originating from the nuclei of termination of the VIII cranial nerve in the toad have been studied by means of silver impregnation techniques. In addition to lesions of the nuclei of termination of the VIII nerve, a complete hemisection of the spinal cord was made and the position of all descending fibers within the spinal cord ascertained.

It was found that the vestibulospinal tract most probably originates only from the ventral nucleus of the VIII nerve, descends bilaterally in the ventral funiculi throughout the whole length of the spinal cord and terminates in the medial region of the ventral horn harboring the medial column of motoneurons.

Other descending fibers within the spinal cord were found in the dorsal and lateral funiculi. Fibers coursing in the dorsal funiculus probably belong to the descending roots of the V and VIII cranial nerves. The lateral funiculus contains two different fiber systems: (i) a dorsolateral tract which originates from some supraspinal structure and terminates in the intermediate gray matter of the spinal cord and (ii) a ventrolateral tract which might be of propriospinal origin and terminates in the cervical cord within the region of the lateral column of motoneurons.

The findings are discussed from an anatomical and functional point of view and considered in relation to relevant physiological data.

ACKNOWLEDGEMENTS

This investigation was supported by PHS research grant NB 07685-03, from the National Institute of Neurological Diseases and Blindness, N.I.H., Public Health Service, U.S.A., and by a research grant from the Consiglio Nazionale delle Ricerche, Italy.

REFERENCES

ARIËNS KAPPERS, C. U., HUBER, G. C. AND CROSBY, E. C. (1936) *The Comparative Anatomy of the Nervous System of Vertebrates, Including Man. Vol. 1.* MacMillan Co., New York, pp.180–190, 459–467.

BARALE, F., CORVAJA, N. AND POMPEIANO, O. (1971) Vestibular influences on postural activity in frog. *Arch. ital. Biol.*, **109**, 27–36.

BROOKHART, J. M. AND KUBOTA, K. (1963) Studies of integrative function of the motor neurone. In G. MORUZZI, A. FESSARD AND H. H. JASPER (Eds.), *Progress in Brain Research. Vol. 1. Brain mechanisms*, Elsevier, Amsterdam, pp. 38–64.

EBBESSON, S. O. E. (1970) The selective silver-impregnation of degenerating axons and their synaptic endings in non mammalian species. In W. J. H. NAUTA AND S. O. E. EBBESSON (Eds.), *Contemporary Research Methods in Neuroanatomy.* Springer, Berlin, Heidelberg, New York, pp. 132–161.

EBBESSON, S. O. E. AND HEIMER, L., (1970) Method 7: Silver impregnation of degenerating axon terminals. In W. J. H. NAUTA AND S. O. E. EBBESSON (Eds.), *Contemporary Research Methods in Neuroanatomy.* Springer, Berlin, Heidelberg, New York, p. 154.

FINK, R. P. AND L. HEIMER (1967) Two methods for selective silver impregnation of degenerating axons and their synaptic endings in the central nervous system. *Brain Res.*, **4**, 369–374.

GAUPP, E., (1899) *A. Ecker's und R. Wiedershein's Anatomie des Frosches. Vol. 2.* Von Friedrich Vieweg und Sohn, Braunschweig, pp. 3–41.

JOSEPH, B. S. AND WHITLOCK, D. G. (1968) The morphology of spinal afferent-efferent relationships in vertebrates. *Brain Behav. Evol.*, **1**, 2–18.

KEMALI, M. AND BRAITENBERG, V. (1969) *Atlas of the Frog's Brain.* Springer, Berlin, Heidelberg, New York, pp. 74.

KENNARD, D. W. (1959) The anatomical organization of neurons in the lumbar region of the spinal cord of the frog (Rana temporaria). *J. comp. Neurol.*, **111**, 447–467.

LAND, L. J., EAGER, R. P. AND SHEPHERD, G. M. (1970) Olfactory nerve projections to the olfactory bulb in rabbit: demonstration by means of a simplified ammoniacal silver degeneration method. *Brain Res.*, **23**, 250–254.

LARSELL, O. (1934) The differentiation of the peripheral and central acoustic apparatus in the frog. *J. comp. Neurol.*, **60**, 473–527.

LIU, C. N. AND CHAMBERS, W. W. (1957) Experimental study of anatomical organization of frog's spinal cord. *Anat. Rec.*, **127**, 326.

NAUTA, W. J. H. (1957) Silver impregnation of degenerating axons. In F. W. WINDLE (Ed.), *New Research Techniques of Neuroanatomy.* C. C. Thomas, Springfield, Ill., pp. 17–26.

NEMEC, H. (1951) Über die Ausbildung der grauen Substanz im Frosch-Rückenmark. *Acta Anat.*, **13**, 101–118.

NIEUWENHUYS, R. (1964) Comparative anatomy of the spinal cord. In J. C. ECCLES AND J. P. SCHADÉ (Eds.), *Progress in Brain Research. Vol. 11. Organization of the spinal cord.* Elsevier, Amsterdam, pp. 1–57.

POMPEIANO, O. (1972) Vestibulospinal relations: vestibular influences on gamma motoneurons and primary afferents. In A. BRODAL AND O. POMPEIANO (Eds.), *Progress in Brain Research. Vol. 37. Basic aspects of central vestibular mechanisms.* Elsevier, Amsterdam, pp. 197–232.

POMPEIANO, O. AND BRODAL, A. (1957) The origin of vestibulospinal fibres in the cat. An experimental–anatomical study, with comments on the descending medial longitudinal fasciculus. *Arch. ital. Biol.*, **95**, 166–195.

SILVER, M. L. (1942) The motoneurons of the spinal cord of the frog. *J. comp. Neurol.*, **77**, 1–39.

WALLENBERG, A. VON (1907) Die kaudale Endigung der bulbo-spinalen Wurzeln des Trigeminus, Vestibularis und Vagus beim Frosche. *Anat. Anz.*, **30**, 564–568.

COMMENT TO CHAPTER IV

MLF Fibers Originating from the Lateral Vestibular Nucleus

M. ITO

*Department of Physiology, Faculty of Medicine, University of Tokyo,
Hongo, Bunkyo-ku, Tokyo, Japan*

Kawai, Ito and Nozue (1969) noticed that in cats certain cells located in the very ventral portion of the lateral vestibular nucleus send descending axons through MLF. Recent work by Akaike *et al.* (1972) has revealed that in rabbits the cells of origin of MLF fibers are located in mixture with the ventral Deiters' neurones that contribute to the lateral vestibulospinal tract. These cells of origin of MLF receive monosynaptic activation from primary vestibular afferents, and monosynaptic inhibition from the anterior and posterior lobes of the cerebellum.

REFERENCES

AKAIKE, T., FANARDJIAN, V. V., ITO, M., KUMADA, M. AND NAKAJIMA, H. (1972) Electrophysiological analysis of the vestibulospinal reflex pathway of rabbit. I. Classification of relay cells. Submitted to *Exp. Brain Res.*

KAWAI, N., ITO, M. AND NOZUE, M. (1969) Postsynaptic influences on the vestibular non-Deiters nuclei from primary vestibular nerve. *Exp. Brain Res.*, **8**, 190–200.

V. RELATIONS BETWEEN THE VESTIBULAR NUCLEI AND THE CEREBELLUM

Vestibulocerebellar Input in the Cat: Anatomy

A. BRODAL

Anatomical Institute, University of Oslo, Oslo, Norway

Impulses arising in the vestibular receptors may influence the cerebellum through various routes. In general one is inclined to think of two of these only, the direct vestibulocerebellar fibres and the secondary vestibulocerebellar fibres, arising in the vestibular nuclei. In studies of the activity in the cerebellum following stimulation of vestibular receptors it is, however, important to remember that transmission along other, although less direct, pathways may be responsible for some of the electrical changes recorded. The subject of the anatomy of the vestibulocerebellar input accordingly comprises more than the direct and secondary vestibulocerebellar fibres.

PRIMARY VESTIBULOCEREBELLAR FIBRES

Vestibular nerve fibres passing to the cerebellum were traced in Golgi preparations by Cajal (1896, 1909–11) while Lorente de Nó (1924), using the same method, denies their existence. In normal brains of reptiles, birds and mammals, for example the opossum and the bat, Larsell (1936a, b) followed primary vestibular fibres to the flocculus and nodulus. Some apparently end in the fastigial nucleus.

More decisive information of the presence, course and termination of primary vestibular fibres can be derived from experimental studies. With the Marchi method degenerating primary vestibular fibres were traced to the nodulus and the adjoining folia of the uvula and the nucleus fastigii by Ingvar (1918) in the cat and by Dow (1936) in the rat and cat. According to Dow all these fibres end in the ipsilateral half of the cerebellum. More recently Carpenter (1960b) briefly described in Nauta preparations in the cat and monkey primary vestibular fibres with approximately the same distribution as Dow (1936).

Concerning the *mode of termination* of the primary vestibulocerebellar fibres conclusions have largely been based on indirect evidence (foetal brains, human pathological material). Some authors advocate a termination as mossy fibres, while others favour a termination as climbing fibres. (For a review of the older literature see Jansen and Brodal, 1958). It may be mentioned that Snider (1936) in his study of the termination of the brachium pontis in the cat found only mossy fibre degeneration in a case in which there was accidental damage to the vestibular nerve.

In order to determine the mode of termination of the primary vestibulocerebellar fibres and to map their termination more precisely than could possibly be done with the Marchi method, we (Brodal and Høivik, 1964) undertook an experimental study

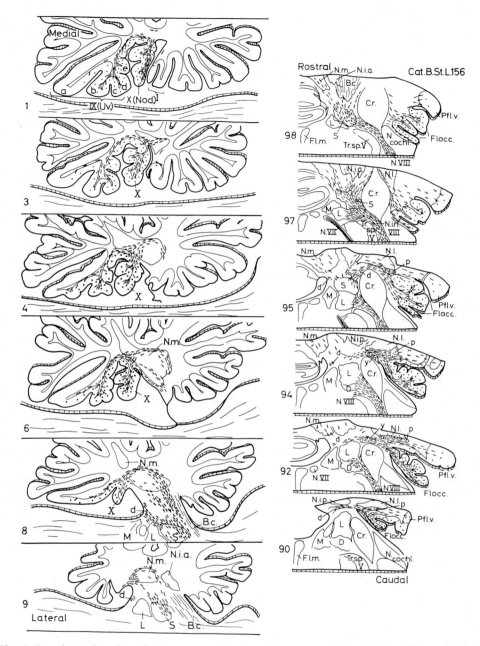

Fig. 1. Drawings of sections from two cats, showing the course and distribution of degenerating primary vestibulocerebellar fibres following interruption of the vestibular nerve. The degeneration in the vestibular nuclei is not entered. To the right a series of transverse sections, to the left some sagittal sections from another animal. Note that most primary vestibulocerebellar fibres pass through or close to the superior vestibular nucleus. Note also the relation to the fastigial nucleus of fibres to the nodulus-uvula. Cp. text. From Brodal and Høivik (1964).

in the cat. Transection of the eighth cranial nerve was performed by an approach through the tympanic bulla in the cat, and the ensuing degenerating fibres were traced in Nauta (1957) and Glees (1946) impregnated sections from the cerebellum. The cerebella were cut in different planes.

Fig. 1 shows the *course and distribution of the primary vestibulocerebellar fibres.* Having entered the brain stem the fibres continue dorsomedially as a fairly well circumscribed bundle. A great number of the fibres penetrate the superior vestibular nucleus, others pass just dorsal to it. (The terminations within the vestibular nuclei will not be considered here, see Walberg, 1972). Then the fibres spread out fanlike into three not entirely separated contingents. The medialmost of these turns medially and dorsally and in part penetrates the fastigial nucleus (drawings 3–9 in Fig. 1). Having curved along or through the nucleus the fibres continue ventrally and enter the white matter of the nodulus and the ventral folia of the uvula (drawings 1–8 in Fig. 1). A lateral group of fibres makes a dorsal bend when the fibres pass laterally. They are found just beneath the fibre bundle of the restiform body before this fans out into the cerebellum. The fibres pass along the ventral aspect of the lateral (dentate) nucleus, some penetrate its ventral part, especially the small-celled region (p in Fig. 1 to the right). This lateral group of fibres enters the flocculus and the ventral paraflocculus (drawings to the right in Fig. 1). An intermediate group of fibres passes ventral to the brachium conjunctivum fibres, continues dorsally through the rostral part of the nucleus interpositus anterior and finally reaches the lateralmost parts of the nodulus and uvula.

The *sites of termination of the primary vestibulocerebellar fibres* are entered in a diagram of the cerebellar surface imagined unfolded in Fig. 2. The termination is restricted to the ipsilateral half of the cerebellum. Most fibres end in the nodulus, the adjoining two–three folia of the uvula and in the flocculus. The ventral paraflocculus receives a fair number of fibres. A few enter the dorsal paraflocculus and the lingula.

On the whole this distribution is in agreement with the observations of Dow (1936) with the exception that Dow did not find terminations in the paraflocculus in his Marchi preparations. In the older studies the flocculus and paraflocculus were often not kept apart as separate lobules.

In the intracerebellar nuclei we (Brodal and Høivik, 1964) found signs of termination only in the small-celled ventral part of the dentate nucleus (labelled p in the illustrations) defined by Flood and Jansen (1961). In the fastigial nucleus we were not able to find convincing signs of terminal degeneration, although many degenerating fibres pass through this nucleus. Only in the ventral regions of the nucleus the picture of degeneration may possibly be interpreted as representing terminations of fibres, but it is not decisive. Our negative evidence does not exclude that primary vestibular fibres actually end in the fastigial nucleus, since it is extremely difficult to verify the presence of terminal degeneration in an area where there are many degenerating fibres of passage. Marchi studies are even less conclusive. Nor do the potentials recorded by Dow (1939) in the fastigial nucleus following stimulation of the vestibular nerve prove the termination of fibres in this nucleus. Matsushita and Iwahori (1971) in a recent Golgi study did not venture definite conclusions as to the termination of primary

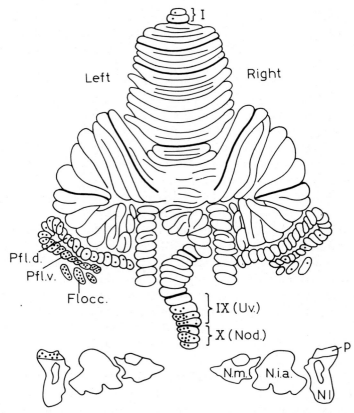

Fig. 2. Diagram of the cerebellar surface of the cat imagined unfolded (above) and of the intra-cerebellar nuclei (adapted from Flood and Jansen 1961). Dots indicate sites of termination of primary vestibulocerebellar fibres from the left vestibular nerve. The relative densities of dots indicate the approximate density of fibres in various parts. Note that the terminal area exceeds the borders of the flocculonodular lobe and includes the ventral paraflocculus and the ventral part of the uvula. The small-celled part p of the lateral nucleus receives primary vestibular fibres. From Brodal and Høivik (1964).

vestibular fibres in the fastigial nucleus, and Larsell (1970) reports that he did not see such fibres in Golgi studies of the rat. On the whole, it is thus still an open question whether primary vestibular fibres end in the fastigial nucleus, as originally suggested by Cajal (1896, 1909–11).

It may be objected that in our material (Brodal and Høivik, 1964) the cochlear division of the VIII nerve was transected, and that therefore some of the cerebellar degeneration found in our cases may be due to interruption of cochleocerebellar fibres. However, this appears not to be the case, since following lesions restricted to the cochlear ganglion no degenerating fibres could be traced into the cerebellum (Osen, 1970).

As concerns the *mode of termination of the primary vestibulocerebellar fibres,* our study (Brodal and Høivik, 1964) leaves no doubt that they terminate as mossy fibres

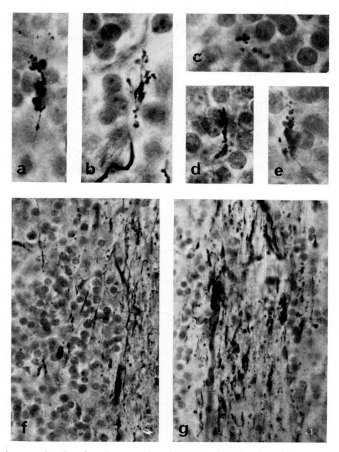

Fig. 3. Photomicrographs showing degenerating fibres (× 410) in the white matter of the nodulus (g) and uvula (f) entering the granular layer, and degenerating mossy fibre terminals (× 1020) in the granular layer of the ventral paraflocculus (a), the nodulus (b and e), the uvula (c) and the flocculus (d). Nauta sections, 9 days following transection of the vestibular nerve. From Brodal and Høivik (1964).

as suggested by Snider (1936). In our experimental cases bundles of degenerating fibres are found in the white matter of the lobules mentioned, and they can be seen to enter the granular layer (Fig. 3f–g). In this argyrophilic fragments (Fig. 3a–e) occur which resemble those seen following interruption of spinocerebellar fibres (Brodal and Grant, 1962) and of fibres from the external cuneate nucleus (Grant, 1962). Even if our study demonstrates that primary vestibulocerebellar fibres end as mossy fibres, they do not permit final conclusions as to whether all of them terminate in this way or whether some may end as climbing fibres. It is well known that the demonstration of degenerating climbing fibres in experimental light microscopic material meets with very great difficulties. In physiological studies Precht and Llinás (1969) confirm the presence of mossy fibre terminations, while they found no electrophysiological evidence for a termination of primary vestibular fibres as climbing fibres in the cat.

The distribution of primary vestibular fibres shown in our study (Brodal and Høivik, 1964) is of relevance for the question of the subdivision of the cerebellum. The *vestibulocerebellum*, if defined as the area of the cerebellum which receives a direct input from the labyrinth, obviously includes more than the flocculonodular lobe of Larsell. In addition it comprises the ventral paraflocculus, the ventral folia of the uvula and the small-celled part of the dentate nucleus. Other data support this notion.

For example, in the regions of the cerebellar cortex which receive primary vestibulocerebellar fibres the mossy fibre terminals differ to some extent morphologically from the "classical" type (Brodal and Drabløs, 1963). With the Golgi as well as the Glees method most of the mossy fibre terminals in the vestibulocerebellum of the cat and rat are seen to be provided with great numbers, and closely packed groups, of terminal boutons. They further appear to be more amply branching and to have shorter branches than the "classical" mossy fibres (Fig. 4). On account of their distribution it appears likely that this special type of mossy fibres are, at least chiefly, terminations of primary

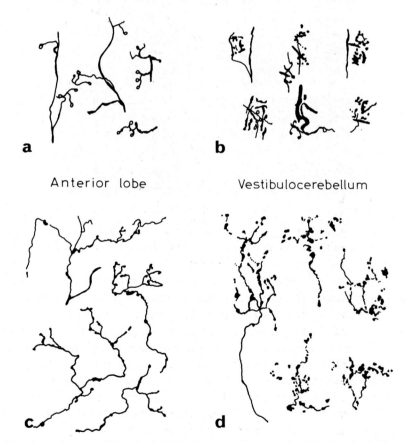

Fig. 4. Drawings of mossy fibre terminals in the cerebellar anterior lobe (to the left) and in the vestibulocerebellum (to the right) of the cat and rat as seen in Glees sections (a and b) and in Golgi sections (c and d). Note ample branching, shorter terminal branches and denser clustering of boutons in the vestibulocerebellum than in the anterior lobe. From Brodal and Drabløs (1963).

vestibular fibres. One may suspect that these terminals will be able to yield a more massive activation of granule cells than the more dispersed endings of the "classical" type. A further indication of morphological, and presumably also functional, peculiarities of the vestibulocerebellum (as defined above) is the presence in this of a greater number of Golgi cells, especially of the larger type (see Brodal and Drabløs, 1963).

SECONDARY VESTIBULOCEREBELLAR FIBRES

Fibres from the vestibular nuclei to the cerebellum have been described in normal silver-impregnated material from reptiles (Weston, 1936), birds (Whitlock, 1952), opossum (Larsell, 1936a), bat (Larsell, 1936b) and man (Larsell, 1947). These authors indicate that the *site of termination* is the same as that of the primary vestibulocerebellar fibres. Experimental studies of these fibres meet with great difficulties. If lesions are made of the vestibular nuclei in order to trace degenerating fibres into the cerebellum, there is great risk of damaging other fibres than those coming from the vestibular nuclei. For example, as mentioned above, the majority of primary vestibulocerebellar fibres pass through the superior vestibular nucleus. Concomitant injury to other fibre bundles, for example, the restiform body, may result in erroneous conclusions. However, some investigations of this kind are available. According to the Marchi studies of Dow (1936) secondary vestibulocerebellar fibres end ipsilaterally in the nodulus, the adjoining folia of the uvula, the flocculus and the fastigial nucleus. Some fibres supply the corresponding regions contralaterally. According to Dow (1936) the secondary fibres appear to be somewhat more abundant than the primary. A termination of secondary vestibular fibres bilaterally in the fastigial nucleus was advocated also by Carpenter, Bard and Alling (1959) and Carpenter (1960a).

Conclusions as to the *origin of the fibres* are difficult to draw on the basis of studies of normal material or following lesions of the vestibular nuclei. While Dow (1936) did not venture any conclusions concerning the origin of the fibres in his material, Carpenter (1960a) following isolated lesions of the descending vestibular nuclei found this to give off fibres to the cerebellum. In normal material of the opossum Voris and Hoerr (1932) give the medial and descending nuclei as sources of the fibres, while Larsell (1936a) in the same animal claims the fibres to come from the superior and lateral vestibular nuclei.

The safest way to establish the origin of secondary vestibular fibres is to look for retrograde cellular changes in the vestibular nuclei following lesions of the cerebellum. Some early authors (for references see Brodal and Torvik, 1957; Brodal, Pompeiano and Walberg, 1962) who used this approach achieved discordant results. They all used adult animals. Since it has been shown that it is often favourable to use very young animals for studies of retrograde cellular changes (modified Gudden method, Brodal, 1940) we decided to study the problem of the origin of the secondary vestibulocerebellar fibres in this way. Following lesions of different parts of the cerebellum in kittens aged 6–21 days, the animals were killed after 4–10 days, and the vestibular nuclei searched for retrograde cellular changes (Brodal and Torvik, 1957). Following lesions of certain parts of the cerebellum (see below) typical retrograde changes could

References pp. 326–327

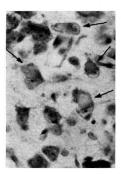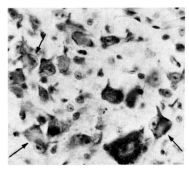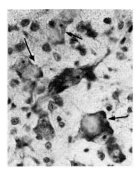

Fig. 5. Photomicrographs (× 350) of Nissl-stained sections through the descending vestibular nucleus in kittens some days following extirpation of the vestibulocerebellum. Many cells (arrows) show typical retrograde changes (tigrolysis and peripheral displacement of the nucleus). Most of the cells are small. To the extreme right a larger affected cell. In between the changed cells there are some normal ones and some which show equivocal changes. From Brodal and Torvik (1957).

be identified in cells in the medial and descending vestibular nuclei (Fig. 5). Cells of this kind were not seen in the lateral and superior nuclei, but were abundant in the small group x, and in the small, rather compact, cell group f in the descending nucleus. It is noteworthy that in the medial and descending nucleus changed cells do not occur over their entire territory. The majority are found in the ventrolateral part of the descending nucleus (including the group f). The more scanty contribution from the medial nucleus comes chiefly from its ventral regions.

In between the definitely changed cells there are always some normal ones and some which show equivocal changes. By restricting the recording of changed cells to those which are typically affected, one records presumably only a certain proportion of those cells which have actually had their axons cut. This drawback is, however, compensated by the fact that no regions are erroneously considered as giving origin to fibres to the cerebellum. It should be noted that the absence of retrograde cellular changes in the superior and lateral vestibular nuclei does not prove that these nuclei do not give origin to cerebellar fibres.

Retrograde cellular changes with the distribution described above were not found following all cerebellar lesions but only in cases where the lesion involved the flocculus, nodulus and the adjoining part of the uvula. Even if our material (Brodal and Torvik, 1957) does not permit definite conclusions as to the sites of termination of the secondary vestibulocerebellar fibres, the observations concerning this point are in agreement with those made by workers using other methods. Concerning possible terminations in the paraflocculus our material does not give any information. However, our findings are compatible with (but do not prove) the presence of secondary vestibulocerebellar fibres to the fastigial nucleus. The majority of the fibres end in the ipsilateral cerebellar half, especially those to the flocculus, while the other contingents appear to have a minor contribution to the contralateral side, as found by Dow (1936). The diagram of Fig. 6 summarizes our findings.

It is interesting to note the preferential distribution of the sites of origin within the

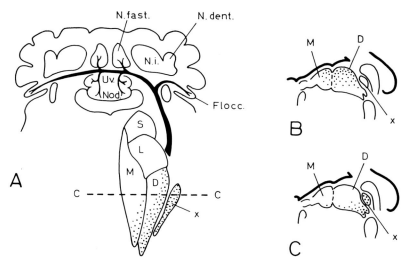

Fig. 6. Diagram (A) showing the sites of origin of secondary vestibular fibres (dotted) as projected on a horizontal section through the vestibular nuclei of the cat. C shows the sites of the origin as seen in a transverse section at the level indicated in A. The sites of termination of the fibres are shown according to Dow (1936). Note restricted site of origin mainly from the caudoventral part of the descending nucleus (D) and the group x and the largely different distribution of primary vestibular fibres within the vestibular nuclei (B). In part from Brodal and Torvik (1957).

vestibular nuclear complex of fibres to the cerebellum. This is but one of many examples which illustrate the fact that even the main nuclear groups can not be separate units from a functional point of view. A further indication for the existence of specific pattern is the observation (Brodal and Torvik, 1957) that the fibres to the flocculus appear to come chiefly from the rostral part of the total area of origin. There may well be further details of this kind which so far remain unknown. This assumption receives some support from the very specific patterns found within the projections of the "vestibulocerebellum" onto the vestibular nuclei (Angaut and Brodal, 1967). I will return to some functional aspects of these findings below.

OTHER POSSIBLE ROUTES FOR VESTIBULAR IMPULSES TO THE CEREBELLUM

In addition to the two fairly direct routes for vestibular impulses to the cerebellum considered above, representing a one-neuron and a two-neuron chain, respectively, there are others which involve chains of three — and possibly even more — neurons. Thus, as studied recently by Ladpli and Brodal (1968), the vestibular nuclei give off fair contingents of fibres to the lateral reticular nucleus and the pontine tegmental reticular nucleus, which both project onto the cerebellum (Brodal, 1943, and others, and Brodal and Jansen, 1946, respectively). Anatomical data suggest that from a functional point of view these nuclei are not identical. For example, the lateral reticular nucleus (nucleus of the lateral funiculus) receives fibres from the ipsilateral lateral vestibular nucleus only, while the reticular tegmental pontine nucleus of Bechterew is supplied by the contralateral superior and lateral vestibular nuclei (Ladpli and Brodal, 1968). Within each of these precerebellar reticular nuclei the fibres from the vestibular nuclei have their preferential sites of termination. However, it appears that vestibular impulses are integrated in the nuclei with impulses from several other sources. This follows from the distribution of various contingents of other afferents within these nuclei (P. Brodal, Maršala and A. Brodal, 1967, and A. Brodal and P. Brodal, 1971, respectively). The cerebellar projections of the two precerebellar reticular nuclei are not known in all details, but there is no evidence to suggest that the parts of the nuclei which receive secondary vestibular fibres project mainly or exclusively to the "vestibulocerebellum". In addition to these there may be other cerebellar projecting nuclei which receive fibres from the vestibular nuclei. There is some evidence, although not conclusive, for a termination of secondary vestibular fibres in the inferior olive (for references see Brodal, 1972b). The perihypoglossal nuclei may receive some secondary vestibular fibres.

It should be noted that there is no good anatomical evidence for a vestibulocerebellar route by way of the main reticular formation. Primary vestibular fibres to this appear to be very scanty, and do not reach those reticular nuclei which project onto the cerebellum.

SOME FUNCTIONAL CONSIDERATIONS

The anatomical data reviewed above are of relevance for physiological studies of the vestibulocerebellar relations. In the first place it is obvious that vestibular impulses passing directly to the cerebellum by way of primary fibres can influence only a restricted part of the cerebellum, even if the proper "vestibulocerebellum" exceeds the limits of the flocculonodular lobe. No anatomical data are available as to the labyrinthine receptors which may influence the cerebellum via this pathway. However, the fact that most of these fibres pass through the superior nucleus may be of interest. According to Stein and Carpenter (1967) and Gacek (1969) the primary fibres ending in the superior nucleus are derived only from the semicircular ducts. This makes it very likely, but does not prove, that at least the majority of vestibular impulses to the cerebellum following this route come from the canals. Physiological studies (Precht and Shimazu, 1965; Shimazu and Precht, 1965; Markham, 1968) have confirmed the presence in the superior nucleus of units responding to stimulation of the canals.

Concerning the secondary vestibular fibres it is very doubtful whether they are at all concerned in the transmission of vestibular impulses to the cerebellum. The areas in the vestibular nuclei found by us (Brodal and Torvik, 1957) to give rise to fibres to the cerebellum (Fig. 6) do not receive an appreciable number of primary vestibular fibres (Walberg, Bowsher and Brodal, 1958; Stein and Carpenter, 1967; Gacek, 1969). The group x as well as the group f in the descending nucleus do not receive such fibres, and in the descending and medial nucleus the regions which project onto the cerebellum are largely different from those which are supplied with primary vestibular fibres (see Fig. 6). Even if there may be some possibilities for dispersion of impulses from the labyrinth within these nuclei by internuncial cells or by recurrent collaterals of axons leaving the nuclei (see Brodal, 1972a), it appears that the main influx to the "vestibulocerebellum" via the vestibular nuclei does not come from the vestibular apparatus. An important source of afferents to these cerebellar projection areas, especially to the group x, is the spinal cord (Pompeiano and Brodal, 1957; Brodal and Angaut, 1967). This anatomical arrangement indicates the presence of *an usually neglected spinocerebellar pathway to the "vestibulocerebellum"*, and makes clear that *the secondary vestibular fibres are scarcely of great concern in transmitting vestibular impulses to the cerebellum*. In fact, the vestibulocerebellar pathways via the precerebellar reticular nuclei (lateral reticular nucleus and tegmental pontine reticular nucleus) appear to be more suited for this purpose. However, from their anatomical organization it appears that these nuclei will influence largely other areas of the cerebellum than the "vestibulocerebellum". Just as the cerebellar projecting parts of the vestibular nuclei mediate mainly non-vestibular impulses to the "vestibulocerebellum", the pathways via the reticular nuclei provide possibilities for vestibular impulses to influence the "non-vestibular" parts of the cerebellum. These are only two examples which show that the separation between functionally different regions of the cerebellum is not as distinct as formerly believed.

SUMMARY

The question of possible pathways for the transmission of vestibular impulses to the cerebellum requires a consideration of more than the traditional primary and secondary vestibulocerebellar connections.

The *primary vestibular fibres* according to recent studies (Brodal and Høivik, 1964) terminate in the nodulus, the adjoining ventral folia of the uvula, the paraflocculus and the ventral paraflocculus. A few fibres end in the lingula and the ventral paraflocculus. Within the intracerebellar nuclei terminations have been established in the small-celled ventral part of the lateral (dentate) nucleus, but a termination in the fastigial nucleus is still conjectural. According to anatomical data (Stein and Carpenter, 1967; Gacek, 1969) it appears that most, if not all, primary vestibular fibres ending in the cerebellum are derived from the semicircular ducts. The primary vestibular fibres end as mossy fibres. These appear to differ in certain respe.ts from the "classical" type (Brodal and Drabløs, 1963).

Secondary vestibular fibres take origin from restricted parts of the vestibular complex only: the group x and the ventrolateral part of the descending vestibular nucleus with a few fibres from the ventral part of the medial nucleus (Brodal and Torvik, 1957). The fibres appear to terminate in the same regions as do the primary vestibular fibres (Dow, 1936). The regions of the vestibular nuclei which give off secondary vestibular fibres receive few or no primary vestibular afferents. A main source of afferents to these regions is the spinal cord (Brodal and Angaut, 1967). Accordingly, the secondary vestibular fibres appear to be mainly a link in a spinocerebellar pathway ending in the "vestibulocerebellum".

Vestibular impulses may reach the cerebellum via *other routes*. For example, fibres from the lateral vestibular nucleus end in the ipsilateral lateral reticular nucleus, fibres from the superior nucleus end bilaterally in the tegmental reticular pontine nuclei (Ladpli and Brodal, 1968). Both these nuclei project to the cerebellum, but there is no evidence that they influence particularly the "vestibulocerebellum".

These anatomical data serve to emphasize the difficulties in distinguishing functionally different subdivisions of the cerebellum.

REFERENCES

ANGAUT, P. AND BRODAL, A. (1967) The projection of the "vestibulocerebellum" onto the vestibular nuclei in the cat. *Arch. ital. Biol.*, **105**, 441–479.

BRODAL, A. (1940) Modification of Gudden method for study of cerebral localization. *Arch. Neurol. Psychiat. (Chicago)*, **43**, 46–58.

BRODAL, A. (1943) The cerebellar connections of the nucleus reticularis lateralis (nucleus funiculi lateralis) in rabbit and cat. Experimental investigations. *Acta psychiat. (Kbh.)*, **18**, 171–233.

BRODAL, A. (1972a) Some features in the anatomical organization of the vestibular nuclear complex in the cat. In A. BRODAL AND O. POMPEIANO (Eds.), *Progress in Brain Research. Vol. 37. Basic aspects of central vestibular mechanisms.* Elsevier, Amsterdam, pp. 31–53.

BRODAL, A. (1972b) Anatomy of the vestibular nuclei and their connections. In H. H. KORNHUBER (Ed.), *Handbook of Sensory Physiology. Vol. VI. Vestibular system.* Springer, Berlin, Heidelberg, New York, in press.

BRODAL, A. AND ANGAUT, P. (1967) The termination of spinovestibular fibres in the cat. *Brain Res.*, **5**, 494–500.

BRODAL, A. AND BRODAL, P. (1971) The organization of the nucleus reticularis tegmenti pontis in the cat in the light of experimental anatomical studies of its cerebral cortical afferents. *Exp. Brain Res.*, **13**, 90–110.

BRODAL, A. AND DRABLØS, P. A. (1963) Two types of mossy fiber terminals in the cerebellum and their regional distribution. *J. comp. Neurol.*, **121**, 173–187.

BRODAL, A. AND GRANT, G. (1962) Morphology and temporal course of degeneration in cerebellar mossy fibers following transection of spinocerebellar tracts in the cat. An experimental study with silver methods. *Exp. Neurol.*, **5**, 67–87.

BRODAL, A. AND HØIVIK, B. (1964) Site and mode of termination of primary vestibulocerebellar fibres in the cat. An experimental study with silver impregnation methods. *Arch. ital. Biol.*, **102**, 1–21.

BRODAL, A. AND JANSEN, J. (1946) The ponto-cerebellar projection in the rabbit and cat. Experimental investigations. *J. comp. Neurol.*, **84**, 31–118.

BRODAL, A., POMPEIANO, O. AND WALBERG, F. (1962) *The Vestibular Nuclei and Their Connections. Anatomy and Functional Correlations.* Oliver and Boyd, Edinburgh, London, pp. VIII-193.

BRODAL, A. AND TORVIK, A. (1957) Über den Ursprung der sekundären vestibulocerebellaren Fasern bei der Katze. Eine experimentell-anatomische Studie. *Arch. Psychiat. Nervenkr.*, **195**, 550–567.

BRODAL, P., MARŠALA, J. AND BRODAL, A. (1967) The cerebral cortical projection to the lateral reticular nucleus in the cat, with special reference to the sensorimotor cortical areas. *Brain Res.*, **6**, 252–274.

CAJAL, S. R. Y, (1896) *Beitrag zum Studium der Medulla oblongata des Kleinhirns und des Ursprungs der Gehirnnerven.* Johann Ambrosius Barth, Leipzig, 139 pp.

CAJAL, S. R. Y, (1909–11) *Histologie du Système Nerveux de l'Homme et des Vertébrés*, Maloine, Paris.

CARPENTER, M. B. (1960a) Fiber projections from the descending and lateral vestibular nuclei in the cat. *Amer. J. Anat.*, **107**, 1–22.

CARPENTER, M. B. (1960b) Experimental anatomical-physiological studies of the vestibular nerve and cerebellar connections. In G. L. RASMUSSEN AND W. WINDLE (Eds.), *Neural Mechanisms of the Auditory and Vestibular Systems.* C. C. Thomas, Springfield, Ill., pp. 297–323.

CARPENTER, M. B., BARD, D. S. AND ALLING, F. A. (1959) Anatomical connections between the fastigial nuclei, the labyrinth and the vestibular nuclei in the cat. *J. comp. Neurol.*, **111**, 1–25.

DOW, R. S. (1936) The fiber connections of the posterior parts of the cerebellum in the cat and rat. *J. comp. Neurol.*, **63**, 527–548.

DOW, R. S. (1939) Cerebellar action potentials in response to stimulation of various afferent connections. *J. Neurophysiol.*, **2**, 543–555.

FLOOD, S. AND JANSEN, J. (1961) On the cerebellar nuclei in the cat. *Acta anat. (Basel)*, **46**, 52–72.

GACEK, R. R. (1969) The course and central termination of first order neurons supplying vestibular endorgans in the cat. *Acta oto-laryng. (Stockh.)*, Suppl. 254, 1–66.

GLEES, P. (1946) Terminal degeneration within the central nervous system as studied by a new silver method. *J. Neuropath. exp. Neurol.*, **5**, 54–59.

GRANT, G. (1962) Projection of the external cuneate nucleus onto the cerebellum in the cat: An experimental study using silver methods. *Exp. Neurol.*, **5**, 179–195.

INGVAR, S. (1918) Zur Phylo- und Ontogenese des Kleinhirns nebst einem Versuche zu einheitlicher Erklärung der zerebellaren Funktion und Lokalisation. *Folia neuro-biol. (Lpz.)*, **11**, 205–495.

JANSEN, J. AND BRODAL, A. (1958) Das Kleinhirn. In v. *Möllendorffs Handbuch der mikroskopischen Anatomie des Menschen. IV/8.* Springer, Berlin, Göttingen, Heidelberg.

LADPLI, R. AND BRODAL, A. (1968) Experimental studies of commissural and reticular formation projections from the vestibular nuclei in the cat. *Brain Res.*, **8**, 65–96.

LARSELL, O. (1936a) The development and morphology of the cerebellum in the opossum. II. Later development and adult. *J. comp. Neurol.*, **63**, 251–291.

LARSELL, O. (1936b) Cerebellum and corpus pontobulbare of the bat (Myotis). *J. comp. Neurol.*, **64**, 275–302.

LARSELL, O. (1947) The development of the cerebellum in man in relation to its comparative anatomy. *J. comp. Neurol.*, **87**, 85–129.

LARSELL, O. (1970) *The Comparative Anatomy and Histology of the Cerebellum from Monotremes Through Apes.* In J. JANSEN (Ed.), The University of Minnesota Press, Minneapolis, pp. 269.

LORENTE DE NÓ, R. (1924) Etudes sur le cerveau postérieur. III. Sur les connexions extra-cérébelleuses des fascicules afférents au cerveau, et sur la fonction de cet organe. *Trab. Lab. Invest. biol. Univ. Madr.*, **22**, 51–65.

MARKHAM, C. H. (1968) Midbrain and contralateral labyrinth influences on brain stem vestibular neurons in the cat. *Brain Res.*, **9**, 312–333.

MATSUSHITA, M. AND IWAHORI, N. (1971) Structural organization of the fastigial nucleus. II. Afferent fiber systems. *Brain Res.*, **25**, 611–624.

NAUTA, W. J. H. (1957) Silver impregnation of degenerating axons. In W. F. WINDLE (Ed.), *New Research Techniques of Neuroanatomy.* C. C. Thomas, Springfield, Ill., pp. 17–26.

OSEN, K. K. (1970) Course and termination of the primary afferents in the cochlear nuclei of the cat. An experimental anatomical study. *Arch. ital. Biol.*, **108**, 21–51.

POMPEIANO, O. AND BRODAL, A. (1957) Spino-vestibular fibers in the cat. *J. comp. Neurol.*, **108**, 353–382.

PRECHT, W. AND LLINÁS, R. (1969) Functional organization of the vestibular afferents to the cerebellar cortex of frog and cat. *Exp. Brain Res.*, **9**, 30–52.

PRECHT, W. AND SHIMAZU, H., (1965) Functional connections of tonic and kinetic vestibular neurons with primary vestibular afferents. *J. Neurophysiol.*, **28**, 1014–1028.

SHIMAZU, H. AND PRECHT, W. (1965) Tonic and kinetic responses of cat's vestibular neurons to horizontal angular acceleration. *J. Neurophysiol.*, **28**, 991–1013.

SNIDER, R. S. (1936) Alterations which occur in mossy terminals of the cerebellum, following transection of the brachium pontis. *J. comp. Neurol.*, **64**, 417–431.

STEIN, B. M. AND CARPENTER, M. B. (1967) Central projections of portions of the vestibular ganglia innervating specific parts of the labyrinth in the rhesus monkey. *Amer. J. Anat.*, **120**, 281–318.

VORIS, H. C. AND HOERR, N. L. (1932) The hindbrain of the opossum, Didelphis virginiana. *J. comp. Neurol.*, **54**, 277–355.

WALBERG, F. (1972) Light and electron microscopical data on the distribution and termination of primary vestibular fibers. In A. BRODAL AND O. POMPEIANO (Eds.), *Progress in Brain Research. Vol. 37, Basic aspects of central vestibular mechanisms.* Elsevier. Amsterdam, pp. 79–88.

WALBERG, F., BOWSHER, D. AND BRODAL, A. (1958) The termination of primary vestibular fibers in the vestibular nuclei in the cat. An experimental study with silver methods. *J. comp. Neurol.*, **110**, 391–419.

WESTON, J. K. (1936) The reptilian vestibular and cerebellar gray with fiber connections. *J. comp. Neurol.*, **65**, 93–199.

WHITLOCK, D. G. (1952) A neurohistological and neurophysiological study of afferent fiber tracts and receptive areas of the avian cerebellum. *J. comp. Neurol.*, **97**, 567–636.

Vestibulocerebellar Input in the Frog: Anatomy

D. E. HILLMAN

Division of Neurobiology, Department of Physiology and Biophysics, University of Iowa, Iowa City, Iowa, U.S.A.

INTRODUCTION

The central projection of the VIII nerve in amphibians is described by Ariëns Kappers, Huber and Crosby (1936) as consisting of two roots which arise from separate anterior and posterior ganglia on the VIII nerve. In the frog, the posterior root enters the medulla dorsally and the anterior root ventrally (Ariëns Kappers and Hammer, 1918) after which they divide to ascend rostrally and descend caudally in the medulla. The dorsal portion is believed to go primarily to the nucleus dorso-magnocellularis while the ventral fiber bundles enter the ventral nucleus of the VIII nerve which has been suggested to be homologous to Deiters' nucleus.

Larsell illustrates primary vestibular fibers as entering the vestibular nucleus at the base of the VIII nerve (Larsell, 1925; Fig. 18). In Golgi preparations a cerebellar projection is shown as a small bundle entering the caudal part of the VIII nerve which divides and sends branches caudally and rostrally to the area of the cerebellar nucleus and granular layer of the auricular lobe (Larsell, 1967; Fig. 142). In a degeneration study (Hillman, 1969), the primary vestibular nerve fibers were found to project for the most part caudal to the vestibular nerve down to the IX–X nerve complex while some fibers projected rostrally to the auricular and marginal region of the cerebellum.

Physiological studies by Ross (1935, 1936) and Gleisner and Henriksson (1964) were the initial studies on the functional relationships in the frog VIII nerve. McNally and Tait (1925) used ablation of specific receptors to determine the function of the various end organs. More recently Llinás, Precht and Kitai (1967) demonstrated in the frog a primary vestibular afferent projection to Purkinje cells which is similar to climbing fiber activation of Purkinje cells in the cat. A morphological study confirmed that primary degenerating afferent fibers in the marginal zone near the auricular lobe not only contacted granule cells but made direct synapses with the Purkinje cells (Hillman, 1969). Precht and Llinás (1969) have studied the functional organization of the vestibular afferents and have confirmed the vestibular relationship to the marginal zone of the cerebellum as described by Goodman (1958). Physiological stimulation of the horizontal canals by angular acceleration produces an increased firing of primary vestibular nerve fibers and type I Purkinje cells during ipsilateral rotation and cessation of firing with contralateral rotation (Precht *et al.*, 1971; Llinás *et al.*, 1971).

In the following the projection of the primary vestibular fibers onto the cerebellum in the frog will be described. The description will be preceded by an account of the vestibular-auditory complex and of the termination of primary vestibular afferents.

MATERIALS AND METHODS

Frogs (*Rana catesbeiana*) were studied for normal histology and following transection of the vestibular nerve cranially. The normal material for light microscopy was obtained by perfusing the animals with a glutaraldehyde solution after which the brain was removed and fixed in osmium tetroxide for a period of 6–8 hours. The brain was embedded in low viscosity nitrocellulose and sectioned at 20 μm with a sliding microtome. The sections were deosmiated with oxalic acid and stained with cresyl violet.

Vestibular nerve lesions were produced under light sodium pentobarbital anesthesia and hypothermia. The cranium was opened and, without injuring the brain, the vestibular nerve was exposed and sectioned at a level just below the VII nerve. After a course of 4–10 days of degeneration, animals were sacrificed by perfusion with a buffered formalin–glutaraldehyde solution and the brains were removed and fixed for 3–7 days. Frozen sections were stained using the Fink and Heimer technique (1967).

RESULTS

Primary afferent degeneration in the VIII nerve following transection proximal to the ganglion cells indicates three main projection sites (Fig. 1). The largest mass of fibers projects to the vestibular-auditory complex while much smaller groups are found in the deep cerebellar nucleus and the cerebellar cortex. With the Fink and Heimer technique (1967) two patterns of degeneration are seen with regard to time. First the projection site can be visualized (2–7 days) as the boutons and small terminal branches break down and become argyrophilic. Later the projection path is observable

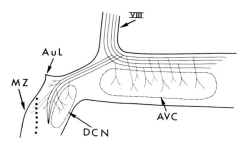

Fig. 1. Diagram to show the primary afferent projection of the vestibular nerve. Primary fibers descend caudally in the medulla to the region of the IX–X nerve complex (to the right) where they give off right angle branches to the auditory-vestibular area. Some fibers ascend towards the cerebellum where they project into the deep cerebellar nucleus (DCN) and other branches continue into the granular layer of the auricular and marginal zone. A few fibers enter the lower part of the molecular layer. MZ, marginal zone. AuL, auricular lobe. AVC, auditory vestibular complex.

(6–15 days) when the large axons of myelinated fibers degenerate. Subsequently, the projection path and site will be considered separately.

Vestibular-auditory complex

The vestibular-auditory complex consists of:

(1) a dorsal concentration of cells known as the dorso-magnocellularis (Fig. 2A and B; DMgC);

(2) ventral to this, a distinct concentration of medium sized neurons set in a lightly myelinated neuropil (Fig. 2C and D; MCN);

(3) caudal to the latter, a group of small neurons;

(4) in the ventral region, scattered large cells between which myelinated fibers are dispersed (Fig. 3E, F and G; VN). This complex extends rostrocaudally from the level of the V nerve down to the IX-X nerve complex. Dorsoventrally it is in the region from the crest of the medulla, which flanks the IV ventricle, extending ventrally to approximately the lower $\frac{1}{4}$ of the vestibular nerve as it enters the brain stem. Laterally it is separated from the outer surface by the massive fiber pathways which occupy the outer half of the medullary wall. Medially it lies close to the ependymal surface but is separated from this by small myelinated bundles.

The large nucleus dorso-magnocellularis extends from the VIII nerve to one half the distance between the IX-X nerve complex (Fig. 2A and B; DMgC). This nucleus is composed of medium sized cells which are embedded in a myelinated fiber mass. Below this is the medium sized cell group (MCN) which has the shape of an elongated column and on which an enlarged head protrudes ventrally at the level of the vestibular nerve (Fig. 2D). This cell group is easily distinguished because of the paucity of myelinated fibers (Fig. 2C and D). Distinctly larger cells (20–30 μm) are present in the rostral enlargement and in the column portion there are small cells (13–20 μm) with only a few large cells. Variation in the light myelin configuration also indicates a separation of the column into these two suggested cell groups. A group of small neurons (13–20 μm) is found caudal to the column nucleus (Fig. 2D). In the ventral portion of the complex, large cells (30–50 μm) are scattered in a myelinated matrix similar to the Deiters neurons. This nucleus has been called the ventral nucleus of the VIII nerve (Ariëns Kappers, Huber and Crosby, 1936), and it is positioned ventral and lateral to the column nucleus and the small cell group.

The *afferent fibers of the VIII nerve* enter the brain stem at an angle of about 30° dorsal. Most of the fibers turn caudally. Those in the caudal portion of the nerve turn with a small radius while those rostrally make a larger arc so that they come to lie on the medial side of the descending bundle of fibers (Figs. 1 and 4A and B). From the arching point, a small number of fibers (either as individual or collaterals) turn rostrally to the cerebellar regions (Figs. 1 and 4A and B).

The silver reaction at 3–4 days shows that the early degenerating *terminal fibers and boutons* form a pattern which outlines the vestibular-auditory complex. These fibers arise from the descending vestibular afferents as right angle branches which pass medially into the nuclear complex (Fig. 5A). The degenerating processes are found

References p. 339

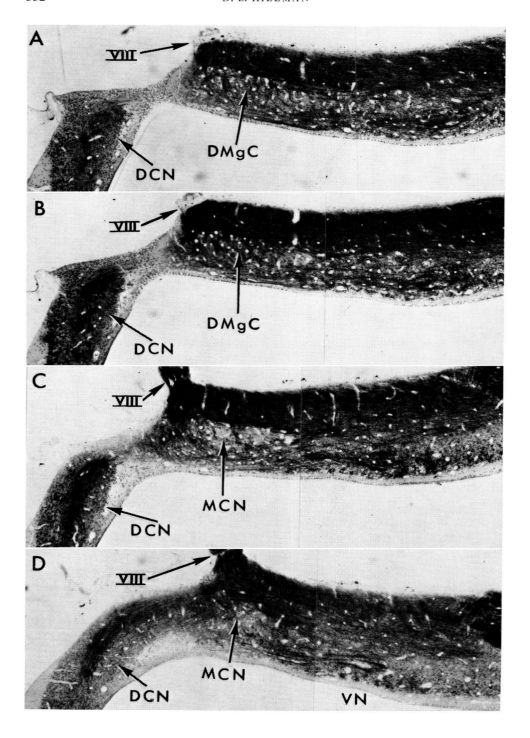

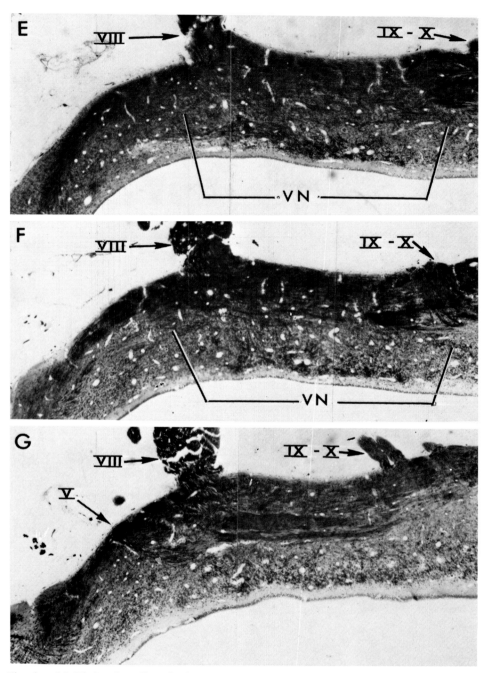

Figs. 2 and 3. Nissl and myelin stained serial sections at 100 μm intervals to illustrate the relationship between the vestibular nerve, auditory-vestibular complex, deep cerebellar nuclei and cerebellum. In A and B the dorsal magnocellular group of cells (DMgC) is visible, while in C and D the medium-sized cell nucleus (MCN) with its enlarged head and descending column is evident because of its light myelin composition. The deep cerebellar nucleus (DCN) extends from A-D and is apparently reaching its most ventral extent in E. At section D the ventral nucleus (VN) is seen and extends from the rostral part of the VIII nerve to the rostral part of the IX–X nerve complex. Its ventral limit seen is in G where the section passes through the descending root of the V. In G the most dorsal part of the V nerve is also visible.

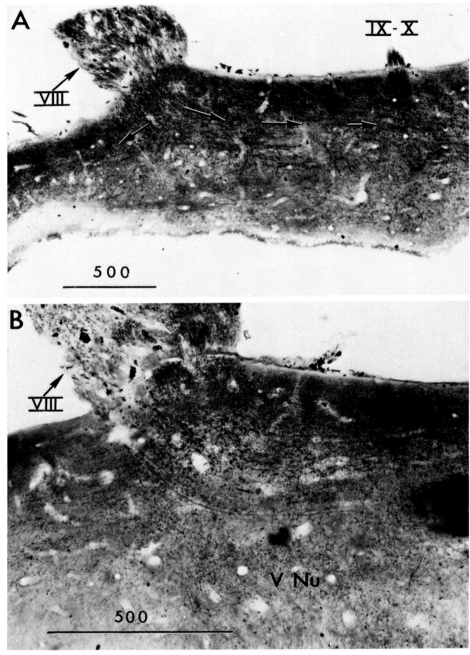

Fig. 4. Primary afferent fiber degeneration 9 days following section of the VIII nerve. The massive descending projection extends down to and slightly beyond the IX nerve. Projecting from this bundle are right angle collaterals which enter the vestibular nuclear region (VNu). In B the ascending part of the VIII nerve is seen as it arises from the incoming root and projects rostrally.

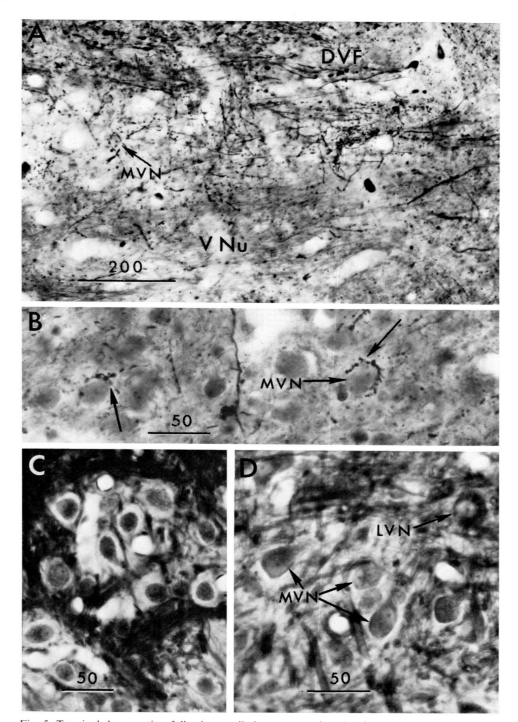

Fig. 5. Terminal degeneration following vestibular nerve section showing the degeneration within the vestibular complex. In A numerous right angle collaterals project from the descending vestibular fibers (DFV) into the vestibular nucleus (VNu). In the background, profiles of neurons can be observed which are outlined by degenerating boutons. The high power picture (B) of primary afferent degeneration to the vestibular nucleus shows medium sized cells from the column nucleus which are contacted directly by primary afferent boutons. C and D show the various types of cells which are found in the vestibular nucleus. C, medium sized cells which are located in the head of the column nucleus. D, medium sized vestibular neurons (MVN) from the column nucleus and a large vestibular neuron (LVN) from the ventral nucleus.

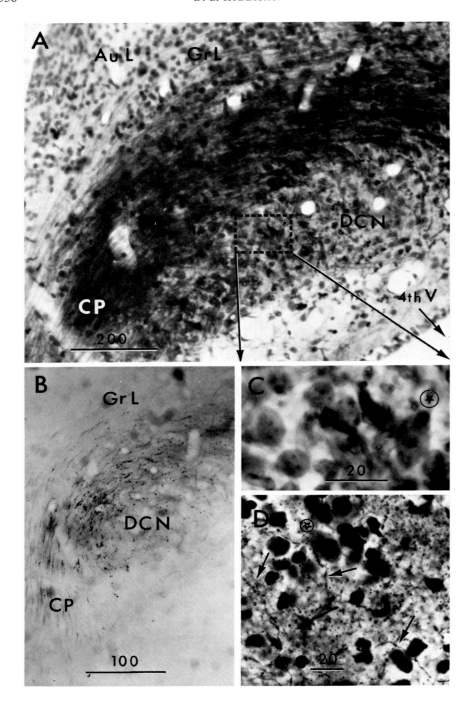

regularly throughout this cellular region where they make contact with the cell bodies many times in a multiple bouton fashion (Fig. 5B) and also with what appears to be dendrites in the neuropil.

Deep cerebellar nuclei

The deep cerebellar nucleus is situated at the junction between the cerebellum and the medulla where it is separated from the granular layer by peduncular fibers as they reach the cerebellum (Figs. 1 and 2A, B and C). The most dorsal part of the nucleus is at the medullary crest of the IV ventricle as it meets the cerebellum (Fig. 2A). From this point the nuclear cells are grouped ventrally and lie medial and caudal to the cerebellar peduncle as it arches to the cerebellum. A part of the nucleus extends below the cerebellum. The predominant cells are 12–18 μm with light nuclear chromatin and a relatively clear cytoplasm (Fig. 5C). A few large cytochromatic cells are distributed in the dorsolateral part of the nucleus and into the peduncular fibers (Fig. 5C). The large cells have not been found in the medial region of the nucleus.

Primary afferent fibers of the VIII nerve ascend in the medullary crest to the cerebellar peduncle. These fibers course lateral to the deep nucleus and turn medially at its rostral border so as to clearly delineate the nuclear margin (Fig. 6B). Within the deep cerebellar nucleus a concentration of degenerating afferents is found in the lateral part of this cell group while only sparse degeneration is seen in the medial zone. The degenerating boutons are occasionally seen near cell bodies of the large neurons; however, the majority appears to be in the neuropil which indicates a dendritic relationship.

Cerebellar cortex

The area of the cerebellum which receives primary vestibular afferents is situated just rostral to the deep cerebellar nucleus and extends dorsally along the marginal region of the cerebellum. The granular layer which is adjacent to the deep nucleus receives most of the fibers while in the marginal zone the number decreases progressively toward the midline. In general, few fibers project to the cerebellum as compared to the vestibular region or even the deep cerebellar nucleus. It could not be determined if this projection originates from collaterals of the deep cerebellar fibers or from separate fibers from the vestibular nerve.

Within the molecular layer a few degenerating processes can be found near the

---

Fig. 6. Photomicrographs to show the deep cerebellar nucleus and the primary afferent projection to this cell region. In A the deep cerebellar nucleus is shown in relationship to the cerebellar peduncle (CP) and the granular layer (GrL) of the cerebellum which is just rostral to this region. This part of the cerebellum is the auricular lobe (AuL) and the adjacent marginal zone. B, Fink and Heimer degeneration at 7 days shows the cerebellar peduncular fibers as they curve around the deep cerebellar nucleus (DCN) which contains numerous degenerating boutons. The greatest amount of degeneration is found in the lateral portion of the nucleus where, in addition to the small sized cells, there are medium sized neurons (C) which are contacted by degenerating primary afferent fibers as shown in D.

References p. 339

Purkinje cell layer (Hillman, 1969). These fibers course at an angle into the molecular layer. Away from the Purkinje cell layer the degenerating fibers break up into a series of dots. Electron microscopical study shows that these fibers are branches of myelinated fibers which synapse on Purkinje cell dendrites without making spine contacts (Hillman, 1969). The vesicular pattern is somewhat like those of climbing fibers in that the vesicles are large, round and have a few dense core vesicles.

DISCUSSION

The primary vestibular projection in lower vertebrates has for the most part been the subject of speculation since the techniques used in their study are unable to distinguish them from secondary vestibular fibers (Ariëns Kappers, Huber and Crosby, 1936; Larsell, 1923, 1925, 1967). The wide extent of the vestibular projection to the auditory-vestibular complex was not expected from a review of the literature as Larsell (1925) mentions only a small vestibular nucleus near the entering vestibular nerve. However, Ariëns Kappers, Huber and Crosby (1936) do mention that the nerve fibers both ascend and descend upon entering the medulla. The nuclear groups which are indicated in earlier studies as being related to the vestibular nerve are the dorso-magnocellularis and the ventral nucleus of the VIII nerve (Ariëns Kappers, Huber and Crosby 1936). The extent of these nuclei and related cell groups, however, has not been fully realized. On the basis of the present material some correlation can be made between the nuclear groups in these lower animals and those of mammals which have been distinguished by Brodal and Pompeiano (1957). For the most part identification of nuclear groups beyond that observable by cyto- and myeloarchitectonics must await further study of the specific primary and secondary projections.

The present study shows that the cerebellar nuclei are located in the caudolateral base of the cerebellum just behind the cerebellar peduncles which separate them from the granular layer. Rüdeberg (1962) was unable to find the cerebellar nuclei in the frog, while Larsell (1923, 1925) consistently outlined this nucleus in the rostral part of the medulla just behind the cerebellum. Very interesting is the finding that this nucleus contains smaller cells which have very light nuclear and cytoplasmic staining. The second type of cell is a larger cytochromatic cell which is scattered throughout the lateral portion of this nucleus. This lateral group of cells appears to be very closely related to the primary vestibular projection, since the degeneration is concentrated in this area and degenerating boutons are found to contact cell bodies of large neurons.

The projection of primary fibers to the cerebellar granular layer of the auricular and marginal zone is an interesting direct connection. The ability of this projection to have a massive effect on Purkinje cells is, however, doubtful since the fibers are not concentrated in any part of the granular layer and its contact is through an intermediary — the granule cells. Direct synapses to Purkinje cells by other fibers may affect very significantly certain Purkinje cells. The number of cells which show direct contacts of a climbing fiber nature is relatively small.

SUMMARY

The projection of the primary fibers in the VIII nerve has been studied in the frog with the Fink and Heimer technique (1967). It was found that the primary fibers project to three main regions of the brain: (i) the auditory-vestibular complex; (ii) the deep cerebellar nuclei; and (iii) the cerebellum. The cyto- and myeloarchitectonics of the auditory-vestibular complex and the deep cerebellar nuclei show distinct cell groupings within these projection sites.

REFERENCES

ARIËNS KAPPERS, C. U. AND HAMMER, E. (1918) Das Zentralnervensystem des Ochsenfrosches (*Rana catesbeiana*). *Psychiat.-neurol. Wschr.*, **22**, 368–415.

ARIËNS KAPPERS, C. U., HUBER, G. C. AND CROSBY, E. C. (1936) *The Comparative Anatomy of the Nervous System of Vertebrates, Including Man. Vol. 1.* MacMillan, New York, pp. XVII–864.

BRODAL, A. AND POMPEIANO, O. (1957) The vestibular nuclei in the cat. *J. Anat. (Lond.)*, **91**, 438–454.

FINK, R. P. AND HEIMER, L. (1967) Two methods for selective silver impregnation of degenerating axons and their synaptic endings in the central nervous system. *Brain Res.*, **4**, 369–374.

GLEISNER, L. AND HENRIKSSON, N. G. (1964) Efferent and afferent activity pattern in the vestibular nerve of the frog. *Acta oto-laryng. (Stockh.)*, **58**, Suppl. 192, 90–103.

GOODMAN, D. C. (1958) Cerebellar stimulation in the unanesthetized bullfrog. *J. comp. Neurol.*, **110**, 321–335.

HILLMAN, D. E. (1969) Light and electron-microscopical study of the relationships between the cerebellum and the vestibular organ of the frog. *Exp. Brain Res.*, **9**, 1–15.

LARSELL, O. (1923) The cerebellum of the frog. *J. comp. Neurol.*, **36**, 89–112.

LARSELL, O. (1925) The development of the cerebellum in the frog (Hyla regilla) in relation to the vestibular and lateral line systems. *J. comp. Neurol.*, **39**, 249–289.

LARSELL, O. (1967) *The Comparative Anatomy and Histology of the Cerebellum from Myxinoids Through Birds.* In J. JANSEN (Ed.), University of Minnesota Press, Minneapolis, pp. VIII-291.

LLINÁS, R., PRECHT, W. AND CLARKE, M. (1971) Cerebellar Purkinje cell responses to physiological stimulation of the vestibular system in the frog. *Exp. Brain Res.*, **13**, 408–431.

LLINÁS, R., PRECHT, W. AND KITAI, S. T. (1967) Climbing fibre activation of Purkinje cell following primary vestibular afferent stimulation in the frog. *Brain Res.*, **6**, 371–375.

MCNALLY, W. J. AND TAIT, J. (1925) Ablation experiments on the labyrinth of the frog. *Amer. J. Physiol.*, **75**, 155–179.

PRECHT, W. AND LLINÁS, R. (1969) Functional organization of the vestibular afferents to the cerebellar cortex of frog and cat. *Exp. Brain Res.*, **9**, 30–52.

PRECHT, W., LLINÁS, R. AND CLARKE, M. (1971) Physiological responses of frog vestibular fibers to horizontal angular rotation. *Exp. Brain Res.*, **13**, 378–407.

ROSS, D. A. (1935) Action potentials from the eighth cranial nerve of the frog. *J. Physiol. (Lond.)*, **84**, 14–15P.

ROSS, D. A. (1936) Electrical studies on the frog's labyrinth. *J. Physiol. (Lond.)*, **86**, 117–146.

RÜDEBERG, S. I. (1962) Formation of the embryonic migration layers in the cerebellar anlage of the reptile *Iguana iguana*. *Acta anat.*, **51**, 329–337.

Vestibulocerebellar Input: Physiology

R. LLINÁS AND W. PRECHT

Division of Neurobiology, Department of Physiology and Biophysics,
University of Iowa, Iowa City, Iowa, U.S.A.
and
Max-Planck-Institute for Brain Research, Frankfurt a.M., G.F.R.

Development of the cerebellar complex was linked, from the early studies in comparative neuroanatomy, to that of the "vestibulo-lateral" system (Herrick, 1924; Larsell, 1967). This close vestibulo-cerebellar relationship remains throughout phylogenetic development; however, its importance has been comparatively reduced in relation to the enormous increase of the other cerebellar afferents in the higher vertebrates. Nevertheless, up to higher primates and man, the vestibulocerebellum occupies a primary role in the functional organization of locomotion and equilibration.

Although we will be primarily concerned with the interactions between the vestibular input and the cerebellar responses which it evokes (*i.e.*, the so-called floccular-nodular area of higher vertebrates), we shall touch briefly on new findings regarding the functional relations between cerebellar cortex and the oculomotor system. As expressed in a recent paper (Llinás, Precht and Clarke, 1971), it is our contention that a proper understanding of the functional characteristics of the vestibular input to the cerebellum will allow quantitative analysis of the properties of cerebellar neurons and, thus, a deeper insight into the functional meaning of "cerebellar control".

We shall divide this paper into four sections: (i) analysis of the electrical responses evoked in the cerebellum of frogs and cats following electrical stimulation of the vestibular nerve: (ii) physiological properties of the vestibular input to the cerebellum studied by means of rotative stimulation of the semicircular canals of frogs; (iii) cerebellar efferent control of the peripheral vestibular system; and (iv) extraocular afferent projection to the cerebellar cortex.

CEREBELLAR FIELD POTENTIALS EVOKED BY ELECTRICAL STIMULATION OF THE VESTIBULAR NERVE

Frog. Basically two types of electrical activity can be recorded in the amphibian cerebellar cortex following vestibular stimulation.

(i) In the auricular area a single electrical activation of the vestibular nerve evokes a negative field potential which increases in amplitude from the surface to 500 μm in depth (Fig. 1B). This response has been shown to be generated by direct terminals of the vestibular nerve on the granule cell layer in the auricular lobe (Precht and Llinás,

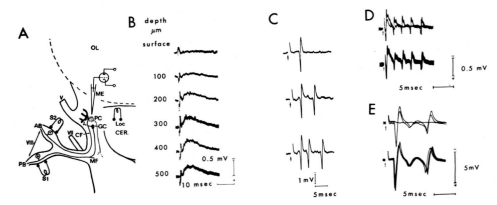

Fig. 1. Field and unitary potentials evoked in the frog auricular lobe following VIII nerve stimulation. A, diagram of frog brain stem and experimental arrangement. CER, cerebellum; CF, climbing fiber; GC, granule cell; Loc, surface stimulating electrode; ME, recording microelectrode;
MF, mossy fiber; OL, optic lobe; PC, Purkinje cell in the auricular lobe; S1 and S2, peripheral nerve
stimulating electrodes; V, trigeminal nerve; VII, facial nerve; VIII, stato-acoustic nerve (AB and
PB, anterior and posterior branches, respectively). In B field potentials recorded at different depths
in the auricular lobe after stimulation in the ipsilateral anterior branch of the VIII nerve. In C,
D and E, unitary Purkinje cell activation following VIII nerve stimulation. In C a Purkinje cell
spike was recorded at 270 μm from the surface. The number of spikes generated increased as the
stimulus amplitude was augmented from the first to last traces. D and E, monosynaptic climbing
fiber activation of Purkinje cells in response to stimulation of the VIII nerve. In D the recording
was obtained 300 μm from the surface and the all-or-none character of the response is shown in the
upper trace. In the lower trace, five records are superimposed. E, another example of monosynaptic
climbing fiber activation of Purkinje cells in response to VIII nerve stimulation. The all-or-none
        nature of the response is illustrated in the upper trace. From Precht and Llinás (1969a).

1969a). The pathway arises, therefore, from the bipolar cells located in the ganglion of
the vestibular nerve and projects to the auricular lobe as mossy fibers (Hillman, 1969).
The graded nature of the Purkinje cell activation and the rather short latency of the
response (Fig. 1C) are in complete agreement with this anatomical finding. A second,
but smaller, input has been found projecting from the vestibular nerve directly to the
molecular layer at the auricular lobe. In this case, however, the synaptic contacts are
made directly with the Purkinje cell in a fashion very similar to the climbing fiber–
Purkinje cell synapse (Hillman, 1969; Precht and Llinás, 1969a) (Fig. 1D and E).
Other pathways projecting on the auricular lobe probably arise from the vestibular
nuclei and may terminate as mossy fibers on the granule cells (Larsell, 1967). It appears, therefore, that the vestibular nerve projects to the auricular lobe in a direct
fashion, either monosynaptically on the Purkinje cells or as a disynaptic input through
the mossy fiber–granule cell system.

    (ii) Regarding the cerebellum proper, electrical activation of the vestibular nerve
evokes clearcut field potentials in the posterior rim of the cerebellar corpus (Llinás
Precht and Clarke, 1971). In this case the latency of the response is much longer than
that found in the auricular lobe. In fact, the latency ranges from 15–18 msec, depending on the place of recording. The field potentials in the frog cerebellar rim can be
categorized as being evoked by the activation of mossy fiber–parallel fiber–Purkinje

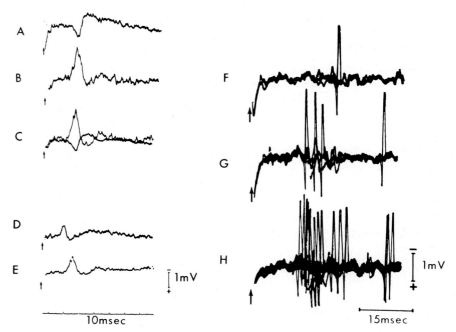

Fig. 2. Field and unitary potentials in the corpus cerebelli evoked by a single electrical stimulation of the VIII nerve in the frog. A and B, field potentials recorded at surface and 300 μm respectively. C, surface and depth recordings as in A and B in another preparation. D and E, field potentials recorded at the Purkinje cell layer at 350 μm distances from the ipsilateral cerebellar peduncle. F, G and H, unitary activity of Purkinje cells evoked by electrical stimulation of the vestibular nerve at increasing amplitude. The action potentials were recorded in the cerebellar corpus. Arrows indicate onset of electrical stimulus. From Llinás, Precht and Clarke (1971).

cell pathways. The potentials recorded near the surface and at the Purkinje cell layer are illustrated in Fig. 2 A–E. These potentials are in every way similar to those described in the frog cerebellar cortex following white matter stimulation and interpreted as generated by the mossy fiber–parallel fiber system (Llinás, Bloedel and Hillman, 1969). Furthermore, the electrical activation of the vestibular nerve generates a potential which seems to propagate along the posterior rim of the cerebellum, from the periphery towards the midline, and extends to reach the contralateral side. Potentials recorded at two different points along the posterior rim illustrate the change in latency as the wavefront of the field potential sweeps across the cerebellar cortex (Fig. 2). The typical unitary Purkinje cell activity evoked by this form of stimulation is shown in Fig. 2, records F, G and H. For the most part, the responses consist of unitary spikes whose firing frequency and latency are related to the vestibular stimulus amplitude. In most cases, two distinct clusters of Purkinje cell spikes can be observed which correspond to the two components of the field potentials shown in Fig. 2 B and C. With very few exceptions, appropriate electrical stimulation of frog vestibular nerve failed to activate the climbing fiber afferent input to the cerebellar corpus (Llinás, Precht and Clarke, 1971).

Cat. Electrical stimulation of the vestibular nerve in the cat evokes field potentials in the floccular and nodular areas of the cerebellar cortex. As in the case of the frog, these field potentials are typical of mossy fiber activation (Eccles *et al.*, 1966a; Eccles *et al.*, 1967). In contraposition with the results in the frog, however, there seems to be a direct input from the vestibular nerve onto both ipsi- and contralateral floccular regions as well as to the ipsi- and contralateral nodulus (Precht and Llinás, 1969a). The potentials evoked in the vestibulo-cerebellum by vestibular nerve stimulation are exemplified in Fig. 3, which illustrates the field potentials evoked in the different layers of the nodulus. As the micropipette penetrates through the nodulus along a slightly para-sagittal track, it records the potentials generated in an alternative manner at molecular (Fig. 3B and D) and granular layers (Fig. 3C and E). The similarity between the field potentials generated in the nodulus as a result of vestibular nerve stimulation and the mossy fiber field potentials (Eccles *et al.*, 1966a; Eccles *et al.*, 1967) assures that the afferent vestibular input to these areas is mainly of a mossy fiber type.

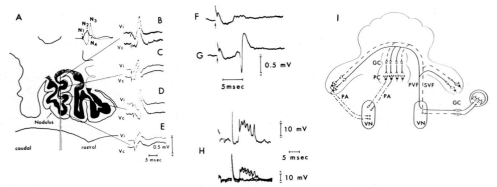

Fig. 3. Field and unitary potentials evoked by VIII nerve stimulation in the nodulus of the cat. A, line drawing of a parasagittal section of the cat cerebellum illustrating the path of the recording electrode. The microelectrode was inserted into the nodulus ventro-dorsally. The dark areas of the drawing correspond to the granular layer, the outer white crossed area the molecular layer of the cerebellum. B to E show averaged field potentials generated by single shocks to the ipsilateral V_i and contralateral V_c stimulation. The sites of recording of field potentials in B to C are indicated by lines in the diagram in A. Field potentials in B and D were recorded in the molecular layer while C and E were taken from the granular layer. Inset line drawing at top of diagram A shows superimposition of field potentials of the molecular layer (dotted line) and in the granular layer (solid line). The various components of the fields at these two sites are marked (N_1–N_4). G illustrates unitary Purkinje cell activity in the nodulus following ipsilateral VIII nerve stimulation. A subthreshold stimulation generated a small field potential in F. In H climbing fiber responses were recorded intracellularly in nodular Purkinje cells following contralateral inferior olive stimulation in the region of the medial accessory olive. The all-or-none character of the response is seen in the lower trace in H. In I, a diagram shows connection of the vestibular system to the cerebellar cortex in the cat. The floccular lobes are shown laterally, nodulus and uvula in the center. Solid and broken lines represent primary (PVF) and secondary (SVF) vestibulo-cerebellar fibers, respectively. Lines of dots and dashes represent Purkinje cell projection to the vestibular nuclei (VN). Afferent connections to the cerebellar cortex on the right of the diagram, the efferent cortico-vestibular projections on the left. The arrows point in the direction of impulse conduction. Vestibulo-cerebellar projection not indicated. GC, granule cells; PA, Purkinje cell axons; PC, Purkinje cells; VN, vestibular nuclei. From Precht and Llinás (1969a).

In the molecular layers of the nodulus the field potentials consisted mainly of a small N_1 and a larger N_3 negative component (Fig. 3 B and D). With records obtained from the granular layer (Fig. 3 C and E), N_1, N_2 and N_4 negative potentials were prominent. In most experiments a small negativity was seen to occur between N_1 and N_2. These different potentials are shown in a superimposed drawing of molecular fields (dotted) and granular fields (solid line) at the top of Fig. 3A.

The field potentials have been interpreted as follows (Precht and Llinás, 1969a). The N_1 potential represents the compound action current generated as the primary vestibular fiber volley reaches the granular layer. This potential is able to follow high frequency stimulation and is resistant to barbiturate anesthesia. The small negative potential interposed between N_1 and N_2 potentials represents the compound action current of secondary vestibulo-cerebellar fibers, although part of it might be generated by primary vestibular fibers having slower conduction velocities. The small amplitude of this second fiber potential does not necessarily imply that the number of secondary vestibulo-cerebellar fibers is small, since it is possible that some of the cells of origin of those fibers do not receive primary vestibular fibers and hence are not excited by vestibular nerve stimulation. The N_2 wave is ascribed to the synaptic and action currents produced by vestibular fibers in the granule and Golgi cells of the granular layer. The N_3 wave represents the action currents in parallel fibers and the synaptic and action currents which these fibers generate in Purkinje cells and in the inter-neurons of the molecular layer. The impulses evoked in Purkinje cells travel down their axons and generate the N_4 potential at the granular layer.

Field potentials of similar configuration were also recorded from the flocculus and ventral parts of the uvula and are in very good agreement with the anatomical distri-bution of the vestibulocerebellar fibers. Likewise the latencies measured from the stimulus artefact to the beginning of the negativity for the different components were in the same range, *i.e.*, 0.6 to 0.75 msec for the N_1, 1.6 to 1.7 msec for the N_2, and 3.3 to 3.5 for the N_3. The short latency of the N_1 potential wave also indicates that this potential must be generated by the action currents of the primary vestibular fibers terminating in the cerebellum, since the earliest transsynaptic activation of neurons in the vestibular nuclei occurs at 0.8–1.0 msec after the stimulus (Precht and Shimazu, 1965).

At single cell level, the two classical types of response have been obtained following electrical stimulation of the vestibular nerve in this animal. As shown in Fig. 3, the typical unitary action potential evoked by the mossy fiber–granule cell system can be seen in the Purkinje cell layer of the nodulus. The responses to vestibular nerve stimulation consisted in all cases of single action potentials with latencies ranging from 3–15 msec. The shortest latency (3 msec), and the occurrence of only one or occasional-ly two action potentials to a single vestibular nerve shock, implies activation of the Purkinje cells via a direct mossy fiber–granule cell pathway. The Purkinje cell spikes were identified by their antidromic generation from the inferior cerebellar peduncle.

On several occasions, vestibular stimulation evoked the all-or-none climbing fiber activation of Purkinje cells. This form of activation was observed both intra- and extra-cellularly and was generated by the classical large, all-or-none EPSP. Vestibular nerve stimulation of the magnitude used for activating vestibular mossy fibers, on the other hand, never evoked any of these Purkinje cell spike bursts. When the stimulus strength was two to three times suprathreshold for vestibular nerve activation (which is known to produce direct activation of structures other than the vestibular nerve), typical all-or-none burst activations of Purkinje cells were occasionally observed, their latencies being between 15–20 msec or longer. These same Purkinje cells usually showed intracellular burst responses evoked monosynaptically from the contralateral inferior olive (Fig. 3H). On the basis of these findings, it may be concluded that primary and secondary vestibulo-cerebellar fibers in the cat project to the cerebellum as a mossy fiber input. On the other hand, the climbing fiber afferents to the vestibulo-cerebellum may be activated either via pathways other than the vestibular nerve or by means of special patterns of afferent activity which cannot be evoked by electrical activation of the nerve. If the first statement is true, then the two afferent systems must carry information from different sources to the cerebellar cortex and, thus, should not be taken as true parallel channel systems. In conclusion, electrical stimulation of the vestibular nerve of cats and frogs strongly suggests that this input is primarily a mossy fiber mediated channel.

PHYSIOLOGICAL STIMULATION OF THE VESTIBULAR INPUT AND ITS ACTION ON THE CEREBELLAR CORTEX

All of the experiments to be described here have been recorded from the cerebellar cortex of frogs. Four types of Purkinje cell responses have been encountered (Fig. 4). Each type of response seems to be related to a particular area of the cortex and we have designated them types I through IV (Precht and Llinás, 1969b).

Type-I Purkinje cells are characterized by increase of activity following ipsilateral horizontal rotation and by decrease of activity following contralateral rotation.

A *type-II* Purkinje cell responds in an opposing manner (*i.e.*, increased activity to contralateral stimulation and little or no response, or a diminution, following ipsilateral rotation).

By far the most common type of Purkinje cell response is that encountered in the posterior rim of the cerebellar corpus. As seen previously, this is a polysynaptic pathway, probably mediated through the vestibular nucleus. This *type-III* response is characterized by an increased firing rate of the Purkinje cell to ipsi- and contralateral stimulation. As in the previous cases, the amplitude of the response is related to the amplitude of the rotative stimulus. *Type-IV* Purkinje cell responses (found rostrally to type-III) are characterized by a pause in their spike activity upon ipsi- and contralateral rotation.

Given the wide distribution of type-III response, a series of studies was undertaken to clarify further the functional properties of this type of Purkinje cell response. It was in fact observed (Fig. 5) that although most of the Purkinje cells in the vestibulo-cerebellum respond to rotation in both directions, a certain degree of asymmetry may be found with respect to their response to identical ipsi- or contralateral rotation. Furthermore, the degree of asymmetry appears to be strongly related to position of

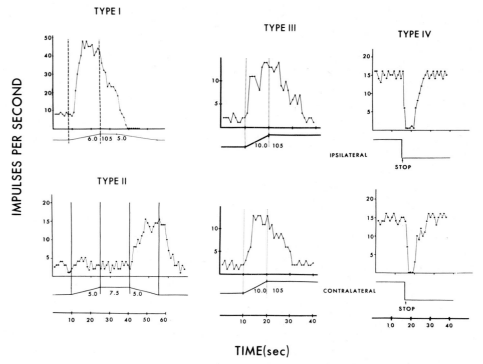

Fig. 4. Frequency diagrams of discharge of type-I, II, III and IV Purkinje cells in response to horizontal angular acceleration. Type-I Purkinje cell was recorded in the auricular lobe. Note that the cell responds by an increase of spike activity during ipsilateral angular aceleration of 6°/sec² and by a marked reduction leading to total silence of the cell following ipsilateral deceleration of 5°/sec². Type-II Purkinje cell also recorded in the ipsilateral auricular lobe shows the opposite response to angular acceleration. Ipsilateral acceleration of 5°/sec² produces no discernible increase of activity but an ipsilateral deceleration of 5°/sec² produces a sizable response. The type-III Purkinje cell responds to both ipsilateral rotation (upper frequency diagram) and to contralateral stimulation (lower frequency diagram) while type-IV Purkinje cell responds with a marked depression of spike activity following sudden arrest from a constant angular velocity of 85°/sec in the ipsilateral and contralateral direction. From Precht and Llinás (1969b).

cells in the cerebellar cortex. Thus, cells located laterally near the auricular lobe are particularly responsive to ipsilateral stimulation and show little or no response to contralateral rotation. As recordings were made closer to the midline, it was found that Purkinje cells became progressively symmetrical such that responses recorded close to the midline during ipsi- or contralateral rotation were rather similar for a given cell. Slightly different responses were encountered, however, when neighboring Purkinje cell responses were compared. Thus, in Fig. 5 twenty Purkinje cells responding to ipsi- and contralateral rotation were illustrated. It is to be noted that while all of the cells respond in a more or less symmetrical manner to ipsi- and contralateral rotation, there seems to be a difference between responses obtained from different cells. In fact, while some are rather phasic in their firing (Fig. 5, left column), others may be rather tonic (extreme right column). A continuous gamut of variations can be found in the central columns.

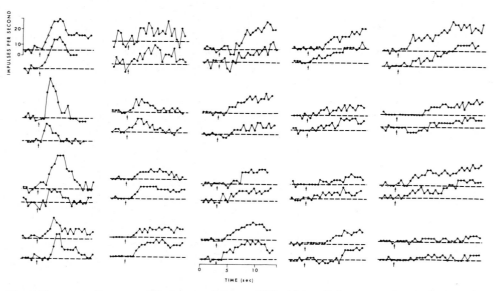

Fig. 5. Frequency diagrams of discharges of 20 type-III Purkinje cells in response to constant angular accelerations in the ipsi- and contralateral directions. Each pair of frequency diagrams represents the responses of individual Purkinje cells to accelerations applied in the ipsi- and contralateral directions at the time indicated by arrows. Broken lines represent the resting level of spontaneous activity. From Llinás, Precht and Clarke (1971).

Finally, it must be noted also that a given Purkinje cell tends to have a similar spike discharge pattern during ipsi- and contralateral rotation. This strongly suggests that the spike discharge pattern observable in a given Purkinje cell may be related not only to the physiological properties of the incoming afferent systems but also to the particular electrophysiological properties of the cell itself.

CEREBELLO-VESTIBULAR EFFERENTS IN THE FROG

Since our study is focused upon the cerebellum, all of the recordings obtained deal with the ipsilateral auricular lobe and the most lateral aspects of the corpus cerebelli itself. This region is known to receive primary and secondary vestibular fibers and corresponds to the flocculus of higher forms (Larsell, 1923; Precht and Llinás, 1969a). At the level of the auricular lobe, electrical stimulation of the vestibular nerve evokes a short latency negative field potential which is followed by a slower negative potential (Fig. 6 B and C) (Llinás and Precht, 1969; Precht, Kitai and Llinás, 1970). At single unitary level, three types of giant extracellular responses can be recorded from the Purkinje cells. As illustrated in Fig. 6 D–E, giant antidromic invasion of action potentials from Purkinje cells can be demonstrated following vestibular nerve stimulation. The minimum latency found was 0.3 msec, the maximum latency being 1.1 msec and the mean value 0.9 msec. On several occasions the units responded both antidromically as well as synaptically with a latency of 2 to 4.5 msec. Intracellular recordings from these neurons (Fig. 6 F) demonstrated an antidromic activation which was followed by a short latency (2 msec) excitatory postsynaptic action potential in that cell. Although other types of synaptic activation of cerebellar units could be obtained in the frog, *i.e.*, the typical Purkinje cell burst evoked by the climbing fiber activation of this cell (Llinás and Bloedel, 1966/1967, 1967; Llinás *et al.*, 1967; Llinás *et al.*, 1969), no such climbing fiber response was ever found following vestibular activation in a cell which responded antidromically to the same stimulus.

Electrical stimulation of the auricular lobe was shown to have an inhibitory action on the spontaneous activity of vestibular afferents. Figure 6G illustrates spontaneous

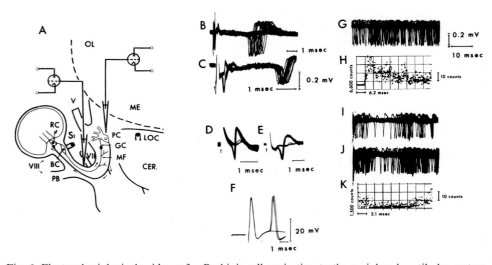

Fig. 6. Electrophysiological evidence for Purkinje cell projection to the peripheral vestibular system in the frog. In A a diagram of the brain stem, labyrinth and experimental arrangement. BC, bipolar ganglion cell; CER, cerebellum; GC, granule cell; LOC, local stimulating electrode; ME, recording microelectrode; MF, mossy fiber; OL, optic lobe; PC, Purkinje cell in the auricular lobe; RC, receptor cell; S, peripheral nerve stimulating electrode; V, trigeminal nerve; VII, facial nerve; VIII, stato-acoustic nerve; PB, posterior branch; arrows indicate the direction of impulse conduction. In B and C, unit responses of peripheral efferent nerve fibers following VIII nerve stimulation. The vestibular receptor organ was removed prior to electrical activation. The electrical stimuli indicated by arrows were applied near the cut end of the VIII nerve and recordings were obtained approximately at the VIII nerve. B and C show the same unit at different speeds. Note the direct activation of efferent fiber followed by the transsynaptic response which shows slightly fluctuating latencies. In D and E are examples of extracellularly recorded antidromic activation of Purkinje cells in the auricular lobe following VIII nerve stimulation. In F Purkinje cells were recorded intra-cellularly at a depth of 300 μm. The antidromic invasion was followed by a synaptic activation, probably through the mossy fiber-granule cell system. In G to K, effects of cerebellar stimulation on vestibular afferent discharge are shown. G illustrates firing of an utricular unit in the absence of any stimulation (25 superimposed traces). H shows the spike interval histogram of the same unit at resting condition. In I and J the auricular lobe of the cerebellum was stimulated at a rate of 3/sec (15 and 25 superimposed traces in I and J respectively). Note depression of spontaneous discharge in response to cerebellar stimulation. In K, post-stimulus histogram of the same unit shows a marked reduction in the probability of spontaneous firing between 5 and about 17 msec after the stimulus. Time and amplitude calibration shown in G is also applicable in I and J. From Llinás and Precht (1969).

firing of an utricular unit. A spike interval histogram is shown in H. The unit was shown to have a minimum interval of 6.2 msec and preferred frequencies at multiples of 6 msec. In Fig. 6 I (15 superimposed traces) following a weak auricular lobe stimulation, a clear inhibition of the spontaneous firing of the unit is seen with a 5 msec latency and a duration of approximately 15 msec. In J with a larger number of superimposed sweeps (25), a smaller gap in the spontaneous firing is observed. In K a post-stimulus histogram shows a marked reduction in the probability of spontaneous firing of this unit commencing at an interval of about 5 msec and lasting for about 17 msec (1500 counts were made). The auricular stimulation was kept at low intensity in order to prevent a direct activation of efferent fibers which could then obscure the true time course of the inhibitory action. It is assumed that the inhibition in this case is produced by the parallel fiber action of Purkinje cells which project directly to the peripheral vestibular organ.

Although our experimentation has been restricted to the cerebellovestibular system, it seems quite feasible following studies by Hillman (1969) that the vestibular efferent system of the frog originates from more than one locus. Transections at different levels of the brain stem, in fact, demonstrate that while some of the fibers are clearly arising from cerebellar structures, a large percentage arise from levels rostral to the V nerve (Hillman, 1969) and most probably are extracerebellar in origin. Direct evidence for a Purkinje cell origin of a portion of these fibers was provided electrophysiologically by the following data.

(i) The antidromic activation of assumed Purkinje cells following vestibular nerve stimulation. These Purkinje cells were characterized by their depth from the surface of the auricular lobe (200–300 μm).

(ii) Their extracellular action potentials were identical to the giant extracellular spikes which can be recorded in the corpus cerebelli after stimulation of the white matter.

(iii) Clear all-or-none burst responses due to climbing fiber activation could be obtained from cells located in the immediate vicinity.

(iv) The units could be synaptically activated by surface activation of the cerebellum, presumably by the activation of parallel fibers.

Given the fact that the cerebellum evolves in close relation to the vestibular system (Larsell, 1923), it seems reasonable to suppose that such a close relation can exist between the vestibular area of the cerebellum and the vestibular apparatus. Since no antidromic activation could be obtained from Purkinje cells located in the corpus cerebelli, it is assumed that the Purkinje cells in question belong to the so-called primordial Purkinje cell group which seems to characterize the type of Purkinje cells found at the level of the auricular lobe (Larsell, 1967).

From these results it can be concluded that following vestibular nerve stimulation, as well as electrical stimulation of the auricular lobe of the cerebellum, inhibition lasting approximately 15 msec can be produced on some of the utricular peripheral units. It deserves mention that many primary vestibular afferent units (particularly those in contact with semicircular canals) were not inhibited by electrical stimulation of either the cerebellum or the vestibular nerve. This may be partly explained by the relatively small number of efferent fibers as compared to the number of afferents (Gacek, 1960), which suggests that only a limited number of sensory cells may be sufficiently supplied with inhibitory efferent fibers to show a clearcut inhibition following single stimulation.

The finding that particularly utricular units are the target of the cerebellar inhibitory fibers suggests that the cerebellum may also have some direct regulatory influence on the structure responsible for the tonic labyrinthine reflex, *i.e.*, the otolith system. This hypothesis is supported indirectly by the demonstration of a monosynaptic inhibitory action of Purkinje axons on Deiters' neurons (Ito *et al.*, 1964) which are known to receive strong excitatory influences from the otolith system (Peterson, 1967; Fujita *et al.*, 1968). An inhibitory action of the flocculus on vestibular neurons related to semicircular canal function has been recently demonstrated by Baker, Precht and Llinás (1972).

In recording from the vestibular nerve of the frog, fibers were occasionally found whose response to horizontal rotation could not be explained on the basis of the cupula-endolymph mechanisms. It is well known from the studies of Lowenstein and Sand (1940a, b) on the isolated labyrinth of fish, that afferent fibers of the horizontal canal increase their discharge frequencies on ipsilateral acceleration, *i.e.*, on utriculopetal deviation of the cupula. The converse, a decrease in firing rate, is found on contralateral angular acceleration which leads to an utriculofugal deviation of the cupula (*cf.* Precht *et al.*, 1971). No exceptions to this rule have been seen in the isolated preparation of the endorgans and the vestibular nerve. On the basis of these findings, it may be assumed that responses other than the ones found in the isolated preparation are derived from efferent vestibular fibers. In the frog the existence of efferent fibers terminating on the sensory hair cells of the labyrinth has been demonstrated both anatomically (Hillman, 1969) and physiologically (Gleisner and Henriksson, 1963; Schmidt, 1963; Llinás and Precht, 1969).

Functionally these vestibular nerve fibers show an increase in discharge frequency during rotation in either direction. This is illustrated by the frequency diagrams of two such fibers shown in Fig. 7. In Fig. 7 A, B and E, F acceleration steps of the same magnitude have been applied in the ipsi- and contralateral directions, resulting in both cases in an increase of firing rate which is correlated with the acceleration and which begins to fall off as soon as the constant velocity is reached. The falling phase of Fig. 7A is considerably irregular and prolonged, a finding which is often observed in efferent nerve fibers. Since these neurons are of central origin and are known to show multisensory convergence, extralabyrinthine inputs might be responsible for the delayed fall-off in frequency of discharge. From the point of view of threshold, significantly higher rates of angular acceleration were necessary to activate these fibers as compared to the afferent fibers. An exceptionally low threshold (approximately $1.0°/sec^2$) was found in one of the units illustrated in Fig. 7 E and F. About half of the units recorded showed spontaneous discharge in the absence of rotatory stimulation (Fig. 7E and F).

The same fiber shown in Fig. 7 A and B was also tested with velocity steps as illustrated in Fig. 7 C and D. Slight asymmetries are noted in the peak responses as

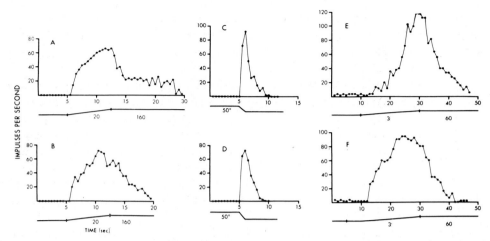

Fig. 7. Frequency diagrams of efferent vestibular fiber in response to angular accelerations. A and B, responses of a vestibular nerve fiber to ipsi- and contralateral horizontal angular accelerations ($20°/\text{sec}^2$) respectively. C and D, responses of same fiber to sudden arrest of ipsi- and contralateral rotations at constant velocities ($50°/\text{sec}$). E and F, responses of another unit to ipsi- and contralateral constant horizontal angular accelerations ($3.0°/\text{sec}^2$), respectively. Note spontaneous activity and low threshold. From Precht, Llinás and Clarke (1971).

well as in the falling phases. Similar asymmetries in the peak responses to ipsi- and contralateral rotation are seen in Fig. 7 E and F. Since the frequency increase caused by contralateral rotation must be generated by impulses arising from the contralateral labyrinth which eventually reach the efferent neuron through multisynaptic chains, such directional asymmetries are not surprising.

Furthermore, the present studies give added information concerning some of the dynamic properties of the efferent fibers in response to horizontal angular acceleration. Since both labyrinths remained intact, most of the efferent units showed an increase in firing on rotation in either direction, indicating that both labyrinths converge onto the cells of origin of efferent fibers. Some of the efferent fibers showed a resting discharge in the absence of stimulation, suggesting that the efferent system is at least partly tonic in nature. Since most of the previous studies were done under anesthesia, the importance of tonic resting discharge may have been underestimated due to the depressor action of anesthesia. The same argument holds true for the threshold for frequency increase in response to rotational stimulation. Although the study of Precht, Llinás and Clarke (1971) confirmed that efferent fibers in general have higher thresholds, it was found that the thresholds of a few units were very close to those of afferent fibers. It has frequently been observed that efferent vestibular fibers respond to stimuli other than labyrinthine, such as passive movement of limbs and cutaneous stimulation (Schmidt, 1963; Llinás and Precht, 1969). Thus, the delayed and irregular decay of the discharge rate of the efferent fiber, which occurs after constant velocity of rotation is reached, may be explained on the basis of concomitant extralabyrinthine stimulation.

Recently another interesting observation was made on the extralabyrinthine activation of efferent vestibular fibers. As described by Dichgans, Wist and Schmidt (1970) and Schmidt, Wist and Dichgans (1970), the discharge frequency of efferent vestibular fibers is modulated in close relationship with saccadic eye movements. The saccadic modulation of efferent discharge is independent of proprioceptive afferents from the eye muscles since it persists after paralyzing the animals and since it commences prior to the onset of the actual eye movement. The coupling of efferent vestibular activity with the central optokinetic mechanisms could be important in the regulation of the interaction between vestibularly and optokinetically-induced eye movements. The fact that the efferent signal occurs about 100 msec prior to the onset of the opto-kinetically-induced or spontaneously-occurring saccades is of particular interest in this respect. At present it is not established whether the fibers that show correlation with saccades are exclusively efferent in nature or if some of them are afferent units. Klinke (1970) has claimed that the recordings he made during optokinetic stimulation originated from afferent fibers. The latter change their discharge rate several seconds after a striped drum, utilized to generate optokinetic nystagmus, has begun to move. This finding may be explained by the action of efferent fibers which change the sensitivity of the receptor cells. The change in discharge frequency of afferent fibers caused by optokinetic activation is such that it would compensate for the change that would have occurred due to labyrinthine stimulation had the animal been allowed to move in response to the visual stimulus. Thus, the efferent system would tend to keep the discharge frequency of a given afferent fiber fairly constant. The direction-dependent changes found in afferent fibers by Klinke (1970) are in keeping with the finding that synchronous electrical activation of the efferent system causes a decrease in spontaneous firing of some afferent fibers, which indirectly suggests that the efferent system is inhibitory in nature as described by Llinás and Precht (1969). It should be emphasized however, that even with electrical stimulation of the efferent vestibular system only a certain percentage of afferent fibers shows significant changes in frequency of firing. This may be caused by the fact that the number of efferent fibers is indeed rather small (Gacek, Nomura and Balogh, 1965; Hillman, 1969).

Although a final conclusion regarding the functional meaning of the vestibular efferent system appears to be premature, it can be stated that various other sensory inputs besides the labyrinthine are able to influence the vestibular system at the receptor level via efferent fibers. Among them, the function of the optokinetically-induced changes may soon be understood. As for the labyrinthine effects on the efferent fiber system, they probably serve as a feedback system which, in the case of the ipsilateral loop, would be partly responsible for the frequency adaptation of some of the afferent fibers. In the case where activation of the inhibitory efferent fibers occurs during contralateral rotation, the efferent system may serve to sharpen the depressor effect produced by the directional sensitivity of the hair cells. The functional description of efferent vestibular fibers by means of physiological stimulation is, finally, very important in deciding whether a particular fiber is indeed efferent in nature. Bracchi (personal communication) has observed that, following peripheral electrical stimulation of the vestibular nerve, a response similar to the dorsal root reflex (Toennies, 1938) may be recorded peripherally after a central delay. This type of phenomenon complicates the identification of efferent fibers when only the latter criterion is utilized.

CEREBELLO-OCULOMOTOR RELATIONSHIPS

In a recent paper, Fuchs and Kornhuber (1969) have indicated that following a rapid stretch of extraocular muscles in the cat there is a clear field potential generated at cerebellar level. This response has a latency of approximately 4 msec from the onset of stimulus and may be recorded in lobules V, VI and VII in the cerebellar vermis. On the other hand, a similar type of study by Rahn and Zuber (1971) has indicated that similar potentials can be recorded at cerebellar level by volume conduction from the brain stem. Their argument is based on the fact that the field potentials mentioned may be recorded in the cerebellar cortex following bilateral cerebellar pedunculotomy. Yet another set of experiments by Wolfe (1971) suggests that, following measurement of field potentials at cerebellar cortex during nystagmus, the cerebellar potential precedes rather than follows the activation of extraocular muscles. It is our feeling that all these authors may be correct since the findings are not mutually exclusive. Thus, Fuchs and Kornhuber could be correct if an afferent system is demonstrated between extraocular muscles and the cerebellar cortex. The fact that, following such stimulation, field potentials can be observed in a pedunculotomized cerebellar cortex does not falsify Fuchs and Kornhuber's findings. It is probable that in Rahn and Zuber's experiments the cerebellar cortex was not responding previous to pedunculotomy (probably because of a very deep state of anesthesia) and thus pedunculotomy did not affect the field potentials recorded at the cerebellar cortex. Wolfe's (1971) results, on the other hand, may be part of another cerebellar mechanism which, as he mentions, precedes saccadic movement of the eye without implying that eye muscle afferents cannot evoke cerebellar activation. Crucial in the issue of cerebellar oculomotor relationships is, therefore, a demonstration of the presence or absence of an afferent system from the extraocular muscles to the cerebellum. To this effect, Baker, Precht and Llinás (1972) have recently demonstrated that following IVth nerve stimulation, which is known to include, besides the motoneuronal axons, the afferents from the extraocular muscles (Winckler, 1937), a clearcut field potential may be recorded in the cerebellar vermis.

In a series of experiments illustrated in Figs. 8 and 9, we have been able to show that following an electrical activation of the IV nerve a field potential can be generated in lobules V, VI and VII of the cerebellar vermis. These potentials can be divided into two different categories. Following ipsilateral stimulation of the nerve, a typical climbing fiber field potential can be recorded ipsi- and contralaterally in these three lobules (Fig. 8A–C) and seems to be especially clear near the junction between lobule VI and the para-vermal zone. On the other hand, microelectrode recordings from the center of lobules V and VII, and especially of lobule VI, show that the afferent input generates an early mossy fiber activation of Purkinje cells followed by a climbing fiber field potential having a latency of 18 to 22 msec (Fig. 9). The mossy fiber component (which

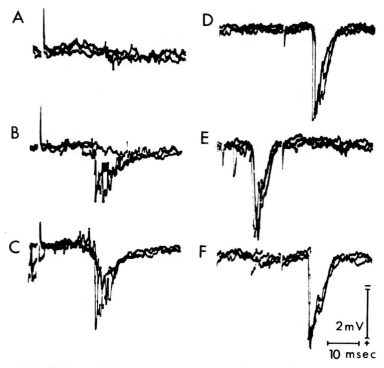

Fig. 8. Extracellular field potentials generated in the molecular layer of the cat cerebellar cortex in vermis lobule VI following electrical activation of trochlear motor nerve at orbital level. In A to C the stimulus was increased in small steps to show the all-or-none nature of the response. This activity could be evoked both ipsi- and contralaterally and was especially clear in the borderline between vermis and paravermal area. D, E and F demonstrate a total blockage of field potential generated by a double orbital stimulation at 15 msec intervals. D and F are controls. From Baker, Precht and Llinás (1972).

has a latency of 5 to 6 msec) can be seen in Fig. 9A–D to generate a series of Purkinje cell spikes with an approximate latency of 5 msec. This potential is followed by an all-or-none burst of Purkinje cell spikes, the typical climbing fiber activation of Purkinje cells (Eccles, Llinás and Sasaki, 1966b; Llinás and Hilman, 1969).

Field potentials evoked in the surface of lobule VI can be followed up to the level of cerebellar nuclei, as described by Fuchs and Kornhuber (1969).

Intracellular recording from Purkinje cells in the midline further substantiates this point. Thus, following IV nerve stimulation, an early and graded EPSP having a latency of 5 to 6 msec was always found in Purkinje cells near the midline. This typical mossy fiber-granule cell-parallel fiber EPSP was followed by the climbing fiber EPSP (Fig. 9 E and F). Climbing fiber activation generally consisted of 1 to 4 action potentials which generated an equivalent number of EPSPs in the Purkinje cell. It can thus be stated that muscle afferents from the extraocular muscles terminate directly as mossy fibers in the granular layer of the cerebellar cortex of lobules V, VI and VII and indirectly as climbing fibers, probably through the olivo-cerebellar system.

References pp. 358–359

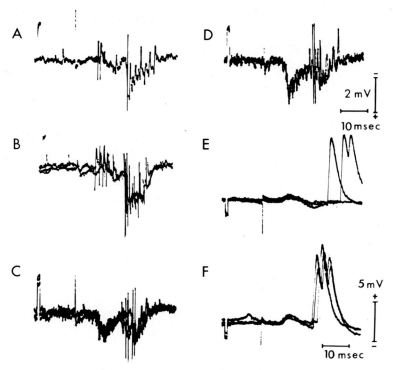

Fig. 9. Unitary potentials recorded in lobule VI following orbital stimulation. A and B, these unitary potentials were recorded at Purkinje cell level near the midline in lobule VI. Orbital stimulation produces in this case activation of Purkinje cells at a short latency (5–6 msec) which is then followed by a clearcut burst of climbing fiber response with a latency of 18 msec. C and D, another set of records taken from midline in vermal lobule VI. Intracellular recordings from Purkinje cells in this area (E and F) demonstrate that orbital stimulation generates a mossy fiber-parallel fiber EPSP followed by the typical climbing fiber EPSP. The records in F are obtained with stimulus amplitude slightly larger than that in E and show an increase in amplitude of the mossy fiber-parallel fiber EPSP and a shortening of the latency of the climbing fiber EPSP. Note the correspondence between the intracellular records shown in F and the extracellular fields illustrated in record D. From Baker, Precht and Llinás (1972).

Of great interest is the finding that mossy and climbing fibers do not seem to be restricted totally to an overlapping area of cerebellar projection. Again this emphasizes the fact that the two main afferents to the cerebellar cortex may operate independently of each other (Llinás, 1970).

DISCUSSION

As stated at the beginning of this paper, it is most probable that, given the complexity of cerebellar circuitry and the rather distant location of the cerebellar cortex with respect to most peripheral inputs, the vestibulo-cerebellum constitutes the most convenient system with which to investigate the true functional properties of the cerebellum. For the most part, we find that as far as the vestibular input is concerned, direct connection to the cerebellar cortex is mainly through the mossy fiber system. With the exception of the climbing fiber activation of auricular lobe cells in the frog cerebellum, the vestibular input to the cerebellum proper in the frog and to the flocculus and nodulus in the cat is almost exclusively a mossy fiber domain, while the climbing fiber input to the same area seems to arise, as suggested some years back (Precht and Llinás, 1969a), from other sources (Maekawa and Simpson, 1971). This particular arrangement is in total agreement with the postulate that climbing and mossy fiber inputs are 'time-sharing' the cerebellar cortex (Llinás, Bloedel and Hillman, 1969) and that they may represent, to a certain degree, phasic and tonic operators respectively.

It is clear that Purkinje cells which respond to vestibular stimulation via the vestibular mossy fiber projection system can also be activated through the climbing fiber system. We have shown this to be the case in the cat (Precht and Llinás, 1969a) and in the frog (Llinás, Precht and Clarke, 1971). This, of course, does not preclude that climbing fiber activation may be involved in the vestibuli-oculomotor physiology when such system is activated in an intact animal. However, in such instances, it is very difficult to differentiate primary afferent projection to the cerebellar cortex from other activity which may be evoked either by activation of afferents other than vestibular, or following spread of activity either centrally or through a peripheral motor response. The latter seems to be especially important, given that neck muscle afferents may evoke a strong activation of the cerebellar cortex in the cat (Berthoz and Llinás, in preparation). The fact that Purkinje cells may be directly involved in vestibular control at the vestibular nuclear, and even at the vestibular receptor level, supports the view that the cerebellum exercises a direct control upon the structuring of motor responses. That such structuring may be initiated at the peripheral receptor level is, however, surprising. Even more intriguing is the fact that the cerebellar cortex may be involved in the "correction" of movement prior to its execution. This predictive type of correction (Llinás, 1970; Kornhuber, 1971), such as implied by Wolfe (1971), may be continuously updated by the presence of a feedback from the muscle spindles themselves (Fuchs and Kornhuber, 1969; Baker, Precht and Llinás, 1972).

SUMMARY

The electrical responses evoked in the cerebellum of frogs and cats following electrical stimulation of the VIII nerve are characterized as mossy and climbing fiber responses in the former and as pure mossy fiber responses in the latter animal.

Four different types of Purkinje cell discharge patterns in response to horizontal constant angular acceleration are described and their functional implications are discussed.

The contribution of the cerebellum of the frog to the efferent vestibular system is described and its inhibitory effects on primary vestibular afferents are demonstrated.

Stimulation of afferents from the extraocular muscles causes short latency activation of Purkinje cells in the posterior vermis *via* mossy and climbing fiber paths. Functional implications of this projection are discussed.

References pp. 358–359

ACKNOWLEDGMENTS

The present research was supported by a special grant from the AMA/ERF Institute
for Biomedical Research and by USPHS Grant 1 R01 NS HD-09916-01.

REFERENCES

BAKER, R., PRECHT, W. AND LLINÁS, R. (1972) Mossy and climbing fiber projections of extraocular
muscle afferents to the cerebellum. *Brain Res.*, **38**, 440–445.
DICHGANS, J., WIST, E. R. AND SCHMIDT, C. L. (1970) Modulation neuronaler Spontanaktivität im
N. vestibularis durch optomotorische Impulse beim Kaninchen. *Pflügers Arch. ges. Physiol.*, **319**,
R154.
ECCLES, J. C., ITO, M. AND SZENTÁGOTHAI, J. (1967) *The Cerebellum as a Neuronal Machine.* Sprin-
ger, Berlin, Heidelberg, New York, pp. 335.
ECCLES, J. C., LLINÁS, R. AND SASAKI, K. (1966a) The mossy fibre-granule cell relay of the cerebellum
and its inhibitory control by Golgi cells. *Exp. Brain Res.*, **1**, 82–101.
ECCLES, J. C., LLINÁS, R. AND SASAKI, K. (1966b) The excitatory synaptic actions of climbing fibres
on the Purkinje cells of the cerebellum. *J. Physiol. (Lond.)*, **182**, 268–296.
FUCHS, A. F. AND KORNHUBER, H. H. (1969) Extraocular muscle afferents to the cerebellum of the
cat. *J. Physiol. (Lond.)*, **200**, 713–722.
FUJITA, Y., ROSENBERG, J. AND SEGUNDO, J. P. (1968) Activity of cells in the lateral vestibular nucleus
as a function of head position. *J. Physiol. (Lond.)*, **196**, 1–18.
GACEK, R. R. (1960), Efferent component of the vestibular nerve. In G. L. RASMUSSEN AND W. F.
WINDLE (Eds.), *Neural Mechanisms of the Auditory and Vestibular Systems.* C. C. Thomas, Spring-
field, Ill., pp. 276–284.
GACEK, R. R., NOMURA, Y. AND BALOGH, K. (1965) Acetylcholinesterase activity in the efferent fibers
of the stato-acoustic nerve. *Acta oto-laryng. (Stockh.)*, **59**, 541–553.
GLEISNER, L. AND HENRIKSSON, N. G. (1963) Efferent and afferent activity pattern in the vestibular
nerve of the frog. *Acta oto-laryng. (Stockh.)*, Suppl. 192, 90–103.
HERRICK, C. J. (1924) Origin and evolution of the cerebellum. *Arch. Neurol. (Chicago)*, **11**, 621–652.
HILLMAN, D. E. (1969) Light and electron microscopical study of the relationships between the
cerebellum and the vestibular organ of the frog. *Exp. Brain Res.*, **9**, 1–15.
ITO, M., YOSHIDA, M. AND OBATA, K. (1964) Monosynaptic inhibition of the intracerebellar nuclei
induced from the cerebellar cortex. *Experientia (Basel)*, **20**, 575–576.
KLINKE, R. (1970) Efferent influence on the vestibular organ during active movements of the body.
Pflügers Arch. ges. Physiol., **318**, 325–332.
KORNHUBER, H. H. (1971) Motor functions of cerebellum and basal ganglia. Cerebellocortical
saccadic (ballistic) clock, cerebellonuclear hold regulator, and basal ganglia ramp (voluntary
speed smooth movement) generator. *Kybernetik*, **8**, 157–162.
LARSELL, O. (1923) The cerebellum of the frog. *J. comp. Neurol.*, **36**, 89–112.
LARSELL, O. (1967) *The Comparative Anatomy and Histology of the Cerebellum from Myxinoids
Through Birds.* In J. JANSEN (Ed.), University of Minnesota Press, Minneapolis, pp. VIII–291.
LLINÁS, R. (1970) Neuronal operations in cerebellar transactions. In F. O. SCHMITT (Ed.), *The Neuro-
sciences. Second Study Program.* Rockefeller Univ. Press, New York, pp. 409–426.
LLINÁS, R. AND BLOEDEL, J. R. (1966/67) Climbing fibre activation of Purkinje cells in the frog
cerebellum. *Brain Res.*, **3**, 299–302.
LLINÁS, R. AND BLOEDEL, J. R. (1967) Frog cerebellum: absence of long-term inhibition upon Purkinje
cells. *Science*, **155**, 601–603.
LLINÁS, R., BLOEDEL, J. R. AND HILLMAN, D. E. (1969) Functional characterization of the neuronal
circuitry of the frog cerebellar cortex. *J. Neurophysiol.*, **32**, 847–870.
LLINÁS, R. AND HILLMAN, D. E. (1969) Physiological and morphological organization of the cerebellar circuits in various vertebrates. In R. LLINÁS (Ed.), *Neurobiology of Cerebellar Evolution
and Development.* Amer. Med. Ass., Chicago, pp. 43–73.
LLINÁS, R. AND PRECHT, W. (1969) The inhibitory vestibular efferent system and its relation to the
cerebellum in the frog. *Exp. Brain Res.*, **9**, 16–29.
LLINÁS, R., PRECHT, W. AND CLARKE, M. (1971) Cerebellar Purkinje cell responses to physiological
stimulation of the vestibular system in the frog. *Exp. Brain Res.*, **13**, 408–431.

LLINÁS, R., PRECHT, W. AND KITAI, S. T. (1967) Climbing fibre activation of Purkinje cell following primary vestibular afferent stimulation in the frog. *Brain Res.*, **6**, 371–375.

LOWENSTEIN, O. AND SAND, A. (1940a) The mechanism of the semicircular canal. A study of the responses of single-fibre preparations to angular accelerations and rotation at constant speed. *Proc. roy. Soc. B*, **129**, 256–275.

LOWENSTEIN, O. AND SAND, A. (1940b) The individual and integrated activity of the semicircular canals of the elasmobranch labyrinth. *J. Physiol. (Lond.)*, **99**, 89–101.

MAEKAWA, K. AND SIMPSON, J. I. (1971) Climbing fiber responses evoked in the flocculus by visual pathway stimulation in the rabbit. *Proc. XXV int. Congr. physiol Sci.*, Munich, IX, n. 1060, 358.

PETERSON, B. W. (1967) Effect of tilting on the activity of neurons in the vestibular nuclei of the cat. *Brain Res.*, **6**, 606–609.

PRECHT, W., KITAI, S. T. AND LLINÁS, R. (1970) Vestibular input to the cerebellum. In W. S. FIELDS AND W. D. WILLIS, JR. (Eds.), *The Cerebellum in Health and Disease*. Warren H. Green Publ., St. Louis, pp. 292–311.

PRECHT, W. AND LLINÁS, R. (1969a) Functional organization of the vestibular afferents to the cerebellar cortex of frog and cat. *Exp. Brain Res.*, **9**, 30–52.

PRECHT, W. AND LLINÁS, R. (1969b) Comparative aspects of the vestibular input to the cerebellum. In R. LLINÁS (Ed.), *Neurobiology of Cerebellar Evolution and Development*. Amer. Med. Ass., Chicago, pp. 677–702.

PRECHT, W., LLINÁS, R. AND CLARKE, M. (1971) Physiological responses of frog vestibular fibers to horizontal angular rotation. *Exp. Brain Res.*, **13**, 378–407.

PRECHT, W. AND SHIMAZU, H. (1965) Functional connection of tonic and kinetic vestibular neurons with primary vestibular afferents. *J. Neurophysiol.*, **28**, 1014–1028.

RAHN, A. C. AND ZUBER, B. L. (1971) Cerebellar evoked potentials resulting from extraocular muscle stretch: evidence against a cerebellar origin. *Exp. Neurol.*, **31**, 230–238.

SCHMIDT, R. F. (1963) Frog labyrinthine efferent impulses. *Acta oto-laryng. (Stockh.)*, **56**, 51–64.

SCHMIDT, C. L., WIST, E. R. AND DICHGANS, J. (1970) Alternierender Spontannystagmus, optokinetischer und vestibulärer Nystagmus und ihre Beziehungen zu rhythmischen Modulationen der Spontanaktivität im N. vestibularis beim Goldfisch. *Pflügers Arch. ges. Physiol.*, **319**, R155.

TOENNIES, J. F. (1938) Reflex discharges from the spinal cord over dorsal roots. *J. Neurophysiol.*, **1**, 378–390.

WINCKLER, G. (1937) L'innervation sensitive et motrice des muscles extrinsèques de l'oeil chez quelques ongulés. *Arch. Anat. (Strasbourg)*, **23**, 219–234.

WOLFE, J. W. (1971) Relationship of cerebellar potentials to saccadic eye movements. *Brain Res.*, **30**, 204–206.

Cerebellovestibular Relations: Anatomy

F. WALBERG

Anatomical Institute, University of Oslo, Oslo, Norway

The fibers from the cerebellum to the vestibular nuclei constitute the largest contingent of afferents to this complex. The fibers are derived from three regions within the cerebellum: They come from the 'vestibular part', from the 'spinal part', and from the fastigial nucleus. The three groups of afferents will be considered separately.

THE PROJECTION FROM THE 'VESTIBULOCEREBELLUM'

The 'vestibulocerebellum' is generally considered to correspond to the flocculo-nodular lobe. This concept is, however, scarcely tenable, since Brodal and Høivik (1964) have clearly shown that the primary vestibular fibers, in addition to the above mentioned part, also are distributed to the caudal (ventral) part of the uvula, the ventral paraflocculus and the ventralmost small celled part of the lateral cerebellar nucleus. All these areas together should therefore be regarded as the 'vestibulocerebellum'.

Only few experimental studies have been done on the efferent projections of these cerebellar subdivisions. The reason for this are the great technical difficulties encountered in operations on the areas. The classical studies in this area are those of Dow (1936, 1938), who used the Marchi method, and who studied the cat, rat and monkey. Dow concluded from his observations that the nodulus as well as the uvula send fibers to all four main vestibular nuclei on the homolateral side. He could find no evidence for a projection from the pyramis. His conclusions were supported by subsequent studies of Jansen and Brodal (1940, 1942), who also used the Marchi method, and Voogd (1964) using the Häggqvist and Nauta methods, came to the same conclusion, although he was unable to trace fibers to the lateral vestibular nucleus.

The first detailed study where a specific pattern in the projection was revealed was that made by Angaut and Brodal (1967). This study was made in the cat, and with silver impregnation techniques.

We will first consider the projection from the *flocculus*. Two distinct fiber bundles leave this cerebellar area to project to the vestibular complex. The first, and smallest, bundle corresponds to Löwy's 'angular bundle', and spreads out in a rostrocaudal direction to supply the superior and medial vestibular nucleus, the latter only rostrally. The second bundle passes ventrally and more laterally than the 'angular bundle',

References pp. 375–376

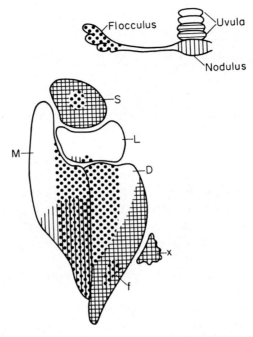

Fig. 1. Diagram showing the distribution within the vestibular nuclei of fibers from the flocculus, nodulus and uvula. For details, see text. Abbreviations, see legend of Fig. 2. From Angaut and Brodal (1967).

and gives off fibers to all the four main vestibular nuclei and group f (see Fig. 1). Thus, fibers from the flocculus terminate in all vestibular nuclei.

The *nodulus and uvula* differ in their projections from the flocculus. Although it was impossible for Angaut and Brodal (1967) to make isolated lesions of the nodulus or of the uvula, a comparison of several cases nevertheless made it possible to make a fairly precise analysis of the projection from the two lobules. These projections turned out to differ. Both regions project to the ipsilateral vestibular complex only, and many of the efferent fibers pass through the fastigial nucleus, most of them caudoventrally. Others follow a curved course through the nucleus. A few fibers also pass through the medialmost part of the nucleus interpositus (for details see Courville and Brodal, 1966), but all the fibers were found to leave the cerebellum through the inferior cerebellar peduncle.

The *uvular* efferent fibers are derived mainly from its ventral (caudal) part. The vestibular areas in receipt of such fibers are the superior vestibular nucleus, chiefly peripherally, the group x, and the descending nucleus, particularly its caudal half. The lateral vestibular nucleus probably receives some fibers, but no uvular efferents were found in the medial vestibular nucleus.

The *nodulus* projects to the superior nucleus, especially peripherally, to the medial nucleus, mainly caudally and medially, and to the descending nucleus, mostly ventrocaudally. The group f and the group x also receive some fibers, and a few fibers were traced to the caudodorsal part of the lateral vestibular nucleus.

As mentioned above, the ventral paraflocculus is included in the 'vestibulocerebellum'. Angaut and Brodal (1967) did, however, not find signs of a projection from this region to the vestibular complex. Their observations thus confirm the conclusions reached by most previous workers, that the paraflocculus does not project onto the vestibular complex.

The fibers from the 'vestibulocerebellum' were found to be rather thin, and since most of the argyrophilic particles were found in the neuropil, Angaut and Brodal (1967) conclude that the cerebellar afferents from the 'vestibulocerebellum' probably terminate with axodendritic synapses.

If one summarizes these findings, it is evident that the lateral vestibular nucleus is the one which is poorest supplied with fibers from the 'vestibulocerebellum'. Within the projection to the other nuclei there is a differential distribution. Thus, although there is some overlapping between the terminal regions of the fibers from the flocculus, the nodulus and the uvula, the terminal areas for the fibers from these three regions are in part separate.

The anatomical details given here provide another example of the clearcut differentiation within the vestibular nuclear complex. One important feature is that afferents from the flocculus end preponderantly in areas receiving primary vestibular fibers, while afferents from the nodulus and uvula reach areas which are supplied from the contralateral fastigial nucleus. This convergence is another example of the intriguing complexity of connections of the vestibular nuclei.

THE FASTIGIOVESTIBULAR PROJECTION

The second great input to the vestibular complex from the cerebellum comes from the fastigial nucleus. Since, however, the fastigial nucleus receives fibers from the 'spinal' part of the cerebellum, the pathway consists of two links, the Purkinje cell axons to the fastigial nucleus and the axons from the cells in this nucleus passing to the vestibular complex. Many details have been revealed in this pathway, not least in the physiological studies of Moruzzi and Pompeiano. (For references see Brodal et al., 1962).

The first link in the pathway, the *cerebellofastigial fibers*, was studied by Jansen and Brodal many years ago (1940, 1942). They concluded from their experimental Marchi studies in rabbit, cat and monkey, that only the vermis proper of the cerebellar cortex projects onto the fastigial nucleus. They demonstrated a rather schematic longitudinal subdivision in the projection, which is now well known. This concept has proved to be correct in principle, even if the pattern is less simple than originally suggested. The authors further provided evidence for a fan-like arrangement in the sagittal plane within the cortical nuclear projection. The anterior parts of the vermis, according to this principle, send fibers to the anterior region of the fastigial nucleus, the posterior part to the posterior region. More detailed studies, and studies where silver methods have been used (Vachananda, 1959; Eager, 1963, 1966; Goodman *et al.*, 1963; Walberg and Jansen, 1964; Voogd, 1964) have revealed further details, but they have not invalidated the conclusions made in the now classical papers by Jansen and Brodal.

The cortico-nuclear fibers terminate on somas and dendrites of the receiving neurons in the fastigial nucleus. This is clear from Eager's (1966) studies with the electron microscope, as well as from corresponding investigations by Mugnaini and Walberg (1967). The situation is the same for the terminations of Purkinje cell axons in the lateral vestibular nucleus (see below).

The second link in the pathway, the *fastigiovestibular fibers*, have been mapped by several authors. All these studies with lesions in the cerebellar nuclei have led to the conclusion that most of the crossing fibers of the hook bundle come from the caudal part of the fastigial nucleus, but that the majority of the ipsilateral fibers are derived from the rostral part (Allen, 1924, Rasmussen, 1933; Jansen, 1956; Thomas *et al.*, 1956; Carpenter *et al.*, 1958; Cohen *et al.*, 1958; Voogd, 1964). Studies with the modified Gudden method (Brodal, 1940) have confirmed these findings, and show that about equal proportions of fibers leave along the two routes (Jansen and Jansen Jr., 1955; Flood and Jansen, 1966).

Although the above mentioned studies of lesions in the fastigial nucleus give valuable information concerning the afferent projection, several details remained unknown. We therefore decided some years ago to attempt a more detailed study of the efferent fastigial projection. We made very small lesions in various parts of the nucleus, and studied the ensuing degeneration in silver stained preparations. However, a study of this projection meets with considerable difficulties. Not only do direct cerebello-cortical fibers to the vestibular complex pass through the rostrolateral part of the fastigial nucleus, but the course of the fastigiofugal fibers also complicates the picture. One contingent of these passes in the ipsilateral inferior cerebellar peduncle. Other fibers cross the midline in the cerebellum, and leave it on the contralateral side to join the hook bundle (fasciculus uncinatus). This bundle courses around the superior cerebellar peduncle. Some fibers ascend within the fastigial nucleus in which they originate, before they cross. This complex anatomy makes it impossible to reach definite conclusions without comparing the findings made in several cats where stereotactic lesions are produced in different parts of the fastigial nucleus. In addition, the electrode has to be introduced through folium VI, which has been shown to give off very few, if any, fibers to the vestibular nuclei. Some main finding made in this study (Walberg *et al.*, 1962) will be reviewed.

Cases with total lesions of the fastigial nucleus show the distribution of the crossed fastigiovestibular fibers, as this appears in silver stained sections. The crossing fibers end in circumscribed regions of the vestibular nuclei (Fig. 2). The distribution is as follows: The crossed fastigiovestibular fibers terminate in the peripheral zone of the superior nucleus, in the ventralmost part of the medial nucleus, in the central half of the lateral nucleus, in the ventrolateral part of the descending nucleus, and in the groups f and x. The small nucleus parasolitarius receives a heavy contribution of fibers. The findings confirm the previous observation that the majority of the crossed

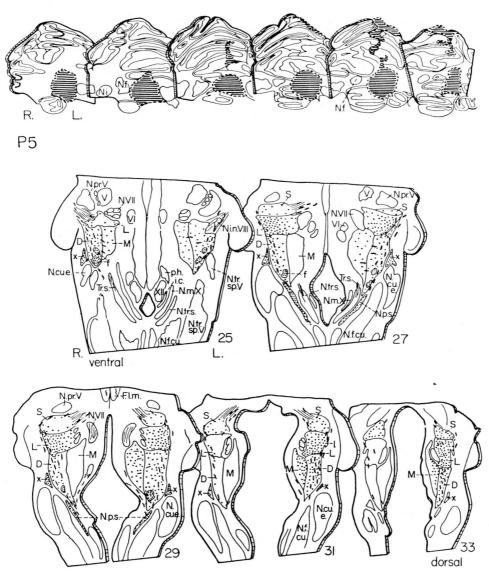

Fig. 2. Diagram showing the distribution of terminal degeneration within the vestibular nuclei follow-ing a total lesion of the left fastigial nucleus. Above, drawings through the cerebellum showing the lesion; below, drawings of horizontal sections through the vestibular nuclei. The lesion in the cere-bellum is indicated by horizontal lines. The fibre degeneration is shown as wavy lines, the field of termination of these fibres as dots. The distribution of the degenerating fibres is not identical on the two sides. For details, see text. Abbreviations: B.C.: brachium conjunctivum, D: descending vesti-bular nucleus, F.l.m.: fasciculus longitudinalis medialis, Flocc.: flocculus, f: cell group f, I.c.p.: inferior cerebellar peduncle, i.c.: nucleus intercalatus, L: lateral vestibular nucleus, L.: left, L. ant.: anterior lobe, L.p.m.: paramedian lobule, l: small-celled group 1, M: medial vestibular nucleus, N.cu.e.: external cuneate nucleus, N.d.: nucleus dentatus, N.f.: nucleus fastigii, N.f.c.: cuneate nucleus, N.f.cu.: cuneate nucleus, N.f.g.: gracile nucleus, N.i.: nucleus interpositus, N.i.n. VIII: interstitial nucleus of vestibular nerve, N.m. X: dorsal motor vagal nucleus, Nod.: nodulus, N.p.s.: nucleus parasolitarius, N.pr. V: principal sensory nucleus of fifth nerve, N.tr.s.: nucleus tractus solitarii, N.tr.sp. V: spinal trigeminal nucleus; N. VII: seventh nerve, P.fl.: paraflocculus, p.h.: nucleus prae-positus hypoglossi, R.: right, S: superior vestibular nucleus, Tr.s.: tractus solitarius, x: cell group x, V: motor nucleus of fifth nerve, VI: motor nucleus of sixth nerve, XII: motor nucleus of twelfth nerve. From Walberg et al. (1962).

fibers are derived from the caudal part of the fastigial nucleus. The group x, however, receives fibers mainly from the middle area of the fastigial nucleus.

An exact analysis of the ipsilateral fastigio-vestibular projection is very difficult. Lesions of one fastigial nucleus will always interrupt crossing fibers from the nucleus on the other side. In addition, lesions of the lateral part of the fastigial nucleus will interrupt the direct cerebellar corticovestibular fibers, to be described below. When these complicating factors are taken into account, a comparison of the distribution of degeneration in the vestibular complex on the two sides, following lesions of one fastigial nucleus in several cases, leads to the conclusion that the ipsilateral fastigial efferents supply most of the medial vestibular nucleus except its ventralmost strip. The ipsilateral fibers, furthermore, appear to end in the peripheral regions of the superior vestibular nucleus, the dorsal half of the lateral nucleus, and the dorsomedial part of the descending nucleus. The uncrossed fibers are derived almost solely from the rostral part of the fastigial nucleus, in agreement with previous observations.

These findings show that the ipsilateral and contralateral fastigiovestibular fibers supply different regions within the lateral, medial, and descending vestibular nuclei. Furthermore, the ipsilateral fibers are derived from the rostral part of the fastigial nucleus, while the contralateral fibers originate in the caudal part of the nucleus. The two contingents of fibers have a common territory only in the superior vestibular nucleus.

Even if our study has extended our knowledge of the projection from the fastigial nucleus to the vestibular complex many details are still unknown. For example, it has not been possible to determine anatomical differences between the projection of the lateral and medial regions of the rostral and caudal parts of the fastigial nucleus. Such differences exist, and the very interesting physiological observations made by Pompeiano and his group is a challenge to anatomists. His findings give evidence of an extremely complex organization of this pathway. Furthermore, the experimental anatomical studies done so far, have been made with the light microscope, and findings concerning synaptic relations, obtained by light microscopy in silver stained sections are not conclusive. Examples of this will be given below. Dr. Corvaja in Pompeiano's laboratory has recently started an experimental electron microscopical study of the fastigial hook bundle projection to the lateral vestibular nucleus. This, we hope, will provide information concerning the synaptic patterns in this projection.

THE CEREBELLAR CORTICOVESTIBULAR PROJECTION

The direct cerebellovestibular fibers are derived from the 'spinal' part of the cerebellar cortex. Fibers from the vermis to the vestibular nuclei have been known for many years (for references see Brodal, Pompeiano and Walberg, 1962). Most of the early observations were made with the Marchi method. They showed that the fibers were ipsilateral and reached the vestibular complex via the inferior cerebellar peduncle.

Walberg and Jansen (1961) re-examined this projection in the cat (Fig. 3). The greatest contribution of fibers to the vestibular complex was found to be derived from

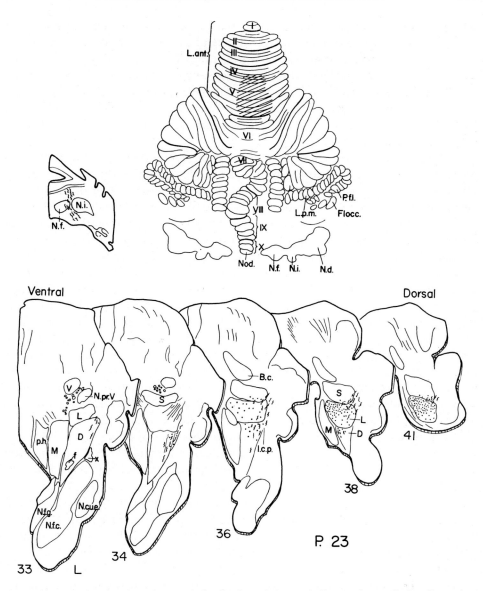

Fig. 3. Diagram showing the course and distribution of the cerebellar corticovestibular fibres. A, a drawing showing the lesion (hatchings) in the anterior cerebellar lobe; B, drawings of horizontal sections through the vestibular nuclei. The fibre degeneration is shown as wavy lines, the field of termination as dots. Degeneration is found only in the dorsal parts of the lateral and descending vestibular nuclei and adjacent part of the superior vestibular nucleus. The inset shows the course of the degenerating fibres on their way through the cerebellum. For details, see text. Abbreviations, see legend to Fig. 2. From Walberg and Jansen (1961).

the vermis of the anterior lobe. A certain number of fibers were also given off from the posterior lobe vermis (chiefly the pyramis and rostral part of the uvula). The middle part of the vermis, especially Larsell's lobule VI, gave off very few, if any, fibers. The most remarkable finding was, however, that the sites of termination for the fibers were restricted to two of the nuclei: the corticovestibular fibers terminate only in the lateral and descending vestibular nucleus. Furthermore, only the dorsal parts of these nuclei receive such fibers (see, however, Voogd, 1964, who claims that some fibers also reach the superior nucleus).

The projection onto the lateral vestibular nucleus is especially interesting. The area of termination is restricted to the dorsal part, and within this, the heaviest degeneration was found rostrally. The projection, therefore, covers neither the entire forelimb, nor the entire hindlimb region of the nucleus of Deiters, since the ventral border of the terminal area runs across the border between the somatotopical regions in the nucleus. Another interesting observation is that the projection from the vermis of the anterior lobe is somatotopically arranged. Lesions of the 'forelimb' region of the cerebellar anterior lobe result in a degeneration with its maximum in the 'forelimb' region of the nucleus. Lesions extending further anteriorly in the anterior lobe vermis, give degeneration also in the dorsocaudal part of the nucleus. A similar pattern in the projection from the posterior lobe vermis could not be shown, but this may be due to the fact that the projection from this vermal area is very sparse. It should be emphasized that anatomical studies of this type can only establish the main pattern in a projection. The physiological studies of Pompeiano and his group have also within this projection revealed an astonishingly sharp localization, since single units in the nucleus of Deiters respond to galvanic stimulation of one folium only of the cerebellar cortex, but not from immediately neighbouring folia.

The intriguing complexity in the projections from the cerebellum to the vestibular complex is especially well illustrated in the nucleus of Deiters. We will for a moment consider this projection. The ventral half of the nucleus receives fibers from the contralateral fastigial nucleus (caudal part), the dorsal half from the rostral part of the ipsilateral fastigial nucleus. The dorsal half of the nucleus of Deiters also receives direct fibers from the anterior lobe vermis. The dorsal half of the nucleus of Deiters is, therefore, influenced by two parallel cerebellar routes, one indirect and one direct. We have already seen that the two contingents of the fastigial fibers from the caudal and rostral parts of the nucleus, respectively, supply the fore- as well as the hindlimb regions of the nucleus of Deiters. Furthermore, we have seen that the direct cerebellovestibular fibers are somatotopically organized in the nucleus of Deiters. The experimental study by Walberg et al. (1962), furthermore, gave evidence of a topographical pattern within both components of the fastigiovestibular projection. Since in addition there is an orderly pattern in the cerebellar corticofastigial projection, as shown by Jansen and Brodal (1940, 1942), the following conclusion in permissible: Both components of the projection from the cerebellar vermis to the nucleus of Deiters are somatotopically organized. The dorsal part of the forelimb region in the nucleus of Deiters is acted upon from the forelimb region of the vermis of the anterior lobe (directly and via the fastigial nucleus). The ventral part of the forelimb region is acted upon from the posterior lobe via the same pathways, and the same principle is valid for the hindlimb region.

As stressed several times, experimental light microscopical studies can only indicate the area of termination of a fiber tract within the nucleus. Many of the argyrophilic fragments seen in silver stained sections in the light microscope are probably only degenerating fibers. Nothing can, therefore, be said concerning the distribution of the boutons of the afferent fibers on various parts of the neurons in the nuclei, and nothing can be stated concerning synaptic arrangements. Electron microscopical studies are necessary if such details shall be revealed.

The recent experimental electron microscopical study by Mugnaini and Walberg (1967) deals with this problem. The authors studied the degenerating fibers and boutons in the nucleus of Deiters following lesions of the anterior cerebellar lobe (Fig. 4). The Purkinje cell axons and boutons react with a marked hypertrophic filamentous degeneration following the injury. This reaction differs markedly from that found in the primary vestibular fibers, which were found initially to shrink and darken during the degeneration. The filamentous degeneration is well developed already after 3 days of survival. From the 4th day the degenerating fibers and boutons are transformed into the dark type.

The study showed that the boutons of the Purkinje cell axons establish synaptic contacts with cells of all sizes in the nucleus of Deiters, and that they are apposed to all parts of the neuronal surface, including spines. The synapses are of the sym-

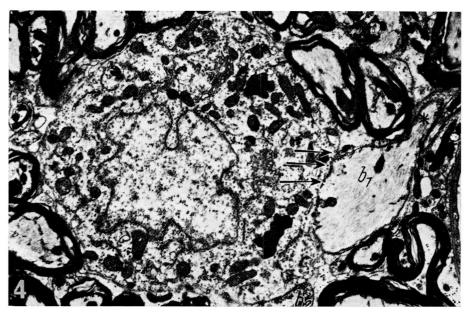

Fig. 4. A degenerating filamentous bouton (b_1) is at the arrows in synaptic contact with the soma of a small cell. The asterisk shows the stalk of the degenerating bouton. Part of a normal bouton is present at b_2. The cat had a lesion of the vermis of the anterior lobe and was killed after 3 days. × 9000. From Mugnaini and Walberg (1967).

References pp. 375–376

metrical as well as of the asymmetrical type. Some of the degenerating boutons appear to belong to thin fibers, which are seen in Golgi sections to end with small swellings. Others appear to be degenerating boutons of the large rounded type seen in normal material (Mugnaini, Walberg and Hauglie-Hanssen, 1967). The findings thus suggest that the Purkinje cell axons establish synaptic contacts by boutons of different types.

The observation that the boutons of the Purkinje cell axons establish contact with all parts of neurons in the Deiters nucleus is of considerable interest. In a remarkable series of physiological studies, Ito and co-workers have shown that the Purkinje cells are inhibitory. These findings made it of interest to clarify whether the synaptic vesicles in the boutons of the Purkinje cell axons are flattened or round. The experimental electron microscopical study performed in our laboratory showed that many of the synaptic vesicles in the degenerating boutons of the Purkinje cell axons are flattened (Mugnaini and Walberg, 1967). However, round vesicles may acquire a flattened shape in degenerating boutons (see Holländer, Brodal and Walberg, 1969). Very early stages of bouton degeneration must therefore be studied, if statements

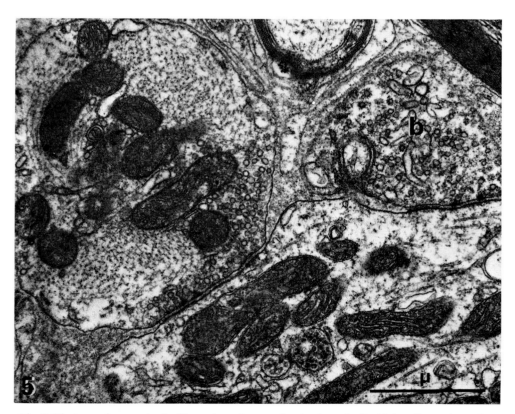

Fig. 5. Electron micrograph of a filamentous degenerating bouton of a Purkinje cell axon in nucleus interpositus posterior of the cat 3 days after a lesion of the overlying cerebellar cortex. The synaptic vesicles in this degenerating bouton are round. b is a normal bouton. Courtesy of Dr. Pierre Angaut.

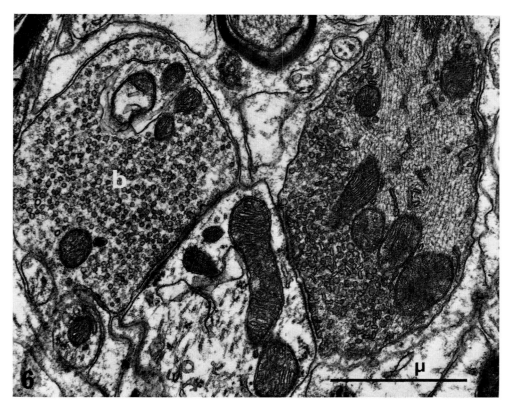

Fig. 6. Electron micrograph of another degenerating bouton of a Purkinje cell axon with a majority of round synaptic vesicles in the same animal as shown in the preceding figure. Note that a certain amount of the vesicles are flattened. Round synaptic vesicles may acquire a flattened shape in degenerating boutons, and it can therefore not be excluded that all the synaptic vesicles in the bouton prior to degeneration have been of the round variety. b is a normal bouton. Courtesy of Dr. Pierre Angaut.

concerning the nature of the synaptic vesicles are to be made. In this connection it is of considerable interest that Angaut (unpublished observations), studying the terminal degeneration in the cerebellar nuclei following lesions of the cerebellar cortex, recently found that degenerating Purkinje cell axon terminals can have round vesicles (Figs. 5 and 6). This furnishes a warning against generalizations concerning the relation between the nature of transmitter substances and the shape of the synaptic vesicles.

We have probably no reason to doubt that inhibitory transmitters can be related to boutons with flattened vesicles. On the other hand, there is no substantial evidence that such transmitters cannot be present together with round synaptic vesicles. A fruitful discussion of this interesting and difficult problem is at present not possible. Histochemical, and more problaby microchemical studies, where by ultracentrifugation in continuous sucrose density gradients a separation can be made between the two types of vesicles, may prove to be valuable in future studies (see especially Kuhar et al., 1971). However, the fact that the aldehyde concentration in the fixative influences the shape of the synaptic vesicles (see *e.g.*, Holländer *et al.*, 1969) considerably complicates the situation.

Ito's finding that the Purkinje cells are inhibitory prompted a collaboration between biochemists and morphologists in Oslo. The result of this was a microchemical study on the possible presence of GABA in boutons of Purkinje cell axons terminating in the dorsal half of the nucleus of Deiters. Observations following Ito's physiological studies had shown that GABA mimicked the natural transmitter action in the lateral vestibular nucleus (Obata, *et al.*, 1967). Our observations were made on small pieces dissected out from the dorsal part of the nucleus of Deiters where the Purkinje cell axons terminate. This dissection was made on freeze-dried sections following lesions of the cerebellar anterior lobe vermis and in normal animals (Fonnum *et al.*, 1970). Samples were also dissected from the ventral halves of the lateral vestibular nucleus on the two sides, and these were compared with those dissected from the dorsal part in normal and operated animals.

The biochemical investigation was based on a quantitative estimate of GAD in the samples. This enzyme, glutamate decarboxylase, synthethizes GABA. A high concentration of GAD in the samples is, therefore, an indication of a similar high concentration of GABA.

The study showed that GAD is concentrated in axons and nerve terminals in the dorsal part of the lateral vestibular nucleus, and that the level of GAD activity is 2.5 times higher in the dorsal than in the ventral part of the normal nucleus. A lesion of the anterior cerebellar lobe vermis which destroys the Purkinje cells sending their fibers to the dorsal part of the nucleus of Deiters, was followed by a great loss of GAD activity in this part of the nucleus (Table 1). The distribution of other enzymes, examined either by histochemical staining (lactate dehydrogenase, succinic dehydrogenase and acetyl cholinesterase) or by chemical assay (choline acetyltransferase), did not change significantly as a result of the operation.

TABLE 1

GAD ACTIVITY IN DORSAL AND VENTRAL PART OF
LATERAL VESTIBULAR NUCLEUS IN UNOPERATED (C1, C6 AND C7) AND
OPERATED (C2, C3, C4) CATS

The operated cats had a lesion of the vermis of the anterior cerebellar lobe. Note the great decrease in enzyme activity in the dorsal part of the nucleus in the operated cats.

Cat No.	Side	Dorsal (D)	Ventral (V)	Ratio (D/V)
C1, C6 and C7	R and L	16.1 ± 3.4	6.4 ± 1.5	2.54
C2	L	9.6 ± 2.0 (4)	7.7 ± 1.4 (6)	1.25
C2	R	6.7 ± 1.6 (6)	6.1 ± 0.9 (7)	1.10
C3	L	9.8 ± 3.5 (5)	7.0 ± 1.2 (5)	1.40
C3	R	6.5 ± 2.9 (5)	7.4 ± 1.2 (6)	0.88
C4	L	11.1 ± 2.7 (3)	6.4 ± 0.6 (4)	1.73
C4	R	5.6 ± 1.4 (4)	6.2 ± 0.6 (4)	0.90

After Fonnum *et al.* (1970).

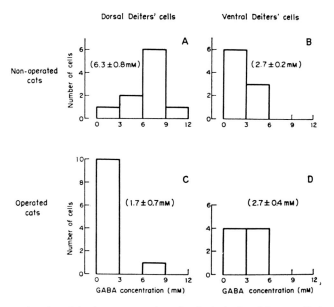

Fig. 7. Histograms showing GABA concentrations in single isolated large cells in the dorsal and ventral parts of lateral vestibular nucleus in the cat. A and B are from normal cats, C and D from cats with lesions of the anterior cerebellar lobe vermis. Note that the GABA concentration in operated cats is greatly reduced in the dorsal part of the nucleus. For details, see text. From Otsuka *et al.* (1971).

Other biochemical observations support these findings. The most elaborate microchemical study done so far on this fiber system is that by Otsuka *et al.* (1971). These authors have developed a very sensitive method for measuring GABA, which permits the measurement of as little as 2×10^{-14} mol. The authors used this method on single isolated nerve cells in the Deiters nucleus and found that the concentration in the ventral part of the nucleus in the large cells was 2.7 mM. The large cells in the dorsal part had a concentration of 6.3 mM. A lesion of the cerebellar anterior lobe vermis reduced the concentration of GABA in the large cells in the dorsal part of the nucleus to 1.7 mM (Fig. 7). The results of this excellent study, in addition to those obtained in our laboratory, make it highly probable that GABA is concentrated in the axon terminals of the Purkinje cells. They extend the information obtained in the microiontophoretical studies mentioned above (Obata *et al.*, 1967). A further interesting observation is that the inhibition produced by the microiontophoretically applied GABA is strychnine resistant, that by glycine not (Bruggencate and Engberg, 1969a). Further studies by these authors have shown that picrotoxin often can prevent the inhibitory action of GABA when applied electroosmotically, but that this interaction does not occur with glycine applied iontophoretically (Bruggencate and Engberg, 1969b, 1971). These observations are in agreement with a similar study by Obata and Highstein (1970), and extend a previous observation by Ito *et al.* (1970). They showed that the inhibition of the vestibular nuclei following stimulation of the cerebellar flocculus, could be blocked by systemic injection of picrotoxin. All these physiological and chemical studies are thus in support of the original observation by Ito, that the Purkinje cells are inhibitory, and favour the hypothesis that GABA is the natural inhibitory transmitter released from the endings of the Purkinje cell axons (Obata *et al.*, 1967).

Let us finally consider a purely morphological problem. Experimental electron microscopical studies have shown that there are two types of reaction when axons and boutons degenerate in the mammalian central nervous system. One is the dark type of reaction. A typical example of this is the degenerating primary vestibular fibers. The other type of reaction is the filamentous degeneration, which occurs in the Purkinje cell axons and boutons. In fortunate situations it is possible to demonstrate both these types of reaction in the same nucleus. The nucleus of Deiters is a favourable region for this demonstration. Although the primary vestibular fibers terminate in the ventral part of the nucleus and those from the cerebellum in the dorsal part, there is a small zone of overlap between the two fiber systems in the middle part of the nucleus. Degenerating boutons of fibers of the two types can be found in this central zone in cats with double operations and a suitable survival time (Walberg and Mugnaini, 1969). Convergence of excitatory and inhibitory fiber systems on the same cell can thus be demonstrated in the electron microscope (see also Eccles *et al.*, 1967). However, we have hitherto not had a silver impregnation method to stain the filamentous degenerating fiber systems. The Nauta modifications and the Fink-Heimer techniques stain only the dark degenerating fibers and boutons. Eager (1970) has recently introduced a new silver stain which is a modification of the previous methods. The technique is easy, and the sections can be counterstained with cresylviolet which gives a very good possibility for an exact demarcation of nuclei. Electron microscopy of silver stained sections made recently in our laboratory have revealed that the Eager method, in addition to staining dark degenerating fiber systems, also is capable of staining the filamentous ones. We have thus for the first time now a silver method to stain both dark and filamentous degenerating fiber systems, and this method may in the future prove very valuable, since it also is capable of staining unmyelinated fibers. The observations made in our laboratory so far show that the degenerating fibers of both types are heavily stained, but that the degenerating boutons are only occasionally impregnated (Walberg, 1972). Our observations have been made in the cerebellar nuclei following lesions of the cerebellar cortex. We need more electron microscopical studies of silver stained sections to reach definite conclusions whether degenerating boutons can be well impregnated in Eager stained sections. If this will turn out to be the case, we will then have a silver impregnation technique more generally applicable than the Fink-Heimer method.

SUMMARY

The origin, course and vestibular termination of the fibres from the (a) 'vestibulo-cerebellum', the (b) fastigial nucleus, and the (c) 'spinal' part of the cerebellum are described, and reference is made to older and recent experimental studies of these connections. Details in the distributions within the vestibular complex of the tracts are considered, and it is stressed that the afferent fibres partly share, but partly also have their own areas of termination within the nuclei. The pattern of termination is very complicated, and a detailed description of the location of stimulating and recording electrodes should therefore always be given in physiological studies where reference is made to morphology.

Recent experimental microchemical studies in support of the suggestion that GABA is an inhibitory transmitter of the Purkinje axon terminals are mentioned, and reference is also made to experimental electron microscopical studies which show that filamentous degenerating boutons of the inhibitory Purkinje cells can have round synaptic vesicles.

REFERENCES

ALLEN, W. F. (1924) Distribution of the fibers originating from the different basal cerebellar nuclei. *J. comp. Neurol.*, **35**, 399–439.

ANGAUT, P. AND BRODAL, A. (1967) The projection of the 'vestibulocerebellum' onto the vestibular nuclei in the cat. *Arch. ital. Biol.*, **105**, 441–479.

BRODAL, A. (1940) Modification of Gudden method for study of cerebral localization. *Arch. Neurol. (Chicago)*, **43**, 46–58.

BRODAL, A. AND HØIVIK, B. (1964) Site and mode of termination of primary vestibulocerebellar fibres in the cat. An experimental study with silver impregnation methods. *Arch. ital. Biol.*, **102**, 1–21.

BRODAL, A., POMPEIANO, O. AND WALBERG, F. (1962) *The Vestibular Nuclei and Their Connections. Anatomy and Functional Correlations.* Oliver and Boyd, Edinburgh, London, pp. VIII–193.

BRUGGENCATE, G. TEN AND ENGBERG, I. (1969a) The effect of strychnine on inhibition in Deiters' nucleus induced by GABA and glycine. *Brain Res.*, **14**, 536–539.

BRUGGENCATE, G. TEN AND ENGBERG, I. (1969b) Is picrotoxin a blocker of the postsynaptic inhibition induced by GABA (γ-aminobutyric acid)? *Pflügers Arch. ges. Physiol.*, **312**, R121.

BRUGGENCATE, G. TEN AND ENGBERG, I. (1971) Iontophoretic studies in Deiters' nucleus of the inhibitory actions of GABA and related amino acids and the interaction of strychnine and picrotoxin. *Brain Res.*, **25**, 431–448.

CARPENTER, M. B., BRITTIN, G. M. AND PINES, J. (1958) Isolated lesions of the fastigial nuclei in the cat. *J. comp. Neurol.*, **109**, 65–89.

COHEN, D., CHAMBERS, W. W. AND SPRAGUE, J. M. (1958) Experimental study of the efferent projections from the cerebellar nuclei to the brainstem of the cat. *J. comp. Neurol.*, **109**, 233–259.

COURVILLE, J. AND BRODAL, A. (1966) Rubrocerebellar connections in the cat. An experimental study with silver impregnation methods. *J. comp. Neurol.*, **126**, 471–485.

DOW, R. S. (1936) The fiber connections of the posterior parts of the cerebellum in the rat and cat. *J. comp. Neurol.*, **63**, 527–548.

DOW, R. S. (1938) Efferent connections of the flocculo-nodular lobe in *Macaca mulatta. J. comp. Neurol.*, **68**, 297–305.

EAGER, R. P. (1963) Efferent cortico-nuclear pathways in the cerebellum of the cat. *J. comp. Neurol.*, **120**, 81–103.

EAGER, R. P. (1966) Patterns and mode of termination of cerebellar corticonuclear pathways in the monkey (*Macaca mulatta*). *J. comp. Neurol.*, **126**, 551, 565.

EAGER, R. P. (1970) Selective staining of degenerating axons in the central nervous system by a simplified silver method: spinal cord projections to external cuneate and inferior olivary nuclei in the cat. *Brain Res.*, **22**, 137–141.

ECCLES, J. C., ITO, M. AND SZENTÁGOTHAI, J. (1967) *The Cerebellum as a Neuronal Machine.* Springer, Berlin, Heidelberg, New York, pp. 335.

FLOOD, S. AND JANSEN, J. (1966) The efferent fibres of the cerebellar nuclei and their distribution on the cerebellar peduncles in the cat. *Acta anat. (Basel)*, **63**, 137–166.

FONNUM, F., STORM-MATHISEN, J. AND WALBERG, F. (1970) Glutamate decarboxylase in inhibitory neurons. A study of the enzyme in Purkinje cell axons and boutons in the cat. *Brain Res.*, **20**, 259–275.

GOODMAN, D. C., HALLETT, R. E. AND WELCH, R. B. (1963) Patterns of localization in the cerebellar corticonuclear projections of the albino rat. *J. comp. Neurol.*, **121**, 51–67.

HOLLÄNDER, H., BRODAL, A. AND WALBERG, F. (1969) Electronmicroscopic observations on the structure of the pontine nuclei and the mode of termination of the corticopontine fibres. An experimental study in the cat. *Exp. Brain Res.*, **7**, 95–110.

ITO, M., HIGHSTEIN, S. M. AND FUKADA, J. (1970) Cerebellar inhibition of the vestibulo-ocular reflex in rabbit and cat and its blockage by picrotoxin. *Brain Res.*, **17**, 524–526.

JANSEN, J. (1956) On the efferent connections of the cerebellum. In J. ARIËNS KAPPERS (Ed.), *Progress in Neurobiology*. Elsevier, Amsterdam, pp. 232–239.

JANSEN, J. AND BRODAL, A. (1940) Experimental studies on the intrinsic fibers of the cerebellum. II. The cortico-nuclear projection. *J. comp. Neurol.*, **73**, 267–321.

JANSEN, J. AND BRODAL, A. (1942) Experimental studies on the intrinsic fibers of the cerebellum. III. The cortico-nuclear projection in the rabbit and the monkey. *Norske Vid.-Akad. Oslo, Avh. I, Math.-Naturv. Kl.*, **3**, 1–50.

JANSEN, J. AND JANSEN, J., JR. (1955) On the efferent fibers of the cerebellar nuclei in the cat. *J. comp. Neurol.*, **102**, 607–632.

KUHAR, M. J., SHASKAN, E. G. AND SNYDER, S. H. (1971) The subcellular distribution of endogenous and exogenous serotonin in brain tissue: comparison of synaptosomes storing serotonin, norepinephrine, and γ-aminobutyric acid. *J. Neurochem.*, **18**, 333–343.

MUGNAINI, E. AND WALBERG, F. (1967) An experimental electron microscopical study on the mode of termination of cerebellar corticovestibular fibres in the cat lateral vestibular nucleus (Deiters' nucleus). *Exp. Brain Res.*, **4**, 212–236.

MUGNAINI, E., WALBERG, F. AND HAUGLIE-HANSSEN, E. (1967) Observations on the fine structure of the lateral vestibular nucleus (Deiters' nucleus) in the cat. *Exp. Brain Res.*, **4**, 146–186.

OBATA, K. AND HIGHSTEIN, S. M. (1970) Blocking by picrotoxin of both vestibular inhibition and GABA action on rabbit oculomotor neurones. *Brain Res.*, **18**, 538–541.

OBATA, K., ITO, M., OCHI, R. AND SATO, N. (1967) Pharmacological properties of the postsynaptic inhibition by Purkinje cell axons and the action of γ-aminobutyric acid on Deiters' neurones. *Exp. Brain Res.*, **4**, 43–57.

OTSUKA, M., OBATA, K., MIYATA, Y. AND TANAKA, Y. (1971) Measurement of γ-aminobutyric acid in isolated nerve cells of cat central nervous system. *J. Neurochem.*, **18**, 287–295.

RASMUSSEN, A. T. (1933) Origin and course of the fasciculus uncinatus (Russell) in the cat, with observations on other fiber tracts arising from the cerebellar nuclei. *J. comp. Neurol.*, **57**, 165–197.

THOMAS, D. M., KAUFMAN, R. P., SPRAGUE, J. M. AND CHAMBERS, W. W. (1956) Experimental studies of the vermal cerebellar projections in the brain stem of cat (fastigiobulbar tract). *J. Anat., (Lond.)*, **90**, 371–385.

VACHANANDA, B. (1959) The major spinal afferent systems to the cerebellum and the cerebellar corticonuclear connections in Macaca mulatta. *J. comp. Neurol.*, **112**, 303–351.

VOOGD, J. (1964) *The Cerebellum of the Cat. Structure and Fibre Connexions*. Van Gorcum, Assen, 215 pp.

WALBERG, F. (1972) Further studies on silver impregnation of normal and degenerating boutons. A light and electron microscopical investigation of a filamentous degenerating system. *Brain Res.*, **36**, 353–369.

WALBERG, F. AND JANSEN, J. (1961) Cerebellar corticovestibular fibers in the cat. *Exp. Neurol.*, **3**, 32–52.

WALBERG, F. AND MUGNAINI, E. (1969) Distinction of degenerating fibres and boutons of cerebellar and peripheral origin in the Deiters' nucleus of the same animal. *Brain Res.*, **14**, 67–75.

WALBERG, F., POMPEIANO, O., BRODAL, A. AND JANSEN, J. (1962) The fastigiovestibular projection in the cat. An experimental study with silver impregnation methods. *J. comp. Neurol.*, **118**, 49–76.

Cerebellar Control of the Vestibular Neurones: Physiology and Pharmacology

M. ITO

Department of Physiology, Faculty of Medicine, University of Tokyo, Hongo, Bunkyo-ku, Tokyo, Japan

Intimate relationship between the vestibular afferents and the cerebellum has long been pointed out (*cf.* Herrick, 1924). Investigations in recent years have been fruitful in revealing the neuronal connections and synaptic actions involved in the vestibulocerebellar system. Various types of vestibular nuclei cells have been distinguished and synaptic actions upon them of primary vestibular afferents, cerebellar Purkinje cells, spinobulbar afferents and fastigial neurones, have been identified. On the basis of these efforts a further attempt is being made to work out the neuronal diagrams which may represent the essential features of the vestibulocerebellar system. Since the vestibulocerebellar system involves the phylogenetically oldest parts of the cerebellum, it may be expected to represent a prototype of the cerebellar motor controlling. From this point of view, very recent physiological and pharmacological investigations on the vestibulocerebellar system will be reviewed below.

SYNAPTIC ACTION OF PRIMARY VESTIBULAR AFFERENTS

Primary vestibular afferent fibers innervate various types of secondary vestibular neurones and then pass into certain portions of the cerebellum, *i.e.*, the vestibulocerebellum. The vestibulo-cerebellum includes the flocculus as its hemispheral part and the nodulus as its vermal part (Jansen and Brodal, 1954). The ventral paraflocculus and the ventral parts of the uvula may also be included, since primary vestibular fibers end in these cerebellar areas as well (Brodal and Høivik, 1964). The primary vestibular fibers terminate in the cerebellar cortex as mossy fibers. They also make synaptic contact with cells in the small celled part, called *p* (Flood and Jansen, 1961) or pars rotunda (Van Rossum, 1969) of the cerebellar lateral nucleus (Brodal and Høivik, 1964).

Synaptic actions of primary vestibular afferent fibers have been studied by intracellular and extracellular recording from various types of secondary vestibular neurones during electric stimulation of the VIII nerve; in the lateral vestibular nucleus (Ito *et al.*, 1964a, 1969a; Wilson, Kato, Peterson and Wylie, 1967a), in the superior, descending and medial vestibular nuclei (Precht and Shimazu, 1965; Wilson *et al.*, 1968; Kawai *et al.*, 1969), in the cerebellar nuclei (Precht and Llinás, 1968), and in cerebellar cortex (Precht and Llinás, 1969). It is now known that the primary vestibular impulses evoke excitatory postsynaptic potentials (EPSPs) mono-synaptically in their direct target neurones. In the ventral Deiters neurones, single primary vestibular impulses produce small unitary EPSPs of 0.2 mV in amplitude (Ito *et al.*, 1969a). Synchronous excitation of the whole vestibular nerve fibers usually causes EPSPs twenty-five times as large as the unitary EPSPs, indicating that about twenty-five primary vestibular fibers converge onto each ventral Deiters neurone. Similar tests in superior and descending vestibular nuclei revealed that sizes of unitary EPSPs are relatively large up to 3 mV, and inversely that the number of the primary vestibular fibers converging onto these cells is in general relatively small (fifteen, Kawai *et al.*, 1969). There seems to be a variety of the mode of convergence of excitatory synapses from the primary vestibular afferents; one extreme, in the ventral Deiters neurones, may be called the "integrative type", since each fiber contributes to a minute synaptic action. The other extreme may be called the "relaying type", since impulses in a relatively small number of primary vestibular fibers effectively cause firing of the postsynaptic cells.

Some pharmacological studies have been performed on the excitatory action of acetylcholine (Steiner and Weber, 1965; Yamamoto, 1967; Obata, 1970) and noradrenaline (Yamamoto, 1967) on Deiters neurones. Since the level of choline–acetyl–transferase is higher in the ventral than in the dorsal part of the lateral vestibular nucleus (Fonnum *et al.*, 1970) and since the primary vestibular afferents impinge onto the the ventral but not the dorsal Deiters neurones (*cf.* Brodal *et al.*, 1962), it might be expected that primary vestibular fibers should have cholinergic properties. However, since primary afferents in the spinal cord are non-cholinergic, this possibility appears to be unlikely. As yet there is no clue for identifying the nature of the excitatory transmitter substance liberated from the primary vestibular afferent terminals.

SYNAPTIC ACTION OF SECONDARY VESTIBULAR NEURONES

Any neurones which are supplied with synapses by primary vestibular afferents will here be called collectively secondary vestibular neurones, even when they are located outside the vestibular nuclei, for example, in the lateral cerebellar nucleus. Histologically, secondary vestibular neurones are usually named according to the structures to which they belong, *i.e.*, superior (SV), medial (MV), lateral (LV) and descending (DV) vestibular nuclei cells etc. (*cf.* Brodal *et al.*, 1962). The term Deiters neurones will be used as synonym for all lateral vestibular nucleus neurones.

Apart from their histological location, the secondary vestibular neurones can be classified according to the sites of destination of their axons. The expression vestibulo-ocular relay cells (VOR) will here be used for those cells which project to oculomotor neurones in the III, IV and VI nuclei. In recent investigations on rabbits, several different types of VOR neurones have been distinguished, as shown in Fig. 1. Certain neurones in the rostral two-thirds of MV convey excitatory impulses through the medial longitudinal fasciculus (MLF), while SV neurones mediate inhibitory impulses through MLF to the III and IV nuclei (Highstein, 1971; Highstein and Ito, 1971; Highstein *et al.*, 1971). However, inhibitory impulses to cat's VI nucleus appear to

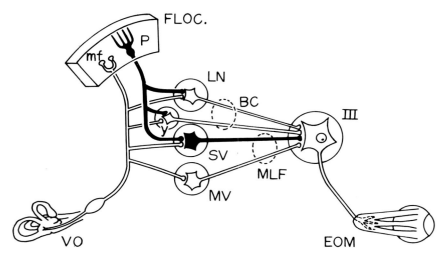

Fig. 1. Neuronal connections in the vestibulo-ocular reflex arcs related to the flocculus. VO, vestibular organ. Floc., flocculus. mf, mossy fiber terminal. P, Purkinje cell. LN, lateral cerebellar nucleus. Y, group *y* of the vestibular nuclear complex. SV, superior vestibular nucleus. MV, medial vestibular nucleus. BC, brachium conjunctivum. MLF, medial longitudinal fasciculus. III, III nucleus. EOM, extra-ocular muscles. From Fukuda *et al.* (1972).

be mediated by the rostral portion of MV but not SV (Baker *et al.*, 1969). There is another group of VOR cells which send excitatory impulses through the brachium conjunctivum (BC) to III nucleus (Highstein *et al.*, 1971). The cells of this BC pathway appear to be located in the cerebellar lateral nucleus (Carpenter and Strominger, 1964) and also in the group *y* of Brodal and Pompeiano (1957) of the vestibular nuclear complex (Highstein, 1971).

Another prominent population of vestibular nuclei cells are those which give origin to the vestibulospinal tract (VST) and send axons down to the spinal cord. Two bundles of VST fibers have been distinguished, the lateral (LVST) and medial (MVST) vestibulospinal tract fibers (*cf.* Nyberg–Hansen, 1964). LVST passes through the ventrolateral corner of the cervical segments, while MVST fibers pass through the MLF. The cells of origin of LVST are located in LV. However, since organization of the vestibular and cerebellar inputs to Deiters neurones differs significantly between the ventral and dorsal portions of LV (*cf.* Brodal *et al.*, 1962), it is reasonable to divide LVST cells into two groups, v-LVST, arising from ventral Deiters neurones and d-LVST, arising from dorsal Deiters neurones. The action of d-LVST is indicated to be excitatory on certain motoneurones and segmental interneurones as studied in the lumbosacral cord (Lund and Pompeiano, 1968; Grillner *et al.*, 1970). The synaptic action of v-LVST on motoneurones appears also to be excitatory (Wilson and Yoshida, 1969b). Concerning the origin of MVST, there have been controversial arguments. Nyberg–Hansen (1964) indicated that MVST arises in the rostral portion of MV. According to recent works by Wilson and Yoshida (1969a) and Wilson *et al.*, (1970), synaptic action of relatively slowly conducting MVST fibers is inhibitory for cervical (C_2–C_3) and thoracic back motoneurones. Existence of another source of MVST fibers has been indicated in physiological investigations (Wilson *et al.*, 1967b; Kawai *et al.*, 1969). Recent investigations on rabbits (Akaike *et al.*, 1972a, b) revealed the existence of three separate groups of VST fibers which mediate the descending secondary vestibular impulses; (1) excitatory, relatively fast conducting LVST; (2) excitatory, relatively fast conducting MVST, and (3) inhibitory, relatively slowly conducting MVST. The cells of origin of these three groups of fibers are located in mixture in the ventral portion of LV (corresponding to Dt (*α*) and Dt (*β*) divisions by Meessen and Olszewski, 1949).

Certain cells in DV respond to stimulation in the cerebellum, near the fastigial nucleus (Kawai *et al.*, 1969). These cells should be the origin of the secondary vestibulocerebellar fibers (Brodal and Torvik, 1957). The vestibular nuclear complex also contains those cells which serve commissural connections between the right and left sides (Mano *et al.*, 1968), and also for intra- and inter-nuclear connections on the same side (Kawai *et al.*, 1969). Cells of origin of these connections are less well specified.

Pharmacological tests so far carried out have revealed that the postsynaptic inhibition of III nucleus neurones by SV cells is blocked very effectively by systemic injection of picrotoxin but not by strychnine (Ito *et al.*, 1970b; Highstein *et al.*, 1971). The SV inhibition was mimicked by gamma-aminobutyric acid (GABA) electrophoretically applied to III nucleus neurones (Obata and Highstein, 1970). It is probable that the inhibitory transmitter substance utilized by SV neurones is GABA or a related substance.

SYNAPTIC ACTION OF CEREBELLAR PURKINJE CELLS

Axons of cerebellar Purkinje cells provide the output of the cerebellar cortex. Purkinje cells of the flocculus project to the small celled part *p* of the lateral cerebellar nucleus and certain portions of the vestibular nuclei (Angaut and Brodal, 1967). Purkinje cells of the nodulus and uvula send axons to certain portions of the vestibular nuclei (Angaut and Brodal, 1967). Purkinje cells in the vermal cortex of the anterior and posterior lobes other than nodulus and uvula also contribute synapses to certain vestibular nuclei cells, particularly to dorsal Deiters neurones (Walberg and Jansen, 1961, 1964; Eager, 1963).

The synaptic action of cerebellar Purkinje cells was first studied in the cat's dorsal Deiters neurones and was shown to be inhibitory (Ito and Yoshida, 1964, 1966; Ito *et al.*, 1966, 1968a); inhibitory postsynaptic potentials (IPSPs) were produced monosynaptically in dorsal Deiters neurones during stimulation of ipsilateral vermal cortex of the anterior and posterior lobes of cerebellum. In recent investigation on rabbits, similar inhibition from the anterior and posterior lobes of cerebellum was found to occur in LV neurones including MVST cells (Akaike *et al.*, 1972c). A possible contribution by the nodulus and uvula to the inhibition of VST cells has been difficult to ascertain because of difficulties in stimulating these areas in isolation from other portions of the posterior lobe. However, since no projection was found from the nodulus and uvula to LV and its ventral region (Van Rossum, 1969), this contribution may not be expected. Monosynaptic inhibition from the flocculus has recently been demonstrated to occur in SV neurones which serve for vestibulo-ocular inhibition (Ito *et al.*,

1970a; Fukuda *et al.*, 1972). There is indirect evidence indicating that stimulation of the flocculus causes similar inhibition in VOR cells of the lateral cerebellar nucleus.

An inhibitory action of cerebellar Purkinje cells has been observed in all of the three divisions (fastigial, interpositus and lateral) of the cat's intracerebellar nuclei (Ito *et al.*, 1964, 1970d). An inhibitory action of Purkinje cells is also apparent in the indirect effect of cerebellar cortical stimulation upon the red nucleus neurones (Toyama *et al.*, 1967) and ventral Deiters and reticular formation cells (Ito *et al.*, 1970c); inhibition of cerebellar nuclear neurones which have an excitatory action resulted in removal of the tonic background excitation, *i.e.*, disfacilitation, of these brainstem neurones.

Purkinje cell axons issue collaterals in the cerebellar cortex and innervate cortical cells, particularly basket cells and Golgi cells. There is evidence indicating that these Purkinje cell collaterals have inhibitory action (Eccles *et al.*, 1967). There are also interesting examples of Purkinje cell action in lower vertebrates. In teleost fish, Purkinje cells exert inhibition monosynaptically upon oculomotor neurones (Kidokoro, 1968). In the frog, Purkinje cell axons pass into the VIII nerve and make synaptic contact with hair cells of vestibular organ, and thereby inhibit initiation of afferent discharges in primary vestibular fibers (Llinás and Precht, 1969).

To establish the postulate that cerebellar Purkinje cells are inhibitory neurones, it is necessary to exclude the following two possibilities. First, the same Purkinje cells may have a dual action which can be excitatory or inhibitory, depending upon the target neurones or upon the discharge frequency in presynaptic spikes, as seen in Aplysia ganglia (Kandel *et al.*, 1967; Blankenship *et al.*, 1971). However, since the transmitter liberated from Purkinje cells is related to gamma-aminobutyric acid (see below) and since there is no known case in which GABA displays excitatory action, this first possibility is very unlikely. Second, a certain population of Purkinje cells may be differentiated as excitatory neurones. Initiation of EPSPs instead of IPSPs, in Deiters neurones during cerebellar stimulation was seen on certain occasions and was explained as being mediated by axon collaterals of cerebellar afferent fibers (Ito *et al.*, 1969b). Occurrence of a kind of axon reflex via collaterals of primary vestibular afferents was clearly demonstrated by Fukuda *et al.* (1972) by systematic mapping within the flocculus with a monopolar stimulating electrode; stimulation at the medioventral portion of flocculus excite vestibular nuclear cells via primary vestibular afferent fibers, whereas stimulation at dorso-lateral portion of flocculus causes purely inhibitory effect upon SV cells. This axon reflex activation as well as the disinhibition (inhibition of inhibitory Purkinje cells via intracortical mechanisms, Ito *et al.*, 1968b) appear to account satisfactorily for the facilitatory effect of cerebellar stimulation upon muscle tone which has been observed under certain experimental conditions (*cf.* Moruzzi, 1950; Brookhart, 1960). Thus, there is no evidence suggesting any excitatory action of Purkinje cells.

Pharmacological investigations were performed on Deiters neurones (Obata, 1965; Obata *et al.*, 1967). This was the first occasion where electrophoretic application of GABA was shown to produce a significant membrane hyperpolarization. GABA produced hyperpolarization has its reversal potential at the same membrane potential as

References pp. 387–390

that for cerebellar-induced IPSPs and also is accompanied by an increase of the membrane conductance as with IPSPs (Obata et al., 1970). Blockage of Purkinje cell inhibition by systemically injected picrotoxin (10–15 mg per kg) was first recognized on the flocculus inhibition of VRO neurones (Ito et al., 1970). In Deiters neurones it was confirmed that picrotoxin blocks both the Purkinje cell inhibition and the depressant action of electrophoretically applied GABA (Obata et al., 1970; Ten Bruggencate and Engberg, 1971). Recently, Purkinje cell inhibition of Deiters neurones was shown to be blocked by bicuculline similarly to other inhibitory synapses related to GABA (Curtis et al., 1970).

In addition to these physiological and pharmacological observations, there is neurochemical evidence indicating that the inhibitory transmitter liberated by cerebellar Purkinje cells is GABA.

(1) GABA is contained in Deiters neurones, particularly in dorsal Deiters neurones (Otsuka et al., 1970). This GABA content is reduced significantly when the cerebellar cortex is removed chronically and GABA hence appears to be contained in Purkinje cell axon terminals.

(2) GABA is released to the fourth ventricle during repetitive stimulation of the cerebellar cortex, presumably being liberated from Purkinje cell axon terminals in the cerebellar and vestibular nuclei (Obata and Takeda, 1969).

(3) The activity of glutamate decarboxylase, the enzyme that synthesizes GABA, is high in dorsal Deiters neurones. This activity is reduced in those animals whose relevant cerebellar cortex was removed chronically (Fonnum et al., 1970).

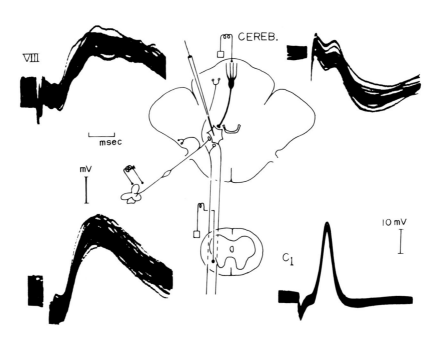

SYNAPTIC ACTION OF SPINAL AND BULBAR AFFERENT INPUTS TO VESTIBULAR NUCLEI NEURONES

Deiters neurones receive synapses from collaterals of some of the cerebellar afferents which pass through the restiform body (Pompeiano and Brodal, 1957; Hauglie-Hanssen, 1968). This connection accounts for the monosynaptic initiation of EPSPs in cat's Deiters neurones during stimulation of C_{2-3} spinal segments (Ito et al., 1964b, 1969b). Similar EPSPs were produced in rabbit's VST cells by stimulating the lateral funiculus of the C_1 segment (Fig. 2) (Akaike et al., 1972c).

Investigation in cat's Deiters neurones also revealed that excitatory synapses are supplied to them through collaterals of certain bulbocerebellar fibers (Ito et al., 1969b). These fibers appear to arise from the medio-dorsal portion of medulla, probably from the region of perihypoglossal nuclei and/or paramedian reticular formation, and project bilaterally into the anterior and posterior lobes of the cerebellum.

SYNAPTIC ACTION OF CEREBELLAR NUCLEAR NEURONES

In addition to the direct connections to the secondary vestibular neurones from the cerebellar afferents and from the cerebellar Purkinje cells, there are indirect connections; certain secondary vestibular neurones in DV project to the cerebellum and terminate in the flocculus, nodulus and fastigial nucleus (Brodal and Torvik, 1957). Spinocerebellar fibers also have synaptic connections with fastigial neurones (Eccles et al., 1967; Matsushita, 1970). Fastigial neurones are under the influence of cerebellar Purkinje cells and in turn project to vestibular nuclei cells (cf. Brodal et al., 1962).

Microelectrode recordings from Deiters neurones and reticular formation cells have revealed that the fastigiobulbar axons, decussating through the hook bundle (Rasmussen, 1933; Jansen and Jansen, 1955), have an excitatory action upon medullary neurones (Ito et al., 1970c). The uncrossed fastigiovestibular projection also appears to have an excitatory action (Shimazu and Smith, 1971). The projection from the interpositus nucleus to the red nucleus (Toyama et al., 1967), that from the interpositus and lateral nuclei to the ventrolateral nucleus of thalamus (Uno et al., 1970) and that from the lateral nucleus to III nucleus (Highstein, 1971) are all shown to have excitatory action. Hence, it is proposed that the cerebellar nucleofugal projection is excitatory in action in contrast to the inhibitory action of the cerebellar corticofugal projection by Purkinje cells.

Fig. 2. Synaptic connections to vestibulospinal tract cells. Center diagram indicates recording microelectrode and stimulating electrodes on transverse sections of the medulla and cerebellum and C_1 spinal segment. Records are EPSPs evoked by ipsilateral VIII nerve stimulation (upper left), IPSPs by ipsilateral vermal stimulation (upper right), EPSPs by stimulation at the ipsilateral ventrolateral corner of C_1 segment (lower left), and antidromic spikes with the same C_1 stimulation (lower right). In the lower left record, C_1 stimulation was weaker than the threshold for evoking antidromic spikes. From Akaike, Fanardjian, Ito and Nakajima (1972c).

VESTIBULO-OCULAR REFLEX AND THE CEREBELLUM

The vestibulo-ocular reflex arc is a well defined trineuronal chain composed of primary vestibular afferents, secondary vestibular neurones, and oculomotor neurones. The vestibulo-ocular reflex can be elicited by electric pulse stimulation of VIII nerve and be recorded in oculomotor nuclei as the secondary vestibular volleys, EPSPs and IPSPs in oculomotor neurones (Sasaki, 1963; Richter and Precht, 1968; Baker et al., 1969; Ito et al., 1970b; Highstein et al., 1971). It has thus been shown that the second link of this trineuronal chain to III and IV nuclei has three major fractions, as shown in Fig. 1; excitatory FLM component arising from MV, inhibitory FLM component originating from SV, excitatory BC component derived from the lateral cerebellar nucleus as well as probably from the group y of the vestibular nuclear complex (Highstein et al., 1971; Highstein, 1971).

Electric stimulation of the flocculus produces prominent inhibition in SV- and BC-mediated vestibulo-ocular reflexes, but no significant effect could be detected on the MV-mediated reflex (Ito et al., 1970a; Fukuda et al., 1972). No significant inhibition could be produced in vestibulo-ocular reflexes by stimulating the vermal zone of the cerebellum, including nodulus and uvula. Even though the possibility still remains that the inhibitory effect of the nodulus-uvula stimulation is so weak that the transmission from the primary vestibular afferents to the secondary vestibular neurones is not effectively blocked, it is clear that the flocculus is the major source of the cerebellar action upon the vestibulo-ocular reflexes. It is of interest in this connection that according to Angaut and Brodal (1967) the flocculus supplies the central part of SV as do the primary vestibular fibers while the fibers from the nodulus-uvula end in the peripheral part of SV. Fig. 1 summarizes the major neuronal connections in the vestibulo-ocular reflex arc. Movement or position changes of the head will evoke discharges of the primary vestibular impulses which will be forwarded through the trineuronal chain and finally cause the compensatory movement of the eyes. The flocculus receives primary afferent impulses, and on the basis of information processing performed there, it will send inhibitory signals to secondary vestibular neurones to achieve an exact compensatory movement of the eyes. Di Giorgio and Giulio (1949) and Manni (1950) demonstrated that lesions in the flocculus cause an abnormal performance of the vestibulo-ocular reflex function. The construction of this system suggests that it acts as a feed-forward control system (Ito, 1970a, b).

The correct compensation of the head movements by eye rotation to prevent blurring of the visual images, can be obtained only when the flocculus knows how much inhibitory signals should be superposed on the incoming primary vestibular impulses. Considerations along this line lead to the postulate that the vestibulo-ocular reflex system is equipped with a kind of checking line which informs the flocculus about the correctness of the compensation, presumably through the visual pathway (Ito, 1970b). Lorente de Nó (1931) described previously that a newborn rabbit displays an abnormal vestibulo-ocular reflex and that the normal reflex is completed only after four weeks during which vision appears to play an important role. Recently, Maekawa and Simpson (1972) found that electrical stimulation of the optic nerve or photic stimulation of the retina causes excitation of Purkinje cells in the flocculus via the inferior olive. This is the climbing fiber pathway impinging upon Purkinje cells with a high transmission efficacy (Eccles *et al.*, 1966), while the primary vestibular afferents make another type of endings in the cerebellar cortex, mossy fiber terminals (Brodal and Høivik, 1964), which are linked with Purkinje cells only via granule cells.

VESTIBULOSPINAL REFLEX AND THE CEREBELLUM

The vestibulospinal reflex arc is a trineuronal chain composed of primary vestibular afferents, secondary vestibular neurones and alpha motoneurones. Vestibulospinal reflexes through MVST can be elicited by electrical pulse stimulation of the VIII nerve and recorded in the ventral horn of cervical segments as a vestibulospinal volley (Cook *et al.*, 1969) and as EPSPs or IPSPs in C_1 neurones (Wilson and Yoshida, 1969a; Wilson *et al.*, 1970; Akaike, Fanardjian, Ito, Kumada and Nakajima, 1972a). Electrical stimulation of the deep lamellae of the cerebellar anterior and posterior lobes caused depression in the vestibulospinal volleys (Akaike, Fanardjian, Ito and Nakajima, 1972c). Intracellular recording from vestibular nuclear cells indicated that MVST neurones in the ventral portion of LV indeed receive IPSPs from deep lamellae of the cerebellar anterior and posterior lobe. These cerebellar areas, however, receive affer-

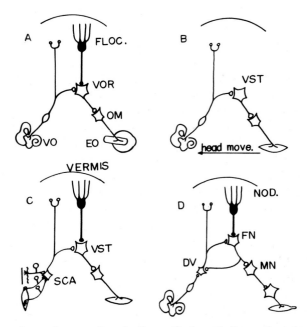

Fig. 3. Prototypes of neural connections in the vestibulocerebellar system. A, vestibular-operated feed-forward control system. B, vestibular-operated feedback control system. C, spinal-operated feed-forward control system. D, involvement of fastigial nucleus. VO, vestibular organ. OVR, vestibulo-ocular relay cell. OM, oculomotor neurones. EO, extra-ocular muscles. VST, vestibulospinal tract cell. SCA, spino-cerebellar afferent. FN, fastigial nucleus cell. DV, descending vestibular nucleus cell. Floc., flocculus. Nod., nodulus-uvula.

ents of spinobulbar origin (Grant, 1962; Van Rossum, 1969) but not primary vestibular afferents. There is no evidence indicating that the vestibulocerebellum has an inhibitory projection to VST cells.

Consequently, the cerebellar control of VST cells should be considered in connection with the spinocerebellar and bulbocerebellar afferents and the relevant cerebellar cortex, but not with the primary vestibular afferents and the vestibulocerebellum. As shown in Figs. 2 and 3C, a feed-forward control system would be composed of the spinocerebellar afferents and vestibulospinal efferents on which the cerebellar vermis is superposed. Positional change or movement in limbs and trunk will provoke compensatory adjustment in certain combination of muscles through the spino-vestibulo-spinal reflexes which will be optimized by the cerebellar action.

The primary vestibular afferent inputs to certain VST cells, not combined with the Purkinje cell inhibition from the vestibulo-cerebellum, may serve for a classic feed-back control system: the output of the vestibulospinal reflexes will readily be fed back to the vestibular organ through movement and positional change of the head (Fig. 3B). It is corollary that a feed-back control system does not need the cerebellar inhibition. Convergence of primary vestibular afferents and vermal Purkinje cell axons onto certain VST cells (Ito *et al.*, 1969a; Walberg and Mugnaini, 1969; Akaike, Fanardjian, Ito and Nakajima, 1972c) would thus be accounted for by assuming that the same VST cells participate in both the spinal-operated feed-forward control system and the vestibular-operated feedback control system.

POSSIBLE ROLE OF FASTIGIAL NUCLEUS

Cerebellar nuclear cells and certain brainstem neurones have reciprocal projections: between fastigial nucleus and the descending vestibular nucleus or paramedian reticular formation, between the interpositus nucleus and red nucleus or pontine nucleus, and between the lateral cerebellar nucleus and pontine nucleus (*cf*. Brodal *et al.*, 1962). The possibility of reverberation through these connections has been pointed out (Brodal *et al.*, 1962; Eccles *et al.*, 1967; Ito, 1969). Recently, Tsukahara and Bando (1970) demonstrated the excitatory circular connections between the interpositus nucleus and pontine nucleus. When Purkinje cell inhibition is blocked by picrotoxin, reverberation indeed occurs, and a steady depolarization as large as 50 mV is built up in the red nuclear neurones by impulse discharges along the interposito-rubral projection (Tsukahara *et al.*, 1971).

It is possible that the interconnections between the fastigial nucleus and DV and between the fastigial nucleus and paramedian reticular formation are such that a reverberating circuit is formed within the vestibulocerebellar control system (Fig. 3D). It can be imagined that this reverberation, if it occurs, provides the background activity which keeps the control system at optimum operating conditions. However, the role of the fastigial nucleus on the vestibulocerebellar control system can be more than to provide the background activity as assumed above. This inference is based on the fact that the direct innervation by Purkinje cells of brainstem neurones as in the vestibular system is rather exceptional and in phylogenetically new parts of the cerebellum there is only an indirect innervation by Purkinje cells through the cerebellar nuclei. The significance of the neuronal diagram involving fastigial nucleus has to be considered in future investigations.

SUMMARY

The neuronal organization in the vestibulo-cerebellar system appears to be a mixture of the following four prototypes: (i) vestibular-operated feed-forward control system (for example, vestibulo-ocular reflex arc combined with the flocculus); (ii) vestibular-operated feed-back control system (vestibulo-spinal reflex arc); (iii) spinal- and bulbar-operated feed-forward control system (spino-vestibulo-spinal reflex arc combined with vermis); (iv) indirect control by fastigiovestibular projection, either operated by secondary vestibular afferents or by spinal afferents. In certain vestibular nuclear cells, these principal connections are combined.

Histological data indicate that Purkinje cells in the vestibulocerebellum project to a fairly wide area of the vestibular nuclear complex (Angaut and Brodal, 1968; Van Rossum, 1969). At the present time, however, the action of the vestibulocerebellum has been revealed only with inhibition from the flocculus on the superior nucleus and the cerebellar lateral nucleus. No information is available about the action of the nodulus and uvula which in previous ablation experiments appeared to exert inhibitory action upon vestibular centers (Fernandez, 1960). Investigation on other types of secondary vestibular neurones than VOR and VST cells is desirable to reveal the action of the nodulus and uvula on vestibular nuclear cells.

REFERENCES

AKAIKE, T., FANARDJIAN, V. V., ITO, M., KUMADA, M. AND NAKAJIMA, H. (1972a) Electrophysiological analysis of the vestibulospinal reflex pathway of rabbit. I. Classification of relay cells. Submitted to *Exp. Brain Res.*

AKAIKE, T., FANARDJIAN, V. V., ITO, M. AND NAKAJIMA, H. (1972c) Cerebellar control of the vestibulospinal relay neurones in rabbit. In preparation.

AKAIKE, T., FANARDJIAN, V. V., ITO, M., AND OHNO, T. (1972b) Electrophysiological analysis of the vestibulospinal reflex pathway of rabbit. II. Synaptic actions upon spinal neurones. Submitted to *Exp. Brain Res.*

ANGAUT, P. AND BRODAL, A. (1967) The projection of the vestibulo-cerebellum onto the vestibular nuclei in the cats. *Arch. ital. Biol.*, **105**, 441–479.

BAKER, R. G., MANO, N. AND SHIMAZU, H. (1969) Postsynaptic potential in abducens motoneurons induced by vestibular stimulation. *Brain Res.*, **15**, 577–580.

BLANKENSHIP, J. E., WACHTEL, H. AND KANDEL, E. R. (1971) Ionic mechanisms of excitatory, inhibitory, and dual synaptic actions mediated by an identified interneuron in abdominal ganglion of Aplysia. *J. Neurophysiol.*, **34**, 76–92.

BRODAL, A. AND HØIVIK, B. (1964) Site and mode of termination of primary vestibulocerebellar fibers in the cat. *Arch. ital. Biol.*, **102**, 1–21.

BRODAL, A. AND POMPEIANO, O. (1957) The vestibular nuclei in the cat. *J. Anat. (Lond.)*, **91**, 438–454.

BRODAL, A., POMPEIANO, O. AND WALBERG, F. (1962) *The Vestibular Nuclei and Their Connections. Anatomy and Functional Correlation*. Oliver and Boyd, Edinburgh, London, pp. VIII-193.

BRODAL, A. UND TORVIK, A. (1957) Über den Ursprung der sekundären vestibulocerebellaren Fasern bei der Katze. Eine experimentelle anatomische Studie. *Arch. Psychiat. Z. ges. Neurol.*, **195**, 550–567.

BROOKHART, J. M. (1960) The cerebellum. In J. FIELD, H. W. MAGOUN AND V. E. HALL (Eds.), *Handbook of Physiology. Section 1. Neurophysiology. Vol. II.* Amer. Physiol. Soc., Washington, D.C., pp. 1245–1280.

CARPENTER, M. B. AND STROMINGER, N. L. (1964) Cerebello-oculomotor fibers in the Rhesus monkey. *J. comp. Neurol.*, **123**, 211–230.

COOK, W. A., JR., CANGIANO, A. AND POMPEIANO, O. (1969) An electric investigation of the efferent pathways from the vestibular nuclei. *Arch. ital. Biol.*, **107**, 235–274.

CURTIS, D. R., DUGGAN, A. W. AND FELIX, D. (1970) GABA and inhibition of Deiters' neurones. *Brain Res.*, **23**, 117–120.

EAGER, R. P. (1963) Efferent cortico-nuclear pathways in the cerebellum of the cat. *J. comp. Neurol.*, **120**, 81–104.

ECCLES, J. C., ITO, M. AND SZENTÁGOTHAI, J. (1967) *The Cerebellum as a Neuronal Machine.* Springer Berlin, Heidelberg, New York, pp. 335.

ECCLES, J. C., LLINÁS, R. AND SASAKI, K. (1966) The excitatory synaptic action of climbing fibers on the Purkinje cells of the cerebellum. *J. Physiol. (Lond.)*, **182**, 268–296.

FERNANDEZ, C. (1960) Interrelations between flocculonodular lobe and vestibular system. In G. L. RASMUSSEN AND W. F. WINDLE (Eds.), *Neural Mechanisms of the Auditory and Vestibular System.* C. C. Thomas, Springfield, Ill., pp. 285–296.

FLOOD, S. AND JANSEN, J. (1961) On the cerebellar nuclei in the cat. *Acta Anat.*, **46**, 52–72.

FONNUM, F., J. STORM-MATHISEN AND F. WALBERG (1970) Glutamate decarboxylase in inhibitory neurons. A study of the enzyme in Purkinje cell axons and boutons in the cat. *Brain Res.*, **20**, 259–275.

FUKUDA, J., HIGHSTEIN, S. M. AND ITO, M. (1972) Cerebellar inhibitory control of the vestibulo-ocular reflex investigated in rabbit IIIrd nucleus. *Exp. Brain Res.*, **14**, 511–526.

GIORGIO DI, A. M. AND GIULIO, L. (1949) Riflessi oculari di origine otolitica ed influenza del cervelletto. *Boll. Soc. ital. Biol. sper.*, **25**, 145–146.

GRANT, G. (1962) Spinal course and somatotopically localized termination of the spinocerebellar tracts. An experimental study in the cat. *Acta physiol. scand.*, **56**, Suppl. 193, 1–45.

GRILLNER, S., HONGO, T. AND LUND, S. (1970) The vestibulospinal tract. Effects on alpha-motoneurones in the lumbosacral spinal cord in the cat. *Exp. Brain Res.*, **10**, 94–120.

HAUGLIE-HANSSEN, E. (1968) Intrinsic neuronal organization of the vestibular nuclear complex in the cat. *Ergebn. Anat. Entwickl.-Gesch.*, **40**, 1–105.

HERRICK, C. J. (1924) Origin and evolution of the cerebellum. *Arch. Neurol. (Chicago)*, **11**, 621–625.

HIGHSTEIN, S. M. (1971) Organization of the inhibitory and excitatory vestibulo-ocular reflex pathways to the third and fourth nuclei in rabbit. *Brain Res.*, **32**, 218–224.

HIGHSTEIN, S. M. AND ITO, M. (1971) Differential localization within the vestibular nuclear complex of the inhibitory and excitatory cells innervating IIIrd nucleus oculomotor neurons in rabbit. *Brain Res.*, **29**, 358–362.

HIGHSTEIN, S. M., ITO, M. AND TSUCHIYA, T. (1971) Synaptic linkage in the vestibulo-ocular reflex pathway of rabbit. *Exp. Brain Res.*, **13**, 306–326.

ITO, M. (1969) Neurons of cerebellar nuclei. In M. A. B. BRAZIER (Ed.), *The Interneuron.* Univ. of California Press, Berkely, Los Angeles, pp. 309–327.

ITO, M. (1970a) The cerebello-vestibular interaction in the cat's vestibular nuclei neurons. In *Fourth Symposium on the Role of the Vestibular Organs in Space Exploration. NASA SP-187*, 183–199.

ITO, M. (1970b) Neurophysiological aspects of the cerebellar motor control system. *Int. J. Neurol.*, **7**, 162–176.

ITO, M., HIGHSTEIN, S. M. AND FUKUDA, J. (1970a) Cerebellar inhibition of the vestibulo-ocular reflex in rabbit and cat and its blockage by picrotoxin. *Brain Res.*, **17**, 524–526.

ITO, M., HIGHSTEIN, S. M. AND TSUCHIYA, T. (1970b) The postsynaptic inhibition of rabbit oculomotor neurones by secondary vestibular impulses and its blockage by picrotoxin. *Brain Res.*, **17**, 520–523.

ITO, M., HONGO, T. AND OKADA, Y. (1969a) Vestibular-evoked postsynaptic potentials in Deiters neurones. *Exp. Brain Res.*, **7**, 214–230.

ITO, M., HONGO, T., YOSHIDA, M., OKADA, Y. AND OBATA, K. (1964a) Intracellularly recorded antidromic responses of Deiters neurones. *Experientia (Basel)*, **20**, 295–296.

ITO, M., HONGO, T., YOSHIDA, M., OKADA, Y. AND OBATA, K. (1964b) Antidromic and transsynaptic activation of Deiters' neurones during stimulation of the spinal cord. *Jap. J. Physiol.*, **14**, 638–658.

ITO, M., KAWAI, N. AND UDO, M. (1968a) The origin of cerebellar-induced inhibition of Deiters neurones. III. Localization of the inhibitory zone. *Exp. Brain Res.*, **4**, 310–320.

ITO, M., KAWAI, N., UDO, M. AND MANO, N. (1969b) Axon reflex activation of Deiters' neurones from the cerebellar cortex through collaterals of the cerebellar afferents. *Exp. Brain Res.*, **8**, 249–268.

ITO, M., KAWAI, N., UDO, M. AND SATO, N. (1968b) Cerebellar-evoked disinhibition in dorsal Deiters' neurones. *Exp. Brain Res.*, **6**, 247–264.

ITO, M., OBATA, K. AND OCHI, R. (1966) The origin of cerebellar-induced inhibition of Deiters' neurones. II. Temporal correlation between the trans-synaptic activation of Purkinje cells and the inhibition of Deiters neurones. *Exp. Brain Res.*, **2**, 350–364.

ITO, M., UDO, M., MANO, N. AND KAWAI, N. (1970c) Synaptic action of the fastigiobulbar impulses upon neurones in the medullary reticular formation and vestibular nuclei. *Exp. Brain Res.*, **11**, 29–47.

ITO, M. AND YOSHIDA, M. (1964) The cerebellar-evoked monosynaptic inhibition of Deiters' neurones. *Experientia (Basel)*, **20**, 515–516.

ITO, M. AND YOSHIDA, M. (1966) The origin of cerebellar-induced inhibition of Deiters' neurones. I. Monosynaptic inhibition of the inhibitory postsynaptic potentials. *Exp. Brain Res.*, **2**, 330–349.

ITO, M., YOSHIDA, M. AND OBATA, K. (1964c) Monosynaptic inhibition of the intracerebellar nuclei induced from the cerebellar cortex. *Experientia (Basel)*, **20**, 575–576.

ITO, M., YOSHIDA, M., OBATA, K., KAWAI, N. AND UDO, M. (1970d) Inhibitory control of intracerebellar nuclei by the Purkinje cell axons. *Exp. Brain Res.*, **10**, 64–80.

JANSEN, J. AND BRODAL, A. (1954) *Aspects of Cerebellar Anatomy*. Johan Grundt Tanum, Oslo, pp. 423.

JANSEN, J. AND JANSEN, J., JR. (1955) On the efferent fibers of the cerebellar nuclei in the cat. *J. comp. Neurol.*, **102**, 607–632.

KANDEL, E. R., FRAZIER, W. T. AND COGGESHALL, R. E. (1967) Opposite synaptic actions mediated by different branches of an identifiable interneuron in Aplysia. *Science*, **155**, 346–349.

KAWAI, N., ITO, M. AND NOZUE, M. (1969) Postsynaptic influences on the vestibular non-Deiters nuclei from primary vestibular nerve. *Exp. Brain Res.*, **8**, 190–200.

KIDOKORO, Y. (1968) Direct inhibitory innervation of teleost oculomotor neurones by cerebellar Purkinje cells. *Brain Res.*, **10**, 453–456.

LLINÁS, R. AND PRECHT, W. (1969) The inhibitory vestibular efferent system and its relation to the cerebellum in the frog. *Exp. Brain Res.*, **9**, 16–29.

LORENTE DE NÓ, R. (1931) Ausgewählte Kapitel aus der vergleichenden Physiologie des Labyrinthes. Die Augen Muskelreflexe beim Kaninchen und ihre Grundlagen. *Ergebn. Physiol.*, **32**, 73–242.

LUND, S. AND POMPEIANO, O. (1968) Monosynaptic excitation of alpha motoneurones from supraspinal structures in the cat. *Acta physiol. scand.*, **73**, 1–21.

MAEKAWA, K. AND SIMPSON, J. I. (1971) Climbing fiber responses evoked in the flocculus by visual pathway stimulation in the rabbit. *Proc. XXV int. Congr. physiol. Sci., Munich*, IX, n. 1060, 358.

MANNI, D. E. (1950) Localizzazioni cerebellari corticali nella cavia. 2. Effetti di lesioni delle "parti vestibulari" del cervelletto. *Arch. Fisiol.*, **50**, 110–123.

MANO, N., OSHIMA, T. AND SHIMAZU, H. (1968) Inhibitory commissural fibers interconnecting the bilateral vestibular nuclei. *Brain Res.*, **8**, 378–382.

MATSUSHITA, M. AND IKEDA, M. (1970) Spinal projection to the cerebellar nuclei in the cat. *Exp. Brain Res.*, **10**, 501–511.

MEESSEN, H. AND OLSZEWSKY, J. (1949) *A Cytoarchitectonic Atlas of the Rhombencephalon of the Rabbit*. S. Karger, Basel, New York, pp. 52.

MORUZZI, G. (1950) *Problems in Cerebellar Physiology*. C. C. Thomas, Springfield, Ill., pp. VI–116.

NYBERG–HANSEN, R. (1964) Origin and termination of fibers from the vestibular nuclei descending in the medial longitudinal fasciculus. An experimental study with silver impregnation methods in the cat. *J. comp. Neurol.*, **122**, 355–367.

OBATA, K. (1965) Pharmacological study on postsynaptic inhibition of Deiters' neurons. *Proc. XXIII int. Congr. physiol. Sci., Tokyo*, n. 958, 406.

OBATA, K. (1970) Inhibitory transmitter of cerebellar Purkinje cells (Japanese). *Advanc. Neurol. Sci.*, **13**, 828–837.

OBATA, K. AND HIGHSTEIN, S. M. (1970) Blocking by picrotoxin of both vestibular inhibition and GABA action on rabbit oculomotor neurones. *Brain Res.*, **18**, 538–541.

OBATA, K., ITO, M., OCHI, R. AND SATO, N. (1967) Pharmacological properties of the postsynaptic inhibition by Purkinje cell axons and the action of γ-aminobutyric acid on Deiters' neurones. *Exp. Brain Res.*, **4**, 43–57.

OBATA, K. AND TAKEDA, K. (1969) Release of γ-aminobutyric acid into the fourth ventricle induced by stimulation of the cat's cerebellum. *J. Neurochem.*, **16**, 1043–1047.

OBATA, K., TAKEDA, K. AND SHINOZAKI, H. (1970) Further study on pharmacological properties of the cerebellar-induced inhibition of Deiters' neurones. *Exp. Brain Res.*, **11**, 327–334.

OTSUKA, M., OBATA, K. MIYATA, Y. AND TANAKA, Y. (1970) The measurement of gamma-amino-butyric acid in isolated nerve cells in cat central nervous system. *J. Neurochem.*, **18**, 287–295.

POMPEIANO, O. AND BRODAL, A. (1957) Spino-vestibular fibers in the cat. An experimental study. *J. comp. Neurol.*, **108**, 353–381.

PRECHT, W. AND LLINÁS, R. (1968) Direct vestibular afferents to cat cerebellar nuclei. *Proc. XXIV int. Congr. physiol. Sci., Washington, D.C., VII*, n. 1063, 355.

PRECHT, W. AND LLINÁS, R. (1969) Functional organization of the vestibular afferents to the cerebellar cortex of frog and cat. *Exp. Brain Res.*, **9**, 30–52.

PRECHT, W. AND SHIMAZU, H. (1965) Functional connections of tonic and kinetic vestibular neurones with primary vestibular afferents. *J. Neurophysiol.*, **28**, 1014–1028.

RASMUSSEN, A. T. (1933) Origin and course of the fasciculus uncinatus (Russell) in the cat with observations on the other fibre tracts arising from the cerebellar nuclei. *J. comp. Neurol.*, **57**, 165–197.

RICHTER, A. AND PRECHT, W. (1968) Inhibition of abducens motoneurones by vestibular nerve stimulation. *Brain Res.*, **11**, 701–705.

SASAKI, K. (1963) Electrophysiological studies on oculomotor neurons of the cat. *Jap. J. Physiol.*, **13**, 287–302.

SHIMAZU, H. AND SMITH, C. M. (1971) Cerebellar and labyrinthine influences on single vestibular neurons identified by natural stimuli. *J. Neurophysiol.*, **34**, 493–508.

STEINER, F. A. AND WEBER, G. (1965) Die Beeinflussung labyrinthär erregbarer Neurone des Hirnstammes durch Acetylcholin. *Helv. physiol. Acta*, **23**, 82–89.

TEN BRUGGENCATE, G. AND ENGBERG, I. (1971) Iontophoretic studies in Deiters' nucleus of the inhibitory actions of GABA and related aminoacids and the interactions of strychnine and picrotoxin. *Brain Res.*, **25**, 431–448.

TOYAMA, K., TSUKAHARA, N. AND UDO, M. (1967) Nature of the cerebellar influences upon the red nucleus neurons. *Exp. Brain Res.*, **4**, 292–309.

TSUKAHARA, N. AND BANDO, T. (1970) Red nuclear and interposate nuclear excitation of pontine nuclear cells. *Brain Res.*, **19**, 295–298.

TSUKAHARA, N., BANDO, T., KITAI, S. T. AND KIYOHARA, H. (1971) Cerebello-pontine reverberating circuit. *Brain Res.*, **33**, 233–237.

UNO, M., YOSHIDA, M. AND HIROTA, I. (1970) The mode of cerebello-thalamic relay transmission investigated with intracellular recording from cells of the ventrolateral nucleus of cat's thalamus. *Exp. Brain Res.*, **10**, 121–139.

VAN ROSSUM, J. (1969) *Corticonuclear and Corticovestibular Projections of the Cerebellum.* Van Gorcum and Comp., Leiden, 170 pp.

WALBERG, F. AND JANSEN, J. (1961) Cerebellar corticovestibular fibers in the cat. *Exp. Neurol.*, **3**, 32–52.

WALBERG, F. AND JANSEN, J. (1964) Cerebellar corticonuclear projection studied experimentally with silver impregnation method. *J. Hirnforsch.*, **6**, 338–354.

WALBERG, F. AND MUGNAINI, E. (1969) Distinction of degenerating fibres and boutons of cerebellar and peripheral origin in the Deiters' nucleus of the same animal. *Brain Res.*, **14**, 67–75.

WILSON, V. J., KATO, M., PETERSON, B. W. AND WYLIE, W. (1967a) A single-unit analysis of the organization of Deiters' nucleus. *J. Neurophysiol.*, **30**, 603–619.

WILSON, V. J., WYLIE, R. M. AND MARCO, L. A. (1967b) Projection to the spinal cord from the medial and descending vestibular nuclei of the cat. *Nature (Lond.)*, **215**, 429–430.

WILSON, V. J., WYLIE, R. M. AND MARCO, L. A. (1968) Synaptic inputs to cells in the medial vestibular nucleus. *J. Neurophysiol.*, **31**, 176–185.

WILSON, V. J. AND YOSHIDA, M. (1969a) Monosynaptic inhibition of neck motoneurones by the medial vestibular nucleus. *Exp. Brain Res.*, **9**, 365–380.

WILSON, V. J. AND YOSHIDA, M. (1969b) Comparison of effects of stimulation of Deiters' nucleus and medial longitudinal fasciculus on neck, forelimb, and hindlimb motoneurons. *J. Neurophysiol.*, **32**, 743–758.

WILSON, V. J., YOSHIDA, M. AND SHOR, R. H. (1970) Supraspinal monosynaptic excitation and inhibition of thoracic back motoneurons. *Exp. Brain Res.*, **11**, 282–295.

YAMAMOTO, C. (1967) Pharmacologic studies of norepinephrine, acetylcholine and related compounds on neurons in Deiters' nucleus and the cerebellum. *J. Pharmacol. exp. Ther.*, **156**, 39–47.

Cerebellar Control of the Vestibular Pathways to Spinal Motoneurons and Primary Afferents

O. POMPEIANO

Institute of Physiology II, University of Pisa, Pisa, Italy

As nerve impulses arrive at the spinal cord and enter the central endings of the afferent fibers, they are subjected to presynaptic mechanisms which may alter the membrane potential of the terminal parts of the fibers. The postsynaptic excitatory effectiveness of an orthodromic impulse is determined by the presynaptic membrane potential. Depolarization of the terminal arborization decreases the postsynaptic effect of arriving impulses (Howland *et al.*, 1955; Wall *et al.*, 1955; Frank and Fuortes, 1957; Eccles, 1961), whereas hyperpolarization of the terminal arborization increases the effectiveness of the impulses (Mendell and Wall, 1964; Wall, 1964).

It has been postulated that in the spinal cord there is continuous depolarization of the primary afferents, attributed to tonic bombardment of the terminal arborizations by afferent impulses (Mendell and Wall, 1964). This tonic mechanism leading to depolarization of the primary afferents is in part at least due to somatic sensory volleys, in part it depends upon tonic activity of supraspinal mechanisms. It is of interest that while transmission from the flexor reflex afferents to the flexor reflex afferents is tonically inhibited in the decerebrate state, the dorsal root potentials (DRPs) evoked by volleys in group I muscle afferents are either identical in the decerebrate and spinal states (Kuno and Perl, 1960; Carpenter *et al.*, 1963; *cf.* Holmqvist and Lundberg, 1961) or else only a slight decrease occurs following transection of the spinal cord. This does not mean however, that supraspinal structures, in particular the cerebellum, are unable to affect primary afferent depolarization (PAD) in the Ia pathway to spinal motoneurons.

It has been mentioned in a previous report (Pompeiano, 1972) that orthodromic labyrinthine volleys are able to depolarize not only the ipsilateral extensor motoneurons but also the group I primary afferents. It was also reported that the nucleus of Deiters exerts an excitatory influence on the ipsilateral extensor motoneurons (Brodal *et al.*, 1962; Lund and Pompeiano, 1965, 1968). On the other hand the medial (and descending) vestibular nuclei produce negative DRPs in the lumbar spinal cord (Carpenter *et al.*, 1966; Cook *et al.*, 1969a). The last effect is due to PAD of different systems of spinal afferents, including the group I pathway from extensor muscles (Carpenter *et al.*, 1966; Pompeiano and Morrison, 1966; Cook *et al.*, 1969b). A segregation, therefore, exists within the vestibular nuclei of those neurons which depolarize the extensor motoneurons and those which depolarize the primary afferents

(Barnes and Pompeiano, 1969, 1970a, b). The experiments reported in the present article indicate that both these vestibular mechanisms are under the control of the cerebellum.

EFFECTS ON MOTONEURONS EVOKED FROM THE FASTIGIAL NUCLEUS

The close anatomical relationship between the fastigial nucleus of the cerebellum and the vestibular nuclei suggests that both the vestibular mechanisms affecting spinal motoneurons and primary afferents may be modified by the fastigial nucleus.

Two efferent projections originate from the fastigial nucleus, namely the crossed and the uncrossed fastigiobulbar pathways; the uncrossed pathway, which originates from the rostral part of the fastigial nucleus, impinges upon the lateral vestibular nuclei (Brodal et al., 1962; Walberg et al., 1962a) and the reticular formation (Walberg et al., 1962b) of the ipsilateral side; the crossed pathway, which constitutes the bulk of Russell's hook bundle, originates from the caudal part of the fastigial nucleus (Jansen and Jansen, 1955; Batini and Pompeiano, 1955, 1957) and impinges upon the vestibular structures (Brodal et al., 1962; Walberg et al., 1962a) and the reticular formation (Walberg et al., 1962b) of the contralateral side.

Experiments of stimulation and destruction of the rostral part of the fastigial nucleus in some instances may affect not only rostro-fastigial neurons, but also direct corticocerebellar-vestibular fibers originating from the ipsilateral vermis of the cerebellar anterior lobe as well as crossed fastigiobulbar fibers originating from the contralateral fastigial nucleus, which both pass through this rostral fastigial region (Brodal et al., 1962). Detailed experiments of localized lesions, however, clearly indicate that the rostral part of the fastigial nucleus exerts a tonic facilitatory influence on the extensor mechanisms of the ipsilateral side (Fig. 1C, D), probably via the ipsilateral fastigio-vestibular projection to Deiters' nucleus (see Pompeiano, 1967, for references).

On the other hand an acute (Moruzzi and Pompeiano, 1955, 1956a, b, 1957b) or chronic (Batini and Pompeiano, 1955, 1957; Cohen et al., 1958) electrolytic lesion limited to the caudal third of one fastigial nucleus reduces or abolishes the extensor tonus of the contralateral limbs. The opposite posture, i.e., crossed facilitation of extensor tonus was observed when the caudal pole of one fastigial nucleus was electrically stimulated (Moruzzi and Pompeiano, 1955, 1956a, b). It was concluded, therefore, that the caudal pole of the fastigial nucleus exerts a tonic facilitatory influence on the extensor mechanisms of the contralateral side, probably via crossed fastigio-vestibular projections (Moruzzi and Pompeiano, 1955, 1956a, b, 1957b).

Further experiments support the view that this effect is mediated by Deiters' nucleus (Pompeiano, 1961, 1962). It appears in fact that when a lesion involved the rostral part of the caudal region of the fastigial nucleus, the ensuing atonia was limited to the contralateral forelimb, while the hindlimbs did not show any postural asymmetry (Fig. 1E, F). On the other hand, destruction of the extreme caudal pole of the fastigial nucleus abolished the extensor rigidity in the contralateral hindlimb only (Fig. 1G, H). Discrete effects, but opposite in character, were elicited after localized stimulation

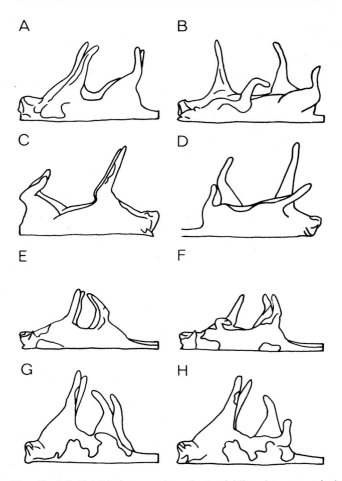

Fig. 1. Effects of localized fastigial lesions on decerebrate rigidity. A: symmetrical distribution of extensor rigidity after chronic electrolytic destruction of the caudal half of both fastigial nuclei followed, 16 days later, by intercollicular decerebration. B: ipsilateral increase and contralateral decrease of extensor rigidity after electrolytic lesion of the rostro-lateral part of the left fastigial nucleus, where the long cerebellar cortico-vestibular fibers course. From Batini and Pompeiano (1958). C: symmetrical distribution of extensor rigidity after chronic electrolytic destruction of the caudal half of both fastigial nuclei followed, 14 days later, by intercollicular decerebration. D: the same cat after electrolytic lesion of the rostro-medial part of the left fastigial nucleus. Note marked decrease in extensor rigidity on the left side and increase of extensor rigidity on the right side. From Batini and Pompeiano (1958). E: symmetrical distribution of extensor rigidity after precollicular decerebration. F: disappearance of extensor rigidity of the right foreleg after lesion of the rostral part of the caudal third of the left fastigial nucleus. From Pompeiano (1962). G: another experiment showing symmetrical rigidity after precollicular decerebration. H: disappearance of extensor rigidity of the right hindleg following lesion of the caudal pole of the left fastigial nucleus. From Pompeiano (1962).

of the same nuclear regions. The somatotopical pattern in the postural responses to local stimulation, or destruction, of the caudal part of the fastigial nucleus is in complete accord with the pattern of localization of the anatomical projection of the caudal part of the fastigial nucleus on the contralateral Deiters' nucleus (Walberg *et al.*, 1962a).

394   O. POMPEIANO

These findings, therefore, support the conclusion that the excitatory influence exerted from the caudal part of the fastigial nucleus on the extensor motoneurons of the contralateral side is mediated via Deiters' nucleus.

The general conclusion of all these experiments namely that the fastigial nucleus exerts an excitatory influence on the vestibular nuclei is supported by recent experiments showing that second order vestibular neurons receive a monosynaptic excitatory impingement during fastigial stimulation (Eccles *et al.*, 1967; Ito, 1970, 1972; Ito *et al.*, 1970a).

PRIMARY AFFERENT DEPOLARIZATION EVOKED FROM THE
FASTIGIAL NUCLEUS

The fastigial nucleus produces not only contraction of the extensor muscles but also *negative* DRPs in the lumbar cord (Cook *et al.*, 1968c; Cangiano *et al.* 1969a). In precollicular decerebrate cats stimulation of the caudal part of the contralateral fastigial nucleus with stimuli 2–3 times the threshold (T) for the increase of the forelimb rigidity, evoked a contraction of the gastrocnemius-soleus (GS) muscle which occurred at a threshold frequency varying from 50 to 100 per sec in different preparations. The response increased in amplitude with increasing frequency of stimulation and the peak tension was reached at the stimulus frequency of 400–500 per sec (Fig. 2A, left diagram). The right diagram in Fig. 2 shows the progressive increase in muscle tension evoked by increasing the intensity of stimulation (at 500/sec) delivered to the fastigial nucleus. The same preparations were also submitted to ventral rhizotomy (L6 to S2). Stimulation of the contralateral fastigial nucleus at 2–3 T evoked a negative DRP which occurred at a threshold frequency varying from 10 to 50 per sec. The amplitude of the responses increased with increasing frequencies of stimulation and reached peak values at 400–500 per sec (Fig. 2B, left diagram). The right diagram in Fig. 2 shows the development of the DRP elicited by stimulating the fastigial nucleus at 500/sec as a function of the stimulus intensities used: both DRP and tension developed together.

The DRPs evoked by fastigial stimulation were not due to proprioceptive reverberation resulting from muscle contraction since both hindlimbs had been completely deafferented.

Since negative DRPs represent a depolarization of the terminal arborization of some of the fibers in the dorsal roots, experiments were performed to identify which type of primary afferents contribute to these potentials. Stimulation of the contralateral fastigial nucleus (500/sec, 2.0–3.0 T) resulted in an increase in amplitude of the antidromic group I volley recorded from the GS nerve. The time course of this effect is shown in Fig. 3B, left diagram. For the parameters of stimulation indicated above the facilitation of the antidromic response (180–200%) was generally smaller than that elicited on the same group I terminals of GS nerve by maximal stimulation of the group I afferents in the ipsilateral hamstring nerve. When the intensity of fastigial stimulation was held at 2.0–3.0 T the excitability of the group I afferents from GS muscle started to increase at about the same threshold frequency of the DRPs.

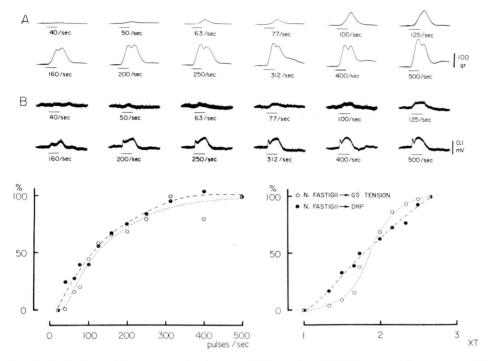

Fig. 2. Contraction of the gastrocnemius-soleus (GS) muscle and DRPs evoked from the caudal part of the contralateral fastigial nucleus. Precollicular decerebrate cat. A: contraction of the left GS muscle recorded isometrically at an initial extension of 6 mm in an intact preparation. The caudal part of the right fastigial nucleus was stimulated repetitively with 400 msec tetanus, 2.0 times the threshold (T) for the increase in the extensor rigidity of the contralateral forelimb, 0.5 msec pulse duration and at the frequencies indicated below each record. Horizontal bars denote duration of the tetanus. B: same experiment as in A. DRPs recorded from the most caudal dorsal rootlet in L6 of the left side on repetitive stimulation of the caudal part of the right fastigial nucleus, with the same parameters of stimulation used in A. In this and the following figures an upward deflection indicates negativity at the central electrode. The amplitudes of the muscle tension (circles) and the DRPs (dots) illustrated in A and B are plotted in the left diagram as percentages of the maximum evoked responses. In this and following diagrams each symbol corresponds to the average of 3–4 responses. The right diagram illustrates the result of another experiment in which the fastigial nucleus was stimulated at 500/sec, 0.2 msec pulse duration and at different strengths. Note the parallel development of the muscle tension and the DRPs by progressively increasing the intensity of stimulation. From Cangiano, Cook and Pompeiano (1969a).

The right diagram in Fig. 3 shows the progressive increase in amplitude of the antidromic group I volley with increasing frequencies of stimulation.

Stimulation of the caudal part of the fastigial nucleus produces presynaptic depolarization not only in the group I afferents from extensor but also from flexor muscles of the contralateral hindlimb (Fig. 4). There is evidence that the Ia afferents contribute to the flexor antidromic response which is facilitated by the descending volleys (Fig. 5). Repetitive stimulation of the contralateral fastigial nucleus also increased the excitability of the fast conducting cutaneous afferents.

The effects of stimulation of the contralateral fastigial nucleus on the spinal re-

O. POMPEIANO

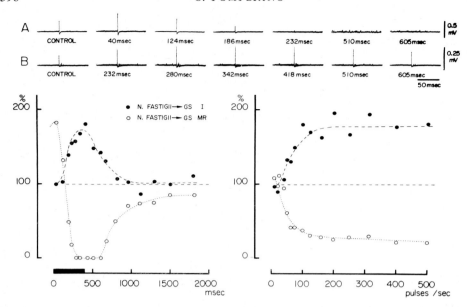

Fig. 3. Changes in amplitude of the gastrocnemius-soleus (GS) monosynaptic reflex and PAD in its group I afferents evoked from the contralateral fastigial nucleus. The right fastigial nucleus was stimulated in A and B at 500/sec, 2.0 T. The effect of fastigial stimulation on the monosynaptic reflex transmission through GS motoneuronal pool of the contralateral side and on the excitability of the group I afferent terminals from the corresponding GS muscle are shown respectively in A and B. The interval between onset of conditioning volleys and test volley is indicated in msec. The amplitudes of the monosynaptic reflex (circles) and the antidromic volley (dots) partially illustrated in A and B are plotted in the left diagram.

In the right diagram the amplitude of the extensor monosynaptic reflex and the group I antidromic volley from GS nerve are plotted as a function of the frequency of stimulation of the contralateral fastigial nucleus. The interval between beginning of the conditioning tetanus and testing shock was 573 msec for the monosynaptic reflex and 415 msec for the antidromic volley. From Cangiano, Cook and Pompeiano (1969a).

flexes have also been investigated. Stimulation of the fastigial nucleus with a 400 msec tetanus generally elicits an early facilitation of the GS monosynaptic reflex, followed 60–100 msec after the beginning of the tetanus by a late depression. This depression or abolition generally lasted about 500–600 msec from the beginning of the tetanus and was followed by a progressive recovery. The time course of the depression of the monosynaptic reflex (Fig. 3A, left diagram) parallels the time course of the increased excitability of the terminal arborization of the group I afferents recorded from the same preparation. The right diagram in Fig. 3 shows the depression of the mono-synaptic reflex as a function of the frequency of stimulation. The curve obtained parallels that of PAD under the same conditions.

The effects of fastigial stimulation have been investigated also on the monosynaptic flexor reflexes (Fig. 4, left diagram). The maximum depression generally occurred at about 300 msec after the beginning of the conditioning tetanus. The early facilitation described for the monosynaptic extensor reflex was rare in its occurrence. However the depression of the monosynaptic flexor reflex resembled that of the monosynaptic

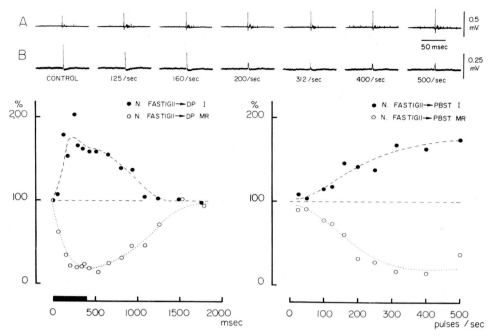

Fig. 4. Depression of the monosynaptic flexor reflexes and PAD in their group I afferents evoked from the contralateral fastigial nucleus. The right fastigial nucleus was stimulated in A and B at 3.0 T and the indicated frequencies. The effect of fastigial stimulation on the excitability of group I afferent terminals from posterior biceps-semitendinosus (PBST) muscle and on monosynaptic reflex transmission through the PBST motoneuronal pool of the contralateral side are shown respectively in A and B. The interval between onset of conditioning stimulation and test volley was 230 msec. The amplitudes of the antidromic volleys (dots) and monosynaptic reflexes (circles) partially illustrated in A and B are summarized in graphic form on the right side. The data plotted to the left were obtained from the same experiment. In this case the effects of fastigial stimulation were studied on the excitability of the group I afferent terminals from the deep peroneal (DP) nerve and on monosynaptic reflex transmission through the corresponding motoneural pool of the contralateral side. The fastigial nucleus was stimulated at 500/sec, 3.0 T, while the interval between beginning of the conditioning stimulus and testing shock was varied. From Cangiano, Cook and Pompeiano (1969a).

extensor reflex except for a more prolonged time course. With stimulation of the fastigial nucleus at 2.0–3.0 T the initial depression of the monosynaptic flexor reflex occurred at the threshold frequency of 66/sec, while the maximum appeared at about 300/sec (Fig. 4B, right diagram). The depression of the monosynaptic flexor reflex was always associated with PAD in the corresponding group I pathway as shown in Fig. 4A, right diagram.

In summary the fastigial stimulation produces not only contraction of the extensor muscles but also negative DRPs in the lumbar cord contralaterally to the side of stimulation. These DRPs are due to depolarization of the terminal arborizations of the primary afferents and involve the group I pathway from both extensor and flexor muscles as well as the cutaneous afferents.

It is very likely that the crossed fastigial influence on the extensor muscles is mediated via Deiters' nucleus, which is known to exert a facilitatory influence on the extensor motoneurons. On the other hand the medial and descending vestibular nuclei are partially involved in the transmission of the fastigial influence on primary afferents. This hypothesis is supported by the findings that: (*i*) crossed fastigio-vestibular fibers derived from the caudal part of the fastigial nucleus terminate within the medial and descending vestibular nuclei (Walberg *et al.*, 1962a) and (*ii*) stimulation of these vestibular nuclei as well as of the VIII cranial nerve is able to produce PAD in different types of primary afferents, including the group Ia pathway (Carpenter *et al.*, 1966; Cook, Cangiano and Pompeiano, 1968a, b, 1969b). This effect is apparently mediated through the descending reticular system (Cook *et al.*, 1969a, b) and the possibility exists that most of the crossed fastigial influences on the primary afferents are mediated by the fastigio-reticular connections which also originate from the caudal part of the fastigial nucleus (Walberg *et al.*, 1962b).

The effects of repetitive stimulation of the fastigial nucleus on the extensor moto-neurons and on the primary afferents closely resemble those elicited by repetitive stimulation of the VIII nerve (Cook *et al.*, 1968a, b, 1969a, b; Barnes and Pompeiano, 1970a, b). However the monosynaptic extensor reflex is facilitated by stimulation of the ipsilateral VIII nerve (Cook *et al.*, 1968a, b; 1969b; Barnes and Pompeiano, 1970a, b), whereas it is depressed by stimulation of the contralateral fastigial nucleus.

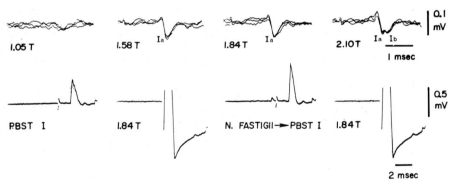

Fig. 5. The composition of the antidromic group I volley facilitated by stimulation of the contra-lateral fastigial nucleus. The upper traces were recorded from the dorsol root entry zone in lower L₇. Ingoing volleys were evoked by single shock stimulation of the ipsilateral posterior biceps-semiten-dinosus (PBST) nerve (0.05 msec pulses). The stimulus intensities are expressed in multiples of the threshold (T) for the group Ia volley. In this series of responses negativity is recorded as a downward deflection and the development of the response with increasing stimulus strengths into its two com-conent parts (Ia and Ib) is labelled. The lower traces should be read from left to right. Traces recorded from PBST nerve following microelectrode stimulation in the motoneuronal pool with 0.1 msec pulses. The first record shows the antidromic test response (PBST I). This response was then preceded by a maximal Ia orthodromic volley (1.84 T) in the PBST nerve and the complete depression of the antidromic response is shown in the second record. The third record shows the facilitation of the antidromic test response during conditioning stimulation of the contralateral fastigial nucleus at 500/sec, 0.3 msec pulse duration, 1.4 T (N. Fastigii → PBST I). The facilitated antidromic volley was then preceded by the orthodromic volley in the PBST nerve at 1.84 T, which abolished the anti-dromic response as shown in the last record. This indicates that fastigial stimulation increases the excitability of the central endings of the group Ia afferents from flexor muscles. From Cangiano, Cook and Pompeiano (1969a).

This last effect is attributed to a more powerful effect from the fastigial nucleus on those reticular structures which control transmission through primary afferents. Although repetitive stimulation of the contralateral fastigial nucleus also causes excitation of the extensor motoneurons, the presynaptic effect is probably sufficient to block the orthodromic transmission of the Ia volley. The role of presynaptic inhibition is supported by the fact that the time course of the depression of the monosynaptic extensor reflex produced by the hook bundle of Russell parallels the time course of the PAD recorded from the Ia extensor afferents under the same stimulation.

The monosynaptic flexor reflex is depressed by fastigial stimulation and this depression is also associated with PAD in the group Ia afferents from flexor muscles. It is of interest however that the depression of the monosynaptic flexor reflex lasts longer than that of the PAD in the corresponding Ia afferents. This effect may be explained by the occurrence of some postsynaptic inhibitory effect.

Stimulation of the rostral fastigial nucleus was not attempted in our experiments since contamination by the long inhibitory corticofugal fibers directed to the vestibular nuclei may occur in these experiments. It is likely but not crucially proved that the uncrossed fastigio-vestibular projection, which originates mainly upon the rostral part of the fastigial nucleus, is also able to influence the primary afferents in the same way as the crossed fastigio-vestibular projection which originates from the caudal part of the fastigial nucleus.

EFFECTS ON MOTONEURONS EVOKED FROM THE VERMAL CORTEX
OF THE CEREBELLUM

It is known that high-frequency electrical stimulation of the vermal cortex of the anterior lobe in a decerebrate animal results in inhibition of the rigidity in the ipsilateral limbs, followed by extensor rebound. After selective lesions of the rostrolateral part of the fastigial nucleus Moruzzi and Pompeiano (1954, 1957a) found that stimulation of the ipsilateral vermis of the anterior lobe did dot yield the typical inhibition of the extensor rigidity in the ipsilateral limbs. The same lesion also produced a postural asymmetry characterized by an ipsilateral increase (and contralateral decrease) of the extensor rigidity (Fig. 1A, B) (Batini and Pompeiano, 1958). This is interpreted as being due to interruption of the cerebellar inhibitory pathways. Since the long corticofugal fibers to the vestibular nuclei, particularly to Deiters' nucleus, from the vermal cortex of the anterior lobe pass through the rostrolateral part of the fastigial nucleus (Walberg and Jansen, 1961), it has been suggested that the long cerebellar cortico-vestibular fibers are inhibitory on Deiters' nucleus thus leading to suppression of the decerebrate rigidity (Brodal, et al., 1962). Observations made by Ito and co-workers (Ito and Kawai, 1964; Ito et al., 1964a, 1965, 1966, 1968a, b, 1969; Ito and Yoshida, 1964, 1966; Eccles et al., 1967; Ito, 1968, 1970, 1972) have clearly shown that stimulation of the vermis of the anterior lobe gives monosynaptic IPSP's in Deiters' cells.

The collapse of the extensor rigidity induced by high-frequency stimulation of the anterior lobe is due to inhibition of Deiters' nucleus, which is responsible for decere-

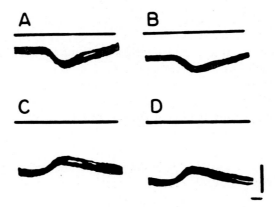

Fig. 6. Absence of reversal of the increase in membrane potential due to cerebellar inhibition during the flow of inward current. A: inhibitory postsynaptic potential recorded from a biceps-semitendinosus motoneuron following stimulation of the quadriceps nerve. Cerebellar inhibition increases the membrane potential (B). In C and D a steady inward current is applied so that a reversal of the inhibitory postsynaptic potential into a depolarizing one is obtained. Cerebellar inhibitory stimulation applied in this condition still increases the membrane potential. The top line is only a reference, and the major displacement in d.c. potential between the upper and the lower pairs of records is not a measure of the hyperpolarization of the membrane due to the flow of inward current. Time: 1 msec. Calibration: 5 mV. From Terzuolo (1959).

brate rigidity. Recent studies using intracellular recording seem to support this hypothesis. It has been observed that stimulation of the vermal cortex of the cerebellum produces hyperpolarization of the membrane of the motoneurons (Terzuolo, 1959; Llinás, 1964), and that this increase in membrane potential is not reversed by passing a hyperpolarizing current through the membrane (Fig. 6), nor is it associated with the conductance changes typical of the IPSPs. The conclusion from these observations was that the cerebellar inhibition is due to suppression of tonic excitatory influences acting upon the motoneurons. Since Deiters' nucleus exerts a monosynaptic excitatory influence on extensor motoneurons (Lund and Pompeiano, 1965, 1968), it has been concluded that the inhibition of the decerebrate rigidity induced by cerebellar stimulation is due to disfacilitation of the extensor motoneurons as a consequence of an abrupt suppression of the vestibulospinal excitatory impingement (Pompeiano, 1967).

PRIMARY AFFERENT HYPERPOLARIZATION EVOKED FROM THE VERMAL CORTEX OF THE CEREBELLUM

Experiments made by Carpenter et al. (1966) have shown that negative DRPs can be evoked from the cerebellar cortex of the anterior lobe and that PAD in group I*b* and cutaneous afferents are responsible for the DRPs. These effects were produced by stimulation of the most lateral strip of the intermediate region on either side. Since this cortical area projects to the interpositus nucleus these effects would not be relayed through the vestibular nuclei. On the other hand no effect on the primary afferents was evoked from the anterior vermis, whereas there was a profound inhibition of ipsilateral extensor motoneurons. The results of these experiments lead to the conclusion that the vermal cortex of the cerebellar anterior lobe does not affect presynaptic transmission through the group I*a* muscle fibers.

It has already been shown that the fastigial nuclei are able to affect the transmission through the I*a* pathway (Cook *et al.*, 1968c; Cangiano *et al.*, 1969a). This effect has been attributed to excitation of the vestibular nuclei and of the descending reticular system, which is also excited by the vestibular nuclei. Since both the fastigial nuclei and the vestibular nuclei are under the control of the cerebellar efferent projections originating from the vermal cortex (Brodal *et al.*, 1962), it was difficult to understand why stimulation of this cortical region was unable to affect the primary afferents. Therefore, experiments were performed to study the effects of stimulation of the cerebellar cortex of the anterior vermis not only on the level of polarization of the intraspinal terminals of the primary afferents, but also on the PAD induced reflexly by orthodromic stimulation of the VIII nerve (Cook *et al.*, 1968c; Cangiano *et al.* 1969b).

Repetitive stimulation of the vermal cortex of the cerebellar anterior lobe performed in precollicular decerebrate cats elicited a *positive* DRP in the ipsilateral dorsal roots of the lumbar cord (Fig. 7). This effect, however, was observed only in some preparations. These positive DRPs were evoked from the medial part of the vermal cortex at stimulus intensities which were effective in evoking DRPs of the opposite polarity from the lateralmost regions of the anterior lobe. The threshold intensity responsible for the positive DRP was always lower than the threshold for the inhibition of the decerebrate rigidity. At the higher intensities of stimulation, the hyperpolarization was followed by a rebound depolarization (Fig. 7). These effects occurred at a threshold frequency of 100–200 per sec and increased with high frequency stimulation of the vermal cortex.

It is generally assumed that the positive DRP is caused by a hyperpolarization of primary afferent terminals. Evidence will by presented indicating that the above

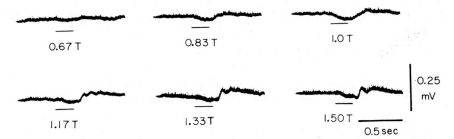

Fig. 7. Positive DRPs evoked from the vermal cortex of the anterior cerebellar lobe. Activity recorded from the most caudal dorsal rootlet of L6 on the left side during stimulation of the ipsilateral vermis of the anterior lobe (with 200 msec trains of 0.2 msec rectangular pulses at 500/sec and different intensities of stimulation, as indicated at the bottom of each record). Cerebellar stimulation elicited hyperpolarization of the central endings of the primary afferents which outlasted the duration of the stimulus (indicated by the horizontal bar). For stimulus intensities at or above the threshold for the inhibition of the ipsilateral decerebrate rigidity (1.0 T), the positive DRP is followed by a negative DRP. From Cangiano, Cook and Pompeiano (1969b).

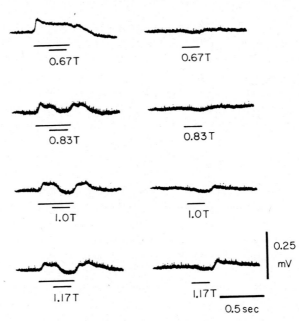

Fig. 8. Inhibition of the negative DRP evoked from the VIII cranial nerve by stimulation of the vermal cortex of the anterior cerebellar lobe. The right column shows the effects of stimulation of the left anterior vermal cortex (with 200 msec trains of 0.2 msec pulses, at 500/sec) on the most caudal dorsal rootlet of L6 on the left side. The strength is indicated for each record in multiples of the threshold (T) responsible for the inhibition of the ipsilateral decerebrate rigidity.

In the left column the same strengths of cerebellar stimulation were applied on a background of negative DRP elicited from the left VIII nerve ipsilateral to the recording side. In each record the VIII nerve was stimulated with 400 msec trains (0.2 msec pulses, 500/sec) at 5.0 times the threshold (T) for the ascending MLF response. The upper and lower horizontal lines below each record indicate the duration of the train of stimuli applied respectively to the VIII nerve and the cerebellum. From Cangiano, Cook and Pompeiano (1969b).

described primary afferent hyperpolarization (PAH) results from inhibition of the vestibular nuclei and suppression of tonic PAD generated by these nuclei. It is very likely that stimulation of the cerebellar vermis evokes PAH only in those decerebrate cats in which there is a large amount of tonic background activity in the vestibular and reticular system leading to tonic depolarization of the terminals.

To create a tonic depolarization of the central terminals of primary afferents on which to test the effects of cerebellar stimulation, the VIII nerve was repetitively stimulated. It has been a regular finding that the negative DRPs evoked from the VIII nerve can be depressed by stimulation of the vermal cortex of the anterior lobe (Fig. 8 left column). This effect occurred either when threshold stimulation of the cerebellar vermis did not evoke any DRP or when stimulation evoked a positive DRP (Fig. 8 right column). It is clear from the records in this figure that the inhibition of the negative DRPs evoked from the VIII cranial nerve did not result from an algebraic summation of the negative and positive DRPs.

Experiments with excitability measurements from different types of afferents have shown that stimulation of the vermal cortex of the anterior lobe did not change the excitability of the central endings of the group I muscular afferents of the GS nerve (Fig. 9A). On the other hand the facilitation of the antidromic group I volley induced by conditioning stimulation of the ipsilateral VIII nerve was depressed during stimulation of the cerebellar inhibitory area (Fig. 9**B**). Similar effects were also obtained on cutaneous afferents. It appears, therefore, that stimulation of the vermal cortex of the anterior lobe produces a repolarization of the types of primary afferents depolarized from the VIII nerve volleys.

We should recall here that repetitive stimulation of the left VIII nerve elicits not only DRPs but also muscle contraction in the ipsilateral hindlimb muscles (Cook

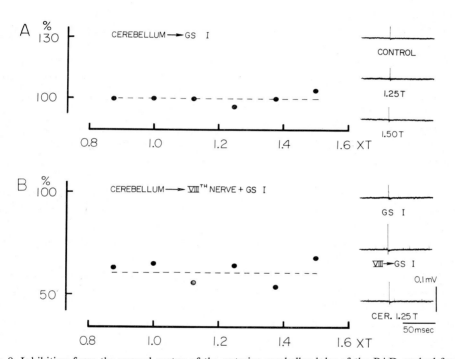

Fig. 9. Inhibition from the vermal cortex of the anterior cerebellar lobe of the PAD evoked from the VIII cranial nerve in group I muscular afferents. A: Diagram showing the excitability changes of the group I muscle afferents produced by cerebellar stimulation. The left cerebellum was stimulated with 400 msec trains of 0.5 msec rectangular pulses at 500/sec. The intensities are indicated in multiples of the threshold (T) responsible for the inhibition of the ipsilateral decerebrate rigidity. The changes in excitability in group I muscle afferents were judged from the traces in which the terminals of group I afferents were stimulated through a microelectrode inserted in the GS motor nucleus and the antidromic discharge recorded peripherally in the GS nerve. The diagram shows no change in the excitability of the tested terminals for intensities of cerebellar stimulation ranging from 0.88 to 1.50 T. B: Diagram showing the effects of cerebellar stimulation on the facilitated antidromic group I volley induced by stimulation of the VIII nerve. 100 percent on the ordinates refers to the amplitude of facilitated antidromic responses. The antidromic group I volley recorded from the gastrocnemius-soleus nerve (GS I) was facilitated by repetitive stimulation of the ipsilateral VIII nerve with 400 msec trains (0.2 msec pulses, 500/sec) at 3.5 times the threshold for the ascending MLF response (VIII → GS I). This effect was depressed by stimulating the anterior cerebellar lobe at the indicated strengths. Samples of the records plotted in the two diagrams are illustrated in the right side. From Cangiano, Cook and Pompeiano (1969b).

et al., 1969a). While the resulting muscle tension is produced by labyrinthine activation of Deiters' nucleus, the DRPs are mainly due to excitation of the medial and descending vestibular nuclei (Barnes and Pompeiano, 1970a, b). It would be of interest to know whether the DRP and muscle tension are equally or differentially affected by the cerebellar stimulation. Our experiments indicate that the evoked tension is more sensitive to the cerebellar inhibition than the DRP. In fact when the intensity of the cerebellar stimuli was increased to 1.13 and 1.25 T, the muscle tension produced by VIII nerve stimulation was almost completely abolished, while the DRP was only partially depressed.

The problem of the cerebellar inhibitory control of the vestibular reflex pathways to primary afferents has been studied not only with stimulation but also with ablation experiments. The negative DRPs elicited by repetitive stimulation of the VIII nerve were greatly enhanced following cerebellar ablation. Fig. 10 shows that cerebellar lesions decrease the threshold frequency required to elicit the DRPs. There is also an increase in the slope of the curve obtained by plotting the amplitudes of the DRPs as a function of the frequency of stimulation applied to the VIII nerve. The critical region responsible for this effect was the vermal cortex of the anterior lobe. Ablation of the intermediate cortex of the anterior lobe or total cerebellectomy did not further increase the amplitude of the DRP. These results suggested that the vermal cortex of the anterior lobe exerts a tonic inhibitory control of the vestibular reflex arc affecting the primary afferents.

Experiments were also performed to find out whether this tonic inhibitory control from the cerebellum affects the vestibular influences on group I muscle afferents. Indeed it was found that the facilitatory effect of conditioning stimulation of the VIII nerve on the antidromic group I volley recorded from the GS nerve was increased after complete cerebellectomy. On the contrary the increased excitability of the group I afferents from the same GS nerve induced by repetitive stimulation of the hamstring nerve was not modified after the cerebellar ablation. This observation further indicates that the cerebellar inhibitory effect on PAD is not exerted at spinal cord level but through the vestibular systems. This inhibitory control is tonic in nature.

In summary the experimental evidence indicates that the vermal cortex of the cerebellar anterior lobe affects primary afferent transmission. While in some of our experiments stimulation of the anterior vermis for the same intensities which inhibited the decerebrate rigidity did not evoke any DRP (*cf.* also Carpenter *et al.*, 1966), in other instances stimulation of the vermal cortex of the anterior lobe resulted in a positive DRP. One may assume that stimulation of the cerebellar vermis of the anterior lobe produces PAH only in those instances in which the spontaneous activity of the supraspinal vestibular and reticular centers responsible for PAD is present. This PAH would then be attributed to cerebellar inhibition of the supraspinal structures exerting some tonic depolarizing influence on the primary afferents.

The results of our stimulation experiments should be correlated with those in which the cerebellum was removed. It is known that decerebrate rigidity is released by complete cerebellectomy or ablation of the vermal cortex of the anterior lobe (*cf.* Batini *et al.*, 1956, 1957; Brodal *et al.*, 1962). The membrane potential of the α-moto-

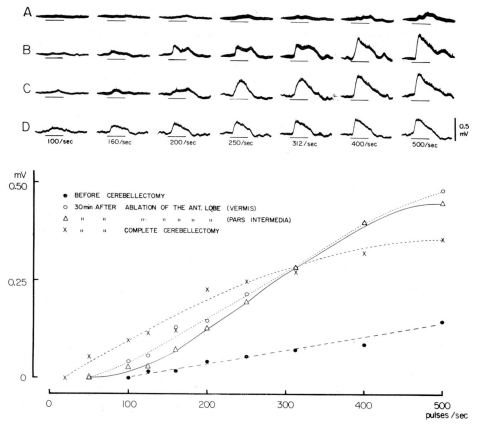

Fig. 10. Effects of cerebellar ablation on the negative DRPs evoked from the VIII cranial nerve. The ipsilateral VIII nerve was stimulated through the experiment with 400 msec trains (0.2 msec pulses, 1.08 T) at the indicated frequencies of stimulation. The horizontal lines below each record indicate the timing and the duration (400 msec) of the train of stimuli applied to the VIII nerve. A: negative DRPs recorded from a decerebrate cat with the cerebellum intact. B: records taken 30 min after bilateral ablation of the vermal cortex of the anterior lobe. C: records taken 30 min after additional bilateral ablation of the intermediate cortex of the anterior lobe. D: the animal was then submitted to complete cerebellectomy. The records were taken 30 min after this lesion. The results obtained have been plotted in the diagram where each point is the average of three responses. The cerebellar lesions decreased the threshold frequency which was effective for eliciting the DRPs and increased the slope of the curve obtained by plotting the amplitudes of the responses (mV) as a function of the frequency of stimulation applied to the VIII nerve (pulses/sec). From Cangiano, Cook and Pompeiano (1969b).

neurons actually depolarizes 10–15 mV during 'release' obtained by removal of tonic inhibition from the cerebellum (Gidlöf, 1968). In our experiments we were unable to show excitability changes of the primary afferents after cerebellar ablation. Investigations made on a larger material would probably have shown, in agreement with stimulation experiments, that at least in some instances the cerebellar ablation might lead to a decrease in membrane potential of the terminal arborizations, due to release of the supraspinal structures exerting a tonic depolarizing influence on the primary afferents.

Experiments were then performed to find out whether there is a direct control of the cerebellum on the vestibular reflex paths to primary afferents. The results reported previously clearly demonstrated that the PAD evoked from the VIII nerve is depressed by the vermal cortex of the anterior lobe. Indeed, in some experiments cerebellar stimulation elicited a positivity of the terminal arborizations, not only with respect to the peak of the large negative DRP produced by labyrinthine volleys, but also with respect to the baseline observed just before labyrinthine stimulation. It is of interest that cerebellar stimulation suppressed the PAD in the group I muscle and the cutaneous afferents elicited by repetitive stimulation of the VIII nerve. Just the opposite effects were obtained following cerebellar ablation.

The cerebellar inhibitory influence on the vestibular mechanisms controlling the primary afferents is part of a more extensive control inhibiting the transmission of labyrinthine volleys to the spinal motoneurons. It is of interest that stimulation of the cerebellar vermis of the anterior lobe with stimulus intensities responsible for inhibition of the decerebrate rigidity abolishes not only the negative DRP but also the contraction of extensor muscles produced by VIII nerve stimulation. It is very likely that both these effects are due to inhibitory control exerted from the cerebellar cortex of the anterior lobe on the vestibular neurons. It is known that stimulation of the vermal cortex of the anterior lobe inhibits not only the spontaneous (de Vito et al., 1956; Pompeiano and Cotti, 1959a), but also the reflex discharge of the vestibular neurons induced by labyrinthine volleys (Pompeiano and Cotti, 1959b, 1960).

An alternative, although not exclusive, explanation is that the cerebellar inhibitory effect is exerted on the fastigial nuclei. It has already been shown that fastigial stimulation produces both contraction of extensor muscles as well as PAD in different systems of primary afferents including the group I muscular and the cutaneous afferents (Cangiano et al., 1969a) and that the activity of the fastigial nuclei can be inhibited by cerebellar stimulation (cf. Brodal et al., 1962). Recent experiments indicate that the Purkinje neurons from the vermis of the anterior lobe produce monosynaptic inhibitory postsynaptic potentials on their target cells located both in the vestibular and the fastigial nuclei (Ito and Kawai 1964; Ito et al., 1964a, b, 1965, 1966, 1968a, b, 1969, 1970b; Ito and Yoshida, 1964, 1966; Eccles et al., 1967; Ito, 1968, 1970, 1972).

Since it appears that neurons in the medial and the lateral vestibular systems influence the primary afferents and the motoneurons, respectively (Pompeiano, 1972), one may suggest that the cerebellar inhibitory control of the vestibular reflex path to primary afferents is exerted through the medial vestibular nucleus, while the cerebellar inhibitory control of the vestibular reflex path to motoneurons is exerted through Deiters' nucleus.

It should be mentioned that the medial vestibular nucleus which controls transmission in the primary afferents seems to receive relatively smaller amount of inhibition from the cerebellar cortex of the anterior vermis than the lateral vestibular nucleus which controls the spinal motoneurons. Since there is both anatomical and physiological evidence indicating that the primary vestibular afferents originating from different receptor organs (the maculae and the cristae) are distributed to particular subdivisions of the vestibular complex, one may conclude that the inhibitory volleys originating from the vermal cortex of the anterior lobe may affect both the labyrinthine positional reflexes as well as the labyrinthine acceleratory reflexes. In the first instance the cerebellar efferent volleys would produce an hyperpolarization of the extensor motoneurons due to suppression of the tonic excitatory influences mediated by Deiters' nucleus. In the second instance the cerebellar efferent volleys would produce a repolarization of the terminal arborization of the primary afferents due to suppression of the depolarizing influence on the primary afferents mediated by the medial vestibular nucleus. The resulting increase in membrane potential of the primary endings would then increase the postsynaptic effectiveness of the orthodromic spinal impulses to the motoneurons. Just the opposite effects would appear in cerebellectomized preparations; in these cases the increase in responsiveness of the vestibular neurons to labyrinthine volleys due to removal of the cerebellar inhibitory pathways, will lead to an enhancement of the depolarizing influences exerted from the different receptor organs (the maculae and the cristae) on spinal motoneurons and primary afferents respectively. The resulting decrease in membrane potential of the primary endings would then decrease the postsynaptic effect of arriving impulses, thus leading to presynaptic inhibition.

SUMMARY

Stimulation of the fastigial nucleus produces not only contraction of the extensor muscles, but also *negative* dorsal root potentials (DRPs) in the lumbar cord. These DRPs are due to depolarization of the terminal arborizations of the primary afferents and involve the group Ia pathway from both extensor and flexor muscles as well as the cutaneous afferents. The fastigial influence on the extensor muscles is mediated via the lateral vestibular nucleus, which is known to exert a facilitatory influence on the extensor motoneurons. On the other hand the medial vestibular nucleus is, in part at least, involved in the transmission of the fastigial influence on primary afferents.

Stimulation of the vermal cortex of the cerebellar anterior lobe with the same intensities which inhibit the decerebrate rigidity may evoke *positive* DRPs in the lumbar cord. The same stimulation is also able to suppress the depolarization in the group Ia muscle and the cutaneous afferents elicited by stimulation of the VIII nerve.

Since it appears that neurons in the lateral and the medial vestibular nuclei influence the motoneurons and the primary afferents respectively, it is concluded that the cerebellar inhibitory control of the vestibular reflex path to motoneurons is exerted through the lateral vestibular nucleus, while the cerebellar inhibitory control of the vestibular reflex path to primary afferents is exerted through the medial vestibular nucleus.

ACKNOWLEDGEMENTS

This work was supported by P.H.S. Research Grant NB 07685-03 from the National Institute of Neurological Diseases and Blindness, N.I.H., Public Health Service, U.S.A. and by a research grant from the Consiglio Nazionale delle Ricerche, Italia.

References pp. 408–410

REFERENCES

BARNES, C. D. AND POMPEIANO, O. (1969) Dissociation of spinal cord effects produced by vestibular volleys. *Physiologist*, **12**, 168.

BARNES, C. D. AND POMPEIANO, O. (1970a) The contribution of the medial and lateral vestibular nuclei to presynaptic and postsynaptic effects produced in the lumbar cord by vestibular volleys. *Pflügers Arch. ges. Physiol.*, **317**, 1–9.

BARNES, C. D. AND POMPEIANO, O. (1970b) Dissociation of presynaptic and postsynaptic effects produced in the lumbar cord by vestibular volleys. *Arch. ital. Biol.*, **108**, 295–324.

BATINI, C., MORUZZI, G. AND POMPEIANO, O. (1956) The release phenomena following cerebellectomy. *Proc. XX int. Congr. physiol. Sci., Bruxelles*, 70–71.

BATINI, C., MORUZZI, G. AND POMPEIANO, O. (1957) Cerebellar release phenomena. *Arch. ital. Biol.*, **95**, 71–95.

BATINI, C. E POMPEIANO, O. (1955) Sugli effetti di distruzioni croniche, parziali o totali, del nucleo del tetto nel gatto. *Boll. Soc. ital. Biol. sper.*, **31**, 805–807.

BATINI, C. AND POMPEIANO, O. (1957) Chronic fastigial lesions and their compensation in the cat. *Arch. ital. Biol.*, **95**, 147–165.

BATINI, C. AND POMPEIANO, O. (1958) Effects of rostro-medial and rostro-lateral fastigial lesions on decerebrate rigidity. *Arch. ital. Biol.*, **96**, 315–329.

BRODAL, A. POMPEIANO, O. AND WALBERG, F. (1962) *The Vestibular Nuclei and Their Connections. Anatomy and Functional Correlations.* Oliver and Boyd, Edinburgh, London, pp. VIII–193.

CANGIANO, A., COOK, W. A. JR. AND POMPEIANO, O. (1969a) Primary afferent depolarization in the lumbar cord evoked from the fastigial nucleus. *Arch. ital. Biol.*, **107**, 321–340.

CANGIANO, A., COOK W. A. JR. AND POMPEIANO, O. (1969b) Cerebellar inhibitory control of the vestibular reflex pathways to primary afferents. *Arch. ital. Biol.*, **107**, 341–364.

CARPENTER, D., ENGBERG, I., FUNKENSTEIN, H. AND LUNDBERG, A. (1963) Decerebrate control of reflexes to primary afferents. *Acta physiol. scand.*, **59**, 424–437.

CARPENTER, D., ENGBERG, I. AND LUNDBERG. A. (1966) Primary afferent depolarization evoked from the brain stem and the cerebellum. *Arch. ital. Biol.*, **104**, 73–85.

COHEN, D., CHAMBERS, W. W. AND SPRAGUE, J. M. (1958) Experimental study of the efferent projections from the cerebellar nuclei to the brainstem of the cat. *J. comp. Neurol.*, **109**, 233–259.

COOK, W. A. JR., CANGIANO, A. AND POMPEIANO, O. (1968a) Vestibular evoked primary afferent depolarization in the lumbar spinal cord. *Proc. XXIV int. Congr. physiol. Sci., Washington, D.C.*, VII, n. 272, 91.

COOK, W. A. JR., CANGIANO, A. AND POMPEIANO, O. (1968b) Vestibular influences on primary afferents in the spinal cord. *Pflügers Arch. ges. Physiol.*, **299**, 334–338.

COOK, W. A. JR., CANGIANO, A. E POMPEIANO, O. (1968c) Controllo cerebellare sulla trasmissione di impulsi spinali lungo le fibre afferenti muscolari di gruppo I. *Boll. Soc. ital. Biol. sper.*, 44, fasc. **20** bis, 85.

COOK, W. A. JR., CANGIANO, A. AND POMPEIANO, O. (1969a) Dorsal root potentials in the lumbar cord evoked from the vestibular system. *Arch. ital. Biol.*, **107**, 275–295.

COOK, W. A. JR., CANGIANO, A. AND POMPEIANO, O. (1969b) Vestibular control of transmission in primary afferents to the lumbar spinal cord. *Arch. ital. Biol.*, **107**, 296–320.

ECCLES, J. C. (1961) The mechanisms of synaptic transmission. *Ergebn. Physiol.*, **51**, 299–430.

ECCLES, J. C., ITO, M. AND SZENTÁGOTHAI, J. (1967) *The Cerebellum as a Neuronal Machine.* Springer-Berlin, Heidelberg, New York, pp. 335

FRANK, K. AND FUORTES, M. G. F. (1957) Presynaptic and postsynaptic inhibition of monosynaptic reflexes. *Fed. Proc.*, **16**, 39–40.

GIDLÖF, A. (1968) Intracellular aspects of 'release' phenomena in α-extensor motoneurones of the cat. *Acta physiol. scand.*, **68**, suppl. 277, 58.

HOLMQVIST, B. AND LUNDBERG, A. (1961) Differential supraspinal control of synaptic actions evoked by volleys in the flexion reflex afferents in alpha motoneurones. *Acta physiol. scand.*, **54**, suppl. 186, 1–51.

HOWLAND, B., LETTVIN, J. Y., McCULLOCH, W. S., PITTS, W. H. AND WALL, P. D. (1955) Reflex inhibition by dorsal root interaction. *J. Neurophysiol.*, **18**, 1–17.

ITO, M. (1968) Two extensive inhibitory systems for brain stem nuclei. In C. VON EULER, S. SKOGLUND AND U. SÖDERBERG (Eds.), *Structure and Function of Inhibitory Neuronal Mechanisms.* Pergamon Press, Oxford, pp. 309–322.

ITO, M. (1970) The cerebellovestibular interaction in the cat's vestibular nuclei neurons. In *Fourth Symposium on the Role of the Vestibular organs in Space Exploration. NASA SP*–187, 183–199.

ITO, M. (1972) Cerebellar control of the vestibular neurones: physiology and pharmacology. In A. BRODAL AND O. POMPEIANO (Eds.), *Progress in Brain Research. Vol. 37. Basic aspects of central vestibular mechanisms*. Elsevier, Amsterdam, pp. 377–390.

ITO, M., HONGO, T. AND OKADA, Y. (1969) Vestibular-evoked postsynaptic potentials in Deiters' neurones. *Exp. Brain Res.*, **7**, 214–230.

ITO, M. AND KAWAI, N. (1964) IPSP-receptive field in the cerebellum for Deiters' neurones. *Proc. Jap. Acad.*, **40**, 762–764.

ITO, M., KAWAI, N. AND UDO, M. (1965) The origin of cerebellar-induced inhibition and facilitation in the neurones of Deiters' and intracerebellar nuclei. *Proc. XXIII int. Congr. physiol. Sci., Tokyo*, 997.

ITO, M., KAWAI, N. AND UDO, M. (1968a) The origin of cerebellar-induced inhibition of Deiters' neurones. III. Distribution of the inhibitory zone. *Exp. Brain Res.*, **4**, 310–320.

ITO, M., KAWAI, N., UDO, M. AND SATO, N. (1968b) Cerebellar-evoked disinhibition in dorsal Deiters neurones. *Exp. Brain Res.*, **6**, 247–264.

ITO, M., OBATA, K. AND OCHI, R. (1964a) Initiation of IPSP in Deiters' and fastigial neurones associated with the activity of cerebellar Purkinje cells. *Proc. Jap. Acad.*, **40**, 765–768.

ITO, M., OBATA, K. AND OCHI, R. (1966) The origin of cerebellar-evoked inhibition of Deiters neurones. II. Temporal correlation between the transsynaptic activation of Purkinje cells and the inhibition of Deiters' neurones. *Exp. Brain Res.*, **2**, 350–364.

ITO, M., UDO, M., MANO, N. AND KAWAI, N. (1970a) Synaptic action of the fastigiobulbar impulses upon neurones in the medullary reticular formation and vestibular nuclei. *Exp. Brain Res.*, **11**, 29–47.

ITO, M. AND YOSHIDA, M. (1964) The cerebellar-evoked monosynaptic inhibition of Deiters' neurones. *Experientia (Basel)*, **20**, 515–516.

ITO, M. AND YOSHIDA, M. (1966) The origin of cerebellar-induced inhibition of Deiters neurones. I. Monosynaptic initiation of the inhibitory postsynaptic potentials. *Exp. Brain Res.*, **2**, 330–349.

ITO, M., YOSHIDA, M. AND OBATA, K. (1964b) Monosynaptic inhibition of the intracellular nuclei induced from the cerebellar cortex. *Experientia (Basel)*, **20**, 575–576.

ITO, M., YOSHIDA, M., OBATA, K., KAWAI, N. AND UDO, M. (1970b) Inhibitory control of intracerebellar nuclei by the Purkinje cell axons. *Exp. Brain Res.*, **10**, 64–80.

JANSEN, J. AND JANSEN, J. K. S. (1955) On the efferent fibers of the cerebellar nuclei in the cat. *J. comp. Neurol.*, **102**, 607–623.

KUNO, M. AND PERL, E. R. (1960) Alteration of spinal reflexes by interaction with suprasegmental and dorsal root activity. *J. Physiol. (Lond.)*, **151**, 103–122.

LLINÁS, R. (1964) Mechanisms of supraspinal actions upon spinal cord activities. Differences between reticular and cerebellar inhibitory actions upon alpha extensor motoneurons. *J. Neurophysiol.*, **27**, 1117–1126.

LUND, S. AND POMPEIANO, O. (1965) Descending pathways with monosynaptic action on motoneurones. *Experientia (Basel)*, **21**, 602–603.

LUND, S. AND POMPEIANO, O. (1968) Monosynaptic excitation of alpha motoneurones from supraspinal structures in the cat. *Acta physiol. scand.*, **73**, 1–21.

MENDELL, L. M. AND WALL, P. D. (1964) Presynaptic hyperpolarization: a role for fine afferent fibres. *J. Physiol. (Lond.)*, **172**, 274–294.

MORUZZI, G. E POMPEIANO, O. (1954) Inversione dell'inibizione paleocerebellare prodotta dalla distruzione parziale del nucleo del tetto. *Boll. Soc. ital. Biol. Sper.*, **30**, 493–494.

MORUZZI, G. E POMPEIANO, O. (1955) Influenze cerebellari crociate sul tono posturale. *Rend. Accad. naz. Lincei, Cl. Sci. fis., mat. nat., Ser. VIII*, **18**, 420–424.

MORUZZI, G. AND POMPEIANO, O. (1956a) Crossed fastigial atonia. *Experientia (Basel)*, **12**, 35.

MORUZZI, G. AND POMPEIANO, O. (1956b) Crossed fastigial influence on decerebrate rigidity. *J. comp. Neurol.*, **106**, 371–392.

MORUZZI, G. AND POMPEIANO, O. (1957a) Effects of vermal stimulation after fastigial lesions. *Arch. ital. Biol.*, **95**, 31–55.

MORUZZI, G. AND POMPEIANO, O. (1957b) Inhibitory mechanisms underlying the collapse of decerebrate rigidity after unilateral fastigial lesions. *J. comp. Neurol.*, **107**, 1–25.

POMPEIANO, O. (1961) Organizzazione somatotopica delle risposte posturali alla stimolazione e alla distruzione della parte caudale del nucleo del tetto. *Boll. Soc. ital. Biol. sper.*, **37**, 916–918.

POMPEIANO, O. (1962) Somatotopic organization of the postural responses to stimulation and destruction of the caudal part of the fastigial nucleus. *Arch. ital. Biol.*, **100**, 259–271.

POMPEIANO, O. (1967) Functional organization of the cerebellar projections to the spinal cord. In C. A. FOX AND R. S. SNIDER (Eds.), *Progress in Brain Research. Vol. 25. The cerebellum.* Elsevier, Amsterdam, pp. 282–321.

POMPEIANO, O. (1972) Vestibulospinal relations: vestibular influences on gamma motoneurons and primary afferents. In A. BRODAL AND O. POMPEIANO (Eds.), *Progress in Brain Research. Vol. 37. Basic aspects of central vestibular mechanisms.* Elsevier, Amsterdam, pp. 197–232.

POMPEIANO, O. E COTTI, E. (1959a) Analisi microelettrodica delle proiezioni cerebello-deitersiane. *Arch. Sci. biol. (Bologna)*, **43**, 57–101.

POMPEIANO, O. E COTTI, E. (1959b) Inibizione cerebellare delle risposte di unità deitersiane a stimolazioni labirintiche. *Rend. Accad. naz. Lincei, Cl. Sci. fis., mat. nat., Ser. VIII*, **27**, 238–241.

POMPEIANO, O. E COTTI, E. (1960) Effetti della stimolazione corticocerebellare sull'attività di singole unità deitersiane provocata da stimolazioni labirintiche. *Boll. Soc. ital. Biol. sper.*, **36**, 303–304.

POMPEIANO, O. AND MORRISON, A. R. (1966) Vestibular influences during sleep. III. Dissociation of the tonic and phasic inhibition of spinal reflexes during desynchronized sleep following vestibular lesions. *Arch. ital. Biol.*, **104**, 231–246.

TERZUOLO, C. A. (1959) Cerebellar inhibitory and excitatory actions upon spinal extensor motoneurons. *Arch. ital. Biol.*, **97**, 316–339.

VITO, R. V. DE, BRUSA, A. AND ARDUINI, A. (1956) Cerebellar and vestibular influences on Deitersian units. *J. Neurophysiol.*, **19**, 241–253.

WALBERG, F. AND JANSEN, J. (1961) Cerebellar corticovestibular fibers in the cat. *Exp. Neurol.*, **3**, 32–52.

WALBERG, F., POMPEIANO, O., BRODAL, A. AND JANSEN, J. (1962a) The fastigiovestibular projection in the cat. An experimental study with silver impregnation methods. *J. comp. Neurol.*, **118**, 49–75.

WALBERG, F., POMPEIANO, O., WESTRUM, L. E. AND HAUGLIE-HANSSEN, E. (1962b) Fastigioreticular fibers in the cat. An experimental study with silver methods. *J. comp. Neurol.*, **119**, 187–200.

WALL, P. D. (1964) Control of impulses at the first central synapse in cutaneous pathways. In J. C. ECCLES AND J. P. SCHADÉ (Eds.), *Progress in Brain Research. Vol. 12. Physiology of spinal neurones.* Elsevier, Amsterdam, pp. 92–118.

WALL, P. D., MC CULLOCH, W. S., LETTVIN, J. Y. AND PITTS, W. H. (1955) Factors limiting the maximum impulse transmitting ability of an afferent system of nerve fibres. In *Third London Symposium on Information Theory*, Butterworth, London, pp. 329–344.

Cerebellar Control of the Vestibular Pathways to Oculomotor Neurons

B. COHEN AND S. M. HIGHSTEIN

*Department of Neurology, Mount Sinai School of Medicine, New York, N.Y., U.S.A. and
Department of Physiology, Faculty of Medicine, University of Tokyo, Hongo, Bunkyo-ku, Tokyo,
Japan*

Two questions will be considered in this review: (*i*) Does the cerebellum participate in oculomotor function, whether vestibular or non-vestibular? (*ii*) What role does the cerebellum play in control of vestibulo-ocular reflexes?

CEREBELLAR PARTICIPATION IN OCULOMOTOR FUNCTION

Anatomic evidence

Carpenter and Strominger (1964) have shown that there are direct cerebello-oculomotor fibers in the brachium conjunctivum. These fibers originate in the dentate nucleus and project to the III nerve nucleus. These are the only known direct motor fibers from the cerebellum. In mammals direct cerebello-oculomotor fibers in the brachium conjunctivum do not originate in the cerebellar cortex, although in the fish Purkinje cell axons project directly on to oculomotor neurons, mediating inhibition (Kidokoro, 1968),

Eye muscle motor nuclei which receive direct cerebellar projections cause the eyes to move up, and rotate (Warwick, 1964). There are no direct cerebellar projections to the abducens nucleus, to the ventral cell group of the oculomotor nucleus which innervates the medial rectus muscle, or to the MLF. Therefore, direct cerebello-oculomotor projections are related to eye movement in planes of space other than horizontal. However, there are also cerebellar projections from the fastigial nuclei through the uncinate fasciculus and juxta-restiform body to regions of the pontine reticular formation (Carpenter *et al.*, 1958; Carpenter, 1959; Walberg *et al.*, 1962b), and vestibular nuclei (Dow, 1936; Jansen and Brodal, 1954; Brodal *et al.*, 1962; Voogd, 1964; Angaut and Brodal, 1967), which project to oculomotor nuclei (McMasters *et al.*, 1966; Tarlov, 1970). These regions, particularly the pontine tegmentum (Bender and Shanzer, 1964; Cohen *et al.*, 1968; Goebel *et al.*, 1971; Cohen, 1971), could cause the eyes to move horizontally.

References pp. 422–425

Stimulation studies

Ferrier (1876) first demonstrated that electrical stimulation of the cerebellar cortex induced eye movements in different spatial planes in a number of mammalian species. Eye movements have also been induced by cerebellar stimulation by Bárány (1914), Hoshino (1921), Mussen (1934), Koella (1955, 1962), Cohen et al. (1965a), and others. In cats horizontal eye muscles were activated at short latencies and high frequencies by stimulation in the region of the fastigial nuclei (Fig. 1A, B; Cohen et al., 1965a).

Stimulation of different parts of the cerebellum induced eye movements in different spatial planes. These eye movements were similar to those induced by semicircular canal nerve (Cohen et al., 1964, 1965b, 1966; Suzuki and Cohen, 1964; Suzuki et al., 1964), or vestibular nucleus stimulation (Tokumasu et al., 1969). Horizontal head and eye movements were induced from the region of the fastigial nuclei and the vermis overlying the fastigial nuclei (Fig. 1C). Induced eye movements from the vermis were mostly ipsilateral, but both ipsilateral and contralateral eye movements were induced from the region of the fastigial nucleus. Stimulation in the region of the juxta-restiform body and uncinate fasciculus at the lateral margins of the 4th ventricle also induced strong ipsilateral horizontal eye movements. Efferent pathways from the cerebellum which carry activity responsible for horizontal eye movements probably lie in these regions.

Horizontal eye movements were not induced by stimulation of the lateral cerebellum or of the dentate or interpositus nuclei. Stimulation of the cortex in the region of the ansate lobes or of the dentate nuclei induced upward rotatory eye movements (Fig. 1D). These movements lay in planes roughly parallel to the plane of the anterior semicircular canal on the same side. When the nodulus or uvula or the interpositus nucleus was stimulated, downward rotatory eye movements were induced (Fig. 1E). These eye movements lay in planes parallel to the plane of the posterior canals. Rotatory eye movements in the coronal plane were induced from the region of the brachium conjunctivum between areas from which upward rotatory and downward rotatory eye movements were evoked (Fig. 1F).

Thus, the cerebellar nuclei exert a powerful influence on all oculomotor motor neurons. There is complex intercrossing of pathways in the region of the cerebellar nuclei (Angaut and Brodal, 1967), and some ambiguity in results would be expected. However, eye movements in different spatial planes were induced from regions of the cerebellum which appeared to be largely separate from each other. Eye movements induced by stimulation are in general agreement with the anatomical studies described in the first section. Neurons from the dentate nucleus project to eye muscle motor neurons which would make the eyes move up, and stimulation in the region of the dentate nucleus caused upward eye movements. The fastigial nuclei project to regions of the pontine reticular formation near where horizontal eye movements are believed to be generated and stimulation of these nuclei also induced horizontal eye movements. In a variety of species (monkeys, cats, dogs, rabbits) it has been shown that stimulation of the fastigial nuclei or of the vermis which overlies the fastigial nuclei mainly induces eye movements in the horizontal plane (Ferrier, 1896; Hoshino, 1921; Mussen, 1934;

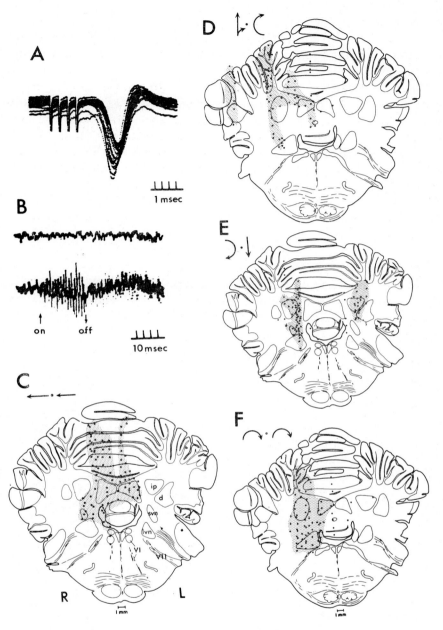

Fig. 1. A: Superimposed traces of potential changes in right lateral rectus (RLR) muscle induced by stimulation of the left fastigial nucleus in its caudal portions. B: Resting and activated EMG of RLR during left fastigial nucleus stimulation at 200/sec. Note synchronous following at stimulation frequency. C–F: Summary of stimulation points from which the following movements were induced. (C), horizontal movements to the right; (D), upward rotatory movements; (E), downward rotatory movements; (F), pure rotatory eye movements. Movements with similar horizontal components to C would be induced by the left lateral semicircular canal, to D by the right anterior canal, to E by the right posterior canal, and to F by the right anterior and posterior canal or by the right utricle. From Cohen et al. (1965a).

Cohen *et al.*, 1965a). These include animals in which the position of the eyes in the head varies widely. This suggests that the function of parts of the fastigial nuclei and overlying vermis may in some way be concerned with eye movements in the horizontal plane. It raises the question of whether eye movements in other planes of space may not be represented in homologous areas of the cerebellum in different species.

Data on vertical eye movements is fragmentary, but in most studies pure horizontal eye movements were not induced by stimulation of the lateral cerebellum. In cat and monkey, downward eye movements were affected by stimulation or lesion of the same region. Stimulation of the nodulus in the cat induced downward eye movements (Cohen *et al.*, 1965a), and lesions of the nodulus caused downward nystagmus in cat (Allen and Fernández, 1960; Fernández, 1960; Fernández *et al.*, 1960; Singleton, 1967), and monkey (Cohen and Komatsuzaki, unpublished data). However, nystagmus in parallel planes was not induced in the rabbit after nodulus lesions (Grant *et al.*, 1964).

Electrophysiological studies

Mossy fibers projecting to the cerebellar vermis, including Larsell's lobules V, VI, and VII, are activated by auditory stimuli (Shofer *et al.*, 1969). These lobules of the cerebellar vermis are also activated by visual and tactile stimuli (Snider and Stowell, 1944)

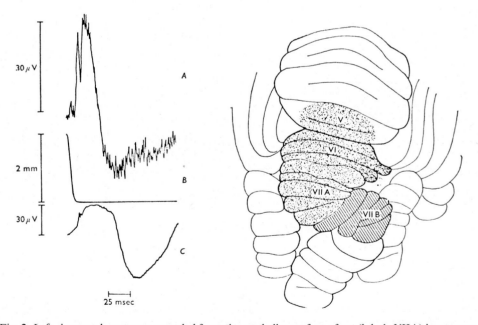

Fig. 2. *Left*. Averaged responses recorded from the cerebellar surface of cat (lobule VIIA) in response to stretching the left lateral rectus muscle. A: recorded under light Nembutal anesthesia, and C: under Nembutal and chloralose anesthesia. B: stretch applied to the left lateral rectus muscle. *Right*. Regions of cerebellar surface from which potential changes were elicited on stretch of extraocular muscles. The dotted region shows the stronger, short latency projection area. Weaker responses were obtained from regions with open shading. From Fuchs and Kornhuber (1969).

as well as by electrical stimulation of the motor and sensory cortex (Hampson *et al.*, 1952; Snider and Eldred, 1952). Recently it has been shown that Purkinje cells in Larsell's lobules V, VI, and VII are activated by eye muscle stretch (Fig. 2; Fuchs and Kornhuber, 1969). This occurs over both mossy and climbing fiber inputs (Baker *et al.*, 1972a). Earliest activation after eye muscle stretch occurred with a latency of approximately 4 msec and individual eye muscles did not have a unique projection (Fuchs and Kornhuber, 1969). Stretching more muscles simultaneously seemed to increase the reliability of the response. Activity responsible for these potential changes arose in eye muscle afferents (Baker *et al.*, 1972a). Similar types of potential changes are associated with spontaneous saccades in fish (Hermann, 1971) and in cat (Wolfe, 1971). Thus, the vermis receives information about the state of eye muscle tension as well as about visual and auditory sensation. In addition, potential changes in the vermis also lead to saccadic eye movements (Wolfe, 1971).

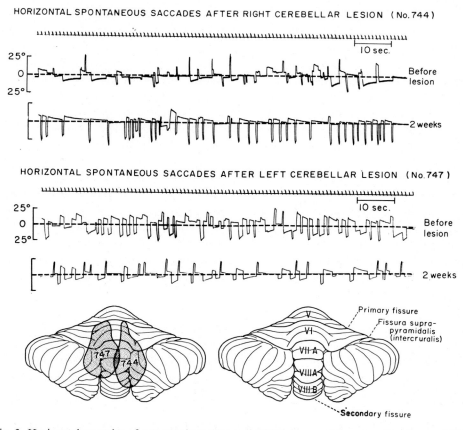

Fig. 3. Horizontal saccades of two monkeys (744 and 747) before and 2 weeks after the cerebellar cortical lesions shown below. The horizontal EOG was recorded with d.c.-coupling. 25° of deviation to the right and left are shown for each trace. The dotted lines represent the approximate midposition determined photographically. Note that after the right cerebellar cortical lesion in 744 there was a strong tendency to move to the left and after the left-sided lesion in 747 to move to the right. From Aschoff and Cohen (1971).

Cerebellar lesions

There is little information about changes in eye movements other than nystagmus after cerebellar lesions. An inability to generate saccadic eye movements of large amplitude has been noted in patients with diffuse cerebellar cortical atrophy (Kornhuber, 1971). When these patients move to lateral targets they do so in a series of smaller jumps, considerably prolonging the duration of the fixation shift. Collewijn (1970) also reported that rabbits do not recenter their eyes during optokinetic nystagmus after cerebellectomy.

Evidence has recently been obtained which implicates parts of the cerebellar cortex in production of ipsilateral saccades or positions of fixation in the ipsilateral hemifield (Aschoff and Cohen, 1971). When parts of the vermis and adjacent paravermis including Larsell's lobules VI and VIIA were ablated, the eyes moved most often from the midposition into the contralateral hemifield (Fig. 3). In four of six animals with one-sided vermian and paravermian lesions, saccades to the contralateral side were larger than to the ipsilateral side after operation. In these monkeys the eyes tended to move from the midline in a series of smaller movements. Amplitude/velocity relationships of saccadic movements, slow pursuit movements, and optokinetic nystagmus were not much affected by these cerebellar cortical lesions. These data are consistent with the hypothesis that the cerebellar cortex of the vermis and paravermis may play a role in producing gaze shifts or positions of fixation to the ipsilateral side.

VESTIBULOCEREBELLAR EFFECTS ON EYE MOVEMENTS

Magnus (1924) noted that compensatory eye movements induced by changes in head position or by rotatory stimulation were preserved after cerebellectomy. He concluded that the cerebellum is not essential for production of either otolith-ocular or semicircular canal-ocular reflexes. Dow (1938) and Ferraro and Barrera (1936, 1938) also reported that cerebellar lesions had little effect on caloric nystagmus. Nevertheless, there is evidence which suggests that the cerebellum may be important in processing activity in the otolith-ocular reflex arcs, and may also control semicircular canal-induced ocular reflexes.

Otolith-ocular reflexes

The saccule and utricle project into the region of the descending vestibular nucleus (DVN) (Stein and Carpenter, 1967; Gacek, 1969) and DVN projects mainly into the cerebellum (Brodal and Torvik, 1957; Carpenter *et al.*, 1959; Carpenter, 1960). There are only meager direct projections from DVN through the brain stem to the oculomotor nuclei (Pompeiano and Walberg, 1957; Carpenter, 1960; Carpenter *et al.*, 1960; Brodal *et al.*, 1962; McMasters *et al.*, 1966; Tarlov, 1970). The presence of direct cerebellar-oculomotor connections have been noted. This suggests that a vestibulo-cerebellar-oculomotor loop may exist which subserves otolith reflexes.

The labyrinth also sends direct primary afferents to the vestibulo-cerebellum as mossy fibers (Precht and Llinás, 1969a), and climbing fibers may also be activated by adequate stimulation of the labyrinthine receptors (Ferin *et al.*, 1971). The fastigial and dentate nuclei of the cerebellum also receive primary vestibular input (Precht and Llinás, 1969b). Thus, the vestibulo-cerebellar cortex as well as the dentate and fastigial nuclei receive information enabling them to monitor incoming vestibular activity.

Manni *et al.* (1965) studied the effects of cerebellar cortical stimulation on III nucleus neurons during spontaneous and labyrinthine-evoked activity in the guinea pig. Sites of cerebellar cortical stimulation were limited to Larsell's lobules V, VI, and VII; the vestibulo-cerebellum was not stimulated. In extracellular recordings ispilateral III neurons were inhibited and contralateral cells were excited. Sometimes patterned firing, *i.e.*, doublets or burst responses occurred after cerebellar stimulation. Efferent activity from Purkinje cells should have been maximally activated by the high rates of stimulation which were employed (200–300 c/sec). The areas of the vermis which were stimulated project to the fastigial and superior vestibular nuclei (SVN) (Van Rossum, 1969) which projects to the III nucleus through the medial longitudinal fasciculus (Szentágothai, 1964; McMasters, *et al.*, 1966; Tarlov, 1970). The fastigial nucleus projects to the contralateral and ipsilateral vestibular nuclei (Walberg *et al.*, 1962a), and the reticular formation. The observed effects on III nucleus neurons could be explained by inhibition of SVN through the fastigial nucleus, or by activation of more complex polysynaptic pathways through the reticular formation.

The effects of cerebellar stimulation on spontaneous oculomotor activity or on that evoked by vestibular stimuli have also been recorded extracellularly in the guinea pig (Azzena and Giretti, 1967). Contralateral dentate stimulation was facilitatory and ipsilateral stimulation inhibitory on these neurons. Interpositus stimulation was consistently facilitatory, regardless of the side stimulated, while fastigial stimulation was reported to be facilitatory in 8 cells regardless of the side stimulated and inhibitory in 2 cells when contralateral stimulation was applied. Field potentials at latencies which were probably monosynaptic were recorded in the contralateral III nucleus after dentate stimulation, while a longer latency field potential was recorded after ipsilateral fastigial stimulation. These results suggests a direct effect of the dentate nucleus and an indirect effect of the interpositus and fastigial nuclei on the III nucleus. Aside from oculomotor effects of interpositus stimulation (Fig. 1E), these are the first data to suggest that the interpositus nucleus is important in the control of eye movements. Pathways carrying information from the ipsilateral dentate to the III nerve nucleus are as yet undefined.

Recent research in the rabbit (Highstein, 1971) has shown that in addition to the dentate nucleus, the group y of the vestibular nuclei (Brodal *et al.*, 1962) also contributes activity carried in the brachium conjunctivum which directly influences III nucleus motor neurons. This work involves both intra- and extracellular recording techniques. Characteristic extra-cellular field potentials were induced in the region of III nucleus by stimulation of the VIII nerve or the medulla at disynaptic and monosynaptic latencies, respectively. These field potentials were associated with EPSP's in motor neurons. Thus, monosynaptic initiation of EPSP's in oculomotor neurons could be determined by extracellular recordings.

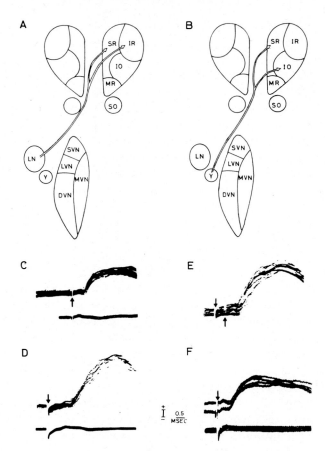

Fig. 4. A: Schematic representation of the projection of the lateral nucleus of the cerebellum (LN) to the oculomotor nucleus in rabbit. B: Schematic representation of the projection of the group y of the vestibular nuclei to the oculomotor nucleus. C–F: Potentials recorded from the inferior oblique subdivision of the oculomotor nucleus. C, Upper traces show intracellularly-recorded EPSP in an inferior oblique neuron after group y stimulation. Lower traces, extracellular field potentials. D, Similar to C except whole VIII nerve was stimulated. E, Combined vestibular nerve and group y stimulation. F, Similar to C except during brachium conjunctivum stimulation. Downward arrows indicate VIII nerve and brachium conjunctivum stimulation, upward arrows, group y stimulation. Abbreviations: SR, superior rectus; IR, inferior rectus; IO, inferior oblique; MR, medial rectus; SO, superior oblique; y, group y of vestibular nuclei; SVN, superior vestibular nucleus; LVN, lateral vestibular nucleus; MVN, medial vestibular nucleus; DVN, descending vestibular nucleus. Calibration, 0.5 msec for all records. Voltage scale, 2 mV in C, D, E, and 1 mV in F. From Highstein (1971).

With a recording microelectrode located in each of the four subdivisions of the IIIrd nucleus, the vestibular nuclei and cerebellum were stimulated monopolarly with limited currents. Short latency field potentials which were evoked by brachium conjunctivum stimulation in the inferior oblique subnucleus were shown to originate in the group y. Those in the cell group which innervated the inferior rectus originated in the dentate nucleus and those in the superior rectus subnucleus came from both the dentate and the group y (see Fig. 4A and B for summary). To confirm the conclusions based on extracellular field potentials, EPSP's with monosynaptic latencies have been recorded from inferior oblique motor neurons following group y stimulation (Fig. 4C). The group y-evoked EPSP's occluded with disynaptic EPSP's evoked by VIII nerve stimulation (Fig. 4D for VIII nerve EPSP's and 4E for the occlusion test). Brachium conjunctivum stimulation also evoked similar EPSP's to those evoked by group y stimulation (Fig. 4F).

It has been shown that the group y receives primary vestibular afferents of saccular origin (Gacek, 1969) and that stimulation of the saccule can produce patterned eye movements (Fluur, 1970) while its ablation leads to a decrease in ocular counter-rolling (Jongkees, 1950). Thus, eye movements induced by the saccule may be mediated at least in part by the group y. The short latency of the evoked EPSP's is surprising, although changes in EMG and contractions have been evoked at equally short latencies after stimulation of the utricular nerve (Suzuki et al., 1969). Since ocular counter-rolling is known to have a fast and slow component the former may be mediated through the short latency pathways. Although both the group y and the dentate project to the superior rectus subgroup of motor neurons, the function of the dentate nucleus has yet to be defined since the peripheral source of its input has not yet been investigated. However, both group y and dentate nucleus participate in the disynaptic excitation produced in the III nucleus by VIII nerve stimulation.

Clinical studies

Evidence that the cerebellum may be important in mediating otolith-ocular reflexes has been available for some time. Manni (1950) reported that compensatory eye movements for head tilt were defective after cerebellar lesions in the guinea pig. In addition, positional nystagmus has been produced by cerebellar lesions in cat, monkey, rabbit and man (Nylén, 1931, 1950; Spiegel and Scala, 1941, 1942; Dix and Hallpike, 1952; Allen and Fernández, 1960; Fernández, 1960; Fernández and Fredrickson, 1964; Aschan et al., 1964; Grant et al., 1964; Cohen et al., 1969; Grand, 1971). Positional nystagmus is nystagmus which appears after a particular head position is assumed (Bárány, 1913; Nylén, 1924), and is a common symptom of damage of the otolith organs or dysfunction in otolith-ocular reflex arcs (Bárány, 1913; Nylén, 1924, 1950; Dix and Hallpike, 1952; Aschan et al., 1956; Jongkees, 1961; Bergstedt, 1961; Jongkees and Philipszoon, 1964). Tests for positional nystagmus were not conducted in most of the early studies on the effects of cerebellar lesions (Ferraro and Barrera, 1936, 1938; Dow, 1938; Dow and Moruzzi, 1958).

An example of apogeotropic or convergent direction-changing positional nystagmus in a monkey of the type seen in PAN II (Aschan et al., 1956; Bergstedt, 1961) is shown in Fig. 5. It was recorded three months after an operative lesion of the fastigial nuclei. There was no nystagmus in light with the animal erect or supine. There was nystagmus to the right when the monkey was on its left side and to the left when its right side was down. After lesions of the cerebellar nuclei, positional nystagmus can persist for long periods of time, and vertigo and positional nystagmus in patients with cerebellar

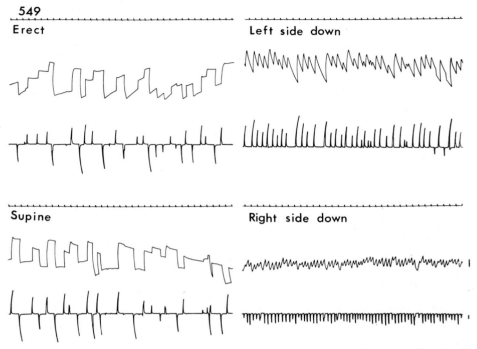

Fig. 5. Convergent direction-changing positional nystagmus after an operative lesion of the fastigial nuclei in monkey. The top trace in each set is the time base at 1 mark/sec. The second trace is the horizontal EOG recorded with d.c.-coupling. The third trace is the differentiated EOG showing the velocity of the eyes. The horizontal bar next to the EOG in the lower right hand corner is 10° and next to the differentiated EOG is 100°/sec.

tumors can be persistent and severe. Positional nystagmus is not induced by lesions of the mesencephalic or pontine reticular formation or by lesions rostral to the mesencephalon (Cohen *et al.*, 1968). It is present after lesions of the posterior fossa (Nylén, 1931), particularly when lesions involve the vestibular nuclei (Aschan *et al.*, 1956; Stahle, 1958; Jongkees *et al.*, 1962; Jung and Kornhuber, 1964; Cohen and Uemura, 1972). To the extent that positional nystagmus represents a disorder of perception of position or movement of the head in various planes of space, it can be said that the cerebellum participates either primarily or directly in control of these reflexes. Specifically what this role might be is not known, however.

Control of semicircular canal-ocular reflexes

The way in which the cerebellum affects nystagmus induced by semicircular canal stimulation is not clear. Bárány (1914) reported changes in post-rotatory nystagmus after lesions of the flocculus. It is certain that horizontal caloric nystagmus is not primarily affected by lesions of the cerebellum (Magnus, 1924; Ferraro and Barrera, 1936, 1938; Dow, 1938; Carpenter *et al.*, 1960), although directional preponderance of caloric nystagmus can be produced by cerebellar nuclear lesions (Jung and Kornhuber,

1964; Komatsuzaki and Cohen, unpublished data). It has been suggested that caloric nystagmus is enhanced or prolonged by cerebellectomy (Bauer and Leidler, 1912) or by cerebellar lesions (Ferraro and Barrera, 1938; Fernández and Fredrickson, 1964; Singleton, 1967). Fernández and Fredrickson (1964) indicate that this is due to lesions of the nodulus, and postulate that this region mediates inhibition on semicircular canal-ocular reflexes. In accord with this, they found that caloric nystagmus was inhibited by electrical stimulation of the nodulus. However, it is not entirely clear how specific this effect might be, and whether stimulation of other areas of the nervous system, would not likewise produce some inhibition of caloric nystagmus.

Recently Ito *et al.* (1970), Fukuda *et al.* (1972) and Baker *et al.* (1972b) have shown that superior vestibular nucleus neurons which project through the MLF are inhibited by Purkinje cell axons from the flocculus. Flocculus stimulation caused dysinhibition of oculomotor and trochlear motor neurons and would facilitate semicircular canal-ocular pathways ending in these motor nuclei.

It has also been suggested that the cerebellum is important for habituation of caloric nystagmus. If caloric stimuli are given repetitively, there is a decrease in the duration and maximum slow phase velocity of the nystagmus which is induced. Halstead (1935, 1937) first demonstrated that head nystagmus in pigeons would not habituate after cerebellectomy. This habituation can be studied only if the state of alertness is carefully controlled and is present for stimulation of single canals and for nystagmus induced in specific directions (Crampton, 1962, 1964; Guedry, 1964; Collins and Updegraff, 1966; Collins, 1969). More recently, Singleton (1967) destroyed the nodulus and indicated that there was no habituation of caloric nystagmus after operation. Wolfe (1968) has reached similar conclusions. However, this would still appear to be a matter for future study.

SUMMARY

In 1964 Dow and Manni concluded that "the cerebellum is not essential for eye movements. As in other motor activity, however, it plays a modifying and influencing role. Abnormalities following cerebellar lesions are readily compensated. They are found most frequently in areas concerned with the vestibular system and areas activated by photostimulation." This conclusion appears to be generally correct, except that positional nystagmus and vertigo may be persistent and severe after cerebellar lesions. There does appear to be an extra-vestibular effect of the cerebellum on eye movements; in part it probably participates in production of saccades or positions of fixation in the ipsilateral hemifield. In addition, there is increasing evidence that the cerebellum probably also is important in modulation or production of otolith-ocular reflexes. The otoliths code information related to head position or to movement of the head in various spatial planes. There is also some evidence to indicate that these planes of space or eye movements in these planes may be represented in different portions of the cerebellum. Specifically it is likely that eye movements in the horizontal plane may be represented in the fastigial nuclei and overlying vermis. Other areas of the cerebellum may be more closely related to movement in vertical vertical or coronal planes.

References pp. 422–425

Evidence to suggest that the cerebellum may participate in controlling responses to caloric stimulation, is still incomplete.

However, the flocculus has been shown to inhibit superior vestibular neurons which mediate inhibition onto trochlear motor neurons. Thus the flocculus dys-inhibits or facilitates some semicircular canal-ocular reflex pathways.

ACKNOWLEDGEMENT

This study was supported by NINDS Grants NS-00294, NS-1 K3-34, 987 (B.C.) and 2F11 NS-2034-03 NSRB (S.M.H.)

REFERENCES

ALLEN, G. AND FERNÁNDEZ, C. (1960) Experimental observations in postural nystagmus. I. Extensive lesions in posterior vermis of the cerebellum. *Acta oto-laryng. (Stockh.)*, **51**, 2–14.

ANGAUT, P. AND BRODAL, A. (1967) The projection of the 'Vestibulocerebellum' onto the vestibular nuclei in the cat. *Arch. ital. Biol.*, **105**, 441–479.

ASCHAN, G., BERGSTEDT, M. AND STAHLE, J. (1956) Nystagmography. *Acta oto-laryng. (Stockh.)*, suppl. **129**, 1–103.

ASCHAN, G., EKVALL, L. AND GRANT, G. (1964) Nystagmus following stimulation in the central vestibular pathways using permanently implanted electrodes. *Acta oto-laryng. (Stockh.)*, Suppl. 192, 63–77.

ASCHOFF, J. C. AND COHEN, B. (1971) Changes in saccadic eye movements produced by cerebellar cortical lesions. *Exp. Neurol.*, **32**, 123–133.

AZZENA, G. B. AND GIRETTI, M. L. (1967) Responses of the oculomotor units to deep cerebellar stimulation. *Brain Res.*, **6**, 523–534.

BAKER, R., PRECHT, W. AND LLINÁS, R. (1972a) Mossy and climbing fiber projections of extraocular muscle afferents to the cerebellum. *Brain Res.*, **38**, in press.

BAKER, R., PRECHT, W. AND LLINÁS, R., (1972b) Cerebellar modulatory action on the vestibulo-trochlear pathway in the cat. *Exp. Brain Res.*, in press.

BÁRÁNY, R. (1913) Dauernde Veränderung des spontanen Nystagmus bei Veränderung der Kopflage. *Mschr. Ohrenheilk.*, **47**, 481–483.

BÁRÁNY, R. (1914) Untersuchungen über Funktion des Flocculus am Kaninchen. *Jber. Psychiat. Neurol.*, **26**, 631–651.

BAUER, J. AND LEIDLER, R. (1912) Ueber den Einfluss der Auschaltung verschiedener Hirnabschnitte auf die vestibulären Augenreflexe. *Arb. Neurol. Inst. Wien Univ.*, **19**, 155–226.

BENDER, M. B. AND SHANZER, S. (1964) Oculomotor pathways defined by electric stimulation and lesions in the brain stem of monkey. In M. B. BENDER (Ed.), *The Oculomotor System*. Hoeber Medical Division, Harper and Row, New York, pp. 81–140.

BERGSTEDT, M. (1961) Studies of positional nystagmus in the human centrifuge. *Acta oto-laryng., (Stockh.)*, Suppl. 165, 1–144.

BRODAL, A., POMPEIANO, O. AND WALBERG, F. (1962) *The Vestibular Nuclei and Their Connections. Anatomy and Functional Correlations*. Oliver and Boyd, Edinburgh, London, pp. VIII–193.

BRODAL, A. AND TORVIK, A. (1957) Über den Ursprung der sekundären vestibulocerebellären Fasern bei der Katze. *Arch. Psychiat. u. Z. ges. Neurol.*, **195**, 550–567.

CARPENTER, M. B. (1959) Lesions of the fastigial nuclei in the rhesus monkey. *Amer. J. Anat.*, **104**, 1–34.

CARPENTER, M. B. (1960) Fiber projections from the descending and lateral vestibular nuclei in the cat. *Amer. J. Anat.*, **107**, 1–22.

CARPENTER, M. B., ALLING, F. A. AND BARD, D. S. (1960) Lesions of the descending vestibular nucleus in the cat. *J. comp. Neurol.*, **114**, 39–49.

CARPENTER, M. B., BARD, D. S. AND ALLING, F. A. (1959) Anatomical connections between the fastigial nuclei, the labyrinth and the vestibular nuclei in the cat. *J. comp. Neurol.*, **111**, 1-26.

CARPENTER, M. B., BRITTEN, G. M. AND PINES, J. (1958) Isolated lesions of the fastigial nuclei in the cat. *J. comp. Neurol.*, **109**, 65–90.

CARPENTER, M. B. AND STROMINGER, W. L. (1964) Cerebello-oculomotor fibers in the rhesus monkey. *J. comp. Neurol.*, **123**, 211–230.

COHEN, B. (1971) Vestibulo-ocular relations. In P. BACH-Y-RITA AND C. C. COLLINS (Eds.), *The Control of Eye Movements*, Academic Press, New York, London, pp. 105, 148.

COHEN, B., GOTO, K., SHANZER, S. AND WEISS, A. H. (1965a) Eye movements induced by electric stimulation of the cerebellum in the alert cat. *Exp. Neurol.*, **13**, 145–162.

COHEN, B., KOMATSUZAKI, A. AND ALPERT, J. (1969) Positional nystagmus after lesions of the cerebellum. *Proc. IX int. Congr. Neurol., Excerpta Med. Int. Congr. Ser.*, **193**, 198–199.

COHEN, B., KOMATSUZAKI, A. AND BENDER, M. B. (1968) Electrooculographic syndrome in monkeys after pontine reticular formation lesions. *Arch. Neurol. (Chicago)*, **18**, 78–92.

COHEN, B., SUZUKI, J. AND BENDER, M. B. (1964) Eye movements from semicircular canal nerve stimulation in the cat. *Ann. Otol. (St. Louis)*, **73**, 153–169.

COHEN, B., SUZUKI, J. AND BENDER, M. B. (1965b) Nystagmus induced by electric stimulation of ampullary nerves. *Acta oto-laryng. (Stockh.)*, **60**, 422–436.

COHEN, B., TOKUMASU, K. AND GOTO, K. (1966) Semicircular canal nerve, eye and head movements: The effects of changes in initial eye and head position on the plane of the induced movement. *Arch. Ophthal. (Chicago)*, **76**, 523–531.

COLLEWIJN, H. (1970) Dysmetria of fast phase of optokinetic nystagmus in cerebellectomized rabbit. *Exp. Neurol.*, **28**, 144–154.

COLLINS, W. E. (1969) Modification of vestibular nystagmus and 'vertigo' by means of visual stimulation. *Trans. amer. Acad. Ophthal. Otolaryng.*, **72**, 962–979.

COLLINS, W. E. AND UPDEGRAFF, B. P. (1966) A comparison of nystagmus habituation in the cat and the dog. *Acta oto-laryng. (Stockh.)*, **62**, 19–26.

CRAMPTON, G. H. (1962) Directional imbalance of vestibular nystagmus in cat following repeated unidirectional angular acceleration. *Acta oto-laryng. (Stockh.)*, **55**, 41–48.

CRAMPTON, G. H. (1964) Habituation of ocular nystagmus of vestibular origin. In M. B. BENDER (Ed.), *The Oculomotor System*. Hoeber Medical Division, Harper and Row, New York, pp. 332–346.

DIX, M. R. AND HALLPIKE, S. C. (1952) The pathology, symptomatology and diagnosis of certain common disorders of the vestibular system. *Ann. Otol. (St. Louis)*, **61**, 987–1016.

DOW, R. S. (1936) The fiber connections of the posterior parts of the cerebellum in the rat and cat. *J. comp. Neurol.*, **63**, 527–548.

DOW, R. S. (1938) Effects of lesions of the vestibular part of the cerebellum in primates. *Arch. Neurol. (Chicago)*, **40**, 500–520.

DOW, R. S. AND MANNI, E. (1964) The relationship of the cerebellum to extraocular movements. In M. B. BENDER (Ed.), *The Oculomotor System*. Hoeber Medical Division, Harper and Row, New York, pp. 280–292.

DOW, R. S. AND MORUZZI, G. (1958) *The Physiology and Pathology of the Cerebellum*. The University of Minnesota Press, Minneapolis, pp. VII-675.

FERIN, M., GRIGORIAN, R. A. AND STRATA, P. (1971) Mossy and climbing fiber activation in the cat cerebellum by stimulation of the labyrinth. *Exp. Brain Res.*, **12**, 1–17.

FERNÁNDEZ, C. (1960) Interrelations between flocculonodular lobe and vestibular system. In G. L. RASMUSSEN AND W. F. WINDLE (Eds.), *Neural Mechanisms of the Auditory and Vestibular Systems*, C. C. Thomas, Springfield, Ill., pp. 285–296.

FERNÁNDEZ, C., ALZATE, R. AND LINDSAY, J. R. (1960) Experimental observations on postural nystagmus. II. Lesions of nodulus. *Ann. Otol. (St. Louis)*, **69**, 94–114.

FERNÁNDEZ, C. AND FREDRICKSON, J. M. (1964) Experimental cerebellar lesions and their effect on vestibular function. *Acta oto-laryng. (Stockh.)*, Suppl. 192, 52–62.

FERRARO, A. AND BARRERA, S. E. (1936) Effects of lesions of the juxta-restiform body (I.A.K. bundle) in *Macacus rhesus* monkeys. *Arch. Neurol. Psychiat. (Chicago)*, **35**, 13–29.

FERRARO, A. AND BARRERA, S. E. (1938) Differential features of 'cerebellar' and "vestibular" phenomena in *Macacus rhesus*. Preliminary report based on experiments on 300 monkeys. *Arch. Neurol. (Chicago)*, **39**, 902–918.

FERRIER, D. (1876) *The Functions of the Brain*. Smith-Elder, London, pp. XV–323.

FLUUR, E. AND MELLSTROM, A. (1970) Saccular stimulation and oculomotor reactions. *Laryngoscope*, **80**, 1713–1721.

FUCHS, A. F. AND KORNHUBER, H. H. (1969) Extraocular muscle afferents to the cerebellum of the cat. *J. Physiol. (Lond.)*, **200**, 713–722.

FUKUDA, J., HIGHSTEIN, S. M. AND ITO, M. (1972) Cerebellar inhibitory control of the vestibulo-ocular reflex investigated in rabbit IIIrd nucleus. *Exp. Brain Res.*, **14**, 511–526.

GACEK, R. R. (1969) The course and central termination of first order neurons supplying vestibular end organs in the cat. *Acta oto-laryng. (Stockh.)*, Suppl. 254, 1–66.

GOEBEL, H. H., KOMATSUZAKI, A., BENDER, M. B. AND COHEN, B. (1971) Lesions of the pontine tegmentum and conjugate gaze paralysis. *Arch. Neurol. (Chicago)*, **24**, 431–440.

GRAND, W. (1971) Positional nystagmus: an early sign in medulloblastoma. *Neurology*, **21**, 1157–1159.

GRANT, G., ASCHAN, G. AND EKVALL, L. (1964) Nystagmus produced by cerebellar lesions. *Acta oto-laryng. (Stockh.)*, Suppl. 192, 78–84.

GUEDRY, F. E., JR. (1964) Visual control of habituation to complex vestibular stimulation in man. *Acta oto-laryng. (Stockh.)*, **58**, 377–389.

HALSTEAD, W. C. (1935) The effects of cerebellar lesions upon habituation of post-rotatory nystagmus. *Comp. Psychol. Monogr.*, **42**, 1–130.

HALSTEAD, W. C., YACORZYNSKI, G. AND FEARING, F. (1937) Further evidence of cerebellar influence in the habituation of after-nystagmus in pigeons. *Amer. J. Physiol.*, **120**, 350–355.

HAMPSON, J. L., HARRISON, C. AND WOOLSEY, C. (1952) Cerebro-cerebellar projections and the somato-topic localization of motor function in the cerebellum. *Res. Publ. Ass. nerv. ment. Dis.*, **30**, 299–316.

HERMANN, H. T. (1971) Saccade correlated potentials in optic tectum and cerebellum of Carassius Auratus. *Brain Res.*, **26**, 293–304.

HIGHSTEIN, S. M. (1971) Organization of the inhibitory and excitatory vestibulo-ocular reflex pathways to the third and fourth nuclei in rabbit. *Brain Res.*, **32**, 218–224.

HOSHINO, T. (1921) Beiträge zur Funktion des Kleinhirnwurmes beim Kaninchen. *Acta oto-laryng. (Stockh.)*, suppl. **2**, 1–72.

ITO, M., HIGHSTEIN, S. M. AND FUKUDA, J. (1970) Cerebellar inhibition of the vestibulo-ocular reflex in rabbit and cat and its blockage by picrotoxin. *Brain Res.*, **17**, 524–526.

JANSEN, J. AND BRODAL, A. (1954) *Aspects of Cerebellar Anatomy*. Johan Grundt Tanum Forlag, Oslo, 423 pp.

JONGKEES, L. B. W. (1950) On the function of the saccule. *Acta oto-laryng. (Stockh.)*, **38**. 18–26.

JONGKEES, L. B. W. (1961) On positional nystagmus. *Acta oto-laryng. (Stockh.)*, suppl. **159**, 78–83.

JONGKEES, L. B. W., MAAS, J. P. M. AND PHILIPSZOON, A. J. (1962) Clinical nystagmography. A detailed study of electronystagmography in 341 patients with vertigo. *Pract. oto-rhino-laryng. (Basel)*, **24**, 65–93.

JONGKEES, L. B. W. AND PHILIPSZOON, A. J. (1964) Electronystagmography. *Acta oto-laryng. (Stockh.)*, suppl. **189**, 1–111.

JUNG, R. AND KORNHUBER, H. H. (1964) Results of electronystagmography in man: The value of optokinetic, vestibular and spontaneous nystagmus for neurologic diagnosis and research. In M. B. BENDER (Ed.), *The Oculomotor System*, Hoeber Medical Division, Harper and Row, New York, pp. 428–482.

KIDOKORO, Y. (1968) Direct inhibitory innervation of teleost oculomotor neurons by cerebellar Purkinje cells. *Brain Res.*, **10**, 453–456.

KOELLA, W. P. (1955) Motor effects from electrical stimulation of basal cerebellum in the unrestrained cat. *J. Neurophysiol.*, **18**, 559–573.

KOELLA, W. P. (1962) Organizational aspects of some subcortical motor areas. *Int. Rev. Neurobiol.*, **4**, 71–116.

MAGNUS, R. (1924) *Körperstellung*. Springer, Berlin, pp. XIII–740.

MANNI, E. (1950) Localizzazioni cerebellari corticali nella cavia. II. Effetti di lesioni delle parti vestibolari del cervelletto. *Arch. Fisiol.*, **50**, 110–123.

MANNI, E., AZZENA, G. B. AND DOW, R. S. (1965) Cerebellar influence on the unitary discharge of oculomotor nuclei and adjacent structures. *Exp. Neurol.*, **13**, 252–263.

MCMASTERS, R., WEISS, A. H. AND CARPENTER, M. B. (1966) Vestibular projections to the nuclei of the extraocular muscles. *Amer. J. Anat.*, **118**, 163–194.

MUSSEN, A. T. (1934) Cerebellum and red nucleus. *Arch. Neurol. (Chicago)*, **31**, 110–126.

NYLEN, C. O. (1924) Some cases of ocular nystagmus due to certain position of the head. *Acta oto-laryng. (Stockh.)*, **6**, 106–137.

NYLEN, C. O. (1931) A clinical study on positional nystagmus in cases of brain tumor. *Acta oto-laryng. (Stockh.)*, Suppl. 15, pp. 1–113.

NYLEN, C. O. (1950) Oto-neurologic diagnosis of tumors of the brain. *Acta oto-laryng. (Stockh.)*, Suppl. 33, 1–151.

POMPEIANO, O. AND WALBERG, F. (1957) Descending connections to the vestibular nuclei: An experimental study in cat. *J. comp. Neurol.*, **108**, 465–503.

PRECHT, W. AND LLINÁS, R. (1969a) Functional organization of the vestibular afferents to the cerebellar cortex of frog and cat. *Exp. Brain Res.*, **9**, 30–50.

PRECHT, W. AND LLINÁS, R. (1969b) Comparative aspects of the vestibular input to the cerebellum. In R. LLINÁS (Ed.), *Neurobiology of Cerebellar Evolution and Development*. Amer. Med. Ass. Press, Chicago, pp. 677–702.

SHOFER, R. S., SAX, D. S. AND STROM, M. G. (1969) Analysis of auditory and cerebrocortically evoked activity in the immature and adult cat cerebellum. In R. LLINÁS (Ed.), *Neurobiology of Cerebellar Evolution and Development*, Amer. Med. Ass. Press, Chicago, pp. 703–721.

SINGLETON, G. T. (1967) Relationships of the cerebellar nodulus to vestibular function: a study of the effects of nodulectomy on habituation. *Laryngoscope*, **77**, 1579–1620.

SNIDER, R. AND ELDRED, E. (1952) Cerebrocerebellar relationships in the monkey. *J. Neurophysiol.*, **15**, 27–40.

SNIDER, R. AND STOWELL, A. (1944) Receiving areas of the tactile, auditory, and visual systems in the cerebellum. *J. Neurophysiol.*, **7**, 331–357.

SPIEGEL, E. A. AND SCALA, N. P. (1941) Vertical nystagmus following lesions of the cerebellar vermis. *Arch. Ophthal. (Chicago)*, **26**, 661–669.

SPIEGEL, E. A. AND SCALA, N. P. (1942) Positional nystagmus in cerebellar lesions. *J. Neurophysiol.*, **5**, 247–260.

STAHLE, J. (1958) Electronystagmography in the caloric and rotatory tests. *Acta oto-laryng. (Stockh.)*, Suppl. 137, pp. 83.

STEIN, B. M. AND CARPENTER, M. B. (1967) Central projections of portions of the vestibular ganglia innervating specific parts of the labyrinth in the rhesus monkey. *Amer. J. Anat.*, **120**, 281–318.

SUZUKI, J. AND COHEN, B. (1964) Head, eye, body and limb movements from semicircular canal nerves. *Exp. Neurol.*, **10**, 395–405.

SUZUKI, J., COHEN, B. AND BENDER, M. B. (1964) Compensatory eye movements induced by vertical semicircular canal stimulation. *Exp. Neurol.*, **9**, 137–160.

SUZUKI, J., TOKUMASU, K. AND GOTO, K. (1969) Eye movements from single utricular nerve stimulation in the cat. *Acta oto-laryng. (Stockh.)*, **68**, 350–362.

SZENTÁGOTHAI, J. (1964) Pathways and synaptic articulation patterns connecting vestibular receptors and oculomotor nuclei. In M. B. BENDER (Ed.), *The Oculomotor System*. Hoeber Medical Division, Harper and Row, New York, pp. 205–223.

TARLOV, E. (1970) Organization of vestibulo-oculomotor projections in the cat. *Brain Res.*, **20**, 159–179.

TOKUMASU, K., GOTO, K. AND COHEN, B. (1969) Eye movements from vestibular nuclei stimulation in monkeys. *Ann. Otol. (St. Louis)*, **78**, 1105–1119.

UEMURA, T. AND COHEN, B. (1972) Vestibulo-ocular reflexes: effects of vestibular nuclear lesions. In A. BRODAL AND O. POMPEIANO (Eds.), *Progress in Brain Research. Vol. 37. Basic aspects of central vestibular mechanisms*. Elsevier, Amsterdam, pp. 515–528.

VAN ROSSUM, J. (1969) *Corticonuclear and Corticovestibular Projections of the Cerebellum*. Van Gorcum and Co., Assen, pp. 170.

VOOGD, J. (1964) *The Cerebellum of the Cat. Structure and Fibre Connexions*. Van Gorcum and Co., Assen, pp. 215.

WALBERG, F., POMPEIANO, O., BRODAL, A. AND JANSEN, J. (1962a) The fastigiovestibular projection in the cat. *J. comp. Neurol.*, **118**, 49–76.

WALBERG, F., POMPEIANO, O., WESTRUM, L. E. AND HAUGLIE-HANSEN, E. (1962b) Fastigio-reticular fibers in the cat. *J. comp. Neurol.*, **119**, 187–199.

WARWICK, R. (1964) Oculomotor organization. In M. B. BENDER (Ed.), *The Oculomotor System*, Hoeber Medical Division, Harper and Row, New York, pp. 173–202.

WOLFE, J. W., (1968) Evidence for control of nystagmic habituation by folium-tuber vermis and fastigial nuclei. *Acta oto-laryng. (Stockh.)*, Suppl. 231, 1–48.

WOLFE, J. W. (1971) Relationship of cerebellar potentials to saccadic eye movements. *Brain Res.*, **30**, 204–206.

VI. EFFERENT CONTROL OF THE LABYRINTHINE RECEPTORS

Efferent Vestibular Fibers in Mammals:
Morphological and Histochemical Aspects

S. IURATO[1], L. LUCIANO[2], E. PANNESE[3]

AND

E. REALE[2]

*Departments of Bioacoustics and of Histology and Embryology, University of Bari, Bari, Italy[1],
Laboratory of Electron Microscopy, Department of Anatomy, University of Hannover, Hannover,
G.F.R.[2] and Institute of Human Anatomy II, University of Milan, Milan, Italy[3]*

In the last fifteen years several researchers have shown the existence in the vestibular sensory areas of two morphologically different systems of nerve fibers and endings, afferent and efferent, suggesting a dual innervation of these organs (Wersäll, 1956; Engström, 1958; Gribenski, 1970). The present review takes into special consideration the morphological and histochemical aspects of the efferent system.

Origin of the efferent vestibular fibers

The results of the degeneration studies are fragmentary and not always in agreement. Petroff (1955), who started the investigations on the efferent vestibular fibers found that the fine fibers in the rami of the vestibular nerve disappeared following eighth nerve section or midline cuts in the floor of the fourth ventricle and concluded that the efferent vestibular fibers were crossed. Carpenter *et al.* (1959) and Carpenter (1960) on the contrary, found that the medial, superior and parts of the descending vestibular nuclei on both sides project efferent fibers to the labyrinth *via* the vestibular nerve and concluded that these fibers are predominantly uncrossed. Also the fastigial nuclei project efferent fibers to the labyrinths which appeared to be both crossed and uncrossed. Rasmussen and Gacek (1958) and Gacek (1960) thought the lateral vestibular nucleus to be the most likely source of uncrossed efferent fibers to the vestibular labyrinth.

More recently, attempts to discover the origin of vestibular efferents were performed with Koelle's histochemical method for acetylcholinesterase (AChE) which stains the efferent fibers. According to Rossi and Cortesina (1962, 1965) three uncrossed efferent bundles participate in the efferent innervation of the vestibular receptors (Fig. 1a): (*i*) the dorsal efferent vestibular bundle which arises from the anterior-inferior part of the lateral vestibular nucleus; (*ii*) the ventral efferent vestibular bundle which was found to arise from the interposed vestibular nucleus, situated between the lateral and the inferior vestibular nuclei, and (*ii*) the reticulo-vestibular bundle which arises

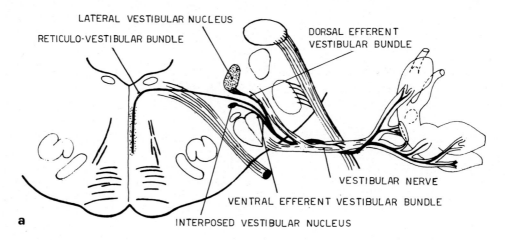

RETICULO-VESTIBULAR BUNDLE

LATERAL VESTIBULAR NUCLEUS

DORSAL EFFERENT
VESTIBULAR BUNDLE

VESTIBULAR NERVE

VENTRAL EFFERENT VESTIBULAR BUNDLE

INTERPOSED VESTIBULAR NUCLEUS

a

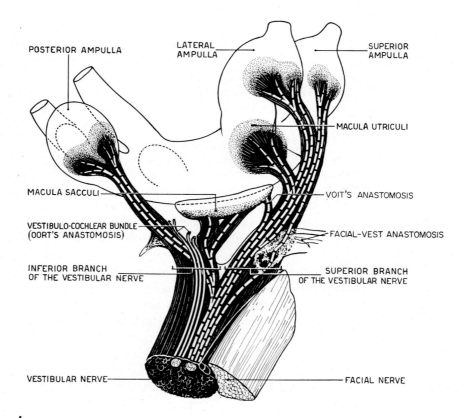

POSTERIOR AMPULLA

LATERAL
AMPULLA

SUPERIOR
AMPULLA

MACULA UTRICULI

MACULA SACCULI

VOIT'S ANASTOMOSIS

VESTIBULO-COCHLEAR BUNDLE
(OORT'S ANASTOMOSIS)

FACIAL-VEST ANASTOMOSIS

INFERIOR BRANCH
OF THE VESTIBULAR NERVE

SUPERIOR BRANCH
OF THE VESTIBULAR NERVE

VESTIBULAR NERVE

FACIAL NERVE

b

Fig. 1. a. Diagram showing the origin and course of the efferent vestibular fibers. The efferents to the cochlea are not shown. Modified after Rossi and Cortesina (1962). b. Diagram showing the course and peripheral distribution in the cat of the efferent (dashed lines) and afferent vestibular fibers (black lines). Efferent cochlear fibers are shown as uninterrupted white lines. Redrawn after Gacek (1960).

from cells scattered at different levels in the reticular substance of the medulla oblongata beside the raphe. According to Ross (1969) the efferent vestibular fibers are part of an AChE positive parasympathetic system which supplies fibers to the facial, vestibular and cochlear nerves. Its preganglionic cells are chiefly organized into four nuclei: one medial to the genu of the facial nerve; one lateral to the genu; the superior salivary nucleus; and a small nucleus lying within the borders of the lateral vestibular nucleus. Additionally, orthosympathetic AChE positive fibers arrive *via* the anterior inferior cerebellar artery (Ross, 1969). Although two of the nuclei described by Rossi and Cortesina (1962, 1965) as the origin of vestibular efferents probably correspond to two of the nuclei found by Ross (1969), it is evident from the above that a wide disagreement prevails in the literature.

Course

The course of the vestibular efferents in the vestibular nerve trunk is that originally described (Gacek, 1960) for a myelinated homolateral vestibular efferent pathway consisting of 150–200 fibers (figures later corrected to 400) (Gacek *et al.*, 1965), having a diameter between 2 and 4 μm (Fig. 1b). In the vestibular root and nerve they travel as a compact bundle just dorsal to the efferent cochlear bundle (Gacek, 1968). The main group then follows the superior (utriculo-ampullar) branch, whereas some fibers leave the parent trunk as scattered fibers to the saccule and posterior ampulla (Gacek, 1960) (Fig. 1b). Gacek (1960) was able to follow these fibers to the basement membrane of the sensory epithelia where some could be seen to turn and course parallel to the membrane before piercing it. Beyond this point the efferent fibers could not be traced further by experimental neuroanatomical techniques. According to Ross (1969) the efferent fibers to the vestibule, as well as those to the cochlea, synapse, perhaps completely, on postganglionic cells located along their peripheral courses.

Peripheral distribution at the light microscopical level

As it is known that in the vestibular sensory areas AChE activity is associated with the efferent fibers and endings (see *Histochemical properties*), the histochemical techniques for the localization of AChE activity have largely been used to trace the peripheral distribution of the efferent system. High AChE activity was found with the aid of Koelle's method below the neuroepithelium of the cristae ampullares and the macula utriculi (Dohlman, 1960) and at the nerve endings between the hair cells (Dohlman *et al.*, 1958). Similar results were obtained by Ireland and Farkashidy (1961). AChE activity at the base of the sensory epithelium was localized on the slopes of the cristae rather than on the crest (Nomura *et al.*, 1965) as seen in Fig. 2a. Marked AChE activity was localized in the neuroepithelium of the macula sacculi and utriculi (Fig. 2b). However, the activity was less in the striola which is located in the middle part of the macula sacculi (Nomura *et al.*, 1965). The presence of efferent nerve fibers and endings in the vestibular sensory areas was confirmed with the methods of Gomori (Ishii *et al.*, 1967b) and Karnovsky (Iurato *et al.*, 1971a, b) (Fig. 3).

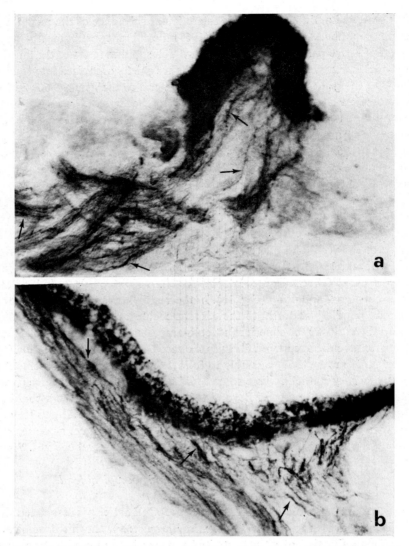

Fig. 2. Peripheral distribution of the efferent vestibular fibers (arrows) traced in the guinea pig by means of histochemical technique for AChE (Gomori). The sites of AChE activity appear black. a, to the superior crista ampullaris; b, to the utricle. Courtesy of Dr. Y. Nomura.

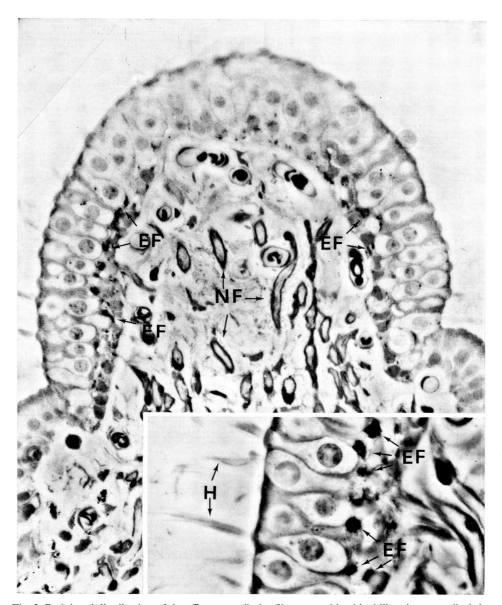

Fig. 3. Peripheral distribution of the efferent vestibular fibers traced in chinchilla crista ampullaris by means of histochemical technique for AChE (Karnovsky). The reaction product is localized at the level of efferent nerve fibers and endings (EF). H, hairs of the sensory cells; NF, myelinated nerve fibers. Phase contrast microscope (310 ×). Inset 1,050 ×.

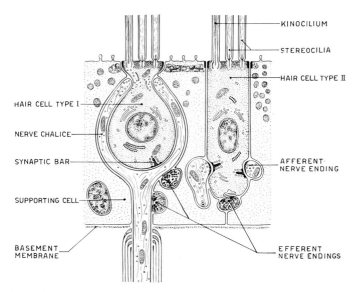

Fig. 4. Schematic drawing of afferent and efferent innervation of hair cells type I and II in mammals. Slightly modified from Wersäll (1967).

Peripheral distribution at the electron microscopical level

After having pierced the basement membrane, the efferent vestibular fibers form a complicated system of branching fibers partly ending at the sensory cells and partly at the afferent nerve fibers (Wersäll, 1956; Engström, 1958). In mammals the hair cell of type I, which is enclosed in an afferent nerve chalice, has no direct contact with the efferent nerve endings (Figs. 4 and 5). However, efferent endings form synapses with the nerve chalices or the afferent fibers and terminals (Fig. 4). The hair cell of type II, on the other hand, has synaptic contacts with both afferent and efferent endings (Fig. 4).

The efferent nerve fibers partly end as true terminal boutons (Wersäll, 1968) and partly show dilated parts or "boutons en passant" along branched presynaptic fibers, which make synaptic contacts with afferent nerve fibers, afferent nerve chalices, hair cells of type II and afferent boutons in contact with hair cells of type II (Iurato and Taidelli, 1964; Smith and Rasmussen, 1968) (Figs. 6 and 7). Probably one presynaptic fiber is in contact with several afferent fibers and hair cells. One efferent in contact "en passant" with a nerve chalice was seen making synapses with an afferent fiber and also with a hair cell of type II (Fig. 6). The efferent presynaptic fibers are slender elements (0.18–0.3 μm in diameter) which run among the supporting cells parallel to the basement membrane. They seem to form a sort of horizontal nerve plexus there (Smith and Rasmussen, 1968) (Fig. 7). They contain a few filaments, some elongated mitochondria and small (300–600 Å) round vesicles (Iurato and Taidelli, 1964).

All efferent endings or synaptic enlargements have the same appearance as the presynaptic endings in other areas of the nervous system (Wersäll, 1960, 1967; Engström,

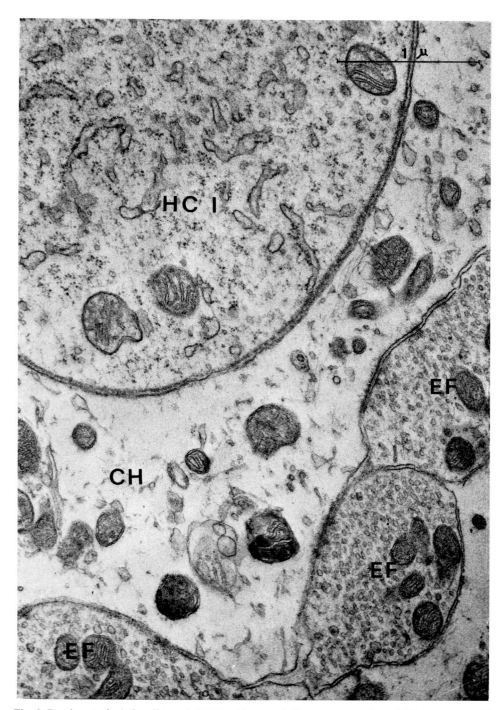

Fig. 5. Basal part of a hair cell type I (HC I) with several efferent nerve endings (EF) in contact with the outside of an afferent nerve chalice (CH). Electron micrograph (37,500 ×).

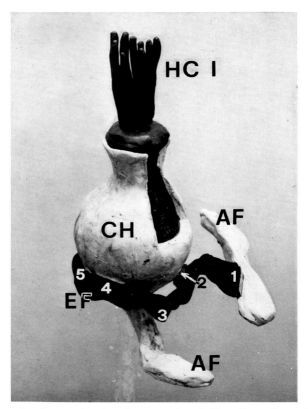

Fig. 6. Three-dimensional reconstruction from a series of 17 sections observed with the electron microscope. A presynaptic efferent fiber (EF) shows 5 synaptic enlargements which are in contact, respectively, (1) with an afferent fiber (AF); (2) (4) (5) with the afferent nerve chalice (CH) of a vestibular cell of type I (HC I); and (3) with a vestibular cell of type II not shown in the reconstruction. From Iurato and Taidelli (1964).

1961; Smith, 1967). They have a diameter between 1 and 2.5 μm, contain a large amount of small round vesicles (Fig. 5), some large (600–1200 Å) vesicles with a dense core and numerous mitochondria at some distance from the presynaptic membrane (Iurato and Taidelli, 1964). Where the efferent endings terminate on the surface of a hair cell of type II a dense substance is visible in the gap and the presynaptic membrane is sometimes thickened. No synaptic bar was found in the sensory cell adjacent to this kind of terminal but Wersäll (1968) observed a subsynaptic cistern surrounded by a thin membrane (Fig. 4). Sometimes this membrane is coated with some ribosomes on the side facing the hair cell (Wersäll, 1968). The efferent nerve endings and branches forming synapses with afferent chalices and dendrites are provided with a simpler synaptic complex formed by a condensation of dense material on both sides of the synaptic membrane and an accumulation of mitochondria and synaptic vesicles on the presynaptic side (Wersäll, 1968).

On the basis of the similarity between the vesiculated nerve endings in the inner ear

Frequency Modulation of Afferent and Efferent Unit Activity in the Vestibular Nerve by Oculomotor Impulses

J. DICHGANS, C. L. SCHMIDT AND E. R. WIST

Department of Neurology and Section of Neurophysiology, University of Freiburg, Freiburg i. Br., G.F.R.

Llinás and Precht (1972) summarized the control of vestibular receptors by efferent fibres activated by stimulation of the contralateral vestibular organ (Ledoux, 1958; Schmidt, 1963; Bertrand and Veenhof, 1964; Sala, 1965). They also described an ipsilateral efferent feedback passing through the vestibular parts of the cerebellum (Llinás *et al.*, 1967; Llinás and Precht, 1969). Furthermore they cited numerous multisensory convergences upon efferent fibres in the vestibular nerve. For example efferent discharge-modulations can be elicited by active and passive movements of the extremities (Schmidt, 1963; Bertrand and Veenhof, 1964). They can also be elicited by stimulation of the skin, mainly in the head region, and by optokinetic stimuli (Klinke and Schmidt, 1970). The functional significance of these latter findings is not yet completely understood.

It will be demonstrated here that saccadic eye movements (spontaneous saccades and the rapid phases of optokinetic and vestibular nystagmus) are associated with phasic discharge-modulations in the vestibular nerve. Most of the modulated neurones are efferent but some are certainly primary afferent fibres. These findings support the assumption that optomotor vestibular integration in animals already takes place at the receptor level.

Single unit activity was recorded with tungsten microelectrodes from the left peripheral vestibular nerve of the goldfish (Carassius aureatus) and the rabbit (Lepus cuniculus). Eye movements were recorded simultaneously by means of photocells. The animals were neither relaxed nor anaesthetized, for it is known that narcotics inhibit the activity of efferent neurones (Schmidt, 1963). The experiments were carried out in encéphale isolé preparations. In order to investigate the neuronal response to adequate vestibular stimuli, the animals were placed on a Tönnies turn-table, and the microelectrode was inserted into the vestibular nerve under visual control with the aid of a microscope.

In the goldfish preparation two electrode positions were selected: (*i*) in the fibres emerging from the horizontal canal; (*ii*) at the point right after the junction of all afferent components of the vestibular nerve. For selective recording of efferent neurones the vestibular nerve was severed and activity was recorded from the proximal stump of the nerve detached from its receptors. The surgical procedures have been described in detail by Schmidt *et al.* (1970, 1972).

References pp. 455–456

In the rabbit the occipital bone was removed. The neuronal activity was recorded from the vestibular nerve in the posterior fossa at its entrance into the internal acoustic meatus (3 mm lateral of the brain stem surface). In some rabbits the ipsilateral cerebellum was ablated by suction.

Since the findings in goldfish and rabbit were almost identical they will be described together. Species differences, where they occurred, will be separately described.

Almost 10 % of the neurones in the peripheral vestibular nerve show modulations of spontaneous activity in correlation with saccadic eye movements. Modulations occur regularly with all rapid eye movements, single saccades as well as the quick phases of optokinetic or vestibular nystagmus.

Types of responses during saccadic eye movements

Four types of neurones could be differentiated.

(i) Bidirectionally activated neurones (type-a). These are activated shortly before and during spontaneous saccades in both horizontal directions. Often the activation lasts longer than the duration of the saccade. In the goldfish most of the type-a neurones exhibit no or only low spontaneous activity (69 % 0–5 imp./sec), while in the rabbit the spontaneous activity averages 35 imp./sec. The activation starts 9–76 msec (mean: 33 msec) before the rapid eye movement. While the activation in the goldfish

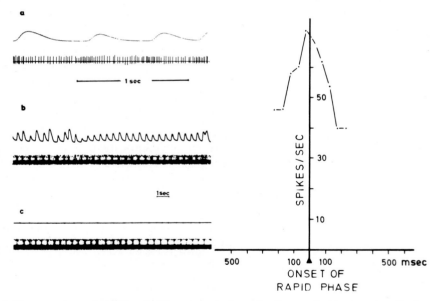

Fig. 1. Type-a neurone (rabbit). a, b: These records show clearly a gradual increase in spike frequency which occurs well before the onset of the saccade. The top line in each record indicates optokinetic nystagmus and the lower represents individual spikes from a single vestibular nerve fibre. c: the record shows that in the same neurone frequency modulation continues after administration of gallamine (lower line) even though no eye movements occur due to paralysis (upper line). On the right: graph showing the relationship between spike frequency (ordinate) and time before and after onset of a saccade (abscissa) averaged over 10 saccades in the same neurone as a–c.

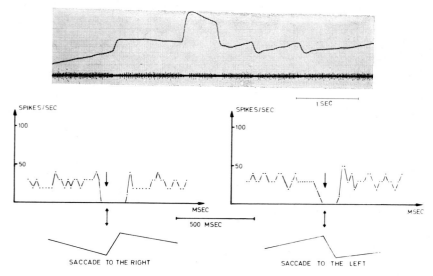

Fig. 2. Type-i neurone (goldfish). Upper record: saccadic eye movements and nystagmus in both directions (top line) preceded by an inhibition of neuronal activity (bottom line). Lower graphs: averaged neuronal activity during 10 beats of nystagmus to the right and to the left as a function of time before and after saccade onset. Arrows indicate onset of rapid phase.

always reaches its peak frequency immediately, the discharge frequency in the rabbit can start up to 110 msec before the saccade with a slow rise and fall (Fig. 1).

(ii) Bidirectionally inhibited neurones (type-i). These are in most cases completely inhibited during saccades in both horizontal directions. The inhibition starts 18–96 msec (mean: 64 msec) before the onset of the saccade and quite clearly outlasts it. The inhibition has a mean duration of 250 msec (Fig. 2).

Type-a neurones were found more frequently than type-i neurones. In the rabbit only the two types mentioned (a, i) were found.* In the goldfish the existence of additional neurone-types (d, p) was established.

(iii) Direction-specific neurones (type-d). These are rare and are inhibited in correlation with saccaces to the ipsilateral side and activated with saccades to the contralateral side (Fig. 3). Here too frequency-modulation starts before the beginning of the saccade.

(iv) Eye position dependent neurones (type-p). Twenty-one percent of the eye movement correlated neurones of the goldfish showed clear tonic frequency-modulations depending upon eye position. A temporal deviation of the eye, ipsilateral to the microelectrode, causes an activation and a nasal deviation an inhibition. Only in this type of neurone did the alteration in frequency start up to 100 msec *after* the change in

---

* The interval between the onset of inhibition and saccade onset in type-i neurones and onset of activation and saccade onset in type-a neurones are not directly comparable due to a measurement artifact associated with the former. The measured interval is about 19 msec greater than its actual duration (Schmidt *et al.*, 1972).

References pp. 455–456

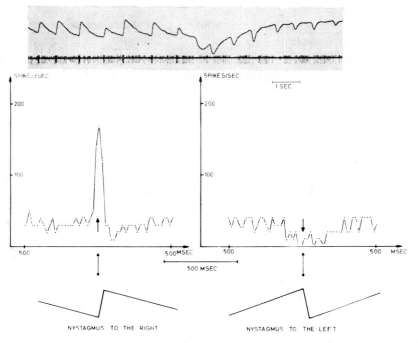

Fig. 3. Type-d neurone (goldfish). Upper record: periodic alternating nystagmus (top line) which is also typically found in intact fish. Activation of vestibular neuronal activity during rapid phases to the right and inhibition to the left (bottom line). Lower graphs: averaged neuronal activity during 10 beats of nystagmus as in Fig. 2. Arrows indicate onset of rapid phase.

eye position. Consequently an initiation of frequency-modulation by proprioceptive afference from the eye muscles seems to be possible. Some of the type-p neurones showed an additional phasic type-a frequency-modulation in correlation with saccadic eye movements (Schmidt et al., 1972).

In type-a, i and d neurones no consistent correlation could be found between the amplitude of eye movements and the degree of frequency-modulation. No relation to the slow phase of nystagmus could be traced. Neither the "crescendo neurones" nor the "decrescendo neurones" described by Duensing and Schaefer (1958) in the vestibular nuclei could be found in the vestibular nerve. Neurones of the macula-organs which can be stimulated by vibratory or acoustic stimuli showed no correlation with eye movements.

Functional considerations

These findings may increase our knowledge about the coordination of eye movements and vestibular afferences. Even though this occurs mainly in the premotorial network of small reticular interneurones of the midbrain- and pontine tegmentum (Kornhuber, 1966), it also occurs in the vestibular nuclei and — as we could demonstrate — at the peripheral vestibular receptor level. Not only vestibular nystagmus but also spontaneous eye movements and optokinetic nystagmus are seen simultaneously with phasic frequency-modulations of neurones in the reticular formation and the vestibular nuclei. Eye movement-correlated neuronal discharges are found in the rabbit's reticular formation near the mid-line of the tegmental rhombencephalon (Duensing and Schaefer, 1957) and in the vestibular nuclei (Eckel, 1954; Duensing and Schaefer, 1958). Similar phenomena in the peripheral vestibular nerve had not until now been discovered.

The eye movement-correlated frequency-modulation of the neuronal types-a, i and d cannot be initiated by proprioceptive afference from the eye muscles, because it starts before the beginning of the saccade and can also be demonstrated after administration of gallamine which produces eye muscle paralysis (Fig. 1). Only the activity of type-p neurones, dependent upon eye position, may be modulated by proprioceptive reafference from the eye muscles. One of our experiments in which the eye was passively moved demonstrated that there exists a relationship between proprioceptive afference and frequency modulation of discharge frequency in the vestibular nerve. This result confirmed the findings obtained earlier by Schmidt (1963). It seems quite probable that the frequency-modulation in type-a, i and d neurones, which starts presaccadically is initiated by collaterals of the supranuclear optomotor centers. It might be interpreted as a kind of supranuclear efference-copy (v. Holst and Mittelstaedt, 1950) or as corollary discharge (Teuber, 1960).

It is unknown where the efferent fibres originate which conduct the information about saccadic eye movements to the peripheral vestibular organ. Among the efferent pathways known the most probable is a fibre-bundle described by Rossi and Cortesina (1965). It originates homolaterally in the region of the pontine supranuclear oculomotor centers but also caudally in the dorsal reticular formation near the midline and goes to the vestibular nerve. At least in the rabbit the cerebellum has no influence upon the eye movement-correlated discharge-modulation in the peripheral vestibular nerve. Ablation of the ipsilateral cerebellum has no effect on the results described. Corresponding investigations in the goldfish were not performed.

The question arises whether some of the neuronal types described can be identified as efferent and others as afferent neurones. Recordings from the proximal stump of the severed vestibular nerve in the goldfish yielded neurones of types-a, i and p. These were therefore identified as efferent neurones. Only the very rare direction-specific neurones (type-d) were not found in the proximal stump. Other neurones (a, i, p) of the intact vestibular nerve were identified as efferent neurones by their reaction to rotatory acceleration. They were activated by ampullofugal acceleration or by acceleration in both horizontal directions (types II and III, described by Duensing and Schaefer, 1958). Such acceleration reactions characterize efferent neurones (Precht et al., 1971). In the goldfish it was not possible to verify that there existed afferent neurones with a frequency-modulation correlated with saccadic eye movements. Further experiments are in progress in which d.c.-recordings are made directly from the receptor layer. Such experiments could make clear the nature of the efferent influence.

In the rabbit some type-a neurones could be identified as being afferent neurones on the basis of their regular spontaneous activity (20–40 imp./sec), and their activation by ampullopetal acceleration. Small doses of barbiturate (2 mg/kg) extinguished the nystagmus-correlated activation, while the spontaneous activity and the response to acceleration were not influenced. The eye movements were abolished with higher dosages of barbiturate (4 mg/kg). Since it is known that efferent fibres are inhibited by narcotics, one can presume that under barbituate influence information about saccades mediated by efferent fibres to the vestibular receptor cells is suppressed. Duensing and Schaefer (1958) drew attention to the narcotic sensitivity of eye movement correlated neurones in the vestibular nucleus also.

The similarity of our results to those of Duensing and Schaefer (1957, 1958) raises the question of whether we recorded from secondary neurones of the nucleus interstitialis vestibularis. Some cells of this nucleus have been found in the most proximal part of the nerve in mammals (Gacek, 1969). In the goldfish similar cells in the peripheral nerve could not be verified histologically. It is quite obvious, however, that the vestibular neurones recorded directly from the ramus ampullaris lateralis in the dogfish were not secondary neurones.

Definite statements about the functional significance of efferent eye movement-correlated frequency-modulation in the peripheral vestibular nerve and the special task of each of the different types of neurones cannot be made at this time. It is striking that *the phasic modulation is always linked with saccadic eye movements but cannot be found in pursuit movements and slow nystagmic phases.* Mainly in the fish and frog, but also in the rabbit, saccadic eye movements are often supplemented by rapid head movements and optokinetic nystagmus by head-nystagmus. Control of vestibular afference during these head movements seems to be reasonable. During passive head-movements the elicited vestibular afference with its direct connection to oculomotor nuclei facilitates the steady fixation of a stationary visual target by inducing eye movements in a direction opposite to that of the head movement. During active head movement with eye movements in the same direction, the reverse afferent vestibular input to the oculomotor nuclei may be counterbalanced by efferent oculomotor impulses as far peripheral as at the vestibular receptor level.

The efferent saccadic discharge-modulation in the vestibular nerve could thus serve as a compensation to the arriving afferent vestibular information during simultaneous head nystagmus in such a way, that the optokinetic nystagmus is not inhibited by opposite impulses for compensatory movements. The same can be assumed for the vestibular nystagmus which under physiological conditions supports the optokinetic nystagmus.

Comparable results from the lateral line-organ were reported by Schmidt (1965). In the mud-puppy about 50 msec before active gill movements efferent discharges are elicited which reach the receptors of the lateral line-organ and might compensate for stimuli produced by the water streaming out of the gill. Contrary to eye movements, gill movements are purely vegetative reflex motions. Duensing and Schaefer (1960) established a descending modulation of reticular neurones linked to motor-efference during active head movements in the rabbit. During passive head movements these neurones were influenced by converging vestibular afferents in the opposite way. The findings cited from the literature support the assumption of compensatory signals mediated by collaterals of the motor centers to the afferent sensory input acting not only in the higher integrating centers of the brain, but also on a more peripheral level.

SUMMARY

1. Single unit activity was recorded from the peripheral vestibular nerve of unrelaxed and unanaesthetized goldfish and rabbits. Eye movements were registered.

2. Nearly 10% of the neurones showed a frequency-modulation starting before the beginning of each spontaneous saccadic eye movement and rapid phase of opto-kinetic and vestibular nystagmus.

3. Bidirectionally activated (type-a) as well as bidirectionally inhibited (type-i) neurones could be established. In the goldfish a few direction-specific neurones with inhibition or activation depending upon the direction of horizontal saccadic eye-movements (type-d) were found.

4. The presaccadic initiated phasic discharge-modulation is supposed to originate from supranuclear optomotor centers.

5. In addition to these phasically modulated neurones found in both the goldfish and rabbit, the goldfish shows neurones whose discharge-frequency depends upon eye position (type-p). These neurones may be influenced by proprioceptive afferents from the eye muscle.

6. Mainly in the goldfish, most of the neurones were identified as being efferent ones. In the rabbit some afferent bidirectionally activated neurones of type-a were verified.

7. The results demonstrate the existence of a vestibular control by oculomotor impulses mediated by efferent fibres to the vestibular receptor level in teleosts and lower mammals. The possible functional significance is discussed.

REFERENCES

BERTRAND, R. A. AND VEENHOF, V. B. (1964) Efferent vestibular potentials by canalicular and oto-lithic stimulations in the rabbit. *Acta oto-laryng. (Stockh.)*, **58**, 515–524.

DUENSING, F. UND SCHAEFER, K. P. (1957) Die Neuronenaktivität in der Formatio reticularis des Rhombencephalons beim vestibulären Nystagmus. *Arch. Psychiat. Nervenkr.*, **196**, 265–290.

DUENSING, F. UND SCHAEFER, K. P. (1958) Die Aktivität einzelner Neurone im Bereich der Vestibulariskerne unter besonderer Berücksichtigung des vestibulären Nystagmus. *Arch. Psychiat. Nervenkr.*, **198**, 224–252.

DUENSING, F. UND SCHAEFER, K. P. (1960) Die Aktivität einzelner Neurone der Formatio reticularis des nicht gefesselten Kaninchens bei Kopfwendungen und vestibulären Reizen. *Arch. Psychiat. Nervenkr.*, **201**, 97–122.

ECKEL, W. (1954) Elektrophysiologische und histologische Untersuchungen im Vestibulariskern-gebiet bei Drehreizen. *Arch. Ohr.- Nas.- u. Kehlk.-Heilk.*, **164**, 487–513.

GACEK, R. R. (1969) The course and central termination of first order neurones supplying vestibular endorgans in the cat. *Acta oto-laryng. (Stockh.)*, Suppl. 254, 1–66.

HOLST, E. V. UND MITTELSTAEDT, H. (1950) Das Reafferenzprinzip (Wechselwirkung zwischen Zentralnervensystem und Peripherie). *Naturwissenschaften*, **37**, 464–476.

KLINKE, R. AND SCHMIDT, C. L. (1970) Efferent influence on the vestibular organ during active movements of the body. *Pflügers Arch. ges. Physiol.*, **318**, 325–332.

KORNHUBER, H. H. (1966) Physiologie und Klinik des vestibulären Systems. In J. BERENDES, R. ZINK AND F. ZÖLLNER (Eds.), *Hals-Nasen-Ohrenheilkunde, ein kurzgefasstes Handbuch. Vol. III/3*, Thieme, Stuttgart, pp. 2150–2351.

LEDOUX, A., (1958) Les canaux semi-circulaires. *Acta oto-rhino-laryng. belg.*, **12**, 109–348.

LLINÁS, R., PRECHT, W. AND KITAI, S. T. (1967) Climbing fibre activation of Purkinje cell following primary vestibular afferent stimulation in the frog. *Brain Res.*, **6**, 371–375.

LLINÁS, R. AND PRECHT, W. (1969) The inhibitory vestibular efferent system and its relation to the cerebellum in the frog. *Exp. Brain Res.*, **9**, 16–29.

LLINÁS, R. AND PRECHT, W. (1972) Vestibulocerebellar input: physiology. In A. BRODAL AND O. POMPEIANO (Eds.), *Progress in Brain Research. Vol. 37. Basic aspects of central vestibular mechanisms.* Elsevier, Amsterdam, pp. 341–359.

ROSSI, G. AND CORTESINA, G. (1965) The efferent cochlear and vestibular system in Lepus cuniculus. *Acta anat. (Basel)*, **60**, 362–381.

PRECHT, W., LLINÁS, R. AND CLARKE, M. (1972) Physiological responses of frog vestibular fibers to horizontal angular rotation. *Exp. Brain Res.*, **13**, 378–407.

SALA, O. (1965) The efferent vestibular system. Electro-physiological research. *Acta oto-laryng. (Stockh.)*, Suppl. 197, 4–34.

SCHMIDT, C. L., WIST, E. R., DICHGANS, J. (1970) Alternating spontaneous nystagmus, optokinetic and vestibular nystagmus and their relationship to rhythmically modulated spontaneous activity in the vestibular nerve of the goldfish. *Pflügers Arch. ges. Physiol.*, **319**, R155–156.

SCHMIDT, C. L., WIST, E. R. AND DICHGANS, J. (1972) Efferent frequency modulation in the vestibular nerve of goldfish correlated with saccadic eye movements. *Exp. Brain Res.*, **15**, 1–14.

SCHMIDT, R. S. (1963) Frog labyrinthine efferent impulses. *Acta oto-laryng. (Stockh.)*, **56**, 51–64.

SCHMIDT, R. S. (1965) Amphibian acoustico-lateralis efferents. *J. cell. comp. Physiol.*, **65**, 155–162.

TEUBER, H. L. (1960) Perception. In J. FIELD, H. W. MAGOUN AND V. E. HALL (Eds.), *Handbook of Physiology. Section 1. Neurophysiology. Vol. III.* Amer. Physiol. Soc., Washington, D.C., pp. 1595–1668.

COMMENT TO CHAPTER VI

Functional Significance of the Efferent Control Mechanisms

O. LOWENSTEIN

Department of Zoology and Comparative Physiology, University of Birmingham, Birmingham, Great Britain

The question of the functional significance of the efferent innervation of the vestibular system is one of the most urgent ones at the present moment. Ever since the ultra-structural evidence of efferent synapses on the hair cell became available my colleagues and I have been pondering this matter. My own first guess was that the efference acts as a setting mechanism of the basic hair cell activity. My results obtained with d.c. polarization (Lowenstein, 1955) which showed that it is possible to shift the working point of a hair cell up and down its S-shaped "characteristic" encouraged me to think that hyperpolarization of the hair cell membrane via the efferent synapse could achieve this very effect at any rate unidirectionally by inhibition. This possibility is still to be taken seriously. Two recent findings show convincingly that the basic activity of the hair cells can be affected by efference. In one case (Russell, unpublished) the activity of the hair cells in the lateral line organ of Xenopus is inhibited whenever the ventral horn cells of the spinal cord are activated for swimming movements. In the other, the same happens in a goldfish immobilized by MS 222 when the animal is subjected to an optokinetic stimulus to which paralysis prevents it from responding by an appropriate motor response (Klinke, 1970). In this connexion I should like to give voice to a warning. In my opinion we shall have to look not for one but for a whole range of functional aspects of sensory efference in accordance with a great variety of biological circumstances and "needs".

REFERENCES

KLINKE, R. (1970) Efferent influence on the vestibular organ during active movements of the body. *Pflügers Arch. ges. Physiol.*, **318**, 325–332.

LOWENSTEIN, O. (1955) The effect of galvanic polarization on the impulse discharge from sense endings in the isolated labyrinth of the thornback ray (*Raja clavata*). *J. Physiol. (Lond.)*, **127**, 104–117.

VII. VESTIBULO-OCULOMOTOR RELATIONS

Structural and Functional Aspects of Extraocular Muscles in Relation to Vestibulo-ocular Function

P. BACH-Y-RITA

Smith-Kettlewell Institute of Visual Sciences,
University of the Pacific, San Francisco, California, U.S.A.

The intimate linkage of the eye muscle control system and the vestibular complex has received the attention of numerous investigators (for reviews see Bach-y-Rita and Collins, 1971). The ready elicitation, reproducibility and characteristics of vestibular nystagmus have made this an invaluable tool for clarification of certain aspects of central nervous system control of eye movements. My own interest has focussed on the determination of the relative contributions of each of the principal nerve and muscle fiber types to the slow and fast phases of vestibular nystagmus. This has been part of our overall objective of studying the physiological and morphological properties of extraocular muscle (EOM) fibers and their innervation. Our studies on EOM properties have been reviewed recently (Bach-y-Rita, 1971a) and will be described here only insofar as they relate to vestibulo-ocular relationships. The present paper will also discuss possible differences in the organization of vestibular and non-vestibular eye movements, and the interaction of muscle proprioceptive activity with vestibular impulses.

EXTRAOCULAR MUSCLE AND NERVE FIBER TYPES

Morphologically there would appear to be as many as five types of muscle fibers in EOMs of cats (Peachey, 1971). However, the majority of investigators studying the physiological properties have been able to distinguish only one or two types. Our own physiological and pharmacological studies in cats have clearly differentiated two types: large, fast singly innervated muscle fibers and smaller, slower multiply innervated fibers. Both of these exhibit twitch properties. The small, slow multi-innervated twitch fibers are located predominantly in the outer (orbital) layers of the muscles. In comparison with limb muscle fibers, these EOM fibers have properties more comparable to intrafusal than extrafusal fibers. However, in the limbs, the intrafusal fibers do not contribute directly to the muscle force or tension. In the EOMs, the small fibers constitute approximately one-third of the tetanic force of each muscle.

Large nerve fibers, with conduction velocities of from 41 to over 100 m/sec innervate the large, fast muscle fibers. Small gamma range fibers, with conduction velocities of from 6 to 40 m/sec, innervate the slow multi-innervated twitch fibers (Bach-y-Rita and Ito, 1966). In our studies, only the small nerve fibers have revealed spontaneous activi-

References pp. 469–470

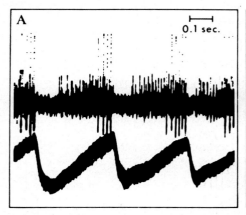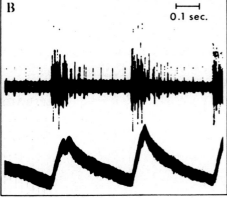

Fig. 1. Responses during vestibular nystagmus. The upper channel presents activity recorded from the VI nerve; the lower channel records lateral rectus muscle tension. A. From the nerve on the same side as the slow phase of nystagmus. Small spikes, representing a slow fiber (CV 25 m/sec) revealed a gradually increasing discharge frequency during the slow phase, with cessation of activity during the fast phase. Large spikes, from a fast fiber (CV 50 m/sec) appeared only during the last half of the slow phase. (The upper portions of the large spikes in A and B have been retouched). The CV of the fiber with very low-amplitude spikes, discharging almost simultaneously with the slow fiber, was not measured. B. From the nerve on the side opposite to the slow phase of nystagmus. Recordings were made from the same nerve fibers as in A, but the direction of nystagmus was reversed. The slow fibers showed a high-frequency burst during the fast (lateral) phase, with a gradual decrease in frequency during the slow phase of nystagmus to the opposite side. The fast fiber (large spikes) was silent during the contralateral slow phase and appeared as a high-frequency burst during the homolateral fast phase. From Yamanaka and Bach-y-Rita, (1968).

ty, which has been recorded when the eyes remain approximately in the mid-position (Yamanaka and Bach-y-Rita, 1968).

During the slow phase of vestibular nystagmus, the early part of the contraction is due to the participation of only the smaller nerve fibers. Activity of the larger fibers is evident only later in the contraction, presumably when the angular deviation of the eye has reached a point reflecting the recruitment of the larger, higher threshold motor neurons (Yamanaka and Bach-y-Rita, 1968). This would appear to be comparable to the development of recruitment in limb motor neuron pools described by Henneman et al. (1965a, b). During the fast phase of nystagmus, apparently both fast and slow fibers discharge simultaneously, as seen in Fig. 1.

TIME-LAG BETWEEN MUSCLES DURING VESTIBULAR NYSTAGMUS

Vestibular nystagmus has been used by physiologists as a model of all conjugate oculomotor activity. The slow phase is generally compared to slow smooth following movements, and the fast to saccades. While these analogies may be valid for the most part, it is possible that the pathways and central structures mediating vestibularly induced nystagmus may differ substantially from those involved in other types of eye movements. One clue to possible differences in organization may be gathered from the fact

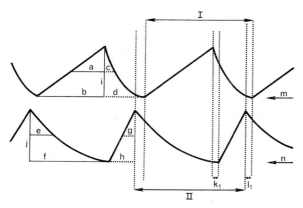

Fig. 2. Schematic representation showing contraction and relaxation of antagonist muscles (upper and lower lines) during each phase of nystagmus; a: half-time of the slow rise; b: time of the slow phase rise; c: half-time of the fast phase decay; d: time of the fast phase decay; e: half-time of the slow phase extension; f: time of the slow phase extension; g: half-time of the fast phase rise; h: time of the fast phase rise; i and j: amplitudes of nystagmus; I: duration of a nystagmus beat of one muscle; II: duration of a nystagmus beat of the antagonist; k_1: 'phase lag' time between beginning of a fast decay of a muscle and beginning of contraction of the antagonist muscle; l_1: 'phase lag' time between beginning of slow extension of a muscle and beginning of a slow contraction of the antagonist; m: tonus level of one muscle; n: tonus level of the antagonist muscle. From Yamanaka and Bach-y-Rita (1970).

that in vestibular nystagmus there is a time lag between the beginning of relaxation (or inhibition) of the antagonist and the initiation of contraction of the agonist (Lorente de Nó, 1934; Yamanaka and Bach-y-Rita, 1970), as shown schematically in Fig. 2. This lag is not present during the 'spontaneous' nystagmus of an encéphale isolé cat (Bach-y-Rita, unpublished results). Time lags of this type have not been found during either following movements or saccades in humans (Collins, personal communication), nor have studies on motoneurons shown it to be present during non-vestibularly induced eye movements in monkeys (Robinson, 1970; Fuchs and Luchei, 1970; Keller, 1971), even during saccades of up to 40 degrees of angular deviation.

Intracellular studies on cat abducens motoneurons have revealed that the quick cessation of nerve discharges associated with the fast decay during vestibular nystagmus is associated not only with a reduction of the excitatory postsynaptic potential but also with the production of an inhibitory postsynaptic potential (Maeda et al., 1971). Maeda and collaborators (1971) noted that the time of onset of the quick hyperpolarization and of the quick depolarization was the same (4.8 msec and 4.7 msec, respectively), and judged that they were therefore synchronous events. However, in their studies, the nerve discharges produced by excitation occurred later than the quick cessation of the antagonist nerve impulses; analysis of their illustration reveals the time lag to be approximately 18 msec. Further information on these studies appear in this volume (Shimazu, 1972). This would be comparable to the 25 msec time lag noted by Lorente de Nó (1934) in the rabbit, and the time lag of up to 29 msec noted in the cat during vestibular nystagmus by Yamanaka and Bach-y-Rita (1968).

Further studies of all types of eye movements are necessary in order to determine the precise conditions under which a time lag occurs. For example, it has not yet been determined whether the lag is found in rotation-induced nystagmus, which involves vestibular stimulation on one side and inhibition of the contralateral side; our results (Yamanaka and Bach-y-Rita, 1968), like those of Lorente de Nó (1934), were obtained following unilateral vestibular stimulation.

If it is found that the time lag is observed only during vestibular nystagmus, this would suggest two interpretations of considerable interest to an understanding of the central nervous system organization of eye movements. (*i*) There would be less of a viscous braking action from antagonist muscles during vestibular nystagmus than during non-vestibular eye movements. Thus a comparable acceleration of the agonists should be effected with less innervational input and with less forceful muscular contraction during vestibular nystagmus than during other types of eye movement. (*ii*) It would be difficult to sustain the concept that the fast phase of nystagmus is identical with a saccadic movement, and thus that the pathway for mediation of saccades passes through the vestibular nuclei.

INTERACTION OF VESTIBULAR AND EXTRAOCULAR MUSCLE PROPRIOCEPTIVE INFLUENCES

The role of proprioception in eye movements has long been a subject of controversy. The subject has been reviewed recently (Bach-y-Rita, 1971). Typical muscle spindles are found in the EOMs of man, chimpanzees, goats and some other species, but not in the eye muscles of cat, dog, rabbit or some monkeys. However, even the latter species have some kind of stretch receptor, as evidenced by the fact that afferent impulses can usually be recorded in response to EOM stretch. Thus far the exception is the squirrel monkey, in which no evidence for true stretch receptors was uncovered by physiological studies of the inferior oblique and lateral rectus muscle (Ito and Bach-y-Rita, 1969).

Until recently it has not been possible to demonstrate actual stretch reflexes in the EOMs of man or animals. However, earlier studies have concentrated on attempts to elicit responses to passive stretch of a muscle. Recently we have demonstrated an inhibitory stretch reflex to be present during active contraction (but not during passive stretch) of the lateral rectus muscle in cats. An example is shown in Fig. 3, with decreased activity of a spontaneously discharging motoneuron during active contraction induced by electrical stimulation of a branch of the VI nerve. The results of this study have been reported at the symposium on "Cerebral Control of Eye Movements and Perception", Freiburg and published elsewhere (Bach-y-Rita, 1972).

EOM stretch receptor responses are of particular interest to an understanding of vestibulo-ocular mechanisms, since there is evidence that afferent impulses from eye movements interact with vestibular impulses in the brain stem. Gernandt (1968) has shown that vestibularly-induced activity recorded in the pontine reticular formation is strongly inhibited by EOM stretch. In the cat, the response of single reticular formation units to vestibular stimulation was depressed following muscle stretch applied

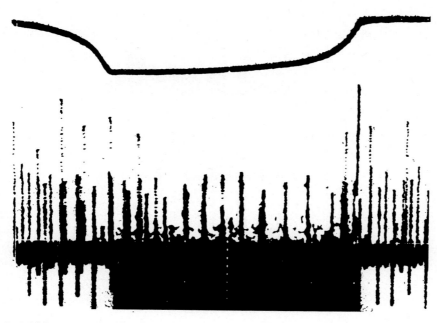

Fig. 3. Inhibitory stretch reflex in cat extraocular muscles (*encéphale isolé* preparation). The VI nerve was exposed at the emergence from the pons, and a small branch cut peripherally and placed over electrodes to record the discharge of motor fibers (upper line). Another bundle of fibers was cut at the emergence of the VI nerve from the brain and placed over stimulating electrodes, through which muscle contraction could be reduced. The major portion of the VI nerve was left intact, since stretch receptor afferents from the lateral rectus muscle reach the brain via this nerve. The homolateral lateral rectus was attached to a strain gauge to record the contraction (lower line). One second of activity is displayed; stimulation at 300 pulses/sec, for 575 msec produced inhibition of some of the discharging motor fibers. Initial tension on the muscle was 16 g, and the amplitude of the contraction was 12 g.

10–30 msec prior to the vestibular stimulation. Gernandt's (1968) experiments indicated that EOM stretch affected only the slower (multi-synaptic) reticular formation pathway from the vestibular nuclei to the extraocular motor nuclei; the faster, more direct pathway involving the medial longitudinal fasciculus remained unaffected by prior muscle stretch.

Comparable evidence was obtained by Ito *et al.* (1969). The effect of electrical stimulation of the lateral semicircular canal on muscle fibers in the contralateral lateral rectus was recorded intracellularly in cats. The latencies of the responses were determined with stretch of the muscle 2, 4 and 6 mm beyond the resting length. A histogram of the responses is presented in Fig. 4. It will be noted that the latencies are short with high initial tension with the longer latency responses virtually eliminated, possibly due to the activation of the stretch receptors due to the muscle contraction (Bach-y-Rita, 1972) induced by the vestibular stimulation. It would therefore seem probable that the slow vestibular influences are indeed inhibited by afferent impulses from EOM stretch receptors, as was concluded by Gernandt (1968).

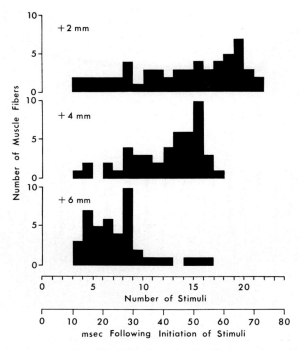

Fig. 4. A histogram of the intracellular discharge latencies for all types of muscle fibers in the lateral rectus muscle fibers of three cats anesthetized with sodium pentothal (35 mg/kg). The contralateral semicircular canal was stimulated electrically (150 msec bursts of 0.1 msec pulses at a frequency of 300/sec). The latencies were measured during the third burst (delivered at 1.5 sec intervals) of stimuli, to the beginning of discharge (lower line). The upper line shows the comparable number of stimuli required to trigger the discharge. From Ito *et al.* (1969).

The functional role of this interaction between EOMs and the vestibular system is not clear. It would be tempting to postulate a mechanism whereby increasing tension development toward the end of the slow phase of nystagmus would inhibit the slow vestibular activity, thus presenting a decreased viscous resistance to the opposite fast phase. However there is no direct evidence in support of this postulation. Indeed, Dusser de Barenne and de Kleyn (1928) showed that neural discharges with nystagmus rhythm could be recorded from the nerves to the extraocular muscles following excision of all six EOMs of one eye, thus eliminating any stretch receptor activity from that orbit. It is not known though, whether there was any change in duration or timing of the neural discharges following excision.

It is conceivable that the inhibition of the slow vestibular component may be related to the time lag between inhibition of the antagonist and contraction of the agonist, discussed above. A further possibility is that inhibition of the slow vestibular pathways might prevent impulses initiating in the vestibular system from arriving at the motoneurons after the end of the slow phase of nystagmus. If impulses were to arrive at this stage over the slow pathways, they would presumably oppose the movement to the opposite direction, thus adding a considerable force requirement to the agonist.

A knowledge of the contributions of the various types of muscle fibers in the EOMs, and of the stretch receptors in these muscles during vestibular-induced eye movements, can contribute greatly to an understanding of both vestibular and oculomotor mechanisms, principally those that use common brain stem structures and integrative mechanisms. The following papers in this session on vestibulo-oculomotor relations will present anatomical, physiological and biophysical data that will help to clarify some of these mechanisms.

SUMMARY

The separate populations of extraocular muscle and nerve fibers were described, and their roles in slow and fast vestibular-induced eye movements was discussed. A time lag between the cessation of contraction of an antagonist eye muscle and the initiation of contraction of the agonist was noted during vestibular-induced eye movements but not in other types of eye movements. The interaction of extraocular muscle proprioceptive activity and vestibular influences was described: the proprioceptive activity has been shown to inhibit vestibular ocular activity arriving in the brain stem via slow (reticular formation) pathways. The functional significance of their interaction was discussed.

ACKNOWLEDGEMENTS

This work was supported by Public Health Service Program Project Research Grant No. 2 PO1 EY-0029 and Research Career Award No. K3 EY-14,094.

REFERENCES

BACH-Y-RITA, P. (1971) Neurophysiology of eye movements. In P. BACH-Y-RITA, C. C. COLLINS AND J. E. HYDE (Eds.), *The Control of Eye Movements*. Academic Press, New York, pp. 7–45.

BACH-Y-RITA, P. (1972) Extraocular muscle inhibitory stretch reflex during active contraction. *Arch. ital. Biol.*, **110**, 1–15.

BACH-Y-RITA, P., COLLINS, C. C. AND J. E. HYDE (1971c) *The Control of Eye Movements*. Academic Press, New York, pp. X–560.

BACH-Y-RITA, P. AND ITO, F. (1966) *In vivo* studies on fast and slow muscle fibers in cat extraocular muscles. *J. gen. Physiol.*, **49**, 1177–1198.

DUSSER DE BARENNE, J. G. UND DE KLEYN, A. (1928) Über vestibulären Nystagmus nach Exstirpation von allen sechs Augenmuskeln beim Kaninchen; Beitrag zur Wirkung und Innervation des Musculus retractor bulbi. *Pflügers Arch. ges. Physiol.*, **221**, 1–14.

FUCHS, A. F. AND LUCHEI, E. S. (1970) Firing patterns of abducens neurons of alert monkeys in relationship to horizontal eye movement. *J. Neurophysiol.*, **33**, 382–392.

GERNANDT, B. E. (1968) Interactions between extraocular myotatic and ascending vestibular activities. *Exp. Neurol.*, **20**, 120–134.

HENNEMAN, E., SOMJEN, G. AND CARPENTER, D. O. (1965a) Functional significance of cell size in spinal motoneurons. *J. Neurophysiol.*, **28**, 560–580.

HENNEMAN, E., SOMJEN, G. AND CARPENTER, D. O. (1965b) Excitability and inhibitability of motoneurons of different sizes. *J. Neurophysiol.*, **28**, 599–620.

ITO, F. AND BACH-Y-RITA, P. (1969) Afferent discharges from extraocular muscle in the squirrel monkey. *Amer. J. Physiol.*, **217**, 332–335.

ITO, F., BACH-Y-RITA, P. AND YAMANAKA, Y. (1969) Extraocular muscle intracellular and motor nerve responses to semicircular canal stimulation. *Exp. Neurol.*, **24**, 438–449.

KELLER, E. L. (1971) *Abducens Unit Activity in the Alert Monkey during Vergence Movements and Extraocular Stretch.* Ph. D. Thesis, Johns Hopkins University, Baltimore, pp. 150.

MAEDA, M., SHIMAZU, H. AND SHINODA, Y. (1971) Inhibitory postsynaptic potentials in the abducens motoneurons associated with the quick relaxation phase of vestibular nystagmus. *Brain Res.*, **26**, 420–424.

LORENTE DE NÓ, R. (1934) Observations on nystagmus. *Acta oto-laryng. (Stockh.)*, **21**, 416–437.

PEACHEY, L. (1971) The structure of the extraocular muscle fibers of mammals. In P. BACH-Y-RITA, C. C. COLLINS AND J. E. HYDE (Eds.), *The Control of Eye Movements.* Academic Press, New York, pp. 47–66.

ROBINSON, D. A. (1970) Oculomotor unit behavior in the monkey. *J. Neurophysiol.*, **33**, 393–404.

SHIMAZU, H. (1972) Vestibulo-oculomotor relations: dynamic responses. In A. BRODAL AND O. POMPEIANO (Eds.), *Progress in Brain Research. Vol. 37. Basic aspects of central vestibular mechanisms.* Elsevier, Amsterdam, pp. 493–506.

YAMANAKA, Y. AND BACH-Y-RITA, P. (1968) Conduction velocities in the abducens nerve correlated with vestibular nystagmus in cats. *Exp. Neurol.*, **20**, 143–155.

YAMANAKA, Y. AND BACH-Y-RITA, P. (1970) Relations between extraocular muscle contraction and extension times in each phase of nystagmus. *Exp. Neurol.*, **27**, 57–65.

Anatomy of the Two Vestibulo-oculomotor Projection Systems

E. TARLOV

Neurosurgical Service, Massachusetts General Hospital, Boston, Mass., U.S.A.

The delicate influences of the vestibular apparatus on coordinated extraocular move-ments depend upon intricate neural mechanisms which are beginning to reveal them-selves to anatomical investigation. In previous studies we have demonstrated two separate systems of vestibulo-oculomotor projections, arising in the rostral part of the medial vestibular nucleus (RMV) and in the superior vestibular nucleus (SV), follow-ing separate courses in the medial longitudinal fasciculus (MLF), and having exten-sively overlapping bilateral distribution among motoneurons innervating the extra-ocular muscles (EOM) (Tarlov, 1970a). We have suggested that these two extensively overlapping fiber projection systems subserve excitatory and inhibitory influences of the semicircular canals on the oculomotor nuclei (Tarlov, 1970b).

The anatomical separation of the two projection systems described is of interest in relation to growing physiological evidence (Baker *et al.*, 1969; Precht and Baker, 1970; Highstein and Ito, 1971) that the SV and RMV each exert differing functional influences on extraocular muscle motoneurons.

Precise anatomical information about the systems of fiber projections which connect the vestibular nuclei with the motor nuclei of the III, IV and VI cranial nerves has been slow to accumulate. Partly because of technical factors and partly because of the limitations of the methods used and the relative difficulties of interpretation of the available data, the numerous schemes which have been previously proposed for these connections have been in disagreement on almost all major points. Regarding the *sites of origin* in the vestibular nuclei of these projections, McMasters, Weiss and Carpenter (1966) have stated that vestibulo-oculomotor projections arise in all four of the main vestibular nuclei; while Gray (1926) found such projections arising only in the medial and superior vestibular nuclei, Buchanan (1937) found the medial, lateral and superior nuclei to be the sources of these fibers; Rasmussen (1932) found them to arise from the medial, superior and descending nuclei.

Regarding the *course of ascending fibers from vestibular nuclei* there has also been divergence of opinion; while it has been agreed that the superior vestibular nucleus projects ascending fibers only in the ipsilateral MLF, the ascending projection from the medial vestibular nucleus has been found to be contralateral by Gray (1926) and Rasmussen (1932) while Buchanan (1937), Ferraro *et al.* (1940) and McMasters *et al.* (1966) found this projection in the MLF to be bilateral. Axons from the descending vestibular nucleus have been said to ascend only in the contralateral MLF by Ras-mussen (1932) while McMasters *et al.* (1966) have found these only in the ipsilateral

MLF. Fibers from the lateral vestibular nucleus are said by Buchanan (1932) to ascend bilaterally, but Gray (1926) and Rasmussen (1937) do not mention their existence.

Regarding the *terminations of secondary vestibular axons* in the extraocular motor (EOM) nuclei there has also been widely divergent opinion, and while some of the differences may be due to the unsuitability of the Marchi method for exact delimitation of preterminal axon distribution, there have been marked differences in the results of authors who have used the Nauta technique. Szentágothai (1964) and McMasters *et al.* (1966) have described projections to differing limited areas within the EOM nuclei. McMasters *et al.* (1966) state that the superior vestibular nucleus projects to the ipsilateral trochlear nucleus and the motoneurons of the ipsilateral inferior rectus. From the medial vestibular nucleus they describe projections to the contralateral trochlear nucleus, the motoneurons innervating the contralateral inferior oblique, and the motoneurons of the ipsilateral medial rectus. Projections from the lateral and descending vestibular nuclei to certain groups of extraocular muscle motoneurons were also stated to exist.

Szentágothai's (1964) studies, on the other hand, indicated that the projection from the superior vestibular nucleus chiefly innervates the motoneurons of the ipsilateral superior and medial rectus. Projections from the other vestibular nuclei were felt by Szentágothai to be unrelated to crista reflexes and perhaps to subserve influence of the otoliths on extraocular function. Our own findings indicate that these connections are considerably more extensive and highly organized than these authors have indicated. These matters will be discussed further below.

Regarding the projections to the interstitial nuclei of Cajal and the nuclei of Darkschewitsch, these terms have not been used in the same sense by all authors and therefore, findings cannot be readily compared. I have previously reviewed this subject in a study of the rostral limits of the secondary vestibular projections (Tarlov, 1969).

Apart from the discrepancies due to the limitations of the Marchi method and those due to the lack of a standarized nomenclature for the vestibular nuclei in earlier studies, the differences among these experimental observations are largely due to varied interpretations of degenerated fibers which result from unrecognized injuries outside the intended target, due either to the electrode track, to the trauma inflicted upon the vestibular nuclei and other structures during open operation within the fourth ventricle, or to slight but significant extension of the lesions into the adjacent vestibular nuclei. Incidental damage outside the intended target may be evaluated by using a variety of approaches in making the lesions, and by examining sections cut in a plane parallel to the course of degenerated fibers being studied. Neither of these techniques has apparently been used in establishing the many differing views summarized above.

In this paper I will present experimental findings on the following points:

(*i*) Origin within the vestibular nuclei of vestibulo-oculomotor projections.

(*ii*) Course of vestibulo-oculomotor projections.

(*iii*) Representation of individual extraocular muscles within the oculomotor nuclei.

(*iv*) Termination of the vestibulo-oculomotor projections.

(*v*) Rostral limit of ascending secondary vestibular projections.

ORIGIN WITHIN THE VESTIBULAR NUCLEI OF VESTIBULO-OCULOMOTOR PROJECTIONS

Discrete unilateral stereotaxic lesions were placed in portions of each of the four main vestibular nuclei in 17 cats. A variety of electrode approaches was used to control the results of electrode passage through surrounding structures. The resulting degenerated axons were stained at appropriate survival times with the Nauta method and in some cases with the Heimer method as well. As shown in Fig. 1, five lesions involving different portions of the superior vestibular nucleus (SV) all resulted in preterminal axon degeneration in the EOM nuclei. Four lesions involving rostral portions of the medial vestibular nucleus (RMV) all produced preterminal axon degeneration in the EOM nuclei. By contrast, extensive lesions adjacent to these regions including lesions in the lateral vestibular nucleus, the descending vestibular nucleus, and caudal portions of the medial vestibular nucleus produced no axon degeneration in any of the EOM nuclei. These findings indicate that direct vestibulo-oculomotor projections arise only

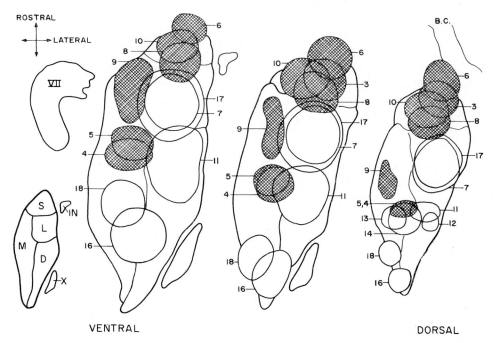

Fig. 1. Origins of vestibulo-oculomotor projections. Diagrams of serial horizontal sections through the right vestibular nuclei as seen from dorsal surface, representing extent of lesions in each case (numbers). Cross-hatched lesions give rise to degenerated fibers in EOM nuclei. Note that these lie in superior vestibular nucleus and rostral portions of medial vestibular nucleus. Lesions in caudal parts of the medial vestibular nucleus and lesions in the lateral and descending vestibular nuclei (not cross-hatched) did not give rise to degenerated axons in the EOM nuclei. Orientation shown in inset. S: superior vestibular nucleus, M: medial nucleus, L: lateral nucleus, D: descending nucleus, VII: genu of facial nerve, IN: interstitial nucleus, X: nucleus x of Brodal and Pompeiano (1958). From Tarlov (1970a).

in the superior vestibular nucleus (SV) and in rostral portions of the medial vestibular nucleus (RMV). Each of the lesions within these nuclei produced a differing pattern of degenerated axons in the EOM nuclei. No direct vestibulo-oculomotor fibers arise in the lateral or the descending vestibular nuclei, or in the caudal portions of the medial vestibular nuclei. Previous findings of vestibulo-oculomotor projections arising in these regions (McMasters *et al.*, 1966) result, in my opinion, from incidental damage to the medial vestibular nuclei, a virtually unavoidable consequence, in my experience, of even the most delicate exposure of the fourth ventricle. Such damage is avoided by stereotaxic approaches to the nuclei in which intended lesions are placed and by using discrete lesions such as those depicted in Fig. 6A and B for the study of anterograde axon degeneration (Fig. 6C and D),

These restricted origins of vestibulo-EOM nuclei projections correlate with physiological data and with certain anatomical data regarding other vestibular connections. Within the vestibular nuclei, the separate distribution of semicircular canal projections and otolithic organ projections described by Lorente de Nó (1933a, b) have recently been studied by Stein and Carpenter (1967) in the monkey and by Gacek (1969) in the cat. These authors have demonstrated that the semicircular canal ganglia project principally to the superior vestibular nucleus and to rostral portions of the medial vestibular nucleus. It is these regions, the present study demonstrates, which project to the EOM nuclei. Gacek (1969) found that within the SV cells lying most medially receive projections from all three semicircular canals, while within central portions of the SV, the anterior and horizontal canals are represented rostrally and laterally while the posterior canal projects caudally and medially. In the medial vestibular nucleus, according to Gacek (1969), the projections of the semicircular canals are not separated. The present study demonstrates differing projections from each of these regions to areas within the EOM nuclei innervating specific muscles.

Both Stein and Carpenter (1967) and Gacek (1969) found sparse projections from the semicircular canal ganglia to rostral portions of the descending vestibular nucleus, and very occasional degenerated fibers, interpreted as preterminals, in the lateral vestibular nucleus. These regions, the present study demonstrates, send sparse projections to the interstitial nuclei of Cajal and the nuclei of Darkschewitsch but do not send axons to the extraocular muscle motor nuclei.

COURSE OF VESTIBULO-OCULOMOTOR PROJECTIONS

Ascending fibers from the SV and RMV take different courses (Fig. 2). From the RMV, fibers pass medially across the midline into medial portions of the contralateral MLF. Fibers arising in more caudal portions of the RMV decussate at the level of the VI nuclei, while those from more rostral parts of the RMV pass across the midline just rostral to the VI nuclei. With respect to their origins, there is thus a topical arrangement within the decussation of the fibers from the RMV.

From the SV, fibers pass rostromedially as a dense bundle into the ipsilateral MLF where they ascend in its lateral portions. A topical arrangement is not so apparent in these fibers as in those of the RMV, perhaps in part because the bundles of ascending fibers from the SV are much closer together than those passing medially from the RMV.

Within caudal portions of the ascending MLF, between the levels of the IV and III nuclei, the fibers from the ipsilateral SV lie in lateral portions of the MLF, while those from the contralateral RMV lie in its medial portions. At higher levels of the MLF, as fibers stream medially into the III nuclei, this arrangement is not clearly apparent. No ascending fibers from the SV were seen in the contralateral MLF, nor were any from the RMV seen ascending in the ipsilateral MLF. In agreement with these findings, crossed projections from the medial vestibular nucleus and ipsilateral ascending pathways from the SV as well as the location of the fibers in the MLF were described by

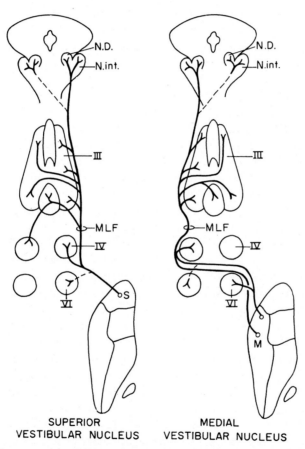

SUPERIOR   MEDIAL
VESTIBULAR NUCLEUS   VESTIBULAR NUCLEUS

Fig. 2. Diagrams of courses of vestibulo-oculomotor fibers. Ascending fibers from superior vestibular nucleus (left) pass in ipsilateral MLF to EOM nuclei bilaterally. Note that fibers to contralateral III and IV nuclei cross midline within III nuclei. In contrast, fibers from medial vestibular nucleus (right) decussate between levels of IV and VI nuclei and ascend entirely in contralateral MLF. Note that distribution of fibers both from superior and medial vestibular nuclei is extensive and bilateral. In MLF, fibers ascending from contralateral medial vestibular nucleus lie medial to fibers ascending from ipsilateral superior vestibular nucleus. Dotted lines indicate sparse projections. From Tarlov (1970a).

Gray (1926). The findings of Ferraro *et al.* (1940) and McMasters *et al.* (1966) of bilateral ascending MLF degeneration following medial vestibular nucleus lesions may well result from their exposure of the fourth ventricle, a procedure likely to traumatize the medial vestibular nuclei bilaterally.

REPRESENTATION OF INDIVIDUAL EXTRAOCULAR MUSCLES WITHIN THE OCULOMOTOR NUCLEI

In light of the highly discrete distribution within the III nerve nuclei of the terminations of secondary vestibular fibers, it is of interest to know where in the oculomotor nuclei the cell bodies innervating each extraocular muscle lie.

The classic studies of Warwick (1950, 1953, 1964) indicated the mode of central representation of the monkey's extraocular muscles, with an entirely crossed representation of the superior rectus, a bilateral representation of the levator palpebrae and an ipsilateral representation in rostrocaudally elongated cell groups of the inferior rectus, inferior oblique, and medial rectus. Warwick (1950) concluded that virtually all neurons in the oculomotor complex in the monkey send axons into the oculomotor nerve. The experimental anatomical evidence available for the cat (Bach, 1899; Abd-El-Malek, 1938), based on the distribution of chromatolysis after section of peripheral branches of the oculomotor nerve, differs widely from the schema proposed by Warwick. These earlier studies of the cat and other species, extensively reviewed by Warwick (1964) are, however, open to considerable criticism on grounds of technique.

Discordant results in the past have also been obtained from experiments in which movements of the globe have been studied after direct stereotaxic stimulation of the oculomotor nuclei. Although these studies (Szentágothai, 1942; Bender and Weinstein, 1943; Danis, 1948) indicated a rostrocaudal arrangement of subnuclei, the findings are somewhat in doubt since such experiments do not permit differentiation between the effects of direct stimulation of cell bodies and stimulation of fibers of passage. Furthermore, since the actions of the extraocular muscles vary with position of the globe, accurate identification of a single muscle "responsible" for any given movement may not be possible. In addition, the stereotaxic technique does not in most cases allow sufficiently precise localization of an electrode within the very small dimensions of the oculomotor nuclei to consistently identify small groups of motoneurons. The former disadvantages have been overcome in the study of Bienfang (1968) who found by recording from oculomotor neurons following antidromic stimulation of the nerves to the superior rectus and inferior oblique an entirely crossed representation in the monkey and cat. With respect to other extraocular muscles represented in the III nuclei, our findings for the cat differ from all previous descriptions for this and other species.

We have examined in the somatic oculomotor nuclei the retrograde neuronal changes following peripheral section of the oculomotor nerve and of its branches to the individual extraocular muscles in newborn kittens (Tarlov and Roffler Tarlov, 1971). The considerable advantages of using newborn animals became evident during the course of this study. Kitten oculomotor neurons examined at appropriate times after peripheral axotomy exhibit far more consistent and widespread retrograde changes than do their adult counterparts. The study of retrograde changes was employed because of its advantages over stimulation techniques in accurately localizing cell bodies innervating each extraocular muscle.

Two series of experiments were made. In one the kittens were sacrificed 4–5 days after orbital evisceration and following removal of each of the five extraocular muscles innervated by the III nerve, and the resulting chromatolysis examined with gallocyanin stains. In a second series of experiments a similar group of lesions was made and areas within the oculomotor nuclei were examined for evidence of atrophic shrinkage of neurons. The two methods gave concordant results.

Orbital evisceration

The distribution of chromatolytic motoneurons in the somatic oculomotor nuclei following orbital evisceration is represented in horizontal sections in Fig. 3, sections 4–6. Following removal of all extraocular muscles on the right side, neurons showing chromatolysis are found in dorsomedial portions of the junction of the rostral and middle thirds. In the caudal central nucleus, chromatolytic neurons are found bilaterally. On the side ipsilateral to the orbital evisceration, neurons showing chromatolysis are found in all portions of the somatic oculomotor cell column, except in its dorsomedial caudal portion, the region which contains chromatolytic neurons on the opposite side. Occasional neurons showing chromatolysis were found slightly ventrolateral to the main portion of the oculomotor nuclei, among fibers of the MLF. The most frequently observed chromatolytic changes were in large neurons; occasional medium sized and small neurons were also found to be chromatolytic in these areas. The interstitial nuclei of Cajal, the nuclei of Darkschewitsch, and the nuclei of the posterior commissure never showed retrograde changes.

It may be seen in Fig. 3, sections 4–6, by comparing the numbers of chromatolytic and normal neurons that the cells showing chromatolysis constitute a relatively small portion of the total number of neurons present in the oculomotor complex. Because of the difficulty in distinguishing, in Nissl stained sections, between very small neurons and glia, and because of difficulties in sampling we are not prepared to advance precise figures for the proportion of cells affected. In contrast to the sporadic occurrence of chromatolysis 5–7 days following orbital evisceration is the widespread occurrence of reduction in neuronal size. Shrinkage of neurons was a widespread and early phenomenon in kittens. Two days after orbital evisceration atrophy was well established in a large population of neurons, and by 12 days postoperatively the changes were very marked. The large number of cells affected may be appreciated in Fig. 7A and C. It is clear that large and medium sized neurons are no longer apparent by 12 days; the extent to which small neurons shrink is more difficult to estimate. Clearly the process of shrinkage involves a larger population of neurons than does chromatolysis. Following evisceration, cell shrinkage was observed throughout the caudomedial two-thirds of the contralateral somatic cell column, among approximately half the neurons in the caudal central nucleus, and throughout the ipsilateral cell column except in its caudo-medial two thirds. These are the same regions in which chromatolytic neurons are observed following orbital evisceration (Fig. 7B, D). The widespread distribution of cellular shrinkage is seen as well in the IV and VI nuclei following orbital evisceration. The marked changes as early as two days are represented in Fig. 7C.

The foregoing experiments show that neurons sending axons into the III nerve lie in the caudomedial two-thirds of the contralateral oculomotor column, in the caudal

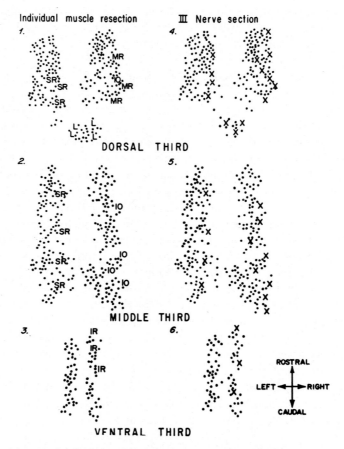

Fig. 3. Tracings from serial horizontal sections parallel to the aqueduct of Sylvius, at three levels (kittens). Dots represent normal cells. In sections 1–3, letters represent chromatolytic cells resulting from resection of individual muscles on the right side; sections 1–3 are composites of tracings from our specimens. In sections 4–6, × marks individual chromatolytic neurons following III nerve section in the right orbit (orbital evisceration) in the kitten.

Note that locations of chromatolytic cells in somatic oculomotor nuclei in sections 4–6, following III nerve section, correspond to the locations of chromatolytic cells in sections 1–3, following resection of individual extraocular muscles.

Following resection of individual muscles, superior rectus motoneurons (SR) are entirely contralateral, while levator palpebrae motoneurons (L) are bilaterally situated in caudal central nucleus. Inferior rectus motoneurons (IR) extend furthest rostrally and are, like the inferior oblique (IO) and medial rectus motoneurons (MR), entirely ipsilateral. From Tarlov and Roffler Tarlov (1971).

central nucleus bilaterally, and throughout the ipsilateral oculomotor cell column except in its caudomedial two-thirds. Extirpation of individual extraocular muscles resulted in retrograde changes in portions of these areas, as follows.

Extirpation of individual extraocular muscles

The locations of chromatolytic neurons following extirpation of individual muscles are indicated in serial horizontal sections in Fig. 3, sections 1–3, and in frontal sections

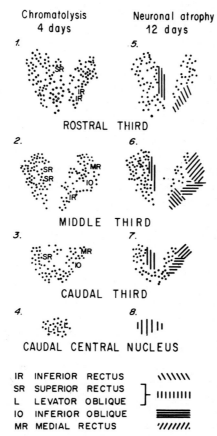

Fig. 4. Tracings from serial frontal sections at three rostro-caudal levels, perpendicular to the aqueduct of Sylvius.

On the left in sections 1–3 are represented the locations of cells showing chromatolysis following individual muscle resection. Dots represent normal cells.

On the right in sections 4–6 are represented the areas in which cellular atrophy was apparent 12 days following resection of individual muscles (see key).

Note that for each muscle the areas showing cellular atrophy at 12 days correspond precisely to the regions in which chromatolytic cells were found 4 days following resection of that muscle.

Note that the medial rectus motoneurons lie dorsolaterally, whereas inferior oblique motoneurons and the inferior rectus motoneurons lie more ventrally. The superior rectus motoneurons are entirely contralateral. From Tarlov and Roffler Tarlov (1971).

References pp. 489–491

in Fig. 4, sections 1–4. The distribution of cellular atrophy following resection of individual muscles is shown in Fig. 4, sections 5–8.

The medial rectus. Four days following total excision of the medial rectus sporadic chromatolytic neurons were found in dorsolateral portions of the ipsilateral cell column, extending nearly from the rostral to the caudal tips of the somatic cell column. The localization of chromatolytic neurons was highly reproducible from case to case. In any given section, the number of chromatolytic neurons represented a small proportion of the neurons in the corresponding portion of the somatic cell column. Profound cellular atrophy was observed 12 days after complete excision of the right medial rectus at age 3 days. No large neurons could be found in dorsolateral portions of the ipsilateral cell column. There appeared to be a shrinkage among all size populations in this region. Cellular atrophy was not apparent in other portions of the oculomotor complex.

The inferior oblique. Four days following total excision of the inferior oblique, chromatolytic neurons were found in lateral portions of the ipsilateral somatic cell column. These were most numerous caudally, and were concentrated at a level ventral to the cells showing changes after medial rectus resection. They were not found at the most rostral levels of the oculomotor columns. Following longer survival times, cellular atrophy was observed in lateral portions of the ipsilateral cell column and affected a much larger population of cells than did chromatolysis.

The inferior rectus. Following resection of the inferior rectus, chromatolytic cells were found in central portions of the ipsilateral oculomotor column, chiefly rostrally (Fig. 3, section 3; Fig. 4, sections 1 and 2). These chromatolytic cells extend further rostrally than those which result from resection of any other muscle. As with the other muscles, large and medium sized cells are predominantly affected. Only occasionally are chromatolytic small cells found. Three days after complete resection of the left inferior rectus, the majority of cells in the most ventral portion of the ipsilateral cell column showed cellular shrinkage (Fig. 4, sections 5 and 6).

The levator palpebrae. Following unilateral resection of the levator palpebrae in the kitten, chromatolytic neurons were found in the caudal central nucleus, distributed on both sides of the midline of this nucleus. Cellular atrophy in the kitten caudal central nucleus was observed 12 days following excision of the levator palpebrae. The number of large neurons in the caudal central nucleus was reduced bilaterally.

The superior rectus. Because of the proximity of the nerves supplying the superior rectus and the levator palpebrae, it was not possible to resect the superior rectus without damaging the nerve supplying the levator, though the converse was accomplished.

In all cases the distribution of chromatolytic cells in the caudal central nucleus following combined resection of the superior rectus and the levator did not differ from that seen following resection of the levator palpebrae alone.

In the remaining portions of the oculomotor nucleus, chromatolytic cells were always contralateral to the side of the muscle resection. In all cases the chromatolytic cells were continued to dorsomedial portions of the contralateral cell column, being most numerous in its caudal portions. Chromatolytic cells were not found in the most

lity is that certain oculomotor neurons may be protected from retrograde changes by the presence of proximal axon collaterals within the oculomotor nuclei. Such axon collaterals have been described in detail in relation to spinal motoneurons by Scheibel and Scheibel (1969) but a detailed study of axon morphology in the oculomotor nuclei has not to our knowledge been made.

Regarding the locations of the cell bodies of motoneurons innervating the cat's extraocular muscles, our findings are similar to those reported by Warwick (1953) for the monkey, except in the cases of the medial and inferior recti where a species difference appears to exist. In the monkey according to Warwick, the medial rectus is represented most ventrally and the inferior rectus most dorsally, an inversion of the arrangement described here for these muscles in the cat. An explanation for the inversion of representation of these two muscles in monkey and cat is not obvious but this arrangement does underscore the risk of extrapolating findings from one species to another.

TERMINATION OF THE VESTIBULO-OCULOMOTOR PROJECTIONS

We have seen that two separate systems of vestibulo-oculomotor projections pass from the vestibular to the oculomotor nuclei. One system of projections arises in the superior vestibular nucleus (SV) and ascends in the lateral portions of the ipsilateral MLF. The other system arises in rostral portions of the medial vestibular nucleus and ascends in the medial portions of the contralateral MLF (Fig. 2). When we consider the preterminal distribution of these projections among extraocular muscle motoneurons, it is clear that the projections of these two systems are extensive, bilateral, and widely overlapping (Fig. 5).

In fact, the projections from each of these regions may be even more extensive than we have indicated; some small portions of the SV and RMV are not involved by lesions (Fig. 1); it may be that if these uninvolved regions were ablated, projections to still other areas of the EOM nuclei would be found. Clearly the projections, even from restricted areas within the superior and medial vestibular nuclei, are not confined to pairs of synergistic muscles but are widely distributed to the motoneurons of both synergists and antagonists.

For example, considering only the medial and lateral recti, a small lesion of the medial vestibular nucleus at the midpoint of its rostrocaudal extent gives rise to axon degeneration in the motor nuclei of the medial and lateral recti bilaterally. A restricted centrocaudal lesion of the superior vestibular nucleus gives rise to axon degeneration in the motor pools of the medial recti bilaterally and the ipsilateral lateral rectus (Fig. 5). In addition, the projections of these two vestibular nuclei overlap each other extensively. Except that we have not found a projection from the SV to the contralateral lateral rectus motoneurons or from the RMV to the ipsilateral superior rectus or superior oblique motoneurons, the projections both from the SV and from the RMV reach all the extraocular motoneurons bilaterally. We have wondered why nature has provided two separate vestibulo-oculomotor fiber projection systems with widely overlapping distributions. In the past we had postulated that the functional significance of these two overlapping vestibulo-oculomotor fiber projection systems

might be that predominantly excitatory vestibulo-oculomotor impulses could be transmitted over one pathway while predominantly inhibitory influences could travel separately over a different pathway (Tarlov, 1970b). The recent findings of Highstein and
Ito (1971) in the rabbit, as least regarding the III nuclei, suggest that such functional
separation exists. Following their earlier finding that stimulation of the rabbit VIII
nerve produced both excitatory and inhibitory post-synaptic potentials in oculomotor
neurons (Ito et al., 1970), Highstein and Ito (1971) have found that excitatory postsynaptic potentials in rabbit oculomotor neurons are induced via the RMV while inhibitory post-synaptic potentials in these neurons are induced via the SV. These
physiological findings indicate that in the rabbit, excitatory and inhibitory vestibular
influences on III nucleus motoneurons are mediated separately via the RMV and
SV, respectively. The anatomical organization described here would allow for a
segregation of such excitatory and inhibitory impulses in the MLF, medial portions of
the MLF carrying the excitatory impulses from the contralateral RMV and lateral
portions of the MLF carrying inhibitory impulses from the ipsilateral SV.

The situation regarding the functional relationship of the SV and RMV to the
trochlear and abducens nuclei in the cat may be more complex. Following stimulation
of the vestibular nerve, Precht and Baker (1970) found disynaptic IPSP's in the ipsilateral IV nucleus while disynaptic EPSP's were recorded in the contralateral IV
nucleus. In a more recent study (Precht, personal communication) stimulation of the
SV produced ipsilateral IV nucleus IPSP's. Further studies of the influence of SV
stimulation on the activity of contralateral trochlear motoneurons are needed to determine whether or not the influence of the SV on trochlear motoneurons is purely
inhibitory. Regarding the abducens nuclei, Baker et al. (1969) found that stimulation
of the RMV in the cat produced monosynaptic IPSP's in ipsilateral abducens and
EPSP's in contralateral abducens motoneurons. These findings indicate that the
RMV mediates both excitatory and inhibitory effects on abducens motoneurons.

It has in the past been tempting to correlate anatomical connections with the predominant influence of stimulation of a given semicircular canal on eye movements in a
certain direction. However, virtually any movement of the globe must require changes
in length of all the extraocular muscles. For example, abduction of the eye must at least
involve the contraction of the lateral rectus and the two obliques with inhibition of
their antagonists. Furthermore, muscle action changes with the position of the globe;
as the globe moves from full adduction to full abduction, the superior oblique is
successively a depressor, an abductor and a rotator of the globe. Past attempts at rigid
correlation of anatomical vestibulo-EOM nuclei pathways with eye movements in
certain directions thus do not seem warranted, and, as noted below, past findings of
limited projections from the SV and RMV to the EOM nuclei may well be the result of
incomplete lesions of these vestibular nuclei. In fact, in their recordings of extraocular
muscle activity during stimulation of any single semicircular canal nerve, Cohen et al.
(1964) found evidence that every eye muscle was activated or inhibited. Such widespread vestibular influences on the extraocular motor nuclei could be conducted over
the two direct vestibulo-EOM nuclei projection systems described here. The require-
ments for delicately balanced excitatory and inhibitory interconnections between the

vestibular nuclei and EOM nuclei may also be met in part through commissural connections between the vestibular nuclei, via multisynaptic connections through the reticular formation, through connections with the interstitial nuclei of Cajal and the nuclei of Darkschewitsch, and even in part through connections with interneurons in the oculomotor nuclei themselves, as discussed above.

In relation to vestibular influences on eye movements in certain directions it is clear from our material that certain regions of the EOM nuclei receive particularly heavy projections from the SV and from the RMV; the number of degenerated axons in any given area is approximately proportional to the density of symbols in Fig. 5. From the SV, particularly extensive projections to the ipsilateral trochlear motoneurons are seen. Heavy projections to the contralateral motoneurons of the superior rectus as well as to those of the ipsilateral superior and lateral recti were found. From the RMV particularly heavy projections to the ipsilateral abducens and contralateral trochlear nuclei were seen. Conversely we have found no projections from the SV to the contralateral lateral rectus motoneurons, or from the RMV to the ipsilateral motoneurons of the superior rectus or superior oblique. Knowledge of the functional significance of these differential projections must, however, await further investigation.

The effects upon eye movement of several types of stimulation of the vestibular nuclei were studied in cats by Tokomasu, Gato and Cohen (1969) who found in cervically transected preparations that stimulation in the "region of the superior vestibular nucleus" produced upward rotatory and occasionally horizontal eye movements. Stimulation in the region of the "junction of the medial and descending vestibular nuclei" produced downward rotatory eye movements. Horizontal eye movements came from pulse train stimulation over an area including the SV, ventral portion of the LV and rostral portions of the MV and descending vestibular nuclei. Strong ipsiversive eye movements were obtained from stimulation of the juxtarestiform body and uncinate fasciculus.

From the findings reported here it is apparent that an extremely high degree of organization is present within the SV nucleus. It seems premature to attempt to correlate the findings of Tokomasu et al. (1969) with anatomical data available now. It is of interest that Tokomasu et al. (1969) found few eye movement responses from stimulation of the lateral vestibular nucleus and the statement is made that no conclusions could be drawn about the stimulation of the caudal portions of the vestibular complex. It would have been of interest to know the incidence with which responses were not obtained from these areas. We found no direct projections from the lateral or descending vestibular nuclei, or from caudal portions of the medial vestibular nuclei, to the EOM nuclei. In keeping with our anatomical findings, in the recent study of Highstein and Ito (1971), no monosynaptic influences on the oculomotor nuclei were found to come from the lateral or descending vestibular nuclei. Since it is known from the studies of Lorente de Nó (1933a, b), Stein and Carpenter (1967) and Gacek (1969) that the otoliths project to these caudal portions of the vestibular complex, it appears that the influences of the otoliths on extraocular movements are not directly mediated over monosynaptic pathways between the vestibular and oculomotor nuclei. Instead, otolithic influences on the extraocular muscles must be mediated over additional

References pp. 489–491

synapses, perhaps between individual vestibular nuclei and the nuclei of Darkschewitsch and Cajal, the reticular formation, the cerebellum or other regions.

The highly organized somatotopic arrangement of these two ascending vestibulo-
oculomotor systems has not been apparent in previous studies, even those using the
sensitive silver methods for demonstrating degenerated axons. In large part this fact
may be due to technical factors. For example, McMasters et al. (1966) exposed the
fourth ventricle in making their lesions. We have repeatedly seen in our material that
the slightest manipulation, even simple exposure alone, of the medial vestibular
nuclei which lie adjacent to the floor of the fourth ventricle, may give rise to axon
degeneration. This subsequently could erroneously be interpreted as resulting from
lesions of the lateral and descending nuclei. As discussed elsewhere (Tarlov, 1970a)
such factors as the length of postoperative survival time (crucial in determining the
stainability of degenerated axons), and the plane of section used (degenerated axons
passing at right angles to the plane of section may be difficult to recognize) also appear
to be important in evaluating the results of such studies.

ROSTRAL LIMIT OF ASCENDING SECONDARY VESTIBULAR PROJECTIONS

Rostral to the oculomotor nuclei, scattered degenerated fibers from all four of the
main vestibular nuclei pass into the interstitial nuclei of Cajal and the nuclei of
Darkschewitsch. From the superior vestibular nucleus the projection to the nuclei of
Darkschewitsch and Cajal is chiefly ipsilateral, while from the medial vestibular nucleus
the projection is chiefly contralateral. Fibers to these regions from the lateral and
descending vestibular nuclei are extremely sparse. No direct secondary vestibular
fibers have been found in our material (Tarlov, 1969, 1970a) to extend rostral to
these nuclei; in particular, none have been found to extend into any portion of the
thalamus. Our experimental data indicate that vestibular sensation which reaches
levels rostral to the posterior commissure must pass over third or higher order neurons
after synapsing at lower levels.

Such synapses may take place at the level of the posterior commissure in the nuclei
of Cajal and Darkschewitsch, or in the mesencephalic or pontine reticular formation.
The functional significance of these regions in relation to the vestibular nuclei (Markham et al., 1966) is discussed elsewhere in this symposium. Since short latency
responses to vestibular stimulation have been recorded in the cortex of monkey
(Frederickson et al., 1966) and cat (Walzl and Mountcastle, 1949; Kempinsky, 1951;
Andersson and Gernandt, 1954; Mickle and Ades, 1954; Massopust and Daigle,
1960) and from subcortical diencephalic regions in the cat (Mickle and Ades, 1954;
Spiegel et al., 1965; Wepsic, 1966) it is of considerable interest to know what pathways
are involved.

Multisynaptic pathways through the reticular formation have been demonstrated
by Lorente de Nó (1933a) and Szentágothai (1964) to be of importance in the rostral
conduction of certain types of vestibular impulses to the oculomotor complex. A
reticulothalamic tract such as that studied by Russell (1954) and Nauta and Kuypers
(1958) may thus provide a vestibulo-reticulo-diencephalic pathway for the rostral

conduction of vestibular sensation. Such a pathway would be compatible with the early experiments of Spiegel (1932, 1934), Aronson (1933) and Price and Spiegel (1937) which suggested that labyrinthine sensation is carried rostrally by pathways independent of connections with the cerebellum and medial longitudinal fasciculus. The precise routes which these multisynaptic pathways ascend is yet to be demonstrated.

SUMMARY

Two separate, direct, somatotopically organized vestibulo-oculomotor fiber projection systems have been demonstrated. One of these arises in the superior vestibular nucleus and ascends in lateral portions of the ipsilateral MLF. The other arises in rostral portions of the medial vestibular nucleus and ascends in medial portions of the contralateral MLF.

The sites of origin of these vestibulo-oculomotor projection systems are the regions where primary vestibular afferents from the ganglia of the semicircular canals have previously been shown to project.

The two vestibulo-oculomotor fiber projection systems each have extensive bilateral projections among the extraocular motoneurons and are widely distributed among motoneurons of both synergistic and antagonistic muscles. Evidence for functional differences in the projection systems from the superior and medial vestibular nuclei in relation to excitation and inhibition of extraocular muscle motoneurons is discussed.

The complex and delicate balance of influences necessary in the fine coordination of head and extraocular movements must depend on such highly organized pathways.

ACKNOWLEDGEMENTS

I am grateful to Dr. John van Buren in Bethesda, Professors Alf Brodal and Fred Walberg in Oslo, and Professor Walle Nauta in Boston for the opportunity to carry out this work in their laboratories. Part of the cost of the research came from the research funds of Dr. William H. Sweet and Dr. H. Thomas Ballantine, Jr.

REFERENCES

ABD-EL-MALEK, S. (1938) On the localization of nerve centres of the extrinsic ocular muscles in the oculomotor nucleus. *J. Anat. (Lond.)*, **72**, 518–523.

ANDERSSON, S., AND GERNANDT, B. (1954) Cortical projection of vestibular nerve in cat. *Acta otolaryng. (Stockh.)*, Suppl. 116, 10–16.

ARONSON, L. (1933) Conduction of labyrinthine impulses to cortex. *J. nerv. ment. Dis.*, **78**, 250–259.

BACH, L. (1899) Zur Lehre von den Augenmuskellähmungen und den Störungen der Pupillenbewegung, *v. Graefes Arch. Ophthalmol.*, **47**, 339–386 and 551–630.

BAKER, R. G., MANO, N. AND SHIMAZU, H. (1969) Postsynaptic potentials in abducens motoneurons induced by vestibular stimulation. *Brain Res.*, **15**, 577–580.

BENDER, M. B. AND WEINSTEIN, E. A. (1943) Functional representation in the oculomotor and trochlear nuclei. *Arch. Neurol. (Chicago)*, **49**, 98–106.

BIENFANG, D. C. (1968) Location of the cell bodies of the superior rectus and inferior oblique motoneurons in the cat. *Exp. Neurol.*, **21**, 455–466.

Brodal, A. (1940) Modification of Gudden method for study of cerebral localization. *Arch. Neurol. (Chicago)*, **43**, 46–53.

Brodal, A. (1969) *Neurological Anatomy in Relation to Clinical Medicine*. Oxford Univ. Press, 2nd. Ed., New York, London, Toronto, pp. XX–807.

Brodal, A. and Pompeiano, O. (1958) The origin of ascending fibers of the medial longitudinal fasciculus from the vestibular nuclei. An experimental study in the cat. *Acta morph. neerl.-scand.*, **1**, 306–328.

Buchanan, A. R. (1937) The course of secondary vestibular fibers in the cat. *J. comp. Neurol.*, **67**, 183–204.

Cohen, B., Suzuki, J. I. and Bender, M. B. (1964) Eye movements from semicircular canal nerve stimulation in the cat. *Ann. Otol. (St. Louis)*, **73**, 153–169.

Danis, P. C. (1948) The functional organization of the third nerve nucleus in the cat. *Amer. J. Ophthal.*, **31**, 1122–1131.

Ferraro, A., Pacella, B. L. and Barrera, S. E. (1940) Effects of lesions of the medial vestibular nucleus. An anatomical and physiological study in *Macacus rhesus* monkeys. *J. comp. Neurol.*, **37**, 7–36.

Frederickson, J., Figge, U., Scheid, P. and Kornhuber, H. H. (1966) Vestibular nerve projection to the cerebral cortex of the rhesus monkey. *Exp. Brain Res.*, **2**, 318–327.

Gacek, R. (1969) The course and central termination of first order neurons supplying vestibular end organs in the cat. *Acta oto-laryng. (Stockh.)*, Suppl., 254, 1–66.

Gray, L. P. (1926) Some experimental evidence on the connection of the vestibular mechanism in the cat. *J. comp. Neurol.*, **41**, 319–356.

Highstein, S. M. and Ito, M. (1971) Differential localization within the vestibular nuclear complex of the inhibitory and excitatory cells innervating III nucleus oculomotor neurons in rabbit. *Brain Res.*, **29**, 358–362.

Ito, M., Highstein, S. M. and Tsuchuiya, T. (1970) The postsynaptic inhibition of rabbit oculomotor neurones by secondary vestibular impulses and its blockage by picrotoxin. *Brain Res.*, **17**, 520–523.

Kempinsky, W. (1951) Cortical projection of vestibular and facial nerves in cat. *J. Neurophysiol.*, **14**, 203–210.

LaVelle, A. and LaVelle, F. W. (1958) Neuronal swelling and chromatolysis as influenced by the state of cell development. *Amer. J. Anat.*, **102**, 219–241.

LaVelle, A. and LaVelle, F. W. (1959) Neuronal reaction to injury during development. Severance of the facial nerve *in utero*. *Exp. Neurol.*, **1**, 82–95.

Lorente de Nó, R. (1933a) Vestibulo-ocular reflex arc. *Arch. Neurol. Psychiat. (Chicago)*, **30**, 245–291.

Lorente de Nó, R. (1933b) Anatomy of the eighth nerve. The central projection of the nerve endings of the internal ear. *Laryngoscope*, **43**, 1–38.

McMasters, R. E., Weiss, A. H. and Carpenter, M. B. (1966) Vestibular projections to the nuclei of extraocular muscles. *Amer. J. Anat.*, **118**, 163–194.

Markham, C. H., Precht, W. and Shimazu, H., (1966) Effect of stimulation of interstitial nucleus of Cajal on vestibular unit activity in cat. *J. Neurophysiol.*, **29**, 493–507.

Massopust, L. and Daigle, H. (1960) Cortical projection of the medial and spinal vestibular nuclei in the cat. *Exp. Neurol.*, **2**, 179–185.

Mickle, W. A. and Ades, H. (1954) Rostral projection pathway of the vestibular system. *Amer. J. Physiol.*, **176**, 243–246.

Nauta, W. J. H. and Kuypers, H. G. J. M. (1958) Some ascending pathways in the brain stem reticular formation. In H. H. Jasper *et al.* (Eds.), *Reticular Formation of the Brain. Henry Ford Hospital Symposium*, Little, Brown and Co., Boston, Toronto, pp. 3–30.

Nyberg-Hansen, R. (1965) Anatomical demonstration of gamma motoneurons in the cat's spinal cord. *Exp. Neurol.*, **13**, 71–81.

Precht, W. and Baker, R., (1970) Field potentials and synaptic potentials in the trochlear nucleus of the cat following labyrinthine stimulation. *Pflügers Arch. ges. Physiol.*, **319**, R 142.

Price, J. and Spiegel, E. (1937) Vestibulocerebral pathways. *Arch. Otolaryng. (Chic.)* **26**, 658–667.

Rasmussen, A. T. (1932) Secondary vestibular fibers in the cat. *J. comp. Neurol.*, **54**, 143–171.

Russell, G. (1954) The dorsal trigemino-thalamic tract in the cat reconsidered as a lateral reticulo-thalamic system of connections. *J. comp. Neurol.*, **101**, 237–263.

Sasaki, K. (1963) Electrophysiological studies on oculomotor neurons of the cat. *Jap. J. Physiol.*, **13**, 287÷302.

Scheibel, M. and Scheibel, A. S. (1969) A structural analysis of spinal interneurons and Renshaw cells. In M. A. B. Brazier (Ed.), *The Interneuron*. University of California Press, Berkeley, Los Angeles, pp. 159–208.

Spiegel, E. (1932) Cortical centers of labyrinth. *J. nerv. ment. Dis.*, **75**, 504–512.

Spiegel, E. (1934) Labyrinth and cortex: electroencephalogram of cortex in stimulation of labyrinth. *Arch. Neurol. Psychiat. (Chicago)*, **31**, 469–482.

Spiegel, E., Szekely, E. and Gildenberg, P. (1965) Vestibular responses in midbrain, thalamus and basal ganglia. *Arch. Neurol.*, **12**, 258–269.

Stein, B. M. and Carpenter, M. B. (1967) Central projections of the vestibular ganglia innervating specific parts of the labyrinth in the rhesus monkey. *Amer. J. Anat.*, **120**, 281–318.

Szentágothai, J. (1942) Die innere Gliederung des Oculomotoriuskernes. *Arch. Psychiat. Nervenkr.*, **115**, 127–135.

Szentágothai, J. (1964) Pathways and synaptic articulation patterns connecting vestibular receptors and oculomotor nuclei. In M. B. Bender (Ed.), *The Oculomotor System*. Hoeber Medical Division, Harper and Row, New York, pp. 205–223.

Tarlov, E. (1969) The rostral projections of the primate vestibular nuclei: an experimental study in macaque, baboon and chimpanzee. *J. comp. Neurol.*, **135**, 27–56.

Tarlov, E. (1970a) Organization of vestibulo-oculomotor projections in the cat. *Brain Res.*, **20**, 159–179.

Tarlov, E. (1970b) Vestibulo-oculomotor organization. Anatomical basis for certain vestibular influences on coordinated eye movements. *Trans. Amer. Neurol. Assoc.*, **95**, 320–322.

Tarlov, E. and Roffler Tarlov, S. (1971) The representation of extraocular muscles in the oculomotor nuclei: experimental studies in the cat. *Brain Res.*, **34**, 37–52.

Tokomasu, K., Gato, K. and Cohen, B. (1969) Eye movements from vestibular nuclei stimulation in monkeys. *Ann. Otol. (St. Louis)*, **78**, 1105–1119.

Walzl, E. and Mountcastle, V. (1949) Projection of vestibular nerve to cerebral cortex of the cat. *Amer. J. Physiol.*, **159**, 595.

Warwick, R. (1950) A study of retrograde degeneration in the oculomotor nucleus of the rhesus monkey, with a note on a method of recording its distribution. *Brain*, **73**, 532–543.

Warwick, R. (1953) Representation of the extraocular muscles in the oculomotor nuclei of the monkey. *J. comp. Neurol.*, **98**, 449–504.

Warwick, R. (1964) Oculomotor organization. In M. B. Bender (Ed.), *The Oculomotor System*. Hoeber Medical Division, Harper and Row, New York, pp. 173–202.

Wepsic, J. (1966) Multimodal sensory activation of cells in the magnocellular medial geniculate nucleus. *Exp. Neurol.*, **15**, 299–318.

Vestibulo-oculomotor Relations: Dynamic Responses

H. SHIMAZU

Department of Neurophysiology, Institute of Brain Research, School of Medicine, University of Tokyo, Hongo, Bunkyo-ku, Tokyo, Japan.

The dynamic vestibulo-oculomotor reactions may be defined here as those induced by canal stimulation during head movements. Under normal conditions the vestibulo-ocular reflex system reacts by rhythmic ocular movements —nystagmus— in response to an asymmetric inflow of steady impulses from the semicircular canals of the two labyrinths. Vestibular nystagmus consists of two phases, *i.e.*, the slow ocular movements in a direction and the quick return to the opposite direction. In some conditions the ocular globe exhibits a static deviation to the direction determined by the canal stimulated, the reaction being called a pseudopostural reflex (Lorente de Nó, 1933).

The slow component of vestibular nystagmus could be equivalent to the static deviation and thus has been attributed to an excitatory action from the labyrinth through the vestibular nuclei (Lorente de Nó, 1933; Dohlman, 1938; Gernandt, 1959). The quick component of vestibular nystagmus has generally been postulated to be central in origin. Spiegel and Price (1939) summarized various hypotheses regarding the origin of the quick component; the cerebral, proprioceptor, ocular muscle nuclei, or labyrinthine theory was refuted by proper reasoning. Thus, the alternative between the vestibular nuclei hypothesis and the reticular substance hypothesis has remained to be studied.

Extensive studies have been performed in order to find the central structures which may be essential for production of vestibular nystagmus. Lorente de Nó (1933) found that the quick component of nystagmus was abolished by destruction of parts of the bulbo-pontine reticular substance. The reticular hypothesis was extended by the striking finding of Lorente de Nó (1934) that the relaxation of an ocular muscle precedes the contraction of the antagonist at the quick phase of vestibular nystagmus. This finding led him to a postulate that in the vestibulo-ocular reflex arc, somewhere in the path towards the motoneuron of the antagonist, time delay circuits must be present. The bulbo-pontine reticular substance would be a path producing this delay according to Lorente de Nó (1938). On the contrary, Spiegel and Price (1939) insisted that the reticular substance is not indispensable for production of nystagmus, and that the origin of the rhythm of nystagmus must lie in the vestibular nuclei. So far these controversial hypotheses appear to have been neither proved nor disproved.

A different approach which would throw light on the central mechanism of production of nystagmus is to elucidate synaptic events in ocular motoneurons underlying their rhythmic activities. There may be two, not necessarily alternative, possibilities that at the quick relaxation phase the ocular motoneurons receive an active inhibition or excitatory effects on the motoneurons are reduced. The latter possibility was considered to be more likely in line with the reticular hypothesis (Lorente de Nó, 1933, 1938). Horcholle-Bossavit and Tyč-Dumont (1969) made an intracellular study on the abducens motoneurons during nystagmus. They have not found evidence for the postsynaptic inhibition of the motoneuron at the silent period of the motor nerve, but suggested a presynaptic inhibitory mechanism. This suggestion would be in line with the above hypothesis that the quick relaxation is caused by reduction of the excitatory action on the ocular motoneuron.

This line of study needs knowledge on the organization of the elementary, three neuron, vestibulo-ocular reflex arc which has been analyzed and substantiated by anatomical and physiological studies (Lorente de Nó, 1933, 1938; Szentágothai, 1950; McMasters et al., 1966; Tarlov, 1970). Recent electrophysiological investigation with intracellular recording techniques has revealed that the vestibulo-ocular reflex arc is composed of excitatory and inhibitory pathways, both of which act on the abducens (Baker et al., 1969a, b), trochlear (Precht and Baker, 1970), and oculomotor (Ito et al., 1970) neurons disynaptically from the primary vestibular nerve. It has been found in these studies that the excitatory and inhibitory actions from one labyrinth are of a reciprocal fashion on the antagonistic pair of ocular motoneurons, excitatory and inhibitory neurons being located in the vestibular nuclei.

On the basis of these analyses of the fundamental vestibulo-ocular reflex pathway, we have made an intracellular study on cat abducens motoneurons in relation to vestibular nystagmus (Maeda et al., 1971a, 1972). This study has led to the conclusion that the quick relaxation phase of nystagmus is attributable not only to a reduction of the excitatory postsynaptic potential (EPSP) but also to a production of the inhibitory postsynaptic potential (IPSP) in the abducens motoneuron.

NATURE OF SYNAPTIC EVENTS IN THE ABDUCENS MOTONEURON IN RELATION TO NYSTAGMUS

Nystagmus was induced by high frequency (400/sec) electric stimulation of the vestibular nerve in the encéphale isolé cat under local anesthesia. It has been established that nystagmus induced by electric stimulation of each canal nerve resembles qualitatively and quantitatively nystagmus induced by angular acceleration (Cohen et al., 1965).

Fig. 1 shows the intracellular potential in a right abducens motoneuron (top) identified by its antidromic response and simultaneously recorded left (middle) and right (bottom) abducens nerve activities in response to repetitive stimulation of the left vestibular nerve. The responses of the abducens nerves consisted of a slow increase and a quick cessation of impulses on the right side followed by a quick initiation of impulses on the left side. These alternating, rhythmic activities in the antagonistic pair of ocular muscle nerves are the neural correlates of the horizontal vector of vestibular nystagmus. Usually the bilateral abducens nerve activities were taken for the indicator of the antagonistic pair of motor nerve discharges, since impulse activities in the left

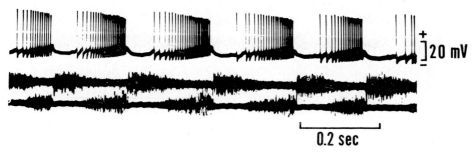

Fig. 1. Rhythmic changes in the intracellular potential of an abducens motoneuron and motor nerve discharges during vestibular nystagmus. Each trace indicates record from right abducens motoneuron (top), left abducens nerve (middle) and right abducens nerve (bottom). High frequency stimulation was applied to left vestibular nerve. From Maeda *et al.* (1972).

abducens nerve and those in the right oculomotor nerve innervating the medial rectus muscle were found to be highly synchronous with respect to their quick occurrence and quick cessation (Maeda *et al.*, 1972).

Rhythmic changes in the intracellular potential in the motoneuron (Fig. 1, top trace) consisted of a slow depolarization generating spikes with gradually increasing firing rates in phase with a slow increase of discharges in the homolateral abducens nerve and a quick hyperpolarization suppressing spikes at the time of quick cessation of nerve impulses. The firing pattern of the motoneuron was in agreement with that observed on unit activities in the abducens nuclei (Schaefer, 1965) or in the abducens nerve (Yamanaka and Bach-y-Rita, 1968). When the slow depolarization did not attain the firing threshold of the cell or the spike generating mechanism had deteriorated some time after penetration, the membrane potential exhibited a typical alternation of a slow depolarization followed by a quick hyperpolarization (Fig. 2A).

Synaptic nature of the quick hyperpolarization was examined by passing hyperpolarizing currents intracellularly through the recording microelectrode during appearance of rhythmic changes in the membrane potential (Fig. 3). Fig. 3D shows a control intracellular potential rhythm which was similar to that in Fig. 1 but recorded with a higher amplification, *i.e.*, a slow depolarization generating spikes followed by a quick hyperpolarization suppressing spikes. The coincidence of the onset of quick hyperpolarization with cessation of nerve discharges is shown by a vertical broken line in Fig. 3G. When hyperpolarizing currents were passed through the recording microelectrode, the spikes were suppressed and the rhythm of the membrane potential associated with the alternating nerve activities exhibited a characteristic pattern (Fig. 3E); the slow depolarization was followed by an additional, steep depolarization instead of the quick hyperpolarization consistently found in the control record. The turning point from the slow to the steep depolarization was coincident with the time of quick cessation of nerve discharges (vertical broken line in Fig. 3H). The IPSP induced by a single shock to the ipsilateral vestibular nerve in the control record (Fig. 3B) was inverted into a depolarizing potential (Fig. 3C) during passage of hyperpolarizing currents with the same amount as in Fig. 3E (*cf.* Baker *et al.*, 1969b). Thus the synaptic

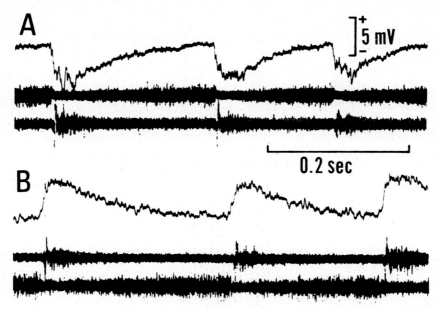

Fig. 2. Membrane potential changes in a left abducens motoneuron associated with rhythmic motor nerve discharges during nystagmus. Each of A and B represents intracellular record (top), left (middle) and right (bottom) abducens nerve discharges. Stimulation was applied to right vestibular nerve in A, and to left vestibular nerve in B. From Maeda *et al.* (1972).

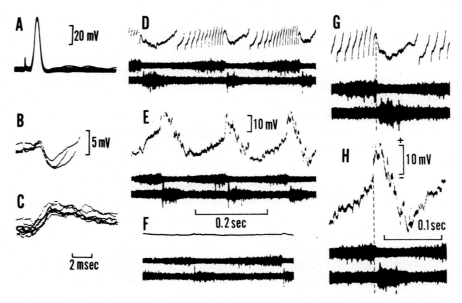

Fig. 3. Effects of intracellular passage of hyperpolarizing currents on quick hyperpolarization recorded from a left abducens motoneuron during nystagmus. A: antidromic response. B: IPSP induced from left vestibular nerve. C: the same stimulation as in B but record made during passage of hyperpolarizing currents of 7.5×10^{-9} A. Calibration for B applies to C. D: control intracellular record in response to high frequency stimulation of right vestibular nerve. E: the same as in D but during reversal of the IPSP to a depolarizing potential due to passage of the hyperpolarizing currents as in C. F: extracellular field potential. G and H: expanded traces of one beat in D and E, respectively, showing the time relation between rhythm of the membrane potential and nerve discharges. Vertical broken line indicates the onset of quick hyperpolarization (G) and that of steep depolarization during reversal of the IPSP (H). In D-H, middle trace indicates left and bottom trace right abducens nerve discharges. Time scale and voltage calibration for E apply to D and F, and those for H to G. From Maeda *et al.* (1971a).

mechanism, having produced a hyperpolarization at the time of quick cessation of nerve discharges in the control, induced a depolarization when the IPSP was inverted into a depolarizing direction.

When the IPSP induced by ipsilateral vestibular nerve stimulation (Fig. 4C) was inverted to a depolarization by electrophoretic injection of Cl⁻ ions into the cell (Fig. 4D) (*cf*. Baker *et al.*, 1969b), the membrane potential rhythm exhibited a pattern which was similar to that observed during intracellular passage of hyper-polarizing currents; the slow depolarization in phase with slow increase in nerve discharges was followed by an additional steep depolarization at the time of quick cessation of nerve impulses (Fig. 4B). When two potential curves obtained before (Fig. 4A) and after (Fig. 4B) Cl⁻ injection were superimposed by taking the moment of quick cessation of nerve discharges as the standard of time in two trials, the onset of the steep depolarization after Cl⁻ injection was found to be coincident with the onset of the quick hyperpolarization in the control trace (Fig. 4E).

From these results it was concluded that there is a production of the IPSP at the phase of quick hyperpolarization. The steep depolarization recorded after Cl⁻ injec-

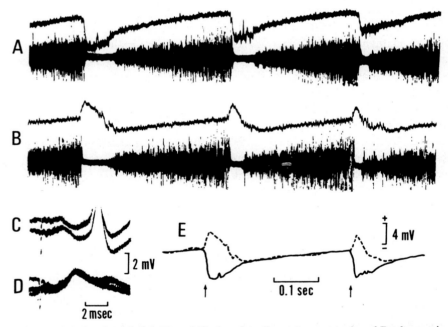

Fig. 4. Effects of electrophoretic injection of Cl⁻ ions into the motoneuron. A and B: changes in the membrane potential of a left abducens motoneuron (top) and left abducens nerve discharges (bottom) in response to right vestibular nerve stimulation. A: control record. B: record obtained during reversal of the IPSP to a depolarizing potential due to Cl⁻ injection. C: IPSP (and rebound excitation) induced in the motoneuron by single shocks to the left vestibular nerve. D: the same as in C but after Cl⁻ injection. E: superimposed traces of intracellular potential curves in A (solid line) and those in B (broken line). Moment of quick cessation of nerve discharges (left arrow) in each trial is taken as the standard of time and the potential at the end of slow depolarization phase is taken as the reference level for superposition. In this particular case the period of the beat in each trial was by chance the same. Calibration and time scale for E apply to A and B. From Maeda *et al.* (1972).

tion (Fig. 4E, broken line) turned relatively slowly into a hyperpolarizing direction and then tended to meet with the slowly depolarizing curve of the control trace at 80–120 msec after the diverging point of two potential curves. These periods may indicate the duration of active inhibition due to production of the IPSP related to the potential rhythm. The later phase of slow depolarization was not affected by reversal of the IPSP (Fig. 4E), indicating that it is caused by a slow increase in the EPSP.

During intracellular passage of hyperpolarizing currents (Fig. 3E and H) or after electrophoretic injection of Cl⁻ ions (Fig. 4B), the membrane potential level at the most hyperpolarized portion was distinctly deeper than the level at the turning point from the slow to the steep depolarization. Therefore the progression of the membrane potential to a hyperpolarizing direction in the control trace was attributed not only to production of the IPSP but also to reduction of the EPSP (disfacilitation). In some neurons the quick hyperpolarization was not inverted to depolarization during reversal of the IPSP, but its downward slope was definitely less steep. The onset of its hyperpolarizing progression was coincident with that of the control quick hyperpolarization before Cl⁻ injection. It was thus postulated that the decrement of the EPSP starts almost simultaneously with the quick production of the IPSP at the time of quick cessation of nerve discharges.

When repetitive stimulation was applied to the vestibular nerve on the side of the motoneuron impaled (Fig. 5), rhythmic changes in the intracellular potential consisted of a quick depolarization generating a burst of spikes in phase with quick discharges of the homolateral abducens nerve followed by a slow hyperpolarization. When spikes were not generated at the phase of quick depolarization, the membrane potential rhythm exhibited a typical alternation of a quick depolarization and a slow hyperpolarization (Fig. 2B). This potential curve was approximately a mirror image of the potential rhythm caused by contralateral vestibular nerve stimulation (Fig. 2A), when nystagmus induced in each direction had a symmetric pattern with the same rate. The quick depolarization was not reversed to a hyperpolarization when the IPSP was inverted to a depolarization by electrophoretic injection of Cl⁻ ions into the motoneuron. Thus, an increase in the EPSP underlies the quick depolarization.

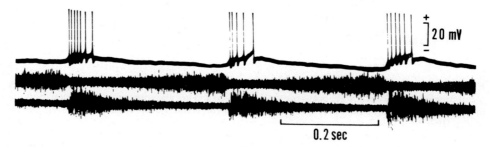

Fig. 5. Rhythmic changes in the intracellular potential of an abducens motoneuron and motor nerve discharges during nystagmus. Each trace indicates record from right abducens motoneuron (top), left (middle) and right (bottom) abducens nerve. High frequency stimulation was applied to right vestibular nerve. From Maeda *et al.* (1972).

However, the slope of the quick depolarization became less steep and its amplitude was decreased during reversal of the IPSP by Cl^- injection, despite the EPSP and the membrane potential being unaltered. This may indicate a contribution of disinhibition to production of the quick depolarization. The later phase of slow hyperpolarization was presumed to be caused not only by a decrease in the EPSP but also by a slow increase in the IPSP (Maeda *et al.*, 1972).

SYNCHRONOUS PRODUCTION OF THE IPSP AND EPSP IN THE ANTAGONISTIC PAIR OF MOTONEURONS AT THE QUICK PHASE

The relaxation of an ocular muscle precedes the contraction of its antagonist at the quick phase of vestibular nystagmus as pointed out above (Lorente de Nó, 1934). This finding was considered to be favorable to the idea that the quick contraction is mediated through a complex neuron chain with a considerable time delay. It has thus been examined if the time delay, clearly existing in motor nerve discharges or muscle activities, could be detected in the postsynaptic potentials in the antagonistic pair of motoneurons.

Fig. 6A shows a part of rhythmic changes in the membrane potential in a right abducens motoneuron (top trace) in response to high frequency stimulation of the

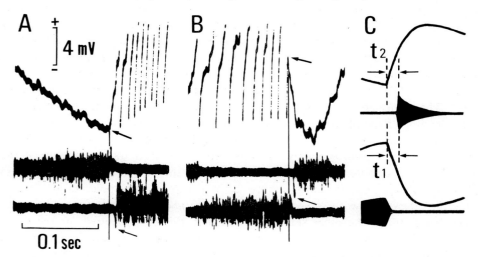

Fig. 6. Comparison between turning point of the membrane potential and onset of quick nerve discharges during vestibular nystagmus. A and B: intracellular records from a right abducens motoneuron (top) and records from the left (middle) and right (bottom) abducens nerves. Repetitive stimulation was applied to the right (A) and left (B) vestibular nerve. In each of A and B, upper arrow indicates turning point of the membrane potential, lower arrow the onset of nerve discharges, and vertical bar the reference line of timing drawn at the turning point of the membrane potential. Calibration and time scale for A apply to B. C: schematic drawing of the membrane potential of left abducens motoneuron (top), left abducens nerve discharges (second), the membrane potential of right motoneuron (third), and right nerve discharges (bottom) at the quick phase of vestibular nystagmus. t_1: interval between onset of quick hyperpolarization and that of contralateral abducens nerve discharges. t_2: interval between onset of quick depolarization and that of ipsilateral abducens nerve discharges. From Maeda *et al.* (1972).

References pp. 505–506

right vestibular nerve together with impulse activities recorded from the left (middle trace) and right (bottom trace) abducens nerves. The quick cessation of nerve discharges on the left side occurred prior to the quick initiation of discharges in the right nerve. A slow hyperpolarization turned quickly to a depolarization which produced a burst of action potentials. The turning point (arrow in top trace) clearly preceded the onset of homolateral abducens nerve discharges (see vertical reference line). Fig. 6B illustrates the same arrangement of records taken from the same motoneuron as in Fig. 6A, but the stimulation was applied to the left vestibular nerve. The slow depolarization generating a spike train turned quickly to a hyperpolarization (arrow in top trace). The turning point was approximately coincident with quick cessation of homolateral abducens nerve discharges (see vertical reference line) and definitely preceded the onset of contralateral nerve discharges.

Fig. 6C schematically shows the membrane potential changes which would occur if simultaneous recordings were made from the left (top trace) and the right (third trace) abducens motoneurons, and the left (second trace) and right (bottom trace) abducens nerves. The quick depolarization in the left motoneuron begins several msec (t_2) before the onset of quick discharges in the homolateral abducens nerve (see Fig. 6A). The quick hyperpolarization in the right motoneuron precedes the onset of quick discharges of the contralateral abducens nerve by several msec (t_1) (see Fig. 6B). Thus, comparison of the interval t_1 with t_2 will solve the question whether the onset of quick depolarization in the left motoneuron is synchronous or asynchronous with the onset of quick hyperpolarization in the right motoneuron in a single event of nystagmus. Both t_1 and t_2 varied relatively widely in each beat during long lasting nystagmus (range: 4–20 msec), but the mean of t_1 was found to be very close to that of t_2 in the same neuron. The differences were usually less than 1 msec and were statistically not significant. There was no tendency of the quick depolarization occurring earlier or later than the quick hyperpolarization in the antagonistic motoneuron.

The first spike in the intracellular record at the quick depolarization phase was found in many cases to be approximately coincident with the onset of quick discharges in the homolateral abducens nerve, whereas the spike at the end of slow depolarization phase was always instantaneously suppressed by the quick hyperpolarization. Therefore, the interval between spike suppression in the abducens nerve on one side and spike initiation on the other side is attributed to the time required for the quick depolarization to reach the firing threshold of the motoneuron (usually 5–10 msec).

With extracellular microelectrodes placed in the bilateral abducens nuclei it was possible to record field potential changes associated with quick production of the IPSP or the EPSP in the antagonistic pair of motoneurons during nystagmus. As shown in Fig. 7A, a relatively steep positive field potential was induced in the left abducens nucleus (top trace) at the time of quick cessation of homolateral abducens nerve discharges (third trace). At the same time the field potential in the right abducens nucleus (second trace) exhibited a negative deflection which was several milliseconds prior to the quick initiation of homolateral nerve discharges (bottom trace). When the direction of nystagmus was changed, the reverse effects were clearly seen as in Fig. 7B. On a large number of beats of nystagmus the onsets of the positive

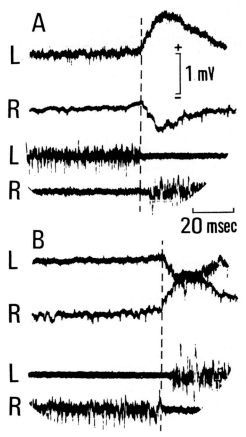

Fig. 7. Simultaneous recording of field potentials in the bilateral abducens nuclei (top and second traces) and of discharges in the bilateral abducens nerves (third and bottom traces). L and R represent recording side, left and right, respectively. Repetitive stimulation was applied to the right (A) and left (B) vestibular nerve. Vertical broken bar indicates the reference line for timing. Time scale and calibration for A apply to B. From Maeda *et al.* (1972).

and the negative deflections of the field potentials in the bilateral abducens nuclei were found to be highly synchronous.

The positive field potential accompanied by the intracellular IPSP at the quick relaxation phase is attributable to inhibitory postsynaptic currents generated in the abducens motoneuron. The negative field potential induced at the time of quick production of the EPSP in the motoneuron is presumably caused by excitatory post-synaptic currents and action currents in the motoneuron. If these explanations are acceptable, the above results provide further evidence that at the quick phase of nystagmus the IPSP is generated in the agonistic motoneuron synchronously with production of the EPSP in the antagonistic motoneuron. On the basis of both the intracellular and the field potential studies, it was concluded that the asynchronism of impulse suppression and initiation in the antagonistic pair of motoneurons at the quick phase is formed at the level of the motoneuron and cannot be attributed to the time delay elapsing somewhere in central pathways.

References pp. 505–506

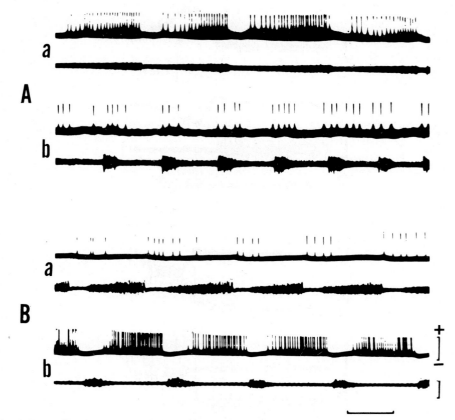

Fig. 8. Recording from axons of vestibular neurons within the left abducens nucleus (top trace in each record) together with left abducens nerve discharges (bottom trace in each record). Repetitive stimulation was applied to the right (Aa and Ba) and left (Ab and Bb) vestibular nerve. A: rhythmic firing of spikes identified as contralaterally activated ones. B: that of ipsilaterally induced spikes. Note that in A the phase of increased firing of unit spikes is consistent with the phase of increased motor nerve discharges, and in B unit spikes are induced at the silent phase of the motor nerve. Time scale: 0.2 sec. Voltage calibration: 0.3 mV for abducens nerve discharges, 8 mV for spikes in A, and 20 mV for those in B. From Maeda *et al.* (1971b).

A POSSIBLE MECHANISM OF RHYTHM FORMATION IN VESTIBULAR NYSTAGMUS

As described in the first section of the present paper, an approximately symmetric configuration of the membrane potential rhythm was observed in the antagonistic pair of motoneurons during vestibular nystagmus (Fig. 2). These potential rhythms were attributed to a rhythmic increase or decrease in the EPSP and the IPSP. It is thus suggested that the excitatory impingements on the agonistic motoneuron and the inhibitory impingements on the antagonistic motoneuron would exhibit a similar pattern of impulse activities.

Rhythmic pattern of unitary activities related to the oculomotor rhythm was observed in the vestibular nuclei (Eckel, 1954; Duensing and Schaefer, 1958; Horcholle and

Tyč-Dumont, 1968), the brain stem reticular formation (Duensing and Schaefer, 1957) and the region around the abducens nucleus (Horcholle and Tyč-Dumont, 1968). In these studies the functional connection of rhythmically firing units with the ocular motor nucleus was not known. It would be notable, however, that many of the vestibular units which exhibited a rhythmic firing related to nystagmus were found in the N. triangularis (the medial nucleus) (Duensing and Schaefer, 1958). This nucleus appears to be one of the main locations of vestibular neurons projecting to the bilateral abducens nuclei (Baker et al., 1969b). If the rhythmic activities of the vestibular neurons exert direct influences on the abducens motoneurons and produce the membrane potential rhythm, the excitatory fibers projecting to the contralateral and the inhibitory fibers to the ipsilateral abducens nucleus (Baker et al., 1969b) would reveal similar activities during vestibular nystagmus.

This possibility has been examined by Maeda et al. (1971b). The axonal spikes were recorded within the abducens nucleus; these spikes were identified by their receiving monosynaptic activation either from the contralateral or from the ipsilateral vestibular nerve and by their receiving commissural inhibition, thus indicating that these axons were presumably efferent fibers of the secondary vestibular neurons. About one third of the identified spikes exhibited rhythmic activities in association with rhythmic motor nerve discharges during vestibular nystagmus. The spikes which were activated by contralateral vestibular nerve stimulation revealed rhythmic activities always in phase with homolateral abducens nerve discharges (Fig. 8A), while the spikes which were activated by ipsilateral vestibular nerve stimulation showed discharge patterns invariably reverse to those of the homolateral abducens nerve (Fig. 8B). These close relations between presynaptic and postsynaptic activities were found not only during the slow phase but also at the quick phase. It was also noted that the discharge pattern of the contralaterally excited units (Fig. 8A) was very similar to that of the ipsilaterally activated units (Fig. 8B). These results appear to be in agreement with the idea that the rhythmic synaptic bombardments producing rhythmic membrane potential changes in the motoneuron originate, at least partly, from the vestibular nuclei.

In the vestibulo-ocular reflex arc there is a mutually inhibiting mechanism between the bilateral vestibular nuclei neurons in the horizontal canal system through the commissural pathway (Shimazu and Precht, 1966; Kasahara et al., 1968; Mano et al., 1968; Shimazu, 1972). Fig. 9 shows a simplified schematic representation of the organization of vestibulo-ocular pathway. Unit-A represents a population of vestibular neurons on one side, sending axons to the contralateral vestibular neurons-B (inhibitory), contralateral abducens motoneuron-C (excitatory), and ipsilateral abducens motoneuron-D (inhibitory). The similar circumstances hold for unit-B which represents a population of vestibular neurons on the other side. If a group of vestibular neurons-A is co-activated during nystagmus, the ipsilateral abducens motoneuron-D would receive an increased IPSP and at the same time the EPSP would be reduced due to inhibition of excitatory neuron in B through the commissural pathway. When the neuron group-B is co-activated in the next stage, the EPSP would be increased in the motoneuron-D and at the same time inhibition coming from the neuron group-A would be decreased due to commissural inhibition. These inferences are in line with

504 H. SHIMAZU

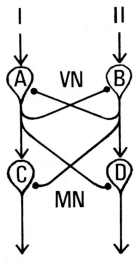

Fig. 9. Simplified schematic representation of the organization of vestibulo-ocular pathway. I and II: labyrinthine input on each side. A and B: population of neurons in the vestibular nuclei (VN) on each side. C and D: abducens motoneuron (MN) on each side. Excitatory synapse is indicated by arrow terminal and inhibitory synapse by filled circle. In the actual organization A and D, likewise B and C, are on the same side, respectively. A and B contain both excitatory and inhibitory neurons, not individually shown.

the results described in the first section of the present paper. Furthermore, if the excitatory and inhibitory neurons in A projecting to the respective motoneuron-C and -D are coactivated during nystagmus, a quick production of the EPSP in the motoneuron-C and that of the IPSP in the antagonistic motoneuron-D would be synchronous. These assumptions meet with the results described in the second section.

The scheme in Fig. 9 is similar to the neural model of mutual inhibition presented by Reiss (1962) except for the existence of inhibitory fibers projecting to the motoneuron in the vestibulo-ocular system. According to simulation experiments of Reiss, a constant-frequency stream of impulses exciting independently (input-I and -II in Fig. 9) a pair of mutually inhibiting units-A and -B can produce alternating, rhythmic bursts of pulses in units-A and -B. The ratio of the number of pulses during a dominance interval in A and B depends on the ratio of input frequency I and II. The firing pattern of axons of vestibular neurons shown in Fig. 8 appears to be in qualitative agreement with the simulation experiments. In accord with a classical hypothesis for production of the spinal rhythm–stepping (Brown, 1911), the mutual inhibition between the bilateral vestibular nuclei would provide a possibility of forming alternating, rhythmic activities in the vestibular neurons on each side.

Lorente de Nó (1933) stressed the importance of integrity of the reticular substance in the brain stem for production of nystagmic rhythm. It is well known that nystagmus is sensitively affected by general conditions or functional states of the brain such as sleep. The reticular substance might be essential for subserving the maintenance of background activities for rhythmic function of the bilateral vestibular nuclei. With respect to the pathways acting on the ocular motor nuclei, the present paper does not exclude the possibility that, besides the medial longitudinal fascicle (MLF), extra-MLF pathways may contribute to propagation of rhythmic impulses from the vestibular nuclei.

SUMMARY

Intracellular recording was made from the abducens motoneurons during vestibular nystagmus in encéphale isolé cats under local anesthesia. Nystagmus was induced by high frequency electric stimulation of the vestibular nerve on each side. Rhythmic changes in both the IPSP and the EPSP in the motoneuron underlie the membrane potential rhythm during vestibular nystagmus. The membrane potential rhythms in the antagonistic pair of motoneurons exhibit an approximately symmetric configuration; a slow depolarization in the agonistic motoneuron and a slow hyperpolarization in the antagonist, which are followed by a quick hyperpolarization in the former and a quick depolarization in the latter. The onset of quick hyperpolarization in the agonistic motoneuron is highly synchronous with the onset of quick depolarization in the antagonistic motoneuron. The asynchronism of impulse initiation and suppression in the antagonistic pair of motor nerves at the quick phase is formed at the level of the motoneuron but not in the path towards the motoneuron. Discharge pattern of axons of the secondary vestibular neurons recorded within the abducens nucleus is closely correlated to the postsynaptic motor activities not only at the slow phase but also at the quick phase. The experimental results appear to be in agreement with the idea that at least a part of the rhythmic synaptic bombardments producing rhythmic membrane potential changes in the motoneuron originates from the vestibular nuclei.

REFERENCES

BAKER, R. G., MANO, N. AND SHIMAZU, H. (1969a) Intracellular recording of antidromic responses from abducens motoneurons in the cat. *Brain Res.*, **15**, 573–576.

BAKER, R. G., MANO, N. AND SHIMAZU, H. (1969b) Postsynaptic potentials in abducens motoneurons induced by vestibular stimulation. *Brain Res.*, **15**, 577–580.

BROWN, T. G. (1911) The intrinsic factors in the act of progression in the mammal. *Proc. roy. Soc.*, *B*, **84**, 308–319.

COHEN, B., SUZUKI, J. AND BENDER, M. B. (1965) Nystagmus induced by electric stimulation of ampullary nerves. *Acta otolaryng. (Stockh.)*, **60**, 422–436.

DOHLMAN, G. (1938) On the mechanism of transformation into nystagmus on stimulation of the semicircular canals. *Acta oto-laryng. (Stockh.)*, **26**, 425–442.

DUENSING, F. AND SCHAEFER, K. P. (1957) Die Neuronenaktivität in der Formatio reticularis des Rhombencephalons beim vestibulären Nystagmus. *Arch. Psychiat. Nervenkr.*, **196**, 265–290.

DUENSING, F. AND SCHAEFER, K. P. (1958) Die Aktivität einzelner Neurone im Bereich der Vestibulariskerne bei Horizontalbeschleunigungen unter besonderer Berücksichtigung des vestibulären Nystagmus. *Arch. Psychiat. Nervenkr.*, **198**, 225–252.

ECKEL, W. (1954) Elektrophysiologische und histologische Untersuchungen im Vestibulariskerngebiet bei Drehreizen. *Arch. Ohr.-, Nas.- u. Kehlk.-Heilk.*, **164**, 487–513.

GERNANDT, B. E. (1959) Vestibular mechanisms. In J. FIELD, H. W. MAGOUN AND V. E. HALL (Eds.), *Handbook of Physiology. Section 1. Neurophysiology. Vol. I.* Amer. Physiol. Soc., Washington, D.C., pp. 549–564.

HORCHOLLE, G. AND TYČ-DUMONT, S. (1968) Activités unitaires des neurones vestibulaires et oculo-
    moteurs au cours du nystagmus. *Exp. Brain Res.*, **5**, 16–31.
HORCHOLLE-BOSSAVIT, G., AND TYČ-DUMONT, S. (1969) Phénomènes synaptiques du nystagmus.
    Exp. Brain Res., **8**, 201–218.
ITO, M., HIGHSTEIN, S. M. AND TSUCHIYA, T. (1970) The postsynaptic inhibition of rabbit oculomotor
    neurones by secondary vestibular impulses and its blockage by picrotoxin. *Brain Res.*, **17**, 520–523.
KASAHARA, M., MANO, N., OSHIMA, T., OZAWA, S. AND SHIMAZU, H. (1968) Contralateral short
    latency inhibition of central vestibular neurons in the horizontal canal system. *Brain Res.*, **8**,
    376–378.
LORENTE DE NÓ, R. (1933) Vestibulo-ocular reflex arc. *Arch. Neurol. Psychiat. (Chicago)*, **30**, 245–291.
LORENTE DE NÓ, R. (1934) Observations on nystagmus. *Acta oto-laryng. (Stockh.)*, **21**, 416–437.
LORENTE DE NÓ, R. (1938) Analysis of the activity of the chains of internuncial neurons. *J. Neuro-
    physiol.*, **1**, 207–244.
MAEDA, M., SHIMAZU, H. AND SHINODA, Y. (1971a) Inhibitory postsynaptic potentials in the ab-
    ducens motoneurons associated with the quick relaxation phase of vestibular nystagmus. *Brain
    Res.*, **26**, 420–424.
MAEDA, M., SHIMAZU, H. AND SHINODA, Y. (1971b) Rhythmic activities of secondary vestibular
    efferent fibers recorded within the abducens nucleus during vestibular nystagmus. *Brain Res.*,
    34, 361–365.
MAEDA, M., SHIMAZU, H. AND SHINODA, Y. (1972) Nature of synaptic events in cat abducens moto-
    neurons at slow and quick phase of vestibular nystagmus. *J. Neurophysiol.*, **35**, 279–296.
MANO, N., OSHIMA, T. AND SHIMAZU, H. (1968) Inhibitory commissural fibers interconnecting the
    bilateral vestibular nuclei. *Brain Res.*, **8**, 378–382.
MCMASTERS, R. E., WEISS, A. H. AND CARPENTER, M. B. (1966) Vestibular projections to the nuclei
    of the extraocular muscles. *Amer. J. Anat.*, **118**, 163–194.
PRECHT, W. AND BAKER, R., (1970) Field potentials and synaptic potentials in the trochlear nucleus
    of the cat following labyrinthine stimulation. *Pflügers Arch. ges. Physiol.*, **319**, R142.
REISS, R. F. (1962) A theory and simulation of rhythmic behavior due to reciprocal inhibition in
    small nerve nets. *Proc. AFIPS Spring Joint Computer Conf.*, **21**, 171–194.
SCHAEFER, K. P. (1965) Die Erregungsmuster einzelner Neurone des Abducens-Kernes beim Kanin-
    chen. *Pflügers Arch. ges. Physiol.*, **284**, 31–52.
SHIMAZU, H. (1972) Organization of the commissural connections: physiology. In A. BRODAL AND
    O. POMPEIANO (Eds.), *Progress in Brain Research. Vol. 37. Basic aspects of central vestibular
    mechanisms.* Elsevier, Amsterdam, pp. 177–190.
SHIMAZU, H. AND PRECHT, W. (1966) Inhibition of central vestibular neurons from the contralateral
    labyrinth and its mediating pathway. *J. Neurophysiol.*, **29**, 467–492.
SPIEGEL, E. A. AND PRICE, J. B. (1939) Origin of the quick component of labyrinthine nystagmus.
    Arch. Otolaryng. (Chicago), **30**, 576–588.
SZENTÁGOTHAI, J. (1950) The elementary vestibulo-ocular reflex arc. *J. Neurophysiol.*, **13**, 395–407.
TARLOV, E. (1970) Organization of vestibulo-oculomotor projections in the cat. *Brain Res.*, **20**,
    159–179.
YAMANAKA, Y. AND BACH-Y-RITA, P. (1968) Conduction velocities in the abducens nerve correlated
    with vestibular nystagmus in cats. *Exp. Neurol.*, **20**, 143–155.

Vestibulo-oculomotor Relations: Static Responses

J.-I. SUZUKI

Department of Otolaryngology, Teikyo University School of Medicine, Tokyo, Japan

It is generally agreed that the otolith organs, the utricle and saccule perceive linear acceleration and gravity (Jongkees, 1968). Because of their role in sensing the position of the head in relation to gravity, Breuer (1891) designated the otolith organs as the organs of the "Statischer Sinn" (static sense). The semicircular canals are generally considered to respond only to angular movement of the head, not to gravity, although this is disputed by several authors (Nito *et al.*, 1964, 1968; Money, 1965.) In this report eye movements induced by stimulation of the utricular nerve will be described, and effects of the semicircular canals on a 'static' vestibulo-ocular reflex, positional alcohol nystagmus, will be demonstrated. The data indicate that the function of the semicircular canals and otolith organs may not be as separate as has been previously assumed.

Oculomotor responses to electrical stimulation of utricular nerves

The sensory cells on the macula of the utricle are polarized and arranged in a radial fashion (Lowenstein and Roberts, 1949; Engström *et al.*, 1962; Spoendlin, 1964; Flock, 1964). Accordingly, different eye movements should be induced if different parts of the utricular macula are stimulated separately. This has been found by Szentágothai (1964) and more recently by Fluur (1970). However, if the utricular nerve is stimulated, eye movements in only one direction are induced. In the cat electrical stimulation of the whole utricular nerve induces countertorsion of both eyes (Fig. 1A). The countertorsion is mixed with slight horizontal and vertical shifts: both eyes move to the contralateral side, while the ipsilateral eye moves upward, and the contralateral eye moves downward (Suzuki *et al.*, 1969). Eye deviations induced by stimulation of the left anterior canal nerve are shown for comparison in Fig. 1B. The rotational component is the same but the contralateral eye does not move downward (Cohen *et al.*, 1964).

Eye deviations induced by utricular nerve stimulation are opposite to the sustained rotation of the eyes after unilateral labyrinthectomy. In both cat and rabbit during the acute and subacute stage the eyes are tilted to the ipsilateral side, and there is an ipsilateral head tilt. After labyrinthectomy the head and eye tilt are much more prominent in the rabbit than in the cat and never show restoration. These findings are consistent with the idea that the utricle is mainly responsible for rotation of the eyes in the coronal plane.

References pp. 513–514

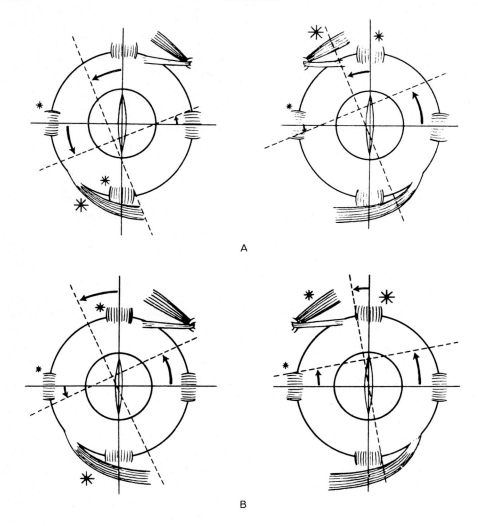

Fig. 1. Eye deviations induced by electrical stimulation of single utricular and anterior canal nerves on the left side in the cat. The diagrams illustrate the cat's eyeball and eye muscles showing eye deviations from left single utricular nerve stimulation (A) and left anterior canal nerve stimulation (B), for comparison. The asterisks indicate the muscles which are activated, the size of the asterisks indicating the intensity of activation. From Suzuki *et al.* (1969).

Two properties of the utriculo-ocular reflex arc suggest that it is capable of compensating for rapid head movements. (*i*) Stimulation of the utricular nerve induces potential changes in eye muscles in about 5 msec (Fig. 2, Ut). This latency is the same as that found after maximal stimulation of the semicircular canal nerves when they are maximally activated. This indicates that maculo-ocular reflexes are equally as fast as those from the semicircular canals (Suzuki, Tokumasu and Goto, 1969). (*ii*) The

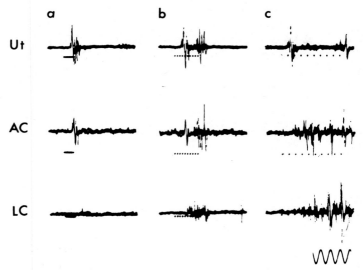

Fig. 2. EMG recording of eye muscles activated by utricular (Ut), anterior canal (AC), and lateral canal (LC) nerve stimulation. EMG recordings were taken from the inferior oblique muscle for Ut and AC stimulation, and from the lateral rectus muscle for LC stimulation. Pulse trains with ten pulses were used. The pulse separation was 1 msec in a (1000 Hz), 2.5 msec in b (400 Hz) and 6.4 msec in c (156 Hz). Calibration 10 msec.

utricular system is able to respond to higher stimulation frequencies in inducing eye muscle contractions than is the canal system. This is shown in Figs. 2 and 3. Changes in tension of eye muscles induced by the same frequencies of stimulation of utricular and lateral ampullary nerves are compared (Fig. 3). The slope of changes of muscle tension, which is comparable to eye speed, induced by utricular nerve stimulation continued to increase as pulse frequencies were increased up to 1000 Hz (Fig. 3, Ut). The maximum slopes induced by lateral canal nerve stimulation did not increase when the nerves were stimulated with frequencies above 400–600 Hz (Fig. 3, LC). There are differences between responses of eye muscles from lateral canal nerve stimulation and those from vertical canal nerve stimulation. The vertical canal system responded to intermediate frequencies, higher than the lateral canal system and lower than the utricular system (Fig. 2) (Suzuki et al., 1969; Tokumasu et al., 1971). This indicates that the utriculoocular reflex arc can respond to very high frequencies of nerve firing, similar to those which might occur in the utricular nerve if the head were moved very rapidly.

Positional alcohol nystagmus

Positional alcohol nystagmus (PAN) is positional nystagmus which develops in many animals and birds including all mammalian species after administration of alcohol (Bárány, 1911; Bárány and Rothfeld, 1914; DeKleijn and Versteegh, 1930; Aschan et al., 1956, 1964; Bergstedt, 1961; Jongkees and Philipszoon, 1964; Suzuki et al., 1968). It is dependent on gravity (Bergstedt, 1961), and is believed to originate in the

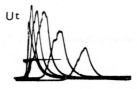

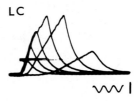

Fig. 3. Eye muscle contractions induced by stimulation of one utricular nerve and lateral canal nerves. Each series of traces are superimposed isometric recordings of eye muscle contractions induced by utricular nerve (Ut) and lateral canal nerve (LC) stimulation on the left side. Successively, pulse trains of constant duration (200 msec) with pulse separations of 0.6, 1.0, 1.6, 2.5, 4.0 and 6.0 msec were used to stimulate each nerve. Recordings were taken from the right inferior oblique for Ut and from the right lateral rectus for LC. The cat was under light pentobarbital anesthesia. Calibrations: 50 msec and 5 gm.

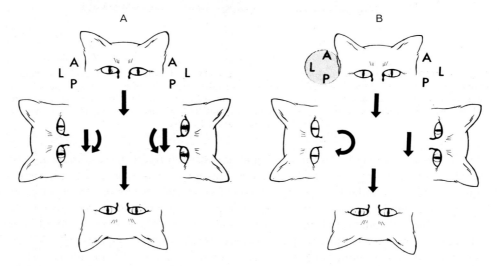

Fig. 4. Diagrams showing the direction of positional alcohol nystagmus in normal cats (A) and in cats after unilateral labyrinthectomy (B). The normal, left and right lateral, and head hanging positions are represented. The arrows indicate the direction of the quick phases of the induced nystagmus. In normal cats (A) the direction of nystagmus is horizontal-rotatory in lateral positions. After the right labyrinth is destroyed (B) the nystagmus is purely rotatory when the right side is down, and purely horizontal when left (normal) side is down.

otolith organs (Bárány, 1911). In cats and rabbits the nystagmus begins about 15 min after a parenteral dose of about 2 cc/kg and lasts approximately 1 h. This is the first phase of positional nystagmus according to Aschan *et al.* (1964). The direction of the quick phases of nystagmus is determined by the position of the head and is geotropic; that is, the quick phases beat towards gravity. Thus they are to the right with the head right side down and to the left with the head left side down (Fig. 4A). In the cat, in the right and left side down positions, however, the horizontal nystagmus is often mixed with varying amounts of rotation. The horizontal components usually predominate, and the rotatory components are less pronounced in most cats. In the upright position, nystagmus is directed vertically towards the chin, and in the head hanging position, it is directed vertically towards the forehead. Namely, the nystagmus is geotropic in the best sense of the meaning. In nose up and nose down position there is no nystagmus, and these positions may be called 'null' positions (Suzuki *et al.*, 1968).

Effects of alcohol on tonic horizontal deviations and nystagmus in the rabbit are shown in Fig. 5B in muscle tension recordings of the horizontal eye muscles. When the

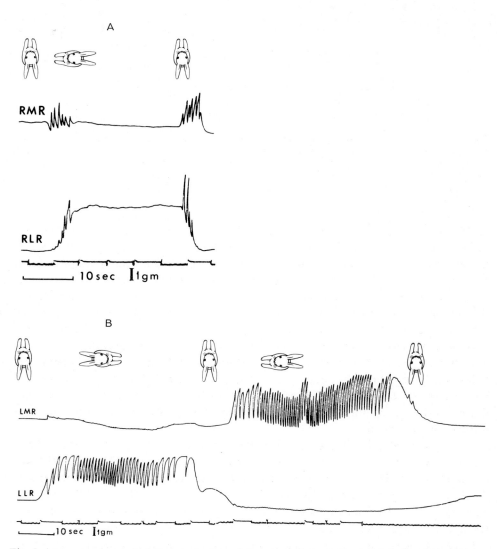

Fig. 5. Apogeotropic eye deviations in the lateral direction in lateral side-positions in rabbits without and with alcohol intoxication. A: The right lateral rectus muscle (RLR) has a sustained increase in tonus when the normal rabbit is put into the left side down position. From Takemori and Suzuki (1969). B: After administration of alcohol the horizontal deviation of the eyes is increased and the tonic movement is interrupted by oppositely-directed quick return movements resulting in nystagmus. RLR and RMR: Right lateral and medial rectus muscles, respectively. LLR and LMR: Left lateral and medial rectus muscles, respectively.

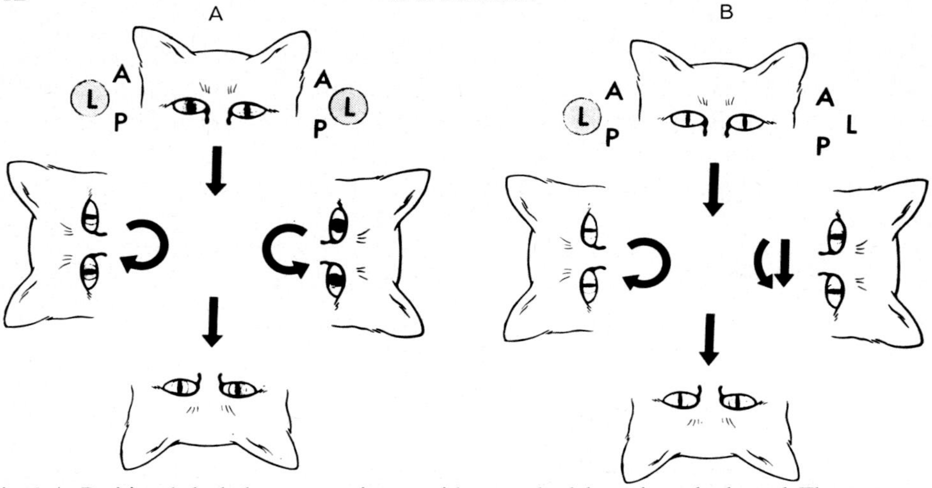

Fig. 6. A: Positional alcohol nystagmus in cats with one or both lateral canals plugged. The nystagmus was purely rotatory in either of the lateral side down positions. However, vertical nystagmus with the head down was not different from that found in normal animals. B: After only one lateral canal was plugged on the right side, the nystagmus in the right side down position was purely rotatory. Normal horizontal-rotatory nystagmus was still induced in the left side down position.

rabbit's head is tilted with one side down before administration of alcohol (Fig. 5A), there is a smaller amount of compensatory lateral deviation of the eyes in the apogeo-tropic direction. There is also a large rotatory shift of the globe in the rabbit without alcohol, however. If alcohol is administered, the horizontal deviation increases and horizontal nystagmus develops, while the rotatory deviation becomes minimal. The slow phases of positional alcohol nystagmus are in the same direction as the horizontal deviations recorded before intoxication. The main differences are that the horizontal deviations are larger after alcohol and the rotatory deviations are less.

In this regard it is of interest that ocular counter-rolling, a static compensatory reflex which probably arises mainly in the utricle (Miller, 1962), also decreases after administration of alcohol (Miller and Graybiel, 1968). However, rotatory components during positional alcohol nystagmus in the cat are opposite to those which occur during counter-rolling.

After unilateral labyrinthectomy, the pattern of response changes so that the direction of the induced nystagmus is no longer entirely geotropic (Fig. 4B). With the operated side down, the nystagmus is purely rotatory, while with the normal side down it is mainly horizontal and shows minimum rotation. This is different from normals. As is well known after bilateral labyrinthectomy, positional alcohol nystagmus can no longer be induced (Aschan et al., 1964).

In 1965 Money came to the conclusion that position alcohol nystagmus is initiated by the action of gravity on the receptors of the semicircular canals. This was based on experiments which showed that the horizontal component of positional alcohol nystagmus disappeared after the lateral canals were inactivated on both sides by plugging them with bone chips. We also studied effects of bilateral and unilateral lateral canal inactivation on positional nystagmus. Both horizontal canals were inactivated in cats which had had strong horizontal positional alcohol nystagmus before operation. After operation the horizontal components of the nystagmus disappeared while the rotatory components remained the same or were even augmented (Fig. 6A).

Findings in cats after only one lateral canal had been inactivated were different in some respects from those reported by Money (1965). In our experiments horizontal components disappeared only if the side of the inactivated lateral canal was down, but not when the intact side was down. These data suggest that the horizontal component of geotropic positional nystagmus in side down positions is dependent on the lateral canals. This provides a challenge to the classical theory that gravity affects only the otolith organs.

While inactivation of both lateral canals caused disappearance of the horizontal component of positional alcohol nystagmus, it did not affect the rotatory component in side down positions, nor did it change the vertical positional nystagmus which appeared in normal and head hanging positions. This shows that other labyrinthine receptors were not inactivated by the operation on the lateral canals. Whether the vertical component is induced from the otolith organs or from the vertical canals has not been tested. In cats with unilateral labyrinthectomy there were no rotatory components during positional nystagmus with the normal side down (Fig. 4B). In contrast, cats with lateral canals inactivated had a prominent rotatory component with the normal side down in the same manner as in normal cats intoxicated (Fig. 6B). This may mean that the rotatory component originates in the opposite labyrinth. It is not yet clear whether it originates in the vertical canals or in the otolith organs.

SUMMARY

Eye deviations were produced in cats and rabbits in side down positions before and after alcohol intoxication. After alcohol, horizontal deviations became dominant and rotatory movements were less prominent. The direction of rotation during positional alcohol nystagmus was contrary to that which occurs during compensatory counter-rolling. In intoxicated cats it was shown that intact lateral canals were necessary to produce the horizontal components of positional alcohol nystagmus in side down positions. There was some indication that the labyrinth on the opposite side induced the rotatory components of this nystagmus. These experiments indicate that gravity acts on both cupular and macular receptors.

REFERENCES

ASCHAN, G., BERGSTEDT, M., GOLDBERG, M. AND LAURELL, L. (1956) Positional nystagmus in man during and after alcohol intoxication. *Quart. J. Stud. Alc.*, **17**, 381–405.
ASCHAN, G., BERGSTEDT, M. UND GOLDBERG, L. (1964) Positional alcohol nystagmus in patients with unilateral and bilateral labyrinthine destructions. *Confin. neurol.*, **24**, 80–102.
BÁRÁNY, R. (1911) Experimentelle Alkoholintoxikation. *Mschr. Ohrenheilk.*, **45**, 959–962.
BÁRÁNY, R. UND ROTHFELD, J. (1914) Untersuchungen des Vestibularapparates bei akuter Alkohol-intoxikation und bei Delirium tremens. *Dtsch. Z. Nervenheilk.*, **50**, 133.

BERGSTEDT, M. (1961) Studies of positional nystagmus in the human centrifuge. *Acta oto-laryng. (Stockh.)*, Suppl. 165, 1–144.

BREUER, J. (1891) Über die Funktion der Otolithen-apparates. *Pflügers Arch. ges. Physiol.*, **48**, 195–306.

COHEN, B., SUZUKI, J. AND BENDER, M. B. (1964) Eye movements from semicircular canal nerve stimulation in the cat. *Ann. Otol. (St. Louis)*, **73**, 153–169.

DEKLEIJN, A. UND VERSTEEGH, C. (1930) Experimentelle Untersuchungen ueber den sogenannten Lagenystagmus während akuter Alkoholvergiftung beim Kaninchen. *Acta oto-laryng. (Stockh.)*, **14**, 356–377.

ENGSTRÖM, H., ADES, H. W. AND HAWKINS, J. E., JR. (1962) Structure and function of the sensory hairs of the inner ear. *J. acoust. Soc. Amer.*, Suppl. 34, 1356–1362.

FLOCK, Å. (1964) Structure of the macula utriculi with special reference to directional interplay of sensory responses as revealed by morphological polarization. *J. Cell Biol.*, **22**. 413–431.

FLUUR, E. (1970) Utricular stimulation and oculomotor reactions. *Laryngoscope*, **70**, 1701–1712.

JONGKEES, L. B. W. (1968) On the otoliths: their function and the way to test them. In *Third Symposium on the Role of the Vestibular Organs in Space Exploration. NASA SP*–152, 307–330.

JONGKEES, L. B. W. AND PHILIPSZOON, A. J. (1964) Electronystagmography. *Acta oto-laryng. (Stockh.)*, Suppl. 189, 1–111.

LOWENSTEIN, O. AND ROBERTS, T. D. M. (1949) The equilibrium function of the otolith organs of the Thornback Ray. *J. Physiol. (Lond.)*, **110**, 392–415.

MILLER, E. F. (1962) Counter-rolling of the human eyes produced by head tilt with respect to gravity. *Acta oto-laryng. (Stockh.)*, **54**, 479–501.

MILLER, E. F. AND GRAYBIEL, A. (1968) Effects of drugs on ocular counterrolling. In *Third Symposium on the Role of the Vestibular Organs in Space Exploration. NASA SP*–152, 341–349.

MONEY, K. E. (1965) Role of semicircular canals in positional alcohol nystagmus. *Amer. J. Physiol.*, **208**, 1065–1070.

NITO, Y., JOHNSON, W. H. AND IRELAND, P. E. (1968) Positional alcohol nystagmus in the cat. *Ann. Otol. (St. Louis)*, **77**, 111–125.

NITO, Y., JOHNSON, W. H., MONEY, K. E. AND IRELAND, P. E. (1964) The non-auditory labyrinth and positional alcohol nystagmus. *Acta oto-laryng. (Stockh.)*, **58**, 65–67.

SPOENDLIN, A. H. (1964) Organization of the sensory hairs in the gravity receptors in utricle and saccule of the squirrel monkey. *Z. Zellforsch.*, **62**, 701–716.

SUZUKI, J.-I., GOTO, K., KOMATSUZAKI, A. AND NOZUE, M. (1968) Otolithic influences on tonus changes of the extraocular muscles. *Ann Otol. (St. Louis)*, **77**, 959–970.

SUZUKI, J.-I., TOKUMASU, K. AND GOTO, K. (1969) Eye movements from single utricular nerve stimulation in cat. *Acta oto-laryng. (Stockh.)*, **68**, 350–362.

SZENTÁGOTHAI, J. (1964) Pathways and synaptic articulation patterns connecting vestibular receptors and oculomotor nuclei. In M. B. BENDER (Ed.) *The Oculomotor System.* Hoeber Medical Division, Harper and Row, New York, pp. 205–223.

TAKEMORI, S. AND SUZUKI, J. (1969) Influence of neck torsion on otolithogenic eye deviations in the rabbit. *Ann. Otol. (St. Louis)*, **78**: 640–647.

TOKUMASU, K., SUZUKI, J. AND GOTO, K. (1971) A study of the current spread with electric stimulation of the individual utricular and ampullary nerves. *Acta oto-laryng. (Stockh.)*, **71**, 313–318.

Vestibulo-ocular Reflexes: Effects of Vestibular Nuclear Lesions

T. UEMURA AND B. COHEN

Department of Neurology, Mount Sinai School of Medicine, New York, N. Y., U.S.A.

Recent studies have shown that primary afferent fibers from the semicircular canals and otolith organs end in portions of the vestibular nuclei which are largely separate from each other (Stein and Carpenter, 1967; Gacek, 1969). This suggests that activity from the semicircular canals and otolith organs may be integrated in different parts of the vestibular nuclei. If so, then lesions of these regions should have different effects on semicircular canal-ocular and otolith-ocular reflexes.

To date there is little information on this subject which is of clinical as well as of physiological interest. There are no studies to our knowledge which describe changes in otolith-ocular reflexes after discrete vestibular nuclei lesions. Several authors (Ferraro *et al.*, 1940; Buchanan, 1940) have reported that there were changes in caloric nystagmus after medial vestibular nucleus lesions, but there is little detail about exactly what these changes might be. Caloric nystagmus was reported to be unaffected when the descending vestibular nucleus was destroyed in the cat (Carpenter *et al.*, 1960).

There is also relatively little detail about spontaneous nystagmus after vestibular nuclei lesions. Contralateral nystagmus has been described after lesions of the vestibular complex (Ferraro *et al.*, 1936; Ferraro and Barrera, 1936; Buchanan, 1940; Cranmer, 1951; Shanzer and Bender, 1959), or after lesions of the medial (Ferraro *et al.*, 1940), or descending vestibular nuclei (Carpenter *et al.*, 1960). After lesions of the supramedullary portion of the juxtarestiform body, nystagmus was to the ipsilateral side (Ferraro *et al.*, 1936).

In earlier studies vestibular testing was generally inadequate by present standards, and there was little attempt at quantitation. Since vestibular response can be strongly inhibited in light, testing should be done in darkness using recording techniques such as electrooculography (EOG) or electronystagmography (ENG) (Henriksson, 1955a, b; Aschan *et al.*, 1956; Stahle, 1958; Jongkees and Philipszoon, 1964; Jung and Kornhuber, 1964; Kornhuber, 1966; Uemura, 1967).

The present study was undertaken to obtain information about effects of vestibular nuclei lesions using EOG. This report will summarize some results of this study. A more complete account will be published subsequently. Other aspects of the vestibulo-ocular reflex arc, namely the relative importance of the pontine reticular formation and median longitudinal fasciculus (MLF) in transmitting some vestibular reflexes to eye muscles has been described in a recent review and will not be discussed here (Cohen, 1971).

References pp. 527–528

METHODS

Juvenile monkeys (Macaca mulatta) were used in these experiments. Electrolytic lesions were made through electrodes implanted in and around the vestibular nuclei. The oculomotor effects of stimulation were used to aid in the final placement of electrodes (Tokumasu, Goto and Cohen, 1969). Changes in eye movements were observed, photographed, and recorded with EOG. Animals received amphetamine (0.5 mg/kg) to maintain alertness. They were tested in light for spontaneous nystagmus, and optokinetic nystagmus (OKN), and in darkness for spontaneous nystagmus, positional nystagmus, positional alcohol nystagmus (PAN), optokinetic after-nystagmus (OKAN), and caloric nystagmus. Techniques of testing using the EOG in monkeys have been described in detail in a previous publication (Komatsuzaki *et al.*, 1969). After lesions animals were followed for one or several months until they had recovered or had reached a plateau of improvement. Then the labyrinth on the side contra-

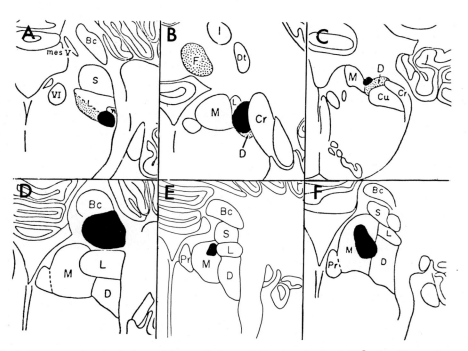

Fig. 1. Diagrams showing lesions of the vestibular nuclei in six animals of this series. The sections are in the vertical stereotaxic plane. The lesions were on the left except in B in which it was on the right. The diagram in B was reversed, however, for uniformity. Areas of destruction are shown in black. Regions with significant gliosis and demyelination are stippled. Lesions were predominantly in the following regions: A, root entry zone. B, rostral portions of descending vestibular nucleus (DVN). C, caudal portion of DVN. D, Superior vestibular nucleus (SVN). E, rostral portion of medial vestibular nucleus (MVN). F, medial portion of MVN.
Abbreviations: S, superior vestibular nucleus; L, lateral vestibular nucleus; M, medial vestibular nucleus; D, descending vestibular nucleus; n, vestibular nerve; Bc, brachium conjunctivum; Cr, restiform body; F, fastigial nuclei; I, interpositus nucleus; Dt, dentate nucleus; Pr, praepositus hypoglossi; VI, abducens nucleus; mes. V, trigeminal mesencephalic nucleus; Cu, cuneate nucleus.

lateral to the lesion was destroyed in most animals and they were retested for another month. The extent of the lesions was determined in histological sections. Diagrams through the center of the lesion in several of the animals are shown in Fig. 1. The subdivision of the vestibular nuclei conforms to the terminology of Brodal *et al.* (1962), with the exception that only four major vestibular nuclei were distinguished and the smaller cell groups were not considered.

Several comments are pertinent about the value or meaning of the various tests which were used:

(i) Positional nystagmus and PAN were considered to test mainly otolith-ocular reflexes. OKN was used as an index of the state of the central oculomotor system since visual-oculomotor pathways were not interrupted by vestibular nuclei lesions.

(ii) Several semicircular canals are activated when one ear is stimulated with hot or cold water although horizontal nystagmus induced by the lateral canal predominates in the observed response.

If both ears are simultaneously stimulated with hot or cold water, strong vertical nystagmus is induced in the monkey (Shanzer and Bender, 1959). Stimulation with cold water with the animal upright induces upward nystagmus, and stimulation with hot water, the reverse. The vertical nystagmus probably comes mainly from activation of the anterior canals which lie close to the lateral canals and the eardrum. The posterior canals lie deeper in the temporal bone in the monkey, and would not be much activated by caloric stimuli if the drums were intact. For these and other reasons it is likely that pathways from anterior and lateral canals to eye muscles, but not from posterior canals were mainly tested in this study.

RESULTS

Labyrinthectomy

To provide a basis for comparison with effects of vestibular nuclei lesions, the peripheral vestibular apparatus was destroyed on one or on both sides. After unilateral labyrinthectomy there was an ipsilateral head tilt and contralateral spontaneous nystagmus. The horizontal component of the spontaneous nystagmus was intensified when the side ipsilateral to the lesion was down and the rotatory component when the contralateral side was down.

Caloric nystagmus was induced to either side by stimulation of the contralateral ear with hot or cold water, but there was preponderance of the nystagmus to the contralateral side. That is, the maximum velocity of slow phases of nystagmus with contralateral quick phases was greater than that of nystagmus with ipsilateral quick phases. This agreed with the direction of the spontaneous nystagmus, and presumably reflected the loss of tonic activity due to the unilateral labyrinthine destruction. Initially there was also directional preponderance of OKN to the contralateral side.

An interesting finding was that OKAN, normally prominent in the monkey (Krieger and Bender, 1956; Komatsuzaki *et al.*, 1969), was dependent on the presence of the labyrinths. This is shown in Fig. 2. The duration of OKAN before labyrinthectomy is

References pp. 527–528

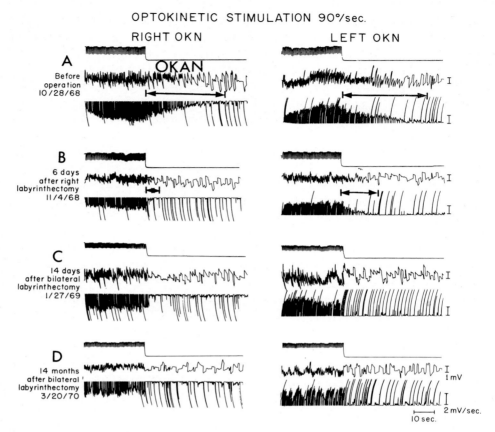

Fig. 2. Changes in OKN and OKAN after unilateral and bilateral labyrinthectomy. The top line in each series is the photocell trace showing the passage of OKN drum stripes. At the downward movement of this trace, the lights were extinguished. For the rest of the recording the monkey was in darkness. The second trace is the horizontal EOG recorded with d.c.-coupling. Eye movements to the right cause an upward trace deflection. The third trace is the rectified slow phase velocity. The speed of drum rotation during OKN was 90°/sec in each instance. The approximate duration of OKAN is shown between the 2nd and 3rd traces in A and B. After unilateral labyrinthectomy (B) the duration of OKAN was reduced to both sides, more to the ipsilateral than to the contralateral side. No OKAN was induced 14 days (C) and 14 months (D) after bilateral labyrinthectomy. The calibrations are shown on the right. 1 mV represents approximately 20° of deviation and 2 mV/sec about 40°/sec.

marked by the arrows in Fig. 2A. After unilateral labyrinthine destruction the duration of OKAN was considerably shortened, more to the ipsilateral than to the contralateral side (Fig. 2B). After bilateral labyrinthectomy OKAN was permanently abolished (Fig. 2C, D). It never recovered although there was vigorous OKN. In the normal monkey OKN is invariably followed by OKAN if alertness is maintained and the animal is put in darkness.

PAN was induced to both sides after labyrinthectomy. If the level of the spontaneous nystagmus was taken as a baseline, then there was an equivalent change in intensity of PAN to either side after unilateral labyrinthectomy. The total magnitude of the response was about half of the response before operation. In the rabbit and cat PAN was induced in only one direction after unilateral labyrinthectomy (DeKleijn and Versteegh, 1930), and it has been questioned whether the otolith organ on one side could induce PAN in both directions. However, the present experiments confirm findings of Aschan *et al.* (1964) that PAN can be induced in both directions if only one labyrinth is present. PAN disappeared after bilateral labyrinthectomy.

Lesions of the root entry zone

An animal with damage of the root entry zone without significant involvement of the vestibular nuclei is shown in Fig. 1A. There was heavy degeneration of fibers project-ing into the ventral part of LVN. There was an ipsilateral head tilt, contralateral horizontal rotatory spontaneous nystagmus, and a preponderance of OKN to the contralateral side. OKAN was strikingly diminished. PAN was not affected by this lesion and was still present after contralateral labyrinthectomy. Therefore, activity necessary for induction of PAN was not seriously reduced by the lesion of this portion of the vestibular nerve roots.

Caloric nystagmus was changed in a characteristic way after root entry zone lesions. The slow phases of nystagmus induced from the ipsilateral ear were of low maximum velocity whether induced by hot or cold stimuli. Furthermore, there was no increase in the velocity of slow phases when more intense cold caloric stimuli were used (Fig. 3A, dotted lines). The duration of the nystagmus was not markedly reduced, however (Fig. 3B, dotted lines). This is similar to findings in humans who are believed to have vestibular nerve lesions (vestibular neuronitis) (Stahle, 1956). It seems probable that faster slow phase velocities could not be recruited because of the reduction in the number of primary afferent fibers reaching the vestibular nuclei.

Lesions of rostral descending vestibular nucleus (DVN)

Rostral portions of DVN were not separately destroyed, but in one animal the major part of the lesions was in rostral DVN (Fig. 1B). The lesion also damaged the posterior portion of the vestibular nerve root causing degeneration of fibers going to ventral LVN, and there was some gliosis and fiber loss in the ipsilateral fastigial nucleus. There was contralateral rotatory spontaneous nystagmus for about one week, and then ipsilateral nystagmus developed. Changes in caloric nystagmus were similar to those found when the lesion was restricted to the nerve root. OKAN was markedly reduced after the rostral DVN lesion and did not recover for 9 weeks.

The most striking changes in this animal were in PAN. Normal PAN is shown in Fig. 4A. Administration of alcohol after lesion induced strong spontaneous nystagmus to the ipsilateral side which was enhanced with the ipsilateral side down and inhibited with the contralateral side down (Fig. 4B, 12 days after lesion). Later nystagmus was induced to both sides during PAN (Fig. 4C, 48 days after lesion). After the contra-lateral labyrinth was destroyed, PAN could no longer be induced by administration of alcohol (Fig. 4D). PAN was not abolished after lesions of other parts of the vestibular

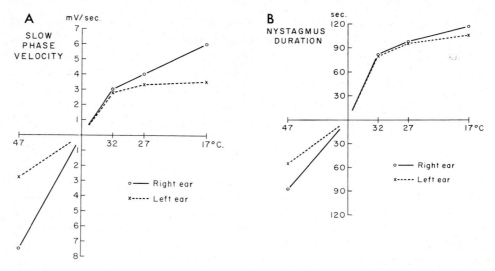

Fig. 3. Maximum slow phase velocity (A) and duration (B) of nystagmus induced by cold and hot stimulation of the right ear (open circles – solid line) and left ear (X's – dotted line). The monkey had a root entry zone lesion on the left which is shown in Fig. 1A.

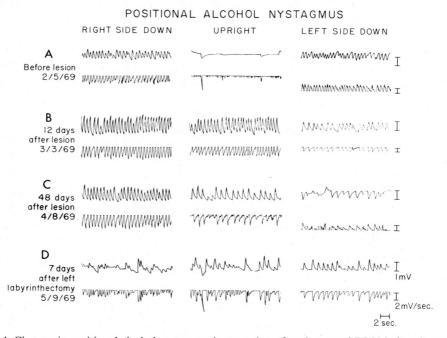

Fig. 4. Changes in positional alcohol nystagmus in a monkey after the rostral DVN lesion shown in Fig. 1B. The lesion was on the right side. The top trace in each series is the horizontal EOG, and the second trace the differentiated rectified EOG, which shows slow phase velocity. After contralateral labyrinthectomy (D) changes in head position had no demonstrable effect on the nystagmus to the right in the upright position induced by administration of alcohol.

nuclear complex and contralateral labyrinthectomy. It would appear that rostral DVN is an important receiving area for afferents from the otolith organs. This would agree with findings of Stein and Carpenter (1967), Gacek (1969) and Peterson (1970).

Lesions of caudal descending vestibular nucleus (DVN)

A lesion of caudal DVN is shown in Fig. 1C. After lesion there was little change in spontaneous nystagmus, OKN, or caloric nystagmus. There were striking postural changes, however. For several days after lesion the animal was unable to sit upright or walk. It lay on the floor with its head tilted to the ipsilateral side. Similar postural changes were described by Ferraro and Barrera (1936) and Carpenter et al. (1960) after DVN lesions.

Convergent direction-changing positional nystagmus was induced on head position change and was prominent throughout the month after lesion, before a contralateral labyrinthectomy was performed. This type of nystagmus is generally associated with central vestibular or cerebellar lesions. An example of convergent direction-changing positional nystagmus after a fastigial nucleus lesion is shown in Fig. 5 of Cohen and Highstein (1972).

PAN was still induced after the caudal DVN lesion and after contralateral labyrinthectomy. Thus, caudal DVN is not essential for processing activity from the ipsilateral labyrinth which induces PAN, although it may control or modulate this reflex. Caudal DVN appeared to have little role in producing caloric nystagmus.

Lesions of superior vestibular nucleus (SVN)

No lesions were restricted solely to SVN, but it was destroyed in two animals along with the adjacent brachium conjunctivum. One of these is shown in Fig. 1D. Brachium conjunctivum lesions without direct involvement of SVN were made in other monkeys, so that it was possible to make some assessment of SVN function. The head was tilted slightly to the contralateral side after SVN lesions. This was opposite to the direction of head tilt after labyrinthectomy and root entry zone lesions.

Upward rotatory spontaneous nystagmus followed SVN lesions which was just the reverse of the nystagmus induced by SVN stimulation (Tokumasu et al., 1968). Cells from SVN project through the lateral wing of the MLF primarily to the ipsilateral IV and III nerve nuclei (McMasters et al., 1966; Tarlov, 1970), mediating inhibition onto ipsilateral trochlear and inferior rectus motor neurons (Ito and Highstein, 1970; Highstein and Ito, 1971; Baker et al., 1972; Fukuda et al., 1972; Precht and Baker, 1972). Inhibition of these eye muscles would cause the eyes to countertort and move up, similar to the movements which were induced by SVN stimulation. After removal of this inhibition it might be expected that the eyes would roll to the ipsilateral side and move down, and this was the direction of the slow phases of spontaneous nystagmus which followed the SVN lesion. Similar nystagmus would be induced by stimulation of the posterior canal on the contralateral side (Suzuki and Cohen, 1964; Suzuki et al., 1964; Cohen et al., 1965). This type of vertical rotatory nystagmus was not produced by lesions confined to the brachium conjunctivum.

References pp. 527–528

CALORIC STIMULATION

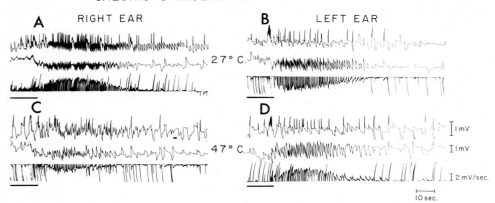

Fig. 5. Changes in caloric nystagmus after the left SVN – brachium conjunctivum lesion shown in Fig. 1D. The top trace is the vertical EOG, the second trace the horizontal EOG, and the third trace the differentiated rectified horizontal EOG showing slow phase velocity. The horizontal bar under the third trace shows the period of stimulation. At the end of stimulation the lights were extinguished, and the rest of the recording was done in darkness. Note the strong upward component of the nystagmus in A, top trace, induced by stimulating the right ear with cold water (27°C), and the downward component in C, top trace, from stimulating the right ear with hot water (47°C). This vertical component was not present when the ipsilateral (left) ear was stimulated (B, D). Note also the prominent horizontal component of nystagmus during cold caloric stimulation of either ear (A, B, middle and bottom traces) or during hot stimulation of the ipsilateral ear (D, middle and bottom traces). The nystagmus in this animal is represented diagramatically in Fig. 6B.

Positional nystagmus was present after SVN lesions. When the ipsilateral side was down, the upward rotatory spontaneous nystagmus was replaced by strong nystagmus to the ipsilateral side. When the contralateral side was down, there was a decrease in the upward rotatory spontaneous nystagmus. Positional nystagmus is considered to be a sign of dysfunction in otolith-ocular reflex arcs. However, few direct afferents have been reported from the utricle or saccule to SVN (Stein and Carpenter, 1967; Gacek, 1969). On the other hand SVN receives a strong afferent input from the fastigial nuclei, the flocculus and the nodulus (Angaut and Brodal, 1967), the flocculus mediating monosynaptic inhibition onto secondary vestibular neurons. Thus, the ipsilateral positional nystagmus was probably related to interruption or destruction of cerebello-SVN pathways or of SVN cells which integrate the cerebellar activity. Lesions of these cerebellar regions also cause positional nystagmus (Spiegel and Scala, 1941; Allen and Fernandez, 1960; see Cohen and Highstein, 1972).

Changes in caloric nystagmus were of interest after SVN lesions. The direction of the quick phases of caloric nystagmus in the normal animal is shown in Fig. 6A. The horizontal components of caloric nystagmus induced by hot and cold caloric stimulation on the lesion side were intact (Figs. 5B, D, 6B). Since the SVN was almost totally destroyed in this animal, activity which induced horizontal slow phases could not have been processed in this region. (Quick phases of nystagmus were not significantly affected by any of the vestibular nucleus lesions.) On the other hand, nystagmus induced by stimulation of the contralateral ear was affected. When the contralateral

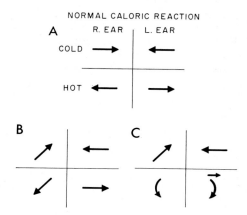

Fig. 6. Diagram of the vertical, horizontal and rotatory components of nystagmus induced by unilateral stimulation with cold (27°C) and hot (47°C) water. Testing was done with the animal upright and the head tipped 30° back. The arrows show the direction of the quick phases as they would appear to the observer. A, direction of caloric nystagmus in the normal monkey. B, after a left SVN lesion cold stimulation of the contralateral (right ear) caused upward oblique nystagmus to the left and hot stimulation the reverse. Nystagmus induced by stimulation of the ipsilateral ear was unchanged. C, after a left rostral MVN lesion only the nystagmus induced by stimulation of the ipsilateral ear with cold water was unaffected.

(right) ear was stimulated with cold water, the nystagmus had a strong upward component (Figs. 5A, 6B), and when it was stimulated with hot water, the nystagmus had a strong downward component (Figs. 5C, 6B). This type of nystagmus induced by unilateral stimulation has been designated as a perverted caloric response. The vertical components probably came from the contralateral anterior canal.

Possible explanations for the perversion include (i) a deficit in handling activity from the lateral canal, or (ii) a loss of an inhibitory mechanism which would normally suppress the response of the anterior canal. Since the horizontal components of the nystagmus from the contralateral side were preserved (Fig. 5A, C, bottom traces), it seemed unlikely that there had been an important change in the impact of lateral canal activity. Rather there appeared to have been a release of the response of the contralateral anterior canal, *i.e.*, a loss of suppression.

Commissural fibers which originate in SVN distribute to the contralateral vestibular nuclei (Ladpli and Brodal, 1968). Commissural fibers are known to mediate inhibition onto cells in the contralateral vestibular nuclei (Shimazu and Precht, 1966). Results which show that SVN mediates inhibition in most of its known connections (Ito and Highstein, 1971; Ito, 1972) are in accord with the postulated loss of suppression after SVN lesions.

Lesions of medial vestibular nucleus (MVN)

A lesion which destroyed rostral MVN is shown in Fig. 1E. Spontaneous nystagmus was present for a short time to the ipsilateral side. Postural changes were slight. Positional nystagmus was not found after rostral MVN lesions in most animals, and there was no loss of PAN after a contralateral labyrinthectomy in one monkey. It is unlikely that activity responsible for otolith-ocular reflexes is mediated to any great extent through rostral MVN.

Changes in caloric nystagmus were produced in each of the animals with rostral MVN lesions. Stimulation of the contralateral (right) ear with cold water initially caused upward oblique nystagmus (Figs. 6C, 7A), and stimulation with hot water caused downward counterclockwise nystagmus (Figs. 6C, 7C). In addition, stimulation of the left (ipsilateral) ear with hot water also induced downward clockwise nystagmus (Figs. 6C, 7D). Nystagmus with these vertical and rotatory components could originate only in the anterior canals. In each of the animals with rostral MVN lesions the horizontal nystagmus induced by stimulation of the ipsilateral ear with cold water was unaffected by the lesion (Figs. 6C, 7B).

If animals were turned upside down the directions of nystagmus induced by stimulation with cold and hot water were just the reverse of those found with the animal upright. The nystagmus was still perverted but now the major perversion was caused by cold, not by hot stimuli. Similar changes in caloric nystagmus were not produced by lesions of the central portion of MVN (Fig. 1F) or by destruction of the medullary reticular formation medial to MVN.

Thus, rostral MVN lesions caused similar perversion in caloric nystagmus as did the SVN lesions with two exceptions: (i) The horizontal component of nystagmus induced by stimulation of the contralateral ear with hot water after SVN lesions was generally absent or was weak after rostral MVN lesions.

(ii) The nystagmus induced by ipsilateral hot stimuli was predominantly vertical rotatory after rostral MVN lesions, and the horizontal component of this nystagmus was reduced.

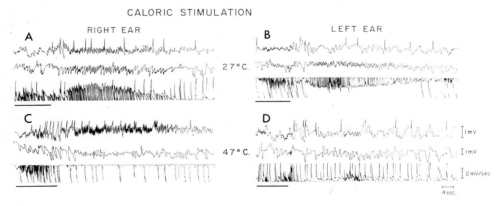

Fig. 7. EOG's showing caloric nystagmus after a left rostral MVN lesion shown in Fig. 1E. The top trace is the vertical EOG, the second trace the horizontal EOG and the bottom trace the horizontal slow phase velocity. The period of stimulation is marked by the horizontal bar under the lower trace. A, note the upward component from right cold (27°C) stimulation and C, D, the downward component from right and left hot (47°C) stimulation. B, the horizontal component of the nystagmus from left cold (27°C) stimulation was maintained despite the rostral MVN lesion. There was little horizontal component when either side was stimulated with hot water. This nystagmus is shown diagramatically in Fig. 6C.

Taken together with the findings after SVN lesions, the data suggest that in the normal animal activity arises in or passes through SVN and rostral MVN which projects across the brain stem to suppress contralateral anterior canal and enhance lateral canal responses. The projections from SVN to the lateral wing of the MLF could not have caused the perverted caloric responses since the rostral MVN lesions did not interrupt these fibers.

A common finding after both SVN and rostral MVN lesions was that there was no demonstrable change in horizontal slow phases induced by stimulation of the ipsilateral ear with cold water. The stimulus would reduce activity in the lateral canal nerve and while stimulation with hot water would do the reverse (Lowenstein and Sand, 1940; Lowenstein, 1956; Cohen et al., 1965). Thus, there was a differential effect of rostral MVN lesions on ipsilateral and contralateral slow phases induced by an increase or decrease of afferent activity from the ipsilateral lateral canal. Whether this implies a different locus for processing the increase or decrease of activity responsible for these eye movements in the vestibular nuclei or different central pathways to the oculomotor nuclei is not clear at present.

Midline sections

To further determine whether commissural fibers were responsible for the perverted caloric responses which have been described, midline sections were made through the brain stem above and below the level of the VI nerve nuclei (Cohen and De Jong, unpublished data). The vestibular nuclei were not directly involved by these lesions. If commissural fibers just caudal to the decussation of the MLF were cut, animals developed perverted caloric responses similar to the responses described above. That is, stimulation of one ear with cold water induced horizontal or horizontal upward nystagmus while stimulation with hot water caused predominantly downward rotatory nystagmus with a much smaller horizontal component.

If the decussation of the MLF was also cut, perverted nystagmus was still produced, but in addition there was bilateral paralysis of ocular adduction for all types of eye movements. However, even after midline sections through the decussation of the MLF, fast phases of caloric nystagmus which were induced by cold stimulation and were mediated through the contralateral abducens nucleus remained intact, and the beats of nystagmus in both eyes were synchronous. Thus, activity primarily responsible for contralateral quick phases of nystagmus in the abducting eye could not have crossed the brain stem in the vestibular commissural system (Maeda et al., 1971; Shimazu, 1972). A more likely possibility is that activity from the vestibular system projected into the pontine reticular formation (Ladpli and Brodal, 1968), into regions where conjugate horizontal saccades and nystagmus are believed to originate (Cohen, 1971) and from there reached the contralateral abducens nucleus.

SUMMARY

1. Postural changes caused by vestibular nuclei lesion in monkeys were to the ipsilateral side after lesions of lateral or caudal parts of the vestibular nuclear complex and

to the contralateral side after SVN or rostral MVN lesions. Postural changes after central MVN lesions were slight. The direction of the slow phases of spontaneous nystagmus agreed with the direction of the postural change in each of the animals.

2. OKN was little affected by vestibular nuclear lesions. There was some transient preponderance of OKN after lesions in the direction of the spontaneous nystagmus. OKAN was reduced to both sides after unilateral labyrinthectomy, ipsilateral $>$ contralateral, and was abolished by bilateral labyrinthectomy. The vestibular system appears to play an important role in supporting or maintaining OKAN. Quick phases of nystagmus were not affected by vestibular nuclear lesions.

3. Activity responsible for horizontal divergent direction-changing positional nystagmus of PAN which probably arises in the otolith organs appears to be mediated through rostral DVN. Rostral DVN does not seem to be of primary importance for production of caloric nystagmus. On the other hand, rostral MVN does not appear to play an important role in otolith-ocular reflexes.

4. Convergent direction-changing positional nystagmus of the type commonly associated with central vestibular or cerebellar lesions was found after caudal DVN lesions. Positional nystagmus was also produced by SVN lesions. Both caudal DVN and SVN have prominent vestibulo-cerebellar or cerebello-vestibular projections. Positional nystagmus is also produced by lesions of portions of the cerebellum where these projections originate or end. This is in accord with the hypothesis that the cerebellum may play an important role in controlling utriculo-ocular or sacculo-ocular reflex arcs.

5. The velocity of slow phases of caloric nystagmus induced by ipsilateral stimulation was reduced by lesions of portions of the vestibular nerve root which project strongly to ventral LVN. Similar changes in slow phases induced by cold caloric stimuli were not found after lesions of rostral MVN or SVN, which are also heavily supplied by semicircular canal afferents. This raises the possibility that the ventral part of LVN may mediate activity important for producing ipsilateral slow phases of caloric nystagmus.

6. SVN lesions caused changes in nystagmus induced by stimulation of the *contralateral* ear. *Ipsilateral* responses were intact after SVN lesions. The perverted responses from the contralateral side could have been due to a loss of suppression of anterior canal responses on the contralateral side.

7. Rostral MVN lesions caused perverted nystagmus similar to that produced by SVN lesions with the exception that the nystagmus induced by ipsilateral hot stimuli was also perverted after the rostral MVN lesions. Central MVN lesions did not cause perverted nystagmus.

8. Midline sections which interrupted the commissural system between the vestibular nuclei also caused perverted responses to caloric stimulation. Neither the synchrony of nystagmus in the two eyes nor the horizontal abductive components of nystagmus in the contralateral eye were abolished by midline section. Therefore, the vestibular commissural system could not be of primary importance in carrying activity which produces quick phases of nystagmus. Instead this activity probably utilizes pathways through the pontine reticular formation.

ACKNOWLEDGEMENTS

This study was supported by NINDS Grant NS-00294 and Career Research Development Award 1 K 3-34, 987 (B.C.) from the National Institute of Neurological Diseases
and Stroke.

We thank Mr. D. Borras, Mrs. D. Cabrera and Mr. E. Murray for assistance in
these studies.

REFERENCES

ALLEN, G. AND FERNANDEZ, C. (1960) Experimental observations in postural nystagmus. I. Extensive
    lesions in posterior vermis of the cerebellum. *Acta oto-laryng. (Stockh.)*, **51**, 2–14.
ANGAUT, P. AND BRODAL, A. (1967) The projection of the 'vestibulocerebellum' onto the vestibular
    nuclei in the cat. *Arch. ital. Biol.*, **105**, 441–479.
ASCHAN, G., BERGSTEDT, M. AND STAHLE, J. (1956) Nystagmography. *Acta oto-laryng. (Stockh.)*,
    Suppl. 129, 1–103.
ASCHAN, G., BERGSTEDT, M. AND GOLDBERG, L. (1964) Positional alcohol nystagmus in patients with
    unilateral and bilateral labyrinthine destructions. *Confin. neurol.*, **24**, 80–102.
BAKER, R., PRECHT, W. AND LLINÁS, R. (1972) Cerebellar modulatory action on the vestibulo-
    trochlear pathway in the cat. *Exp. Brain Res.*, in press.
BRODAL, A., POMPEIANO, O. AND WALBERG, F. (1962) *The Vestibular Nuclei and Their Connections.
    Anatomy and Functional Correlations.* C. C. Thomas, Springfield, Ill., pp. VIII–193.
BUCHANAN, A. R., (1940) Nystagmus and eye deviations in guinea pigs with lesions in the brain stem.
    Laryngoscope, **50**, 1002–1011.
CARPENTER, M. B., ALLING, F. A. AND BARD, D. S. (1960) Lesions of the descending vestibular
    nucleus in the cat. *J. comp. Neurol.*, **114**, 39–50.
COHEN, B. (1971) Vestibulo-ocular relations. In P. BACH-Y-RITA, C. C. COLLINS AND J. E. HYDE
    (Eds.), *The Control of Eye Movements*. Academic Press, New York, pp. 105–148.
COHEN, B. AND HIGHSTEIN, S. M. (1972) Cerebellar control of the vestibular pathways to oculomotor
    neurons. In A. BRODAL AND O. POMPEIANO (Eds.), *Progress in Brain Research. Vol. 37. Basic aspects
    of central vestibular mechanisms*. Elsevier, Amsterdam, pp. 411–425.
COHEN, B., SUZUKI, J. AND BENDER, M. B., (1965) Nystagmus induced by electric stimulation of
    ampullary nerves. *Acta oto-laryng. (Stockh.)*, **60**, 422–436.
CRANMER, R. (1951) Nystagmus related to lesions of the central vestibular apparatus and the cere-
    bellum. *Ann. Otol. (St. Louis)*, **60**, 186–196.
DEKLEIJN, A. UND VERSTEEGH, C. (1930) Experimentelle Untersuchungen über den sogenannten
    Lagennystagmus während akuter Alkoholvergiftung beim Kaninchen. *Acta oto-laryng. (Stockh.)*,
    14, 356–377.
FERRARO, A. AND BARRERA, S. E. (1936) Effects of lesions of the juxtarestiform body (I.A.K. bundle)
    in *Macacus rhesus* monkeys. *Arch. Neurol. Psychiat. (Chicago)*, **35**, 13–28.
FERRARO, A. AND BARRERA, S. E. (1938) Differential features of 'cerebellar' and vestibular phenomena
    in *Macacus rhesus*. Preliminary report based on experiments on 300 monkeys. *Arch. Neurol.
    Psychiat. (Chicago)*, **39**, 902–918.
FERRARO, A., BARRERA, S. E. AND BLAKESLEE, G. A. (1936) Vestibular phenomena of central origin.
    Brain, **59**, 466–482.
FERRARO, A., PACELLA, B. L. AND BARRERA, S. E. (1940) Effects of lesions of the medial vestibular
    nucleus. An anatomical and physiological study in *Macacus rhesus* monkeys. *J. comp. Neurol.*, **73**,
    7–36.
FUKUDA, J., HIGHSTEIN, S. M. AND ITO, M. (1972) Cerebellar inhibitory control of the vestibulo-
    ocular reflex investigated in rabbit IIIrd nucleus. *Exp. Brain Res.*, **14**, 511–526.
GACEK, R. R. (1969) The course and central termination of first order neurons supplying vestibular
    end organs in the cat. *Acta oto-laryng. (Stockh.)*, Suppl. 254, 1–66.
HENRIKSSON, N. G. (1955a) An electrical method for registration and analysis of the movements of
    the eyes in nystagmus. *Acta oto-laryng. (Stockh.)*, **45**, 25–41.

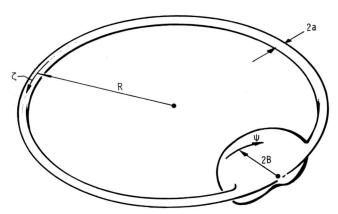

Fig. 1. Assumed hydromechanical model for semicircular canal.

stiffness and the mode of its deflection (linear, angular, or both), the steady state pressure difference is directly related to the stimulus torque and is independent of assumptions made about the cupula, and the source and magnitude of the flow velocity dependent countertorques which result from endolymph motion. The only assumptions required to calculate the steady state pressure differences concern the moment of inertia of the ring of endolymph, and the surface area of the cupula.

When the head is turned so that, say, the horizontal semicircular canal is stimulated, what volume of endolymph is effected? This has been the subject of some discussion (Groen, 1961; Money et al., 1969), but it does not seem unreasonable to model the canal duct as a torus of large radius R and small radius a, as shown in Fig. 1. The increased volume in the utricle and the ampulla may be approximated by a two radian section of a torus whose large and small radii are equal to the radius of the cupula B. Hence:

$$\text{Membranous canal volume} \cong 2\pi^2 a^2 R + 2\pi B^3 \tag{1}$$

Igarishi's (1966) study suggests that representative values for the human morphology are: a = 0.015 cm, B = 0.06 cm, and R = 0.3 cm.

This indicates that the utriculo-ampullary volume is at least equal, in man, to the volume of fluid in the horizontal canal duct. Therefore,

$$\text{Canal volume} \cong 2\pi^2 K' R a^2 \tag{2}$$

where $K' \cong 2$ in humans.

It is possible that the utricular volume has been underestimated somewhat, i.e., K' is possibly greater than the value of 2.0 assumed here. However, it is not clear how utricular volume should be partitioned, and it is hard to see how errors in K' of 20%–30% could materially effect the fundamental conclusions reached.

The moment of inertia of the endolymph ring about the center of the canal duct is therefore given by

$$\theta \cong 2\varrho\pi^2 K' a^2 R^3 \tag{3}$$

where the assumption is made that the radius of gyration of the endolymph is approximately the torus radius (R) and ϱ is the density of endolymph. In the steady state, since the acceleration of the endolymph eventually equals the acceleration of the head after a step stimulus, the torque balance equation is:

$$\theta a = \pi B^2 PR \text{ (steady state)} \tag{4}$$

where: a = angular acceleration of the head (rad/sec^2), P = pressure difference across cupula (dyne/cm^2).

The steady state relation of cupula pressure to head acceleration in the plane of the canal is therefore:

$$\frac{P}{a} \cong \frac{2\varrho\pi K' a^2 R^2}{B^2} \frac{\text{dyne sec}^2}{\text{rad cm}^2} \tag{5}$$

CALCULATION OF CUPULA PRESSURE AT ACCELERATION THRESHOLD

To calculate the steady state pressure drop across the cupula for subjective threshold, we need only select a reasonable acceleration level for such threshold. Observed values of behavioral thresholds to constant angular acceleration vary widely over the range 0.035°/sec^2 to greater than 2°/sec^2. The literature in this area is reviewed by Clark (1967). The wide variation in results is attributable partly to intersubject variance and partly to differences in experimental protocol. The subjective thresholds vary over the widest range. Oculogyral illusion (OGI) probably is the most sensitive behavioral indicator of vestibular function. Oosterveld (1970) was able to provoke OGI in two of his five subjects at angular accelerations of 0.036°/sec^2. This is roughly consistent with the lowest subjective threshold reported by Mann and Ray (1956) in four subjects. Meiry (1965) found subjective thresholds (75% identification in 3 subjects) to vary from 0.1 to 0.2°/sec^2, with a mean of 0.14°/sec^2. Nystagmus thresholds seem to be slightly more consistent, but higher in value. Buys (1937) and Buys and Rijlant (1939) report 0.8°/sec^2. Montandon and Russbach (1955) and Montandon et al. (1971) indicate similar values.

It is not clear what acceleration levels ultimately reflect the physical threshold of motion of the cupula-endolymph system. It does not seem unreasonable to assume, however, that accelerations of 0.1°/sec^2 are a sufficient stimulus to produce behavioral responses in a substantial percentage of the normal population. Adopting this value as typical of subjective thresholds, one obtains:

$$P_{\text{Subjective threshold}} = 2\varrho\pi K' a^2 R^2 B^{-2} a = 1.25 \times 10^{-4} \frac{\text{dyne}}{\text{cm}^2} \tag{6}$$

One would expect that nystagmus would not be elicited until $P_{\text{nystagmus threshold}} = 10^{-3}$ dyne/cm^2, since nystagmus acceleration thresholds are roughly eight times greater than the assumed subjective threshold.

CALCULATION OF CUPULA PRESSURE AT CALORIC THRESHOLD

An independent method of estimating the threshold pressure difference across the cupula is by considering the pressure and torque involved in caloric stimulation. The figure of 10^{-3} dyne/cm² for nystagmus pressure threshold is consistent with the calculations of Steer *et al.* (1968) of the torque induced on the canal in a uniform temperature gradient field. Steer assumed only a toroidal duct, small radius = 0.015 cm, large radius = 0.3 cm. He measured the temperature coefficient of expansion of human endolymph, and determined:

$$\frac{1}{\varrho} \frac{\partial \varrho}{\partial T} = -0.44 \times 10^{-3}/°C \pm 5\% \qquad (7)$$

Steer found that by integrating the torque about the center of the torus on an elemental volume of fluid, a uniform temperature gradient across the duct gives rise to a torque on the duct which is:

$$M = 4 \times 10^{-8} \text{ g } \cos\Phi\Delta T \text{ dyne cm} \qquad (8)$$

where ΔT is the temperature difference across the canal in degrees centigrade, g is the gravitational constant and Φ is the angle between the plane of the duct and the vertical. ΔT is normally less than the difference between body temperature and the temperature at the tympanic membrane during caloric irrigations. The torque can be expressed in terms of pressure difference across the cupula by the equation $M = P\pi B^2R$. Hence, if the canal is vertical, $(\cos\Phi = 1)$

$$P = 1.16 \times 10^{-2} \Delta T \qquad (9)$$

McLeod and Meek (1962) took caloric threshold measurements using the standard Hallpike 40 second irrigation procedure, and found that 75% of the responses had occurred at $\pm$ 0.5° difference from body temperature. Hence, if we assume that:

$$\Delta T = K_T (T_{\text{temporal bone}} - T_{\text{tympanic membrane}}) \qquad (10)$$

then:

$$P_{\text{nystagmus threshold}} = 5.5 \times 10^{-3} K_T \text{ dyne/cm}^2 \qquad (11)$$

One can be certain that K_T is never greater than unity, so 5.5×10^{-3} represents an upper limit on $P_{\text{nystagmus threshold}}$ Results of *in vivo* experiments by Dohlman (1935) and Cawthorne and Cobb (1954) on this temperature gradient suggest that K_T = 0.1 to 0.2. This brings $P_{\text{nystagmus threshold}}$. into agreement with the valuep reviously calculated from acceleration stimulus.

These calculations can be put in some perspective by the following considerations:

The subjective threshold value of 10^{-4} dyne/cm² constitutes an extremely small pressure. In the normal physiological range of head motions, sustained accelerations greater than 30 °/sec² are only rarely encountered, although brief acceleration impulses of up to 600 °/sec are often associated with step changes in angular velocity of the head

(Hallpike and Hood, 1953). Steady cupula pressure differences should only rarely exceed 3.8×10^{-2} dyne/cm² (less than 4×10^{-5} cm water). The brief moments of high inertial reaction torque associated with impulses of acceleration are balanced almost entirely by the endolymph viscous torques, and not by pressure drop across the cupula.

This result suggests that procedures which involve subjecting the cupula to pressures very much in excess of 10 cm water for more than the briefest instant might well move the cupula far beyond its normal dynamic range of motion, and that damage to the organ might possibly result. We feel this possibility should be carefully considered when evaluating experiments aimed at visualizing the motion of the cupula by the injection of ink or dye, or histological studies in which the membranous wall was punctured in preparation.

PHYSIOLOGICAL RANGE OF CUPULA DEFLECTION

Since the preceding calculations suggest that the semicircular canals sensory areas are enormously sensitive to pressure gradients, one can only assume that experiments directed at observing the range of cupula motions directly by fenestration might easily traumatize the cupula. Unfortunately, the cupula is practically invisible under bright field microscopy.

However, the theoretical model for the canal hydrodynamics can provide a useful estimate of the range of cupula motion. It will be shown that hydrodynamic models which assume that the cupula swings about its crista imply that the actual physiologic range of cupula motions is sufficiently small as to make a small angle approximation valid: the volume swept out by a swinging cupula is practically identical to that obtained by linear displacements of the cupula, although the resulting hair cell bending angles are vastly larger for a sliding cupula (Dohlman, 1971). In other words, it can be shown that if the dynamics of the cupula endolymph system are second order, calculated values of the short time constant of the canal, and observed values of the long time constant imply cupula deflections sufficiently small as to render the dynamic model insensitive to whether the cupula rotates about the crista or the upper margin, deflects like a diaphragm, or displaces linearly in the ampulla. The only assumptions which are really required are that the cupula be somehow capable of supporting a pressure difference by generating forces which oppose its deflection. Following the notation of Van Egmond et al. (1949) the differential equation of motion of the system is:

$$\Theta \ddot{\zeta} = -\Pi \dot{\zeta} - \Delta \zeta + a\Theta \qquad (12)$$

in which: Π = viscous drag coefficient of the cupula/endolymph system; torque about the center of the canal duct per unit of angular velocity of the flow in the duct. (Equal to $16\eta \pi^2 R^3 = 0.05$ gm cm² by simplified Poiseuille Flow analysis of flow in duct). Steer (1967) suggests viscous drag of cupula could increase its value. ζ = endolymph flow deflection in the duct. Δ = torque coefficient on cupula/endolymph system about the center of the canal duct resulting from cupula motion per unit of angular motion of endolymph flow in the duct.

Behavioral responses give every indication that these dynamics are overdamped, and that the long time constant of the response, Π/Δ is approximately 20 seconds (Young and Oman, 1969; Malcolm, 1968). The earlier estimates of Π/Δ from 8 to 10 seconds in man, based on cupulograms or decay of sensation, were probably in error by failing to account for the effect of adaptation.

The value of the short time constant (Θ/Π) appears to be 1/200th sec or less (Steer, 1967; Money et al., 1969). The "exact" values of these time constants as determined from behavioral responses, particularly Θ/Π, have been the subject of some debate. However, it has become increasingly evident that behavioral responses deviate significantly from the second order characteristics of the fluid dynamics because of intervening neurophysiological dynamics. A 0.005 sec time constant is certainly unobservable on a behavioral basis, and it appears that long term subjective and nystagmus responses show consistent evidence of adaptation involving a homeostatic mechanism of different relative strengths for subjective and nystagmus response, respectively. Studies by Nashner (1970) and Benson (1970) also suggest the presence of a rate sensitive component in responses which interpose lead dynamics with a time constant of 0.1 to 0.05 seconds between cupula deflection and behavioral responses. Accepting $\Pi/\Delta = 20$ sec, and $\Theta/\Pi = 0.005$ sec as at least reasonable estimates for the canal time constants, one can determine that Θ/Δ should be equal to the product of the two approximate second order time constants of the system represented by equation 12. Hence:

$$(\Delta \simeq 10\Theta = 2.4 \times 10^{-3} \text{ dyne cm/rad})$$

Now, suppose one were to adopt the assumption, as a tentative working hypothesis, that the cupula rotates as a rigid body about a point at its base. One can then relate the above calculated value of Δ, which is the torque on the endolymph ring per unit radian flow in the duct, to events occurring in the ampulla. In particular, by applying the continuity equation for flow between cross sections at the cupula and in the duct, one obtains

$$\frac{\Psi}{\zeta} = \frac{Ra^2}{B^3} \tag{13}$$

Now, if K = the torque on the cupula about its base per unit cupula angular motion,

$$K = \frac{\Delta B^4}{a^2 R^2} = 1.5 \times 10^{-3} \text{ dyne cm/rad} \tag{14}$$

and, from Eqn. 5 one can determine that cupula angle is:

$$\Psi = \frac{\Pi B^3 \Delta P}{K} = \frac{2\varrho \Pi^2 \, K'a^4 R^4}{\Delta B^3} \, \alpha \tag{15}$$

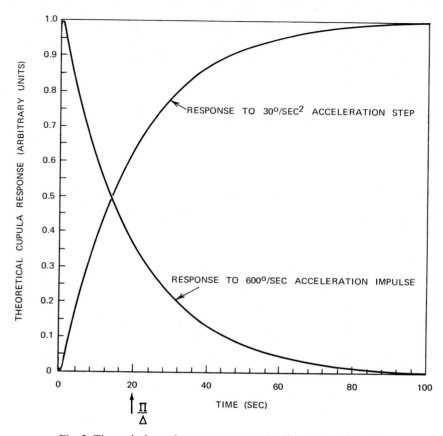

Fig. 2. Theoretical cupula response to acceleration step and impulse.

For accelerations of the 0.1 deg/sec² level associated with behavioral thresholds, the cupula should deflect 0.177×10^{-4} radians (0.001 °). This corresponds to a deflection of the midpoint of the cupula of approximately 10^{-2} μm. This is roughly three orders of magnitude less than the size of the hair cells in the crista, and a thirtieth the diameter of the kinocilium. It is approximately the same dimension as the thickness of the unit membrane in the hair cells.

Another implication of this calculation is that the dynamic range of cupula deflections is constrained to less than a third of a degree for long term accelerations of less than 30°/sec². Actually, almost all long duration dynamic tests of canalicular response to sustained acceleration are performed at acceleration levels considerably less than this. Acceleration levels considerably higher than 30°/sec² are commonly encountered in normal quick head motions, or in the cupulogram impulsive stop. However, the duration of these motions is sufficiently small that large cupula deviations are never achieved. This is understandable because, as is well known, cupula position is approximately proportional to the time integral of the stimulus angular acceleration, over the first several seconds after stimulation. Specifically, solution of the torsion pendulum equation (12) indicates that cupula deviation for unit step increments in angular acceleration are related to deviations for step increments in angular velocity by the factor of Π/Δ, which is taken to be 20. Hence it can be seen that approximately the same peak cupula deflection results for a step in acceleration of 30°/sec² or a velocity step of 600°/sec, as shown in Fig. 2. One can conclude, then, that over the normal range of velocities used in the cupulogram experiment (up to 50°/sec), the cupula should move less than 0.025 deg. The midpoint of the cupula would move less than a quarter of a micron.

The basic implication of the torsion pendulum model is that for sinusoidal stimuli of the frequency range Π/Δ to Π/Θ radians/sec, the cupula should act as a transducer of angular velocity. Tests on human subjects in our laboratory indicate that in this frequency range, human subjects can sustain self induced sinusoidal head motions up to only 600–700°/sec, and only at frequencies below 7–8 Hz. Hence, the linear model represented by equation 12 predicts that cupula deflections would always be less than a third of a degree, and midpoint displacements would be less than 3 μm.

Thus, it can be concluded that although acceleration input amplitudes vary over a range of almost 10^4 above threshold, because of the nature of the frequency distribution of these acceleration stimuli, and the particular way in which the semicircular canal has evolved as a biological transducer, the dynamic range required of the cupula in the linear model appears to be only on the order of 10^2. Perhaps this provides a better match to the dynamic range characteristics of the afferent processes.

DISCUSSION

One obvious criticism of the foregoing argument is that the cupula may exhibit a torque to deflection saturation nonlinearity at larger deflection amplitudes. Another is that, perhaps due to cupula viscous drag, the actual short time constant of the canal is less than the value of 0.005 seconds assumed here (Steer, 1967). However, the effect of both of these errors is to increase the effective value of K, which results in an even smaller, not larger, value for the displacement threshold. Actually, however, the value of cupula stiffness calculated here seems not entirely unreasonable. The Young's modulus of elasticity for a homogeneous cupula of height 2B, thickness B/2, and stiffness coefficient K can be approximated as

$$E \cong \frac{12\,K}{B^4} \tag{16}$$

This calculation does depend on assumptions associated with bending movement of inertia, and hence, on the assumed cupula thickness, so the results are only representative.

For B = 0.06 cm, equation 16 yields a value of 1.4×10^3, which can be compared to values of 10^6 for rubber and unity for mucus found by Philipoff (1966) and 10^3 to 850×10^3 for gelatin found by Pouradier (1967). It is consistent with values calculated by Ten Kate (1969) for the cupula of the pike.

It is important to note, however, that since the calculation range of cupula motions is very small for the actual physiologic range of the cupula, one cannot rule out the hypothesis that the cupula does not deflect about its base at the crista, as was assumed for this calculation, but rather generates equivalent torques on the endolymph due to lateral displacement as well. Some histological justification for this has recently been shown by Dohlman (1971). The volume displaced by a moving cupula is practically the same whether its midpoint traverses linearly, or in an arc, for deflection angles up to about 10 degrees. Obviously, both alternatives have to be considered. Hence, the only conclusion justified from this analysis is that the dynamic range of the motion of the midpoint of the cupula, which displaces nearly identically under either hypothesis, is probably from 10^{-2} μm at threshold up to several μm for maximal self induced head motions, provided amplitude nonlinearities do not limit cupula displacements for the stronger stimuli.

It is interesting to note that the calculated threshold displacement in the semicircular canal is 10^6 larger than that calculated by Lawrence (1968) for displacement of the basilar membrane at the auditory threshold. However, it should be noted that Lawrence's calculation is based on data taken by Von Bekesy at 134 db over threshold. The range of displacement values calculated here for the cupula is generally consistent with the assumed dynamic range of the lateral line organs in fish and amphibians, as reported by Flock (1967). This discrepancy between auditory and vestibular/lateral line displacements is intriguing.

While the calculated thresholds in terms of displacements of the sensory structure are different by a factor of a million, the pressure thresholds for the semicircular canal and the human auditory system are quite similar. The accepted standard for human auditory threshold at the tympanic membrane is 2×10^{-4} dyne/cm^2, essentially the same value found for the semicircular canal.

CONCLUSIONS

The cupula of the human horizontal semicircular canal constitutes an important link in an enormously sensitive biological pressure transducer, one which is probably quite easily subject to trauma in research preparations or otologic surgery. Subjective behavioral thresholds to rotation are likely associated with cupula pressure differences of 10^{-4} dyne/cm^2. This small pressure is approximately equivalent to the acoustic threshold at the tympanic membrane. A pressure difference of 10^{-3} dyne/cm^2 is probably required to produce nystagmic response to rotational or caloric stimuli. In the course of everyday life, peak pressures should rarely exceed 10^{-2} dyne/cm^2. Hence, the application of even 10^{-4} cm of water pressure across the ampulla (10^{-1} dyne/cm^2) would subject the cupula to a distinctly unphysiologic steady state pressure.

Calculations indicate that the dynamic range of motion of the midpoint of the cupula is from about 10^{-2} μm at threshold up to about 3 μm at the upper limit of self induced sinusoidal head motions. The presence of a torque saturating characteristic in the cupula for large displacements could limit the upper end of the dynamic range to smaller values, however. Nonetheless, the dynamic range of motion calculated here is generally consistent with results obtained from the lateral line organs.

No conclusion is reached with respect to whether the cupula moves angularly or linearly or both, except that it should be noted that all modes are possible, because of the small dynamic range of motions required. In any event, describing the cupula as a "swinging door" which normally makes gross displacements within the ampullary lumen is probably a misleading analogy.

SUMMARY

The question of what constitutes the "physiologic" behavior of the cupula has been the subject of debate for some time. Considerations based on calculation of the moment of inertia of endolymph in the membranous semicircular canal and on known behavioral responses to angular accelerations suggest that the pressure across the cupula associated with behavioral thresholds must be less than 10^{-4} dyne/cm^2. Calculation of the density gradient pressures resulting from threshold level caloric stimulation yields results consistent with this figure. These calculations result directly from the known morphology of the canals, and involve no assumptions with respect to cupula stiffness or cupula drag. They suggest that the cupula constitutes a biological pressure transducer with a threshold of the same order as that of the auditory system. The calculations also suggest that it would be extremely easy to traumatize the cupula structure by exposing it to pressure gradients far beyond its normal dynamic range in the course of experimental preparations intended to visualize cupula motion.

An estimate of the range of cupula motion is also obtained from theoretical considerations. Conservative calculations indicate that the cupula midpoint moves only about 10^{-2} μm at the 0.1°/sec^2 acceleration levels commonly associated with behavioral thresholds. Accelerations of 30°/sec^2 or velocity changes of 600°/sec, typical of maximal self-induced head motions should produce cupula midpoint motions no greater than about 3 μm. Because of the small dynamic range of cupula motions, modes of cupula deflection other than rotation about the crista cannot be ruled out, because they are indistinguishable from a dynamic point of view.

ACKNOWLEDGEMENT

This research was supported by Grant NGR 22 009 156 from the National Aeronautics and Space Administration.

REFERENCES

BENSON, A. (1970) Interactions between semicircular canals and gravireceptors. *Recent Advances in Aerospace Medicine*, D. Reidel Co., Dordrecht, Holland, pp. 249–261.
BUYS, E. (1937) Interrogatoire de l'appareil semi-circulaire pour déclanchement d'un nystagmus post-rotatoire 'primaire' au moyen du fauteuil Buys-Rijlant. *Valsalva*, **13**, 139–144.
BUYS, E. ET RIJLANT, P. (1939) Le seuil d'excitation (accélération angulaire) des canaux semi-circulaires. *Arch. int. Physiol.*, **49**, 101–112.

CAWTHORNE, T. AND COBB, W. A. (1954) Temperature changes in the perilymph space in response to caloric stimulation in man. *Acta oto-laryng (Stockh.)*, **44**, 580-588.

CLARK, B. (1967) Thresholds for the perception of angular acceleration in man. *Aerospace Med.*, **38**, 443–450.

DOHLMAN, G. F. (1935) Some practical and theoretical points in labyrinthology. *Proc. roy. Soc. Med.*, **28**, 1371-1384.

DOHLMAN, G. F. (1971) The attachment of the cupulae, otolith, and tectorial membranes to the sensory cell areas. *Acta oto-laryng. (Stockh.)*, **71**, 89–105.

FLOCK, A. (1967) Ultrastructure and function in the lateral line organs. In P. COHN (Ed.), *Lateral Line Detectors*. Indiana University Press, Bloomington, Ind., pp. 163–197.

GROEN, J. J. (1961) Vestibular stimulation and its effects from the point of view of theoretical physics. *Confin. neurol.*, **21**, 380–389.

HALLPIKE, C. S. AND HOOD, J. D. (1953) The speed of the slow component of ocular nystagmus induced by angular acceleration of the head: its experimental determination and application to the physical theory of the cupular mechanism. *Proc. roy. Soc. B*, **141**, 216–230.

IGARASHI, M. (1966) Dimensional study of the vestibular end organ apparatus. In *Second Symposium on the Role of the Vestibular Organs in Space Exploration*. NASA SP–115, 47–54.

LAWRENCE, M. (1968) Dynamic range of the cochlea transducer. *Cold Spr. Harb. Symp. quant. Biol.*, **30**, 159–167.

MALCOLM, R. E. (1968) A quantitative study of vestibular adaptation in humans. In *Fourth Symposium on the Role of the Vestibular Organs in Space Exploration*. NASA SP–187, 369–380.

MANN, C. W. AND RAY, J. T. (1956) Absolute thresholds of perception of direction of angular acceleration. *U.S. Naval School Aviation Med.*, *Research Report NM* 001–110–500, No. 41.

MCLEOD, M. E. AND MEEK, J. C. (1962) A threshold caloric test: results in normal subjects. *U. S. Naval School Aviation Med.*, NASA R-47.

MEIRY, J. L. (1965) The vestibular system and human dynamic space orientation. *NASA CR*-628. pp. 192.

MONEY, K. E., BONEN, L., BEATTY, J., KUEHN, L., SOKOLOFF, M. AND WEAVER, R. (1971) The physical properties of fluids and structures of the vestibular apparatus of the pigeon. *Amer. J. Physiol.*, **220**, 140–147.

MONTANDON, A., HUGUENIN, S., LEHMANN, W. AND JOHN, F. (1971) Comparative study of the rotatory vestibular nystagmus thresholds obtained by means of constant or sinusoidal angular acceleration. *Acta oto-laryng. (Stockh.)*, **71**, 273–277.

MONTANDON, A. AND RUSSBACH, A. (1955) L'épreuve giratoire liminaire. *Pract. oto-rhino-laryng.*, **17**, 224–236.

NASHNER, L. M. (1970) *Sensory Feedback in Human Posture Control*. Sc. D. thesis, MIT, Department of Aeronautics and Astronautics, Man-Vehicle Laboratory, pp. 198.

OOSTERVELD, W. J. (1970) Threshold value for stimulation of the horizontal semicircular canals. *Aerospace Med.*, **41**, 386–389.

PHILIPOFF, W. (1966) Visco-elasticity in the field of biorheology. *Ann. N.Y. Acad. Sci.*, **130**, 970–973.

POURADIER, J. (1967) Contribution à l'étude de la structure des gelatines. IX énergie des liaisons assurant la rigidité des gels. *J. Chim. phys.*, **64**, 1616–1620.

STEER, R. W. (1967) *The Influence of Angular and Linear Acceleration and Thermal Stimulation on the Human Semicircular Canal*. Sc. D. thesis, MIT, Department of Aeronautics and Astronautics, Man-Vehicle Laboratory, pp. 143.

STEER, R. W., JR., LI, Y. T., YOUNG, L. R. AND MEIRY, J. L. (1968) Physical properties of the labyrinthine fluids and quantification of the phenomenon of caloric stimulation. In *Third Symposium on the Role of the Vestibular Organs in Space Exploration*. NASA SP–152, 409–420.

STEINHAUSEN, W. (1931) On the proof of the movement of the cupula in the complete arcade-ampulla of the labyrinth under rotory and caloric stimulation. *Pflügers Arch. ges. Physiol.*, **22**, 322–328.

TEN KATE, J. (1969) *The Oculo-Vestibular Reflex of the Growing Pike*. Ph. D. thesis, Rijksuniversiteit te Groningen, the Netherlands, pp. 167.

VAN EGMOND, A. A. J., GROEN, J. J. AND JONGKEES, L. (1949) The mechanics of the semicircular canal. *J. Physiol. (Lond.)*, **110**, 1–17.

YOUNG, L. R. AND OMAN, C. (1969) Model for vestibular adaptation to horizontal rotation. *Aerospace Med.*, **40**, 1076–1080.

COMMENTS TO CHAPTER VII

Inhibitory and Excitatory Relay Neurons for the Vestibulo-ocular Reflexes

M. ITO

*Department of Physiology, Faculty of Medicine, University of Tokyo, Hongo,
Bunkuo-ky, Tokyo, Japan*

Stimulation of VIII nerve evokes IPSPs or EPSPs disynaptically in III and IV nuclei neurons of rabbits. By systematically tracking through the medulla, the locations of vestibuloocular relay neurons have been determined (Highstein and Ito, 1971; Highstein *et al.*, 1971; Highstein, 1971).

Inhibitory relay cells are concentrated in the superior vestibular nucleus, while excitatory relay cells are contained in the rostral 2/3 of the medial vestibular nucleus, in the lateral cerebellar nucleus and also probably in the group y of the vestibular nuclear complex. These inhibitory and excitatory projections to each subgroup of

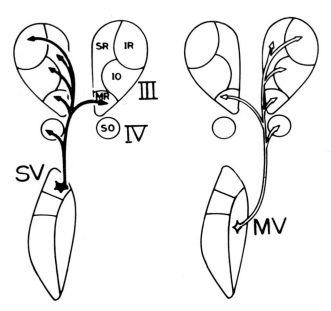

Fig. 1. Diagrams illustrating the synaptic linkage of the vestibular nuclei with III and IV cranial nuclei in rabbit. Thick solid arrows indicate inhibitory projection and hollow ones excitatory. SV, superior vestibular nucleus. MV, medial vestibular nucleus. SR, subgroup of oculomotor neurons innervating superior rectus extraocular muscle. IR, inferior rectus. IO, inferior oblique. MR, medial rectus. SO, superior oblique.

References p. 544

III and IV nuclei innervating different extra-ocular muscles were determined by identifying oculomotor neurons antidromically with separate stimulation of nerve branches in the orbit (Highstein, 1971). It is thus indicated that inhibition from the superior nucleus is exerted ipsilaterally upon all subgroups of III and IV nuclei except for bilateral action upon medial rectus motoneurons (Fig. 1). Excitation from the medial nucleus is on the other hand exerted contralaterally except for bilateral innervation of medial rectus neurons (Fig. 1).

REFERENCES

HIGHSTEIN, S. M. (1971) Organization of the inhibitory and excitatory vestibulo-ocular reflex pathways to the third and fourth nuclei in rabbit. *Brain Res.*, **32**, 218–224.

HIGHSTEIN, S. M. AND ITO, M. (1971) Differential localization within the vestibular nuclear complex of the inhibitory and excitatory cells innervating IIIrd nucleus oculomotor neurones in rabbit. *Brain Res.*, **29**, 358–362.

HIGHSTEIN, S. M., ITO, M. AND TSUCHIYA, T. (1971) Synaptic linkage in the vestibulo-ocular reflex pathway of rabbit. *Exp. Brain Res.*, **13**, 306–326.

Origin of Quick Phases of Nystagmus

B. COHEN

Department of Neurology, Mount Sinai School of Medicine, New York, N.Y., U.S.A.

Although cells in the vestibular nuclei may participate in or reflect neural events associated with nystagmus (Duensing and Schaefer, 1958; Pompeiano, 1972; Dichgans *et al.*, 1972; Shimazu, 1972), there are several reasons for believing that the quick phases of nystagmus are not primarily generated in the vestibular nuclei:

(*i*) Quick phases of optokinetic nystagmus (OKN) and of nystagmus induced by the vestibular system have similar characteristics, and along with saccadic eye movements probably have a common site of origin. Visual-oculomotor pathways do not go through the vestibular nuclei, and neither saccades nor OKN were much affected by vestibular nuclei lesions (Cohen and Uemura, 1972). Therefore, it is unlikely that the vestibular nuclei play a significant role in generating quick phases of OKN or saccades.

(*ii*) Unilateral destruction of almost every part of the vestibular nuclei in two recent studies (McMasters *et al.*, 1966; Cohen and Uemura, 1972) did not abolish quick phases of nystagmus induced by the vestibular system.

(*iii*) After midline section which interrupted commissural fibers between the vestibular nuclei in the monkey, synchronous beats of nystagmus were still induced in the two eyes by vestibular or optokinetic stimuli (Cohen and de Jong, unpublished data). If the decussation of the MLF's was cut, there was paralysis of adduction in both eyes. However, the adductive paralysis was present during all types of eye movements, including saccades and OKN, and probably was due to interruption of axons which originate in the pontine reticular formation, not in the vestibular nuclei (Cohen, 1971).

(*iv*) Neural activity in the pontine reticular formation precedes each rapid eye movement (Cohen and Feldman, 1968; Henn and Cohen, 1971), and lesions of this region cause profound changes in horizontal saccades and quick phases of nystagmus to the ipsilateral side (Bender and Shanzer, 1964; Cohen et al., 1968; Goebel et al., 1970). Lesions of similar size in other parts of the nervous system do not affect rapid eye movements in the horizontal plane in the same way (Cohen, 1971). These and other studies indicate that saccades and quick phases of optokinetic and vestibular nystagmus in the horizontal plane are probably generated primarily in the pontine reticular formation, not in the vestibular nuclei (Cohen, 1971). The site of origin of vertical rapid eye movements is probably in the midbrain in and near the pretectum (Pasik, Pasik and Bender, 1969a, b), although the pontine reticular formation may contribute to production of vertical quick phases (Bender and Shanzer, 1964). Less is known of the supranuclear motor organization for production of rotatory eye movements.

REFERENCES

BENDER, M. B. AND SHANZER, S. (1964) Oculomotor pathways defined by electric stimulation and lesion of the brain stem of monkey. In M. B. BENDER (Ed.), *The Oculomotor System*. Harper and Row, New York, pp. 81–140.

COHEN, B. (1971) Vestibulo-ocular relations. In P. BACH-Y-RITA, C. C. COLLINS AND J. E. HYDE (Eds.), *The Control of Eye Movements*, Academic Press, New York, pp. 105–148.

COHEN, B., KOMATSUZAKI, A. AND BENDER, M. B. (1968) Electrooculographic syndrome after pontine reticular formation lesions. *Arch. Neurol.*, **18**, 78–92.

COHEN, B. AND FELDMAN, M. (1968) Relationship of electrical activity in the pontine reticular formation and lateral geniculate body to rapid eye movements. *J. Neurophysiol.*, **31**, 806–817.

DICHGANS, J., SCHMIDT, C. L. AND WIST, E. R. (1972) Frequency modulation of afferent and efferent unit activity in the vestibular nerve by oculomotor impulses. In A. BRODAL AND O. POMPEIANO (Eds.), *Progress in Brain Research. Vol. 37. Basic aspects of central vestibular mechanisms*. Elsevier, Amsterdam, pp. 449–456.

DUENSING, F. UND SCHAEFER, K. P. (1958) Die Aktivität einzelner Neurone im Bereich der Vestibulariskerne bei Horizontalbeschleunigungen unter besonderer Berücksichtigung des vestibulären Nystagmus. *Arch. Psychiat. Nervenkr.*, **198**, 225–252.

GOEBEL, H., KOMATSUZAKI, A., BENDER, M. B. AND COHEN, B. (1971) Lesions of the pontine tegmentum and conjugate gaze paralysis. *Arch. Neurol.*, **24**, 431–440.

HENN, V. AND COHEN, B. (1971) Pontine neural activity preceding saccades, quick phases of nystagmus, and blinks in alert monkeys. *Fed. Proc.*, **30**, 666.

MCMASTERS, R., WEISS, A. H. AND CARPENTER, M. B. (1966) Vestibular projections to the nuclei of the extraocular muscles. *Amer. J. Anat.*, **118**, 163–194.

PASIK, T., PASIK, P. AND BENDER, M. B. (1969a) The pretectal syndrome in monkeys. I. Disturbances of gaze and body posture. *Brain*, **92**, 521–534.

PASIK, T., PASIK, P. AND BENDER, M. B. (1969b) The pretectal syndrome in monkeys. II. Spontaneous and induced nystagmus, and 'lightning' eye movements. *Brain*, **92**, 871–884.

POMPEIANO, O. (1972), Reticular control of the vestibular nuclei: physiology and pharmacology. In A. BRODAL AND O. POMPEIANO (Eds.), *Progress in Brain Research. Vol. 37. Basic aspects of central vestibular mechanisms*. Elsevier, Amsterdam, pp. 601–618.

SHIMAZU, H. (1972). Vestibulo-oculomotor relations: dynamic responses. In A. BRODAL AND O. POMPEIANO (Eds.), *Progress in Brain Research. Vol. 37. Basic aspects of central vestibular mechanisms*. Elsevier, Amsterdam, pp. 493–506.

UEMURA, T. AND COHEN, B. (1972) Vestibulo-ocular reflexes: effects of vestibular nuclear lesions. In A. BRODAL AND O. POMPEIANO (Eds.), *Progress in Brain Research. Vol. 37. Basic aspects of central vestibular mechanisms*. Elvesier, Amsterdam, pp. 515–528.

Dynamic Oculomotor Reaction

H. SHIMAZU

Department of Neurophysiology, Institute of Brain Research, School of Medicine, University of Tokyo, Hongo, Bunkyo-ku, Tokyo, Japan.

The functional importance of the reticular formation for any motor activities including vestibular nystagmus is obvious. However, I would stress the fact that the EPSP and the IPSP are produced highly synchronously in the antagonistic motoneurons at the quick phase. This indicates that a synchronous arrival of excitatory and inhibitory impulses at the motoneuron determines the onset of the quick phase. The synchronism may not be well explained by multineuronal chains in the reticular formation mediating the quick contraction. Although it is likely that delayed impulses through multineuronal chains intensify the synaptic activities as suggested by Lorente de Nó, we can at present neither accept nor reject the possibility that inhibitory and excitatory reticular neurons project directly to the ocular motoneurons and produce the synchronized IPSP and EPSP in a reciprocal fashion as vestibular nuclei neurons may do.

With respect to Dr. Cohen's discussion on the temporal relation between the ocular movement and neural activity in the pontine reticular formation, we must take it into account that the onset of the EPSP in motoneurons also considerably precedes motor nerve discharges or muscle contraction. The delay of nerve discharges varies in each case (4–20 msec or more), depending on the amplitude and the rising slope of the EPSP, and cannot be estimated uniformly. Therefore the neural activity in a particular structure in the pons preceding muscle contraction might precede in some cases, but might follow in other cases, the onset of the EPSP related to that particular movement.

The hypothesis on the functional role of mutually inhibiting neural elements in production of rhythmic motor activities seems for me to be still worth testing on the fairly well defined vestibulo-ocular system. Although contralateral inhibition of type-I neurons is mediated through the commissural pathway under decerebrate and decerebellate conditions, the possibility has not been excluded that pathways other than the commissural connections might also contribute to it. Comparison between postsynaptic potential changes in the motoneuron and behavior of type-I neurons in the vestibular nuclei under various lesions in the brain stem would be relevant to this point.

We do not know whether the synaptic events in optokinetic nystagmus or saccades are similar to those in vestibular nystagmus.

Static Oculomotor Reactions, Counter-rolling

B. COHEN

Department of Neurology, Mount Sinai School of Medicine, New York, N.Y., U.S.A.

Ocular counter-rolling (CR) is induced when the head is tilted from side to side in the coronal plane (Hunter, 1786; Barany, 1906). The eyes tort or roll to oppose the head movement in an attempt to maintain the original angle of the retina in space. CR against 5° of head and body tilt is barely recognizable, and maximum of about 5–7° of CR is induced by head and body tilts of from 45° to 90° (Woellner and Graybiel, 1959; Miller, 1962; Miller and Graybiel, 1965; Nelson, 1971; Krejcova *et al.*, 1971). Thus CR against head and body tilt is small and does not adequately compensate for the retinal displacement caused by lateral head positions. Examples of compensatory CR in a monkey induced by 45° of head and body tilt are shown in Fig. 1.

In both humans and monkeys CR is the same whether the head is tilted on the neck or the head and body are tilted together (Fig. 2A) (Nelson, 1971; Krejcova *et al.*, 1971). It is also essentially the same whether subjects are in light or in darkness (Krejcova *et al.*, 1971). This indicates that activity which induces CR must come mainly from the labyrinths, and cervical, visual or somato-sensory afferents contribute little to its production.

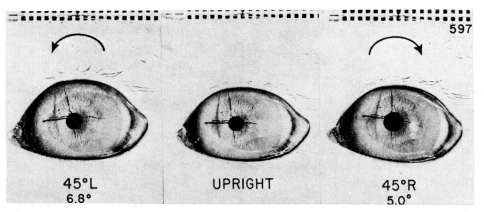

Fig. 1. Photographs showing compensatory counter-rolling in a monkey. When the head and body were tilted 45° to the left (45°L), the eye opposed this by counter-rolling 6.8° in the counterclockwise direction. When the animal was tilted 45° to the right (45°R), the eye opposed this by rolling 5° in the clockwise direction. The arrows over the eyes show the direction of CR. From Krejcova *et al.* (1971).

References p. 549

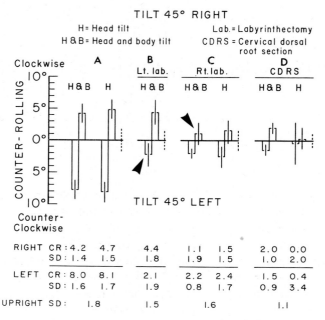

Fig. 2. Graph showing CR induced by head or head and body tilts of 45° of a monkey before and after labyrinthectomy and cervical dorsal root section (CDRS). CR induced by tilts to the right are shown above the abscissa and to the left below the abscissa. The vertical line through each bar shows 2 standard deviations. The dotted lines show 2 standard deviations of angular eye position with the animal upright. Numerical values in degrees are given below. A, CR before operation. B, after left labyrinthectomy (Lt. lab.). C, after right or bilateral labyrinthectomy (Rt. lab.). D, after bilateral cervical dorsal root section (CDRS). The upward arrow in B and the downward arrow in C point to the CR which was reduced by labyrinthectomy. From Krejcova *et al.* (1971).

When one labyrinth is destroyed, CR is no longer induced if the operated side is down (Fig. 2B, upward arrow). On the other hand a normal amount of CR is still induced if the intact ear is down (Fig. 2B, clockwise CR). Others have reported similar findings shortly after labyrinthectomy (Nelson, 1971). This suggests that in the normal subject clockwise CR is mainly induced by the right labyrinth when the right side is down, and vice versa. When both labyrinths are destroyed, most CR disappears. However, small amounts of CR can be induced from extra-labyrinthine sources (Krejcova *et al.*, 1971) (Fig. 2C, D).

Activity which induces CR most probably originates in the otolith organs. CR increases when 'G' forces are increased by centrifugation (Miller and Graybiel, 1965), and disappears during weightlessness (Miller *et al.*, 1966). It is not known for certain which of the otolith organs is responsible for CR. From anatomical considerations it would appear to arise mainly in the utricle (Miller, 1962). However, Nelson (1971) reports that CR is preserved after superior vestibular nerve section. Since the superior vestibular nerve carries afferent fibers from the utricle, he postulates CR might arise in the saccule. There is no information about clinical disorders which might be due to a failure of the eyes to counter-roll. However, CR induced by static head tilt can serve

COMMENTS 549

as one measure of the functional integrity of the reflex arc from the otolith organs to the eye muscle motor nuclei.

REFERENCES

BÁRÁNY, R. (1906) Über die vom Ohrlabyrinth ausgelöste Gegenrollung der Augen bei Normal-horenden Ohrenkranken und Taubstummen. *Arch. Ohr.-, Nas.- u. Kehlk-Heilk.*, **68**, 1–30.

HUNTER, J. (1786) The use of the oblique muscles. In *Observations on Certain Parts of the Animal Oeconomy*. London, pp. 209–212.

KREJCOVA, H., HIGHSTEIN, S. AND COHEN, B. (1971) Labyrinthine and extra-labyrinthine effects on ocular counter-rolling. *Acta oto-laryng. (Stockh.)*, **72**, 165–171.

MILLER, E. F. II (1962) Counter-rolling of the human eyes produced by head tilt with respect to gravity. *Acta oto-laryng. (Stockh.)*, **54**, 479–501.

MILLER, E. F. II AND GRAYBIEL, A. (1965) Otolith function as measured by ocular counterrolling. In *The Role of the Vestibular Organs in the Exploration of Space. NASA SP*–77, 121–131.

MILLER, E. F. II, GRAYBIEL, A. AND KELLOGG, R. S. (1966) Otolith organ activity within earth standard, one-half standard and zero-gravity environments. *Aerospace Med.*, **37**, 399–403.

NELSON, J. R. (1971) The otolith and the ocular counter-torsion reflex. *Arch. Otolaryng. (Chicago)*, **94**, 40–50.

WOELLNER, R. C. AND GRAYBIEL, A. (1959) Counter-rolling of the eyes and its dependence on the magnitude of gravitational or inertial force acting laterally on the body. *J. appl. Physiol.*, **14**, 632–634.

CHAPTER VIII. RELATIONS OF THE VESTIBULAR NUCLEI TO THE RETICULAR FORMATION AND "UPPER LEVELS" OF THE BRAIN

Anatomy of the Vestibuloreticular Connections and Possible 'Ascending' Vestibular Pathways from the Reticular Formation

A. BRODAL

Anatomical Institute, University of Oslo, Oslo, Norway

Our knowledge of the subject indicated in the title of this paper is restricted. In the following I will deal first with the projections of the vestibular nuclei onto the reticular formation (abbreviated RF) and make some comments on the anatomy of the RF. Secondly I will attempt to present the scanty data available on possible pathways ascending from the RF to 'higher levels' of the brain, with particular reference to the question whether these pathways may be concerned in the rostralward transmission of impulses originating in the vestibular nuclei.

VESTIBULORETICULAR CONNECTIONS

Stimulation of the vestibular nerve has been shown to activate extensive parts of the RF (Gernandt *et al.*, 1959; Duensing and Schäfer, 1960; Shimazu and Precht, 1965, and others), but the sites of the responses have not been mapped in detail. *Primary vestibular fibres* to the RF can be concerned in this activation to a very limited extent only since a very small number of primary vestibular fibres have been followed to the RF and appear to have a very restricted distribution: the most dorsolateral part of the RF close to the vestibular nuclei (in the nucleus reticularis parvicellularis).

Important pathways for vestibular impulses to the RF are, however, formed by way of *secondary vestibular fibres*. The presence of these is well known, but information of details in the projections has been scanty. In Golgi preparations axonal branches and collaterals have been traced from all four main vestibular nuclei to the pontomedullary RF, mainly its medial part (Cajal, 1909–11; Lorente de Nó, 1933; Scheibel and Scheibel, 1958). Collaterals of the vestibulospinal tract to the RF were described by Cajal (1909–11), and Valverde (1961) followed axons from the lateral vestibular nucleus to the nucleus reticularis parvicellularis.

In experimental studies of the efferent projections of the vestibular nuclei (for example Gray, 1926; Rasmussen, 1932; Buchanan, 1937; Ferraro *et al.*, 1940; Szentágothai, 1943; Carpenter, 1960; Matano *et al.*, 1964, and others) reference is sometimes made to fibres to the RF, but often the lesions made were large and involved other structures in addition to the vestibular nuclei. Most authors found a bilateral distribution of the projection.

In other studies we have found that the connections of the vestibular nuclei are in general very specifically organized. It is a likely assumption that the same might be the

References pp. 564–565

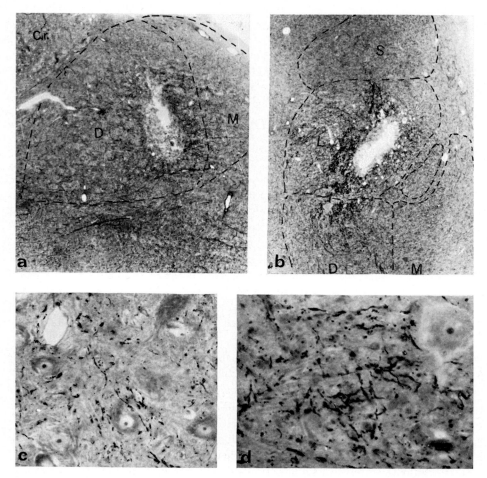

Fig. 1. Above photomicrographs showing a lesion restricted to the descending vestibular nucleus (D) as seen in a transverse section (a) and a lesion restricted to the lateral vestibular nucleus (L) as seen in a horizontal section (b). C.r., restiform body; M and S, medial and superior vestibular nucleus. Below, photomicrographs of Nauta sections showing the degeneration in reticular nuclei following vestibular nuclear lesions. c, From the lateral reticular nucleus (nucleus of lateral funiculus) 6 days after a lesion of the ipsilateral lateral vestibular nucleus (shown in b). × 300. d, From the nucleus reticularis tegmenti pontis 6 days after a lesion of the contralateral superior vestibular nucleus. × 500. From Ladpli and Brodal (1968).

case for the vestibuloreticular projections. In order to test this assumption and, if possible, to determine the projections in greater detail than had been done by previous authors, we (Ladpli and Brodal, 1968) undertook an experimental investigation of the vestibuloreticular projections. Stereotactic lesions of the vestibular nuclei were made in adult cats, and the ensuing degeneration was examined with the Nauta (1957) method after a survival period of 5–8 days. In 15 out of 22 animals we achieved lesions restricted to only one of the main vestibular nuclei. Fig. 1a, b shows the lesions in two of our cases. The evaluation of the degeneration in the RF following such lesions is, however, complicated by the fact that fastigioreticular fibres traverse certain regions of the vestibular nuclear complex. As a necessary preliminary step the course of these fibres was therefore studied. Furthermore, fibres to the RF from one vestibular nucleus may pass through another. The presence of such fibres of passage prevents a complete mapping of the vestibuloreticular projections by the approach used. (Since primary vestibular fibres will often be interrupted by the lesion it is not possible to draw conclusions concerning associational connections in studies like the present one.) Nevertheless, certain points in the projections onto the RF have been clarified. One of the interesting findings is that *the 4 main vestibular nuclei differ with regard to their projections onto the RF.*

Before considering the vestibuloreticular projections it will be appropriate to recall briefly *some features in the anatomical organization of the RF.* In spite of its at first glance diffuse structure it is possible to delineate within it several groups which differ cytoarchitectonically (for a survey see Brodal, 1957). Three of these groups form rather well delimited nuclei, namely the nucleus reticularis tegmenti pontis (N.r.t. in Figs. 2 and 3), the nucleus reticularis lateralis or nucleus of the lateral funiculus (N.r.l. in Fig. 2) and the paramedian reticular nucleus (not shown in the diagrams). These three nuclei all project onto the cerebellum (see Brodal and Jansen, 1946; Brodal, 1943; and Brodal and Torvik, 1954; respectively). Within the main RF other, less clearly delimited groups, may be distinguished. Only a few concern us here. They are all found in the medial two-thirds of the RF. Dorsal to the rostral part of the inferior olive is the nucleus reticularis gigantocellularis (R.gc. in Figs. 2 and 3). This contains numerous giant cells in addition to small and medium-sized cells. The same is the case with the nucleus reticularis pontis caudalis (R.p.c. in Figs. 2 and 3), while its rostral continuation, the nucleus reticularis pontis oralis (R.p.o.) lacks giant cells. These nuclei give off fibres ascending to the brain stem, as well as descending fibres to the spinal cord (see below).

Fig. 2 shows the distribution within the RF of fibres from the *lateral vestibular nucleus.* The lesion in this case is shown in Fig. 1b. Two of the cerebellar projecting reticular nuclei receive such fibres, the ipsilateral lateral reticular nucleus (Fig. 1c) and the contralateral pontine tegmental reticular nucleus. Most of the fibres to the main RF are distributed ipsilaterally to the nuclei containing giant cells (R. gc. and R.p.c. in Fig. 2). It will be seen that many fibres which reach the N.r.l. and R.gc. descend through the descending and medial vestibular nuclei. (For a description of the course of the fibres, the original paper by Ladpli and Brodal, 1968, should be consulted.)

The projection onto the RF from the *superior vestibular nucleus* is somewhat different. Fig. 3 shows that in a case with an isolated lesion of this nucleus there is a projection only to one of the cerebellar projecting nuclei, namely the contralateral reticular tegmental pontine nucleus (N.r.t. in Fig. 3, see also Fig. 1d). This is more heavy than the degeneration in the same nucleus following a lesion of the lateral vestibular nucleus. In the main RF the distribution is mostly the same as for the lateral vestibular nucleus, except that the degeneration extends further rostrally and includes part of the nucleus reticularis pontis oralis (R.p.o., not shown in Fig. 3; see Fig. 2 in Brodal, 1972a).

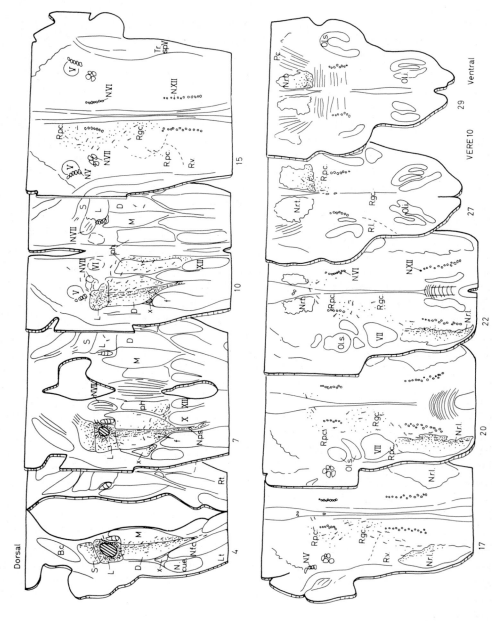

Fig. 2. Diagram showing the course and terminations of degenerating fibres as seen in horizontal sections through the brain stem of a cat, killed 6 days after a lesion restricted to the lateral vestibular nucleus (cf. Fig. 1b). Degenerating fibres shown as wavy lines, sites of termination indicated by dots. Note degeneration in contralateral nucleus reticularis tegmenti pontis (N.r.t.), in ipsilateral lateral reticular nucleus (N.r.l.) and mainly ipsilaterally in main RF in nucleus reticularis gigantocellularis (R.gc.) and pontis caudalis (R.p.c.). From Ladpli and Brodal (1968).

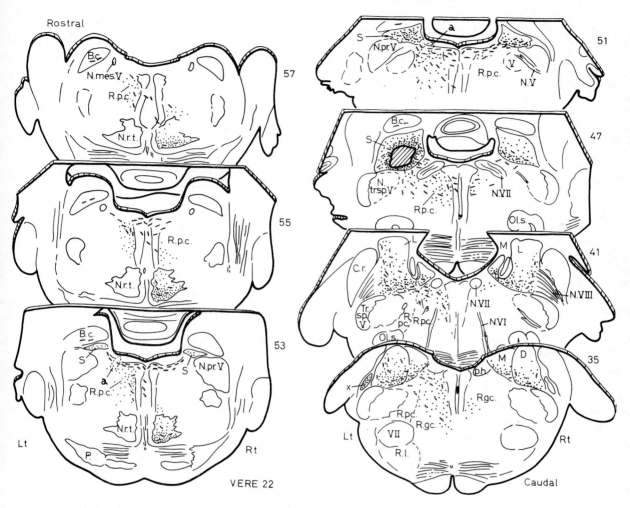

Fig. 3. Diagram of the course and termination of degenerating fibres following a lesion restricted to the superior vestibular nucleus as seen in a series of transverse sections. Symbols and abbreviations as in Fig. 2. In addition to fibres to nuclei in the reticular formation commissural connections are illustrated in Figs. 2 and 3. From Ladpli and Brodal (1968).

The *descending vestibular nucleus* does not supply the cerebellar projecting reticular nuclei (see Table I). Following lesions of the descending nucleus there is degeneration bilaterally in the main RF. Since fibres from the superior and lateral vestibular nuclei as well as fastigioreticular fibres pass through the descending nucleus and end ipsilaterally (see Table I), it is not possible to decide whether the descending nucleus projects onto the ipsilateral RF, except for possibly a few fibres to the R.p.c. However, it may be concluded that the nucleus gives off fibres to the contralateral RF, mainly to the reticularis gigantocellularis and an area between this and the descending nucleus,

TABLE I

SUMMARY OF THE MAIN LOCATIONS OF TERMINAL DEGENERATION IN THE RETICULAR
FORMATION FOLLOWING LESIONS IN VARIOUS VESTIBULAR NUCLEI

Symbols: +, degeneration; ++, heavy degeneration; ?, degeneration present, but may come from
other vestibular nuclei as well; blank, no degeneration. From Ladpli and Brodal (1968).

	Vestibular nuclei							
	Superior		Lateral		Medial		Descending	
	Ipsi	Contra	Ipsi	Contra	Ipsi	Contra	Ipsi	Contra
Retic. pontis oralis		+						
Retic. pontis caudalis	+	+	+	+			+	
Retic. parvocell.	+		+		?	?	?	++
Retic. gigantocell.	+		+		?	?	?	++
Retic. ventralis							?	
Nucl. retic. tegmenti		++		+				
Nucl. retic. later.			++					

the nucleus reticularis parvicellularis. (A diagram of the projections of the descending
nucleus can be found in Fig. 3 in Brodal, 1972a).

The projection of the *medial vestibular nucleus* onto the RF cannot be defined, since
fibres from all the other vestibular nuclei as well as the fastigial nucleus pass through
the medial nucleus on their way to the RF. Golgi studies have shown that there is a
projection. The only conclusion which can be drawn from our findings is that the
fibrse to the RF from the medial vestibular nucleus must terminate within the areas
supplied by the other nuclei, more specifically in the reticularis gigantocellularis,
ponits caudalis and parvicellularis. The findings made concerning the vestibuloreticular projections are summarized in Table I. (See also Fig. 5 in Brodal, 1972a).

It is seen from Table I and from the preceding account that *each of the main
vestibular nuclei has its specific pattern of projection onto the RF.* Some observations
suggest that there may in addition be minor differences between the projections
of different parts of some of the main nuclei. For example, the dorsolateral part
of the lateral vestibular nucleus does not take part in its projection onto the contralateral reticular tegmental pontine nucleus. Correspondingly, the projections
described for the other nuclei can not be taken as being representative of the entire
territory of the particular nucleus. Whether some of the small cell groups project
onto the RF is not known. From his study of the efferent vestibular projections
in the macaque, baboon and chimpanzee, Tarlov (1969) concluded that the projections
to the RF appear to be somewhat more restricted in primates than in the cat.

Further evidence for the specificity within the vestibuloreticular projections is
found when one considers their terminations in the RF in relation to the efferent
projections of the various reticular nuclei involved.

EFFERENT PROJECTIONS FROM THE VESTIBULAR-INFLUENCED RETICULAR NUCLEI

As we have seen, the two large cerebellar-projecting reticular nuclei receive fibres from the vestibular nuclei, more specifically from the superior and the lateral nucleus. There are thus *two different routes via the RF by which vestibular impulses may influence the cerebellum* (see Brodal, 1972b). However, the functional role of these two reticular nuclei cannot be identical. The lateral reticular nucleus receives fibres only from the ipsilateral lateral vestibular nucleus, while the pontine reticular tegmental nucleus is supplied by the contralateral lateral as well as the contralateral superior vestibular nucleus. These two vestibular nuclei receive different afferent inputs from the labyrinth. It is, furthermore, of some interest that within both reticular cerebellar-projecting nuclei there is an extensive overlapping of terminations of vestibular fibres with fibres from other sources, among them the cerebral cortex and the cerebellar nuclei (see P. Brodal, Maršala and A. Brodal, 1967; and A. Brodal and P. Brodal, 1971). The anatomical organization of these two nuclei suggests that they make possible an extensive integration of vestibular impulses with others before they influence the cerebellum. In addition they are links in cerebelloreticular feedback systems, since they receive fibres from the intracerebellar nuclei.

While only the superior and lateral vestibular nucleus have anatomical possibilities to influence the cerebellum via the RF, *all four vestibular nuclei may act on the spinal cord and 'higher levels' of the brain via the RF*. This can be concluded from a correlation of the findings made in the present study with what is known of the efferent connec-

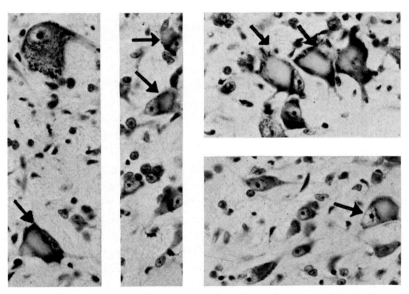

Fig. 4. Acute retrograde changes (arrows) in cells of the reticular formation of kittens subjected to a section above the mesencephalon when 8 days old and killed 6–8 days later. In upper left corner a normal large cell. Note that changes occur in cells of all sizes. Similar changes are seen following lesions of the spinal cord. × 300. From Brodal and Rossi (1955).

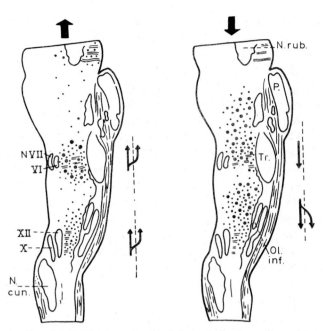

Fig. 5. Diagrams showing the distribution of cells of the reticular formation of the cat sending long axons to the spinal cord (right) and of cells having long axons ascending beyond the mesencephalon (left) as projected on parasagittal sections of the brain stem. Large dots indicate giant cells. In spite of some overlapping the sites giving off the maximal numbers of ascending and descending fibres are not identical. Arrows to the right indicate that the pontine reticulospinal fibres descend homolaterally, while the other contingents are crossed as well as uncrossed. The lower dotted region in the diagram to the right corresponds to the nucleus reticularis gigantocellularis, the upper to the nucleus reticularis pontis caudalis. Based on experimental studies by Brodal and Rossi (1955) and Torvik and Brodal (1957). From Brodal (1957).

tions of the main RF. Some data on these connections are of interest for the subject of this lecture.

Some years ago we studied the origin of these fibres by mapping the retrograde cellular changes which occur following lesions of the mesencephalon (Brodal and Rossi, 1955) or the spinal cord (Torvik and Brodal, 1957). When the modified Gudden method (Brodal 1940) is used, small, medium-sized and large (giant) cells of the RF show characteristic changes (Fig. 4). Even if the sites of origin of ascending and descending fibres overlap considerably, there are certain regions which have predominantly descending, others which give off mainly ascending projections. These regions, shown in the diagrams of Fig. 5, are found within the medial two-thirds of the RF. As is seen there are two main sites of origin for each type of fibres, a medullary and a pontine. The two lower ones cover the nucleus reticularis gigantocellularis, the rostral ones the nucleus reticularis pontis caudalis, that is the regions which receive the majority of the vestibular fibres to the non-cerebellar projecting parts of the RF.

We are here mainly concerned with the ascending fibres, but it is of interest to notice some anatomical features which demonstrate that *the ascending and descending pro-*

jections from the RF must collaborate very intimately. In the first place, from quantitative studies of cells with retrograde changes after rostral or caudal lesions, respectively, it can be concluded that some cells project both ways. This is in complete agreement with observations in Golgi material (Scheibel and Scheibel, 1958; Valverde, 1961, and others). These show that many of the cells of the RF give off an axon which dichotomizes into an ascending and a descending branch. Such cells have been identified also physiologically (Magni and Willis, 1963). Secondly (see Fig. 5), regions which give off many ascending fibres are situated caudal to those projecting mainly to the spinal cord. Since the long axons give off many collaterals during their course, it is likely that by means of such collaterals rostrally projecting cells may influence caudally projecting cells and *vice versa*. These anatomical data, especially the presence of dichotomizing axons, leave no doubt that the influences of the RF on the spinal cord and 'higher levels' are functionally linked together.

As is seen from the diagram in Fig. 5 the ascending fibres from the RF are crossed as well as uncrossed. This is in agreement with the results of Golgi studies (Scheibel and Scheibel, 1958; Valverde, 1961) as well as with experimental tracings of the ascending fibres with the Nauta method (Nauta and Kuypers, 1958). The presence of two main regions of origin of ascending fibres in the RF suggests that they are not identical in a functional respect. It is likely, although little is known about this, that the composition of afferents impinging on the two regions differs to some extent. For example, as seen from Table I, they are not identical with regard to their vestibular influx. A further indication of a functional dissimilarity of the two regions is the absence of rostrally projecting large and giant cells in the medullary region of origin of ascending fibres. (All large and giant cells here appear to project caudally).

A further point, worth recalling, is the confluence of afferents from many sources on these regions of the RF. They receive spinal afferents, fibres from the cerebral cortex, from the fastigial nucleus, the superior colliculi, sensory cranial nerve nuclei and from several other sources, quantitatively probably less important. Even if each of these groups of afferents has its preferential site of termination within the RF, there is considerable overlapping between the terminal areas (see Brodal, 1957; Rossi and Zanchetti, 1957, for particulars). The organization of the RF as seen in Golgi preparations (see Scheibel and Scheibel, 1958) likewise demonstrates the vast possibilities for integration within the RF of impulses from many sources, as has indeed been shown also physiologically (see for example Scheibel *et al.*, 1955; Duensing and Schäfer, 1957; Magni and Willis, 1964). (Spinal impulses may even be integrated with vestibular impulses in the vestibular nuclei).

The data reviewed above make it *extremely unlikely that there are particular routes for impulses from the vestibular nuclei to 'higher levels'* (and to the spinal cord) *via the RF*. On the contrary, what is transmitted rostrally via the RF as a consequence of vestibular stimulation are presumably impulse patterns resulting from an integration of vestibular impulses with impulses from many other sources.

With these qualifications in mind we may turn to the question of the *terminations of the ascending fibres from the reticular formation*, with particular reference to possible pathways along which impulses may reach the somatosensory and the vestibular cortex and stations in the visual pathways. Anatomical studies of these fibre connections meet with great difficulties. Lesions of the RF are likely to interrupt passing fibres. Golgi preparations may be useful but have their limitations. The method of retrograde changes can give information of sites of origin, but are of little value for the study of terminations.

In Golgi preparations and in experimental studies ascending fibres from the RF have been traced to a number of nuclei, especially in the thalamus. It is beyond the scope of this presentation to review this extensive field completely. It appears that most ascending fibres from the pontomedullary RF reach the thalamus, while those from the mesencephalic RF, to which we (Ladpli and Brodal, 1968) found no vestibular projections, mainly supply the hypothalamus and septal region.

Most of the ascending fibres from the RF to the thalamus end in the so-called 'non-specific' thalamic nuclei. The further projections of these nuclei have been difficult to clarify (for some references see Brodal, 1969), but it appears from the Golgi studies of Scheibel and Scheibel (1966, 1967) that their projections to the cerebral cortex are sparse and restricted mainly to the orbitofrontal cortex. However, the original distinction between 'specific 'and 'non-specific' thalamic nuclei can no longer be upheld. Relevant to our problem is the fact that ascending fibres from the RF have been shown to end in several of the 'specific' thalamic nuclei (Nauta and Kuypers, 1958; Scheibel and Scheibel, 1958), among them the nucleus ventralis posterior medialis. These observations, as well as the ample interconnections between 'specific' and 'non-specific' thalamic nuclei emphasized by Nauta and Whitlock (1954) and Scheibel and Scheibel (1967) indicate possible routes by which vestibular stimuli may reach the 'primary vestibular cortex', as outlined by Fredrickson et al. (1966) in the monkey (where it appears to be situated in Brodmann's area 2) and by Mickle and Ades (1954), Landgren et al. (1967) and Sans et al. (1970) in the cat.

There are several possibilities for ascending impulses from the RF to reach stations in the optic system. Collaterals or terminals of ascending fibres have been followed into the superior colliculus in Golgi materal (Scheibel and Scheibel, 1958) as well as experimentally (Nauta and Kuypers, 1958). In Golgi preparations Scheibel and Scheibel (1958) in addition found reticular fibres to the lateral geniculate body.

Above attention has been focused on ascending connections of the RF which may be imagined to be involved when vestibular stimulation produces electrical activity in the 'vestibular cortical area' or stations in visual pathways. These connections are of particular interest since there appears to be no convincing evidence for a direct vestibulo-thalamo-cortical pathway (see Tarlov, 1969, 1970, for particulars). The positive findings reported by some authors appear to be due to encroachments of the lesions of well known thalamic projecting structures, such as the medial lemniscus or the brachium conjunctivum. Nor is there evidence for vestibular nuclear fibres to the geniculate bodies or the tectum.

It should be remembered that in addition to those discussed there may be other indirect vestibulocortical pathways. The nucleus of Darkschewitsch and the interstitial nucleus of Cajal in the mesencephalon receive secondary vestibular fibres (see Tarlov, 1969, 1970) as well as fibres from the reticular formation (Nauta and Kuypers,

1958). The possibility that these small mesencephalic nuclei have projections which may serve as links in pathways for the transmission of vestibular impulses to higher levels cannot be excluded. Other circumvential routes may be imagined, for example by way of primary vestibular fibres to the small-celled group of the dentate nucleus (Brodal and Høivik, 1964) and from this by way of the brachium conjunctivum and the thalamus to the cerebral cortex. This route may perhaps be of particular relevance for transmission to the secondary vestibular area observed in the motor cortex of the monkey (Fredrickson *et al.*, 1966) and the cat (Sans *et al.*, 1970).

Obviously there are several more or less indirect routes by which impulses arising on vestibular stimulation may influence the cerebral cortex. The two components of the ascending fibres from the RF are probably not functionally identical. In all of these pathways there are stations where a convergence of vestibular with somatosensory and visual impulses may take place. All of them involve several synapses and can scarcely be considered as being purely or even mainly vestibulocortical pathways. It may in addition be worth remembering that the widespread efferent connections of the RF provide possibilities for an influence of vestibular stimulation on almost any part of the central nervous system.

SUMMARY

Only very few primary vestibular fibres end in the reticular formation (RF) in its most dorsolateral medullary part.

Secondary vestibular fibres to the RF arise from all four main vestibular nuclei. Experimental studies of the distribution of degenerating fibres following lesions restricted to the particular nuclei (Ladpli and Brodal, 1968) show that each of the main nuclei has its particular pattern of distribution of fibres within the RF, as summarized in Table I. The cerebellar projecting reticular nuclei (the lateral reticular nucleus and the nucleus reticularis tegmenti pontis) are supplied by the superior and lateral vestibular nuclei only. These two reticular nuclei differ with regard to the source of their vestibular afferents. They are presumably chiefly relay stations in cerebello-reticular feedback systems, and are organized so as to make possible an extensive integration of vestibular impulses with impulses from other sources.

The superior, lateral and descending, and probably the medial, vestibular nucleus project to the main RF in somewhat different patterns. The majority of the vestibular efferents end in the nucleus reticularis gigantocellularis in the medulla and the nucleus reticularis pontis caudalis. Both these reticular nuclei give rise to ascending fibres which pass beyond the mesencephalon and to fibres to the spinal cord. Some data on the organization of these nuclei are discussed. It is emphasized that their rostrally and caudally directed influence must be intimately linked. On account of the many other kinds of efferents to the RF its ascending projections cannot be considered as purely or even mainly vestibular pathways.

Little is known of the routes along which impulses ascending from the RF may reach the vestibular cortical area or influence stations in the optic pathways. As to the latter terminations of ascending reticular fibres have been found in the superior colliculus and the lateral geniculate body. Some ascending fibres from the RF reach specific thalamic nuclei, among them the nucleus ventralis posterior. This as well as the ample interconnections between specific and non-specific thalamic nuclei may permit vestibular impulses (integrated with impulses from other sources) to reach the vestibular cortex. Other, incompletely known additional pathways may be imagined to be involved as well when vestibular stimulation influences the cerebral cortex.

REFERENCES

BRODAL, A. (1940) Modification of Gudden method for study of cerebral localization. *Arch. Neurol. Psychiat. (Chicago)*, **43**, 46–58.

BRODAL, A. (1943) The cerebellar connections of the nucleus reticularis lateralis (nucleus funicuil lateralis) in rabbit and cat. Experimental investigations. *Acta psychiat. (Kbh.)*, **18**, 171–233.

BRODAL, A. (1957) *The Reticular Formation of the Brain Stem. Anatomical Aspects and Functional Correlations.* Oliver and Boyd, Edinburgh, London, pp. VII–87.

BRODAL, A. (1969) *Neurological Anatomy in Relation to Clinical Medicine.* 2nd Ed., Oxford Univ. Press, London, pp. XX–807.

BRODAL, A. (1972a) Organization of the commissural connections: anatomy. In A. BRODAL AND O. POMPEIANO (Eds.), *Progress in Brain Research. Vol. 37. Basic aspects of central vestibular mechanisms.* Elsevier, Amsterdam, pp. 167–176.

BRODAL, A. (1972b) Vestibulocerebellar input in the cat: anatomy. In A. BRODAL AND O. POMPEIANO (Eds.), *Progress in Brain Research. Vol. 37. Basic aspects of central vestibular mechanisms.* Elsevier, Amsterdam, pp. 315–327.

BRODAL, A. AND BRODAL, P. (1971) The organization of the nucleus reticularis tegmenti pontis in the cat in the light of experimental anatomical studies of its cerebral cortical afferents. *Exp. Brain Res.*, **13**, 90–110.

BRODAL, A. AND HØIVIK, B. (1964) Site and mode of termination of primary vestibulocerebellar fibres in the cat. An experimental study with silver impregnation methods. *Arch. ital. Biol.*, **102**, 1–21.

BRODAL, A. AND JANSEN, J. (1946) The ponto-cerebellar projection in the rabbit and cat. Experimental investigations. *J. comp. Neurol.*, **84**, 31–118.

BRODAL, A. AND ROSSI, G. F. (1955) Ascending fibers in brain stem reticular formation of cat. *Arch. Neurol. (Chicago)*, **74**, 68–87.

BRODAL, A. AND TORVIK, A. (1954) Cerebellar projection of paramedian reticular nucleus of medulla oblongata in cat. *J. Neurophysiol.*, **17**, 484–495.

BRODAL, P., MARŠALA, J. AND BRODAL, A. (1967) The cerebral cortical projection to the lateral reticular nucleus in the cat, with special reference to the sensorimotor cortical areas. *Brain Res.*, **6**, 252–274.

BUCHANAN, A. R. (1937) The course of the secondary vestibular fibers in the cat. *J. comp. Neurol.*, **67**, 183–204.

CAJAL, S. RAMÓN Y (1909-11) *Histologie du Système Nerveux de l'Homme et des Vertébrés.* Maloine, Paris.

CARPENTER, M. B. (1960) Fiber projections from the descending and lateral vestibular nuclei in the cat. *Amer. J. Anat.*, **107**, 1–22.

DUENSING, F. UND SCHAEFER, K. P. (1957) Die Neuronenaktivität in der Formatio reticularis des Rhombencephalons beim vestibulären Nystagmus. *Arch. Psychiat. Nervenkr.*, **196**, 265–290.

DUENSING, F. UND SCHAEFER, K. P. (1960) Die Aktivität einzelner Neurone der Formatio reticularis des nicht gefesselten Kaninchens bei Kopfwendungen und vestibulären Reizen. *Arch. Psychiat. Nervenkr.*, **201**, 97–122.

FERRARO, A., PACELLA, B. L. AND BARRERA, S. E. (1940) Effects of lesions of the medial vestibular nucleus. An anatomical and physiological study in *Macacus rhesus* monkeys. *J. comp. Neurol.*, **73**, 7–36.

FREDRICKSON, J. M., FIGGE, U., SCHEID, P. AND KORNHUBER, H. H. (1966) Vestibular nerve projection to the cerebral cortex of the Rhesus monkey. *Exp. Brain Res.*, **2**, 318–327.

GERNANDT, B. E., IRANYI, M. AND LIVINGSTON, R. B. (1959) Vestibular influences on spinal mechanisms. *Exp. Neurol.*, **1**, 248–273.

GRAY, L. P. (1926) Some experimental evidence on the connections of the vestibular mechanism in the cat. *J. comp. Neurol.*, **41**, 319–364.

LADPLI, R. AND BRODAL, A. (1968) Experimental studies of commissural and reticular formation projections from the vestibular nuclei in the cat. *Brain Res.*, **8**, 65–96..

LANDGREN, S., SILFVENIUS, H. AND WOLSK, D. (1967) Vestibular, cochlear and trigeminal projections to the cortex in the anterior suprasylvian sulcus of the cat. *J. Physiol. (Lond.)*, **191**, 561–573.

LORENTE DE NÓ, R. (1933) Anatomy of the eighth nerve. I. The central projection of the nerve endings of the internal ear. *Laryngoscope (St. Louis)*, **43**, 1–38.

MAGNI, F. AND WILLIS, W. D. (1963) Identification of reticular formation neurons by intracellular recording. *Arch. ital. Biol.*, **101**, 681–702.

MAGNI, F. AND WILLIS, W. D. (1964) Subcortical and peripheral control of brain stem reticular neurones. *Arch. ital. Biol.*, **102**, 434–448.

MATANO, S., ZYO, K. AND BAN, T. (1964) Experimental studies on the medial longitudinal fasciculus in the rabbit. I. Fibers originating in the vestibular nuclei. *Med. J. Osaka Univ.*, **14**, 339–370.

MICKLE, W. A. AND ADES, H. W. (1954) Rostral projection pathway of the vestibular system. *Amer. J. Physiol.*, **176**, 243–246.

NAUTA, W. J. H. (1957) Silver impregnation of degeneration axons. In W. F. WINDLE (Ed.), *New Research Techniques of Neuroanatomy.* C. C. Thomas, Springfield, Ill., pp. 17–26.

NAUTA, W. J. H. AND KUYPERS, H. G. J. M. (1958) Some ascending pathways in the brain stem reticular formation. In H. H. JASPER, L. D. PROCTOR, R. S. KNIGHTON, W. C. NOSHAY AND R. J. COSTELLO (Eds.), *Reticular Formation of the Brain.* Henry Ford Hospital Symposium, Little, Brown and Co., Boston, pp. 3–30.

NAUTA, W. J. H. AND WHITLOCK, D. G. (1954) An anatomical analysis of the non-specific thalamic projection system. In J. F. DELAFRESNAYE (Ed.), *Brain Mechanisms and Consciousness.* Blackwell, Oxford, pp. 81–104.

RASMUSSEN, A. T. (1932) Secondary vestibular tracts in the cat. *J. comp. Neurol.*, **54**, 143–171.

ROSSI, G. F. AND ZANCHETTI, A. (1957) The brain stem reticular formation. *Arch. ital. Biol.*, **95**, 199–435.

SANS, A., RAYMOND, J. ET MARTY, R. (1970) Réponses thalamiques et corticales à la stimulation électrique du nerf vestibulaire chez le chat. *Exp. Brain Res.*, **10**, 265–275.

SCHEIBEL, M. E. AND SCHEIBEL, A. B. (1958) Structural substrates for integrative patterns in the brain stem reticular core. In H. H. JASPER, L. D. PROCTOR, R. S. KNIGHTON, W. C. NOSHAY AND R. J. COSTELLO (Eds.), *Reticular Formation of the Brain.* Henry Ford Hospital Symposium, Little, Brown and Co., Boston, pp. 31–55.

SCHEIBEL, M. E. AND SCHEIBEL, A. B. (1966) The organization of the ventral anterior nucleus of the thalamus. A Golgi study. *Brain Res.*, **1**, 250–268.

SCHEIBEL, M. E. AND SCHEIBEL, A. B. (1967) Structural organization of nonspecific thalamic nuclei and their projection toward cortex. *Brain Res.*, **6**, 60–94.

SCHEIBEL, M. E., SCHEIBEL, A. B., MOLLICA, A. AND MORUZZI, G. (1955) Convergence and interaction of afferent impulses on single units of reticular formation. *J. Neurophysiol.*, **18**, 309–331.

SHIMAZU, H. AND PRECHT, W. (1965) Tonic and kinetic responses of cat's vestibular neurons to horizontal angular acceleration. *J. Neurophysiol.*, **28**, 991–1013.

SZENTÁGOTHAI, J. (1943) Die zentrale Innervation der Augenbewegungen. *Arch. Psychiat. Nervenkr.*, **116**, 721–760.

TARLOV, E. (1969) The rostral projections of the primate vestibular nuclei. An experimental study in macaque, baboon and chimpanzee. *J. comp. Neurol.*, **135**, 27–56.

TARLOV, E. (1970) Organization of vestibulo-oculomotor projections in the cat. *Brain Res.*, **20**, 159–179.

TORVIK, A. AND BRODAL, A. (1957) The origin of reticulospinal fibers in the cat. *Anat. Rec.*, **128**, 113–137.

VALVERDE, F. (1961) Reticular formation of the pons and medulla oblongata. A Golgi study. *J. comp. Neurol.*, **116**, 71–100.

Vestibular Influences on the Vestibular and the Somatosensory Cortex

H. H. KORNHUBER

Department of Neurology and Section of Neurophysiology, University of Ulm, Ulm/Donau, G.F.R.

For a long time the cortical projection of the vestibular nerve was thought to be in the temporal lobe (Spiegel, 1934; Carmichael *et al.*, 1945; Penfield, 1957). The cortical vestibular area was first identified in the cat by Walzl and Mountcastle (1949) with the evoked potential method. In this animal the vestibular cortex is a small field between the auditory and the second somatic area. The juxtaposition to the auditory cortex was taken by several clinicians as confirmation of the temporal lobe hypothesis. However, just in the region between the second somatic and the auditory field the sylvian fissure has evolved in primates because of the large development of the association cortex. It was uncertain whether the vestibular projection went with the auditory to the temporal or with the somatosensory to the parietal lobe. Therefore a study of the vestibulocortical projection in the Rhesus monkey was made (Kornhuber *et al.*, 1965; Fredrickson *et al.*, 1966).

LOCATION OF THE CORTICAL VESTIBULAR AREA IN THE MONKEY

In the Rhesus monkey, the primary cortical projection area of the vestibular nerve lies in the postcentral gyrus at the lower end of the intraparietal sulcus, at the level of the first somatosensory projection of the mouth. It does not extend into Brodmann's area 1 which borders the central sulcus, but it is confined to a small part of cortex belonging to Brodmann's area 2 according to the map of C. and O. Vogt (1919) (Fig. 1). Afferents from other cranial nerves or from the dura have been excluded as a possible source of the evoked potential by control experiments; the evoked potential following electrical stimulation of the vestibular nerve is present after extirpation of the cochlear, facial and intermediate nerves and remains unchanged after section of the V, IX, X and XI cranial nerves at the brain stem, whereas it is abolished by proximal section of the vestibular nerve. The latency is 5 msec in the Rhesus monkey. The cortical projection is bilateral. However, the ipsilateral projection is more susceptible to deep barbiturate anesthesia.

In agreement with the electrophysiological mapping of the cortical vestibular area the truly vestibular sensations of being turned or tilted (as opposed to diffuse vertigo or dizziness) occur in man more often during stimulation of the parietal than the temporal lobe (Foerster, 1936; Penfield, 1957; Penfield and Jasper, 1954).

References pp. 571–572

568 H. H. KORNHUBER

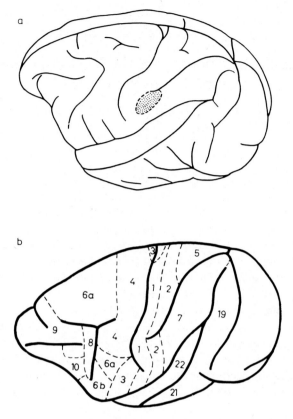

Fig. 1. a, Primary vestibular cortical projection area of the Rhesus monkey according to experiments of Fredrickson and Kornhuber, deep barbiturate anesthesia. b, Mapping of the monkey's cortex by C. and O. Vogt (1919). The vestibular field belongs to Brodmann's area 2 of the postcentral gyrus.

MICROELECTRODE INVESTIGATIONS OF SINGLE UNITS IN THE CAT'S VESTIBULAR CORTEX

Galvanic stimulation of the labyrinths shows several types of neuronal response without any significant relationship between the side of the stimulated labyrinth and the direction-dependence of the responses, which probably means that both cerebral hemispheres are informed about the direction of acceleration by both labyrinths to about the same extent. This is contrary to the situation in the vestibular nuclei as well as in the motor cortex (Kornhuber and Fonseca, 1964). In the motor cortex most neurons responding to labyrinthine polarisation are cathodally activated and anodally inhibited by the ipsilateral labyrinth, and anodally activated and cathodally inhibited by the contralateral labyrinth (Kornhuber and Aschoff, 1964; see Fig. 3). Another difference is the latency; in the primary vestibular cortex the majority of neurons show a short latency (down to 4 msec in the cat, see Fig. 2), in the motor cortex most neurons show a long latency to labyrinthine stimulation.

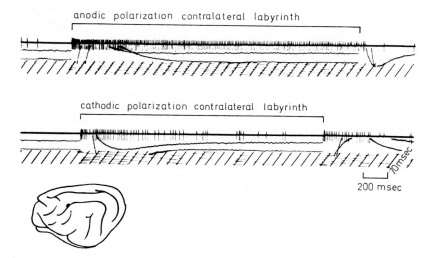

Fig. 2. Responses of a neuron in the vestibular cortex of the cat to labyrinthine polarization. Latency, 4 msec. Insert shows location of the vestibular cortex in the cat. From Kornhuber and Fonseca (1964).

SOMATOSENSORY-VESTIBULAR CONVERGENCE IN THE VESTIBULAR CORTEX, MOTOR CORTEX AND VESTIBULAR NUCLEI

Convergence of vestibular and somatosensory afferents in the vestibular cortex has been found in the cat by Mickle and Ades and in the monkey by Fredrickson *et al.* (1966). Contrary to area 3 of the postcentral gyrus, Brodmann's area 2 receives predominantly deep somatic afferents (Powell and Mountcastle, 1959) and the same is true for the vestibular cortical area of the monkey (Schwarz and Fredrickson, 1971). In contrast to the rest of area 2 which receives unilateral (contralateral) somatic afferents, many neurons of the vestibular cortex receive bilateral deep somatic afferents (Schwarz and Fredrickson, 1971), mainly from the forelegs. There is, however, more influence from the contralateral joints. In addition to afferents from joint receptors there also seem to be muscle afferents in the vestibular cortex of the monkey, judging from responses to deep muscle pressure, predominantly from the proximal flexors and extensors of the contralateral fore- and hindlegs. In the cat, a projection of group I muscle afferents from the contralateral limbs has been found to the region of the vestibular cortex (Landgren *et al.*, 1967).

Similarly a convergence of deep somatic and vestibular afferents has been found in the vestibular nuclei (Fredrickson *et al.*, 1965) and in the motor cortex of the cat (Kornhuber and Aschoff, 1964; see Fig. 3). All these somatic afferents have nothing to do with non-specific arousal reactions according to criteria worked out by the comparison of neuronal responses in several cortical areas using different sensory stimuli (Kornhuber and Fonseca, 1964). The somatic afferents in the vestibular nuclei do not depend on a pathway via the cerebellum. In the vestibular nuclei there are only deep, no superficial somatosensory afferents, predominantly from the neck joint receptors,

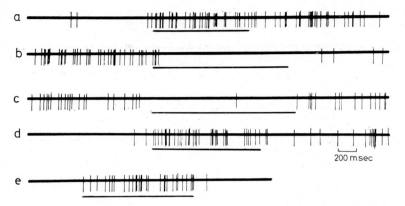

Fig. 3. Convergence of vestibular and deep somatic afferents on a neuron of the cat's motor cortex. a–d, Vestibular responses showing excitation and inhibition dependent on direction of the labyrinthine polarization. Anodal activation (a) and cathodal inhibition (b) during polarization of the contralateral labyrinth; cathodal activation (d) and anodal inhibition (c) from the ipsilateral labyrinth. e, Activation by dorsiflexion of the contralateral forepaws. From Kornhuber and Aschoff (1964).

but also from the limbs. In the motor cortex of the cat about 65 % of the neurons show responses to somatosensory stimuli and about 50 % to vestibular stimuli (Kornhuber and Aschoff, 1964). Although there are many neurons in the motor cortex receiving somatosensory afferents from the skin, only neurons with deep somatic afferents receive direction-specific vestibular afferents (Kornhuber and Aschoff, 1964).

FUNCTIONAL INTERPRETATION OF THE VESTIBULAR CORTEX AND OF VESTIBULOSOMATIC CONVERGENCE

The data just presented show that the vestibular and the proprioceptive somatosensory systems are integrated at all levels of the central nervous system. This is not surprising since functionally the vestibular system belongs to proprioception. The labyrinths, which first evolved in the fish, are in the right place in mammals only for the stabilization of eye position, but they could not stabilize the body position without reference to the afferents from neck receptors. Therefore, the neck reflexes are the opposing partners of the labyrinthine tilting reflexes (Kornhuber, 1966, 1969). The primary vestibular projection area of the cortex does not belong to the oculomotor fields as revealed by stimulation experiments. The directional preponderance of the vestibular nystagmus following hemispheric lesions is not related to the vestibular cortex, but is rather a consequence of the destruction of corticofugal efferents to the brain stem for the visual regulation of eye position (Bader and Kornhuber, 1965).

Obviously the cortical projection of the vestibular nerve serves two functions: first, higher postural motor coordinations and second, conscious orientation in space. Regarding the motor function, area 2 is strongly interconnected with the motor cortex; and the main purpose of the motor cortex seems to be to adjust the motor signal functions generated by the cerebellum and the basal ganglia by means of the tactile analysis provided by the somatosensory cortex so that external objects are appropriately handled (Kornhuber, 1971). On the other hand, the somatosensory cortex (presumably including the vestibular field) projects to the parietal lobe (Jones and Powell, 1969) in which the conscious orientation within space is represented. Parietal lesions result in a tilt of the subjective vertical (Bender and Jung, 1948). In experiments with reversing spectacles, somatosensory and vestibular afferents (and not the visual ones) determine what is up and what is down (Kohler, 1951). Experiments with passive motion show a disturbance of conscious spatial orientation and memory after bilateral labyrinthine loss (Beritoff, 1963).

VESTIBULAR REPRESENTATION IN THE THALAMUS

This, like the representation for the rest of proprioception, should be located in the ventro-caudal part of the lateral thalamus. In the cat, Sans *et al.* (1970) found vestibular responses in the medial part of the VPL. In the monkey, Carpenter and Strominger (1965) found ascending vestibular fibres to the ventralis posterior inferior and ventralis posterior medial nuclei. The long latency vestibular afferents to the motor cortex perhaps go via the basal ganglia, where Segundo and Machne (1956) found vestibular afferents; the few short-latency afferents perhaps come via VL (= V.o. in man), where Sans *et al.* (1970) found vestibular afferents. Recently Deecke, Schwarz and Fredrickson (unpublished observations) found vestibular responses in the VPL of the monkey thalamus which corresponds to a region between the inferior-medial part of the VPL and VPM.

REFERENCES

BADER, W. UND KORNHUBER, H. H. (1965) Grosshirnläsionen und vestibulärer Nystagmus. Vergleichende elektronystagmographische Untersuchungen bei geschlossenen Augen und mit visueller Fixation. *Acta oto-laryng. (Stockh.)*, **60**, 197–206.

BENDER, M. UND JUNG, R. (1948) Abweichungen der subjectiven optischen Vertikalen und Horizontalen bei Gesunden und Hirnverletzten. *Arch. Psychiat. Nervenkr.*, **181**, 193–212.

BERITACHVILI (BERITOFF), J. S. (1963) Les mécanismes nerveux de l'orientation spatiale chez l'homme. *Neuropsychologia*, **1**, 233–249.

CARMICHAEL, D. A., DIX, M. R. AND HALLPIKE, C. S. (1945) Lesions of the cerebral hemispheres and their effects upon optokinetic and caloric nystagmus. *Brain*, **77**, 345–372.

CARPENTER, M. B. AND STROMINGER, N. L. (1965) The medial longitudinal fasciculus and disturbances of conjugate horizontal eye movements in the monkey. *J. comp. Neurol.*, **125**, 41–66.

FOERSTER, O. (1936) Motorische Felder und Bahnen. In O. BUMKE UND O. FOERSTER (Eds.), *Handbuch der Neurologie. Vol. VI.* Springer, Berlin, pp. 1–357.

FREDRICKSON, J. M., FIGGE, U., SCHEID, P. AND KORNHUBER, H. H. (1966) Vestibular nerve projection to the cerebral cortex of the Rhesus-monkey. *Exp. Brain Res.*, **2**, 318–327.

FREDRICKSON, J. M., SCHWARZ, D. AND KORNHUBER, H. H. (1965) Convergence and interaction of vestibular and deep somatic afferents upon neurons in the vestibular nuclei of the cat. *Acta oto-laryng. (Stockh.)*, **61**, 168–188.

JONES, E. G. AND POWELL, T. P. S. (1969) Connections of the somatic sensory cortex of the Rhesus monkey. I. Ipsilateral cortical connections. *Brain*, **92**, 477–502.

KOHLER, I. (1951) Über Aufbau und Wandlungen der Wahrnehmungswelt. *S. Ber. Akad. Wiss. Wien*, IV. hist. Kl., **227**, 1.

KORNHUBER, H. H. (1966) Physiologie und Klinik des zentralvestibulären Systems (Blick- und Stützmotorik). In J. BERENDES, R. LINK UND F. ZÖLLNER (Eds.), *Hals-Nasen-Ohrenheilkunde, ein kurz-gefasstes Handbuch. Vol. III.* Georg Thieme-Verlag, Stuttgart, pp. 2150–2351.

KORNHUBER, H. H. (1969) Physiologie und Klinik des vestibulären Systems. *Arch. Ohr.-Nas.- u. Kehlk. Heilk.*, **194**, 11–148.

KORNHUBER, H. H. (1971) Motor functions of cerebellum and basal ganglia: The cerebello-cortical saccadic (ballistic) clock, the cerebello-nuclear hold regulator, and the basal ganglia ramp (voluntary speed smooth movement) generator. *Kybernetik*, **8**, 157–162.

KORNHUBER, H. H. UND ASCHOFF, J. C. (1964) Somatisch-vestibuläre Integration an Neuronen des motorischen Cortex. *Naturwissenschaften*, **51**, 62–63.

KORNHUBER, H. H. AND FONSECA, J. S. DA (1964) Optovestibular integration in the cat's cortex: a study of sensory convergence on cortical neurons. In M. B. BENDER (Ed.), *The Oculomotor System.* Hoeber, New York, pp. 239–277.

KORNHUBER, H. H., FREDRICKSON, J. M. UND FIGGE, U. (1965) Die corticale Projektion der vestibulären Afferenz beim Rhesus-Affen. *Pflügers Arch. ges. Physiol.*, **283**, R 20.

LANDGREN, S., SILFVENIUS, H. AND WOLSK, D. (1967) Somatosensory paths to the second cortical projection area of the group I muscle afferents. *J. Physiol. (Lond.)*, **191**, 543–559.

MICKLE, W. A. AND ADES, H. W. (1952) A composite sensory projection area in the cerebral cortex of the cat. *Amer. J. Physiol.*, **170**, 682–689.

PENFIELD, W. (1957) Vestibular sensation and the cerebral cortex. *Ann. Otol. (St. Louis)*, **66**, 691–698.

PENFIELD, W. AND JASPER, H. (1954) *Epilepsy and the Functional Anatomy of the Human Brain.* Little Brown, Boston, pp. XV–896.

POWELL, T. P. S. AND MOUNTCASTLE, V. B. (1959) Some aspects of the functional organization of the cortex of the postcentral gyrus of the monkey: a correlation of findings obtained in single unit analysis with cyto-architecture. *Johns Hopk. Hosp. Bull.*, **105**, 133.

SANS, A., RAYMOND, J. ET MARTY, R. (1970) Réponses thalamiques et corticales à la stimulation électrique du nerf vestibulaire chez le chat. *Exp. Brain Res.*, **10**, 265–275.

SCHWARZ, D. W. F. AND FREDRICKSON, J. M. (1971) Rhesus monkey vestibular cortex: a bimodal primary projection field. *Science*, **172**, 280–281.

SEGUNDO, J. B. AND MACHNE, X. (1956) Unitary responses to afferent volleys in lenticular nucleus and claustrum. *J. Neurophysiol.*, **19**, 325–339.

SPIEGEL, E. A. (1934) Labyrinth and cortex. The electroencephalogram of the cortex in stimulation of the labyrinth. *Arch. Neurol. (Chicago)*, **31**, 469–482.

VOGT, C. UND VOGT, O. (1919) Allgemeinere Ergebnisse unserer Hirnforschung. 3. Mitteilung: Die architektonische Rindenfelderung im Lichte unserer neuesten Forschungen. *J. Psychol. Neurol. (Lpz.)*, **25**, 361–398.

WALZL, E. M. AND MOUNTCASTLE, V. B. (1949) Projection of vestibular nerve to the cerebral cortex of the cat. *Amer. J. Physiol.*, **159**, 595.

Interaction of Vestibular and Visual Inputs in the Visual System

O.-J. GRÜSSER AND U. GRÜSSER-CORNEHLS

Institute of Physiology, Free University of Berlin, Berlin, W. Germany

From everyday observations we know that the perception of the visual world is continuously under the control of signals from the vestibular receptors. If we slowly tilt our head or body in any direction in space, the world is still perceived upright, even though the world is now projected 'obliquely' onto the retina with respect to the vertical and horizontal axes of the retina. The processing of the vestibular and visual signals in the perception of the vertical and the horizontal direction of the visual space is probably a mechanism which follows rather strict rules. Some psychophysical data indicating this are mentioned in the first section. In the second section we describe microelectrode findings obtained in the central visual system of the cat, which indicate that the vestibular–visual integration occurs at a rather early stage of the central visual system.

SOME PSYCHOPHYSICAL EXPERIMENTS CONCERNING VISUAL-VESTIBULAR INTERACTION

Steady visual input; variable vestibular input

After we finished the neurophysiological experiments mentioned in the next section we performed in 1959 a simple psychophysical experiment in which the effect of a slow sinusoidal variation of the vestibular input on the perception of visual signals was investigated. The retinal position of the visual signal was kept constant during the variation of the vestibular stimulus. The experimental setup is shown in Fig. 1. The subject was standing at the wall of a cylinder about 6 m in diameter which was rotated at a constant speed (0.2–0.5 rotations per sec, $\omega = \mathrm{d}\,\varphi/\mathrm{dt} = 70–180°\cdot\mathrm{sec}^{-1}$). The cylinder was attached to a movable base which was elevated to a certain position, such that a constant angle α between the axis of the cylinder and the vertical was obtained. At a constant rotation speed ($\mathrm{d}\,\varphi/\mathrm{dt} = \omega = $ constant), the force acting on the otolith and cupula receptors depended on the position of the observer (φ) and the angle α. The force acting in the direction of the axis between both ears was:

$$F_h = k\cdot g\cdot\sin\varphi\cdot\sin\alpha \ [\mathrm{gram\cdot cm\cdot sec^{-2}}] \qquad (1)$$

whereby k is a constant and g is the gravitation constant.

The change of the stimulus acting on the otolith receptors in this experiment was thus a regular function. The constant k was dependent on the direction of the main

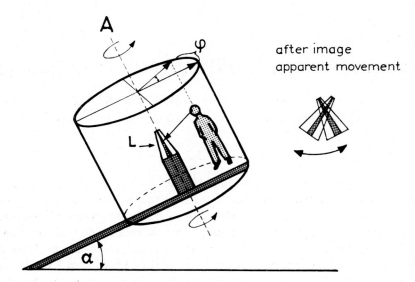

Fig. 1. Schematic drawing of the apparatus used for the psychophysical experiments. The observer was standing in a rotating cylinder. Before the beginning of the rotation he was viewing a bright column of light tubes. During rotation he observed the after-image of this stimulus. The angle (a) of the rotation axis against the vertical was variable.

axis of the otolith receptors and the head position of the subject. The position of the cylinder, at which $\varphi = 0$ for the stimulation of a given receptor, was also dependent on the position of the head with respect to the axis of rotation.

The visual stimulus was a long lasting, bright, positive after-image. This after-image was produced before the rotation by viewing of a bright cone (L), constructed of light tubes located in the center of the rotating cylinder. The described experimental setup was available to us at an extremely low price, as it was used commercially at a fair in Wiesbaden in the late summer of 1959. One 'experimental ride' with this equipment cost 15 cents.

The following results were obtained:

(*i*) The after-image showed a pendular movement around the point of fixation as $a > 0$.

(*ii*) The amplitude of the pendular movement increased approximately with sin a.

(*iii*) The frequency of the pendular movement corresponded to that of the cylinder rotation.

From these observations the following conclusions can be drawn:

(*i*) Visual movement perception can be elicited by vestibular stimulation alone, when the retinal input is exactly stabilized.

(*ii*) The position of the subjective vertical is a regular function of the otolith receptor input. This statement was well known for steady positions in space. The described experiment indicates that it is also true for slow dynamic stimulation ($< 0.5 \cdot \text{sec}^{-1}$) of the vestibular receptors.

Steady vestibular input; variable visual stimuli

The experiment mentioned above is a 'pure' vestibular experiment, because the visual stimulus was constant with respect to the retinal coordinates. Bischof and Scheerer (1970) reported about psychophysical experiments in which the subjective vertical of a human observer was measured at different tilt positions of head and body. Simultaneously a slowly rotating striated visual pattern (0.5 degree·sec^{-1} rotation) was presented in a vertical frontal plane. The subject was asked to indicate his subjective vertical by turning a light line. After one complete measurement of the dependency of the subjective vertical on the direction of the striated pattern, the observer was brought in darkness into a new position in space. The results of these experiments proved that at a constant vestibular input the subjective vertical depends also on the visual input, *i.e.*, the direction of the striation of the visual pattern. This interaction between visual and vestibular signals in the central nervous system was found to contain non-linear components.

The experiments mentioned so far demonstrate that vestibular and visual signals interact in the central nervous system. The experiments described in the next sections indicate possible neuronal mechanisms for such an interaction.

NEUROPHYSIOLOGICAL EXPERIMENTS OF VESTIBULO-VISUAL INTERACTION

Responses of single neurons in the primary visual cortex to electrical polarization of the labyrinth

The experiments described in this section were performed in Freiburg i. Br. (1958). The results and the detailed method are described *in extenso* in earlier papers (Grüsser, Grüsser–Cornehls and Saur, 1959; Grüsser and Grüsser–Cornehls, 1959, 1960a). In these experiments action potentials of single neurons in the primary visual cortex of encéphale isolé cats were recorded extracellularly by means of glass micropipettes (3 M KCl, tip diameter about 0.5 μm). In most experiments a special binocular stimulus apparatus for independent stimulation of each eye with diffuse light was used (Cornehls and Grüsser, 1958; Grüsser and Grüsser–Cornehls, 1965). In a few experiments moving light–dark stripes were projected onto a 60 $\times$ 50° translucent screen placed at a distance of 30 cm from the eyes. The light–dark ratio, the angular velocity and the direction of the movement of the stripes could be varied. The spatial period of the light–dark pattern was limited to a value between 16 and 32°.

For the stimulation of the vestibular receptors of one labyrinth a small silver electrode was placed at the osseus border of the round window; the gross indifferent electrode was fixed in the neck muscles. Direct current of 0.05–0.6 mA was used as a stimulus. At a threshold strength ($<$ 0.1 mA) a *negative polarization* of the different electrode elicited gross conjugate eye movements with a rotatory component to the side of the stimulus electrode, followed by a nystagmus of both eyes into the direction of the stimulating electrode. Turning off the negative labyrinth polarization elicited a conjugate nystagmus to the contralateral side (3–10 sec duration) followed by irregular 'voluntary' eye movements.

References pp. 582–583

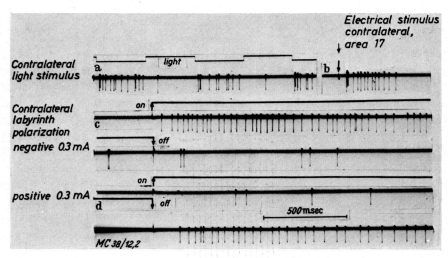

Fig. 2. Off-activated neuron of the primary visual cortex. a, Response to a contralateral diffuse light stimulus. b, Response to electrical stimulation (arrow) of the contralateral visual cortex; latency of the response 45 msec. c, Negative polarization (0.3 mA) of the contralateral labyrinth. The unit was activated after 58 msec. No response at stimulus 'off'. d, Positive stimulation of contralateral labyrinth (0.3 mA). No increase of spontaneous activity at 'on', long latency response (65 msec) at 'off'. From Grüsser, Grüsser–Cornehls and Saur (1959).

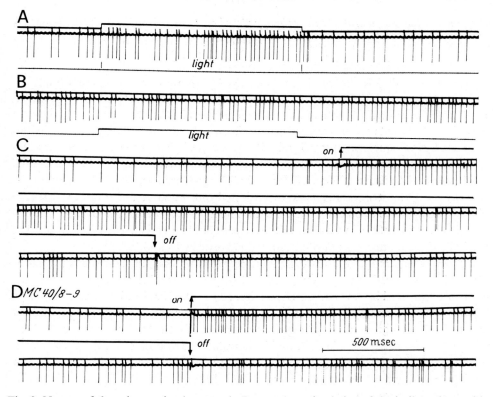

Fig. 3. Neuron of the primary visual cortex. A, Response to stimulation of the ipsilateral eye with 50 Lux, B-neuron (weak on-activation). B, Response to stimulation of the contralateral eye with 50 Lux, C-neuron (weak on-off activation after initial inhibitory periods). C, d.c.-polarization of the ipsilateral labyrinth (0.2 mA, positive). D, d.c.-polarization of ipsilateral labyrinth (0.2 mA, negative). Activation elicited by positive and negative polarization at 'on' and 'off' From Grüsser, Grüsser-Cornehls and Saur (1959).

Positive polarization elicited similar responses but with opposite direction of the nystagmus. No significant differences of the threshold of the nystagmus elicited by positive or negative polarization of the vestibular receptors were found. After the determination of these thresholds, the animals were immobilized by Curarine. Therefore no eye movements were observed during the recording of the neuronal discharges.

Electrical d.c.-depolarization of the vestibular receptors leads to a constant increase or decrease of the impulse rate of the nerve fibers connected with the labyrinth receptors (Lowenstein, 1955) and of the neurons of Deiters' nucleus (De Vito *et al.*, 1956). In both, primary and secondary vestibular neurons, the response type (inhibition or excitation) changes as the direction of the polarizating current is reversed.

The responses of single neurons in the visual cortex to d.c.-polarization of the labyrinth could not be classified according to such simple principles. Four response types of the cortical neurons were found (Figs. 2–4): α) no activation at 'on' or 'off'; β) activation at 'on', no response at 'off'; γ) activation at 'off', no response at 'on'; δ) activation at 'on' and 'off'.

The response type δ was the most frequent one. About 50% of the investigated neurons (70) belonged to this response type. A change of the polarization from negative to positive current did change the response type in a few neurons from β to γ or from γ to β.

The increase of the neuronal impulse rate elicited by labyrinth polarization depended in all investigated neurons on the stimulus strength (Figs. 4, 5). Frequently, the response was a discontinuous increase of the average neuronal impulse rate. Possible

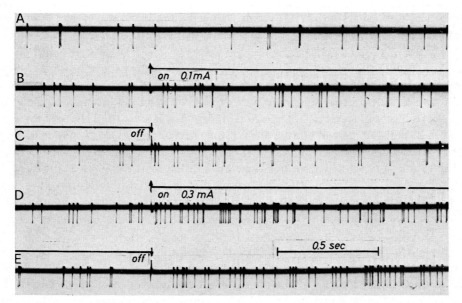

Fig. 4. Neuron from the primary visual cortex; no response to diffuse illumination. A, Spontaneous activity. B, Negative labyrinth polarization (0.1 mA) 'on'. C, Negative labyrinth polarization 'off' (arrow). D, Negative labyrinth polarization (0.3 mA) 'on'. E, Negative labyrinth polarization 'off'.

578   O.-J. GRÜSSER, U. GRÜSSER-CORNEHLS

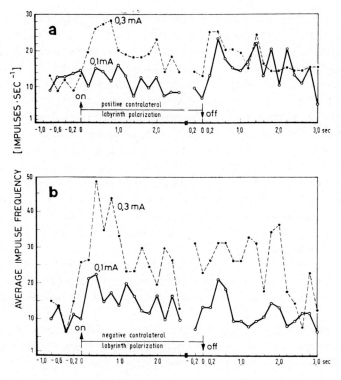

Fig. 5. Monocular dominant on-neuron of the primary visual cortex. Time course of the average impulse rate during and after positive or negative polarization of the contralateral labyrinth. Ordinate: average impulse rate (Impulses· sec⁻¹). Abscissa: time in sec. From Grüsser, Grüsser-Cornehls and Saur (1959).

correlations with the eye nystagmus were not investigated, as the eye movements were suppressed by curarization during all of our recordings.

As a rule, the neuronal activation was strongest during the first second after the electrical labyrinth stimulus was turned on (or off). The latency of the responses varied between 25 and 150 msec in most neurons. Some neurons exhibited even longer latencies up to 250 msec.

The response types a–δ were not correlated to the light response of the neurons (on, off, on–off, on–off inhibition, no response) and were also not correlated to the type of binocular synaptic activation (monocular dominant neurons or neurons with binocular excitation).

Interaction of visual and vestibular signals

The average impulse rate and the response pattern of cortical neurons elicited by stimulation of the retina were changed by vestibular polarization. Fig. 6 shows the response of a light activated cortical unit to brief light flashes projected onto a 60 × 50 degree tangent screen. A weak, rhythmical discharge pattern was obtained; three

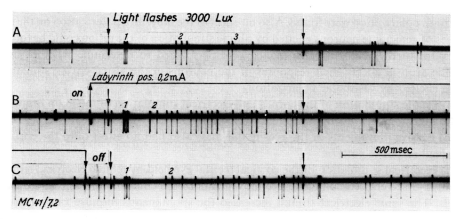

Fig. 6. A, On-activated monocular dominant neuron of the primary visual cortex, which responds after a short diffuse flash of light (arrows) with a weak rhythmical activation of 3 impulse groups (1, 2, 3). B, The flashes (arrows) are combinated with positive polarization of the contralateral labyrinth (0.2 mA). During and after (C) the activation of the labyrinth the response pattern to light flashes is significantly changed. From Grüsser and Grüsser-Cornehls (1960).

excitatory periods separated by inhibitory periods were elicited by each flash. Combination of vestibular polarization with the light flashes enhanced the neuronal impulse rate during the activation periods, but also changed the periodicity of the impulse pattern significantly. In some neurons the instantaneous impulse frequency during the activation period elicited by light flashes or by longer lasting light stimuli increased with simultaneous labyrinth polarization, the duration of the inhibitory periods, however, also increased.

The quantitative analysis of the impulse rate during the excitatory periods elicited by retinal stimulation and the excitation elicited by vestibular stimulation revealed that the specific excitatory visual input and the excitation elicited by vestibular stimulation did not exhibit simple algebraic summation.

The responses of *directionally sensitive cortical neurons* to moving light–dark stripes were also influenced by labyrinth polarization. In most neurons vestibular polarization led to an increase of the neuronal impulse rate during the activation periods elicited by the moving light–dark stripes. The latency of the responses to the moving patterns, however, could be increased; the temporal distribution of the activation periods elicited by the moving patterns was also changed. Some findings in these experiments indicated that the effect of labyrinth polarization also depended on the direction in which the light–dark stripes were moved. However, no systematical analysis of that effect was performed.

Where do visual and vestibular signals interact?

To answer this question we did several control experiments:

(*i*) The occipital and the temporal cortex were removed and action potentials from single nerve cells in the lateral geniculate body were recorded. No responses to

fast nystagmus into the direction of the stimulated labyrinth (negative polarization) or away from it (positive polarization). During the microelectrode recordings, however, this nystagmus was completely interrupted by Curarine injections.

4. Single neurons in the primary visual cortex responded to labyrinth d.c.-polarization either with an on-, off- or on–off activation. The activation was strongest during the first second of labyrinth stimulation. Some grouping of the impulses during the activation periods was found. No correlation between the monocular or binocular light response type and the response type to labyrinth polarization was found.

5. The neuronal response to light stimuli (diffuse light flashes or moving light–dark stripes) was increased by simultaneous polarization of the labyrinth. In some cortical neurons, however, besides an increase of the instantaneous impulse frequency during the light induced excitatory periods also a prolongation of the latency or of the inhibition periods occurred. Hence, the gross electrical stimulus of the labyrinth receptors did not elicit a simple general increase of cortical neuronal activity.

6. The experimental data are believed to indicate a meaningful integration of visual and vestibular signals in the primary visual cortex. Such an integrative mechanism is necessary to guarantee the constancy of the perception of the space independent of the head position. The recent experimental findings of Horn and Hill (1969) support this interpretation. They found a change of the orientation of the receptive field axis of cortical neurons with respect to the axes of the retina, if the animal was tilted around a longitudinal axis (*cf.* Denney and Adorjani, 1972).

REFERENCES

AKIMOTO, H. UND CREUTZFELDT, D. (1958) Reaktionen von Neuronen des optischen Cortex nach elektrischer Reizung unspezifischer Thalamuskerne. *Arch. Psychiat. Nervenkr.*, **196**, 494–519.

BISCHOF, N. UND SCHEERER, E. (1970) Systemanalyse der optisch-vestibulären Interaktion bei der Wahrnehmung der Vertikalen. *Psychol. Forsch.*, **34**, 99–181.

BIZZI, E. AND BROOKS, D. C. (1963) Functional connections between pontine reticular formation and lateral geniculate nucleus during deep sleep. *Arch. ital. Biol.*, **101**, 666–680.

CORNEHLS, U. UND GRÜSSER, O.–J. (1959) Ein elektronisch gesteuertes Doppellichtreizgerät. *Pflügers Arch. ges. Physiol.*, **270**, 78–79.

CREUTZFELDT, O. UND AKIMOTO, H. (1958) Konvergenz und gegenseitige Beeinflussung von Impulsen aus der Retina und den unspezifischen Thalamuskernen an einzelnen Neuronen des optischen Cortex. *Arch. Psychiat. Nervenkr.*, **196**, 520–538.

CREUTZFELDT, O. UND GRÜSSER, O.–J. (1957) Veränderung der Flimmerreaktion (CFF) corticaler Neurone durch elektrische Reizung unspezifischer Thalamuskerne. *C.R. 1er Congr. int. Sci. Neurol., Bruxelles, Vol. III*, 349–355.

DENNEY, D. AND ADORJANI, C. (1972) Orientation specificity of visual neurons after head tilt. *Exp. Brain Res.*, **14**, 312–317.

DE VITO, R. V., BRUSA, A. AND ARDUINI, A. (1956) Cerebellar and vestibular influences on Deitersian units. *J. Neurophysiol.*, **19**, 241–253.

GRÜSSER, O.–J. UND CORNEHLS, U. (1959) Reaktionen einzelner Neurone im primären optischen Cortex der Katze auf elektrische Polarisation des Labyrinths. *Pflügers Arch. ges. Physiol.*, **270**, 31-32.

GRÜSSER, O.–J. UND GRÜSSER–CORNEHLS, U. (1957) Neurophysiologische Grundlagen des Binocularsehens. *Arch. Psychiat. Nervenkr.*, **207**, 296–317.

GRÜSSER, O.–J. UND GRÜSSER–CORNEHLS, U. (1960) Mikroelektrodenuntersuchungen zur Konvergenz vestibulärer und retinaler Afferenzen an einzelnen Neuronen des optischen Cortex der Katze. *Pflügers Arch. ges. Physiol.*, **270**, 227–238.

GRÜSSER, O.–J. UND GRÜSSER–CORNEHLS, U. (1961) Reaktionsmuster einzelner Neurone im Geniculatum laterale und visuellen Cortex der Katze bei Reizung mit optokinetischen Streifenmustern.

In R. JUNG UND H. KORNHUBER (Eds.), *Neurophysiologie und Psychophysik des visuellen Systems.* Springer, Berlin, pp. 313–324.

GRÜSSER, O.-J., GRÜSSER–CORNEHLS, U. UND SAUR, G. (1959) Reaktionen einzelner Neurone im optischen Cortex der Katze nach elektrischer Polarisation des Labyrinths. *Pflügers Arch. ges. Physiol.*, **269**, 593–612.

HORN, G. AND HILL, R. M. (1969) Modifications of receptive fields of cells in the visual cortex occurring spontaneously and associated with bodily tilt. *Nature (Lond.)*, **221**, 186–188.

HORN, G., STECHLER, G. AND HILL, R. M. (1972) Receptive fields of units in the visual cortex of the cat in the presence and absence of bodily tilt. *Exp. Brain Res.*, **15**, 113–132.

HUBEL, D. H. AND WIESEL, T. N. (1959) Receptive fields of single neurones in the cat's striate cortex. *J. Physiol. (Lond.)*, **148**, 574–591.

HUBEL, D. H. AND WIESEL, T. N. (1962) Receptive fields, binocular interaction and functional architecture in the cat's visual cortex. *J. Physiol. (Lond.)*, **160**, 106–154.

LOWENSTEIN, O. (1955) The effect of galvanic polarization on the impulse discharge from sense endings in the isolated labyrinth of the thornback ray (*Raja clavata*). *J. Physiol. (Lond.)*, **127**, 104–117.

MICKLE, W. A. AND ADES, H. W. (1954) Rostral projection pathway of the vestibular system. *Amer. J. Physiol.*, **176**, 243–246.

WALZL, E. M. AND MOUNTCASTLE, V. (1949) Projection of vestibular nerve to cerebral cortex of the cat. *Amer. J. Physiol.*, **159**, 595.

Descending and Reticular Relations to the Vestibular Nuclei: Anatomy

F. WALBERG

Anatomical Institute, University of Oslo, Oslo, Norway

The largest contingent of afferents to the vestibular complex comes from the cerebellum. The other major input to the complex is the fibres of the eighth nerve. A more modest contibution is that from the spinal cord. In addition to these inputs there are some descending and reticular afferents that reach the complex.

Experimental studies made in our laboratory (Pompeiano and Walberg, 1957) have shown that the main source of the *descending fibres* appears to be the interstitial nucleus of Cajal (see, however, Mabuchi and Kusama, 1970). This nucleus is situated ventrolateral to, and partly among, the fibres of the medial longitudinal fasciculus, ventrolateral to the oculomotor nucleus (Fig. 1). Our findings did not give any evidence for a projection from the nucleus of Darkschewitsch, which is located dorsomedial to the middle part of the interstitial nucleus, internal to the lateral border of the periaqueductal grey. Likewise, the nucleus of the posterior commissure lacks a connection with the vestibular complex. This nucleus is situated dorsal to the central grey, associated with the fibres of the posterior commissure.

The observations indicated that the fibres descending to the vestibular complex passed in the medial longitudinal fasciculus, and that they reached only the ipsilateral medial vestibular nucleus, chiefly its dorsal and caudal parts (Fig. 2). Most of the fibres to the medial nucleus are thin, indicating that they probably are collaterals from the interstitio-spinal tract.

Cajal (1909–11), Lorente de Nó (1933) and Scheibel and Scheibel (1958) have described fibres in Golgi material to the vestibular complex *from the reticular formation*. Such fibres reach the nuclei via the medial longitudinal fasciculus as well as directly from the reticular formation.

The reticular afferents are probably given off only at pontine and medullary levels. None of them appear to come from the mesencephalon. This conclusion is substantiated by the observation that we were unable in the operated animals to find degeneration in the vestibular nuclei following extensive lesions of the reticular formation above the level of the pons (Pompeiano and Walberg, 1957). However, we do not know where within the vestibular complex these reticular afferent fibres terminate.

Rotational movements of the head and movements of the eye are considered to be related to pathways via the interstitial nucleus of Cajal. The nucleus receives ascending afferents from the vestibular nuclei, and the feedback from the nucleus reaches the

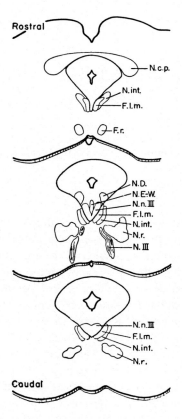

Fig. 1. Diagram showing the nuclei in the periaqueductal region in the cat. Note the location of the interstitial nucleus. Cp. text. From Pompeiano and Walberg (1957). Abbreviations for figures: B.c., brachium conjunctivum; D, descending vestibular nucleus; F.l.m., fasciculus longitudinalis medialis; F.r., fasciculus retroflexus; i.c., nucleus intercalatus; L, lateral vestibular nucleus; M, medial vestibular nucleus; N.c.p., nucleus of the posterior commissure; N.cu.e., external cuneate nucleus; N.D., nucleus of Darkschewitsch; N.E.-W., nucleus of Edinger–Westphal; N.f.c., cuneate nucleus; N.f.g., gracile nucleus; N. int., nucleus interstitialis of Cajal; N.m.d. X, dorsal motor nucleus of vagus; N.n. III, nucleus of third nerve; N.pr. V, principal sensory nucleus of fifth nerve; N.r., nucleus ruber; N.tr.s., nucleus tractus solitarii; N.tr.sp. V, nucleus of spinal tract of fifth nerve; N. III, third nerve; N. V, fifth nerve; N. VII, seventh nerve; N. VIII, eighth nerve; p.h., nucleus praepositus hypoglossi; S, superior vestibular nucleus; Tr. s., tractus solitarius; V, nucleus of fifth nerve; VI, nucleus of sixth nerve; XII, nucleus of twelfth nerve; x, cell group x; z, cell group z.

vestibular complex although the fibres obviously terminate only in a restricted part of the medial vestibular nucleus.

Higher levels of the brain probably influence the interstitial nucleus, but such connections appear to be scarce. Fibres have been described to reach the nucleus from the frontal cortex (Szentágothai, 1943; Szentágothai and Rajkovits, 1958), the occipital cortex (Mettler, 1935; Szentágothai, 1943), the pallidum (Woodburne et al., 1946; Johnsen and Clemente, 1959), and the superior colliculus (Altman and Carpenter, 1961; Matano et al., 1964).

The brief description given here shows that it is highly probably that descending and

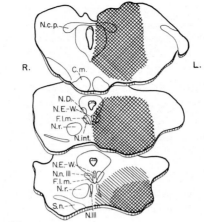

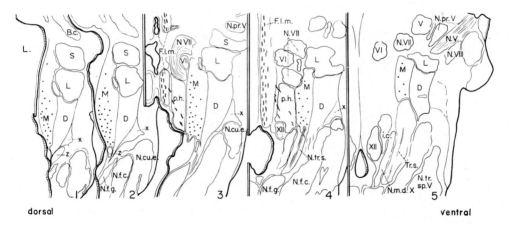

Fig. 2. Diagram showing the descending fibres reaching the vestibular complex from the interstitial nucleus. Degenerating fibres are indicated as wavy lines, the dots show the field of termination for the fibres. Note that the degenerating fibres pass in the medial longitudinal fasciculus, and that they reach only the medial vestibular nucleus. For abbreviations, see Fig. 1. From Pompeiano and Walberg (1957).

reticular afferent fibres to the vestibular complex take their origin only from the interstitial nucleus of Cajal and the pontine and medullary reticular formation. Although a few fibres from the cerebral cortex to the vestibular nuclei have been described (Szentágothai and Rajkovits, 1958), we (Pompeiano and Walberg, 1957) were not able to find such fibres in our study. Neither were we able to trace afferent fibres to the vestibular complex from the basal ganglia, or other parts of the mesencephalon. We may, therefore, conclude that there are probably not important direct descending connections to the vestibular complex from areas rostral to the periaqueductal region of the mesencephalon.

References p. 588

588 F. WALBERG

SUMMARY

A description is given of the descending and reticular afferent fibres to the vestibular nuclei. Experimental light microscopical studies have shown that the descending fibres take their origin in the interstitial nucleus of Cajal, pass in the medial longitudinal fasciculus, and reach chiefly the dorsal and caudal parts of the medial vestibular nucleus. The reticular afferents appear to be derived only from the medullary and pontine reticular formations, but details in the pattern of distribution of the fibres within the various vestibular nuclei are not known.

REFERENCES

ALTMAN, J. AND CARPENTER, M. B. (1961) Fiber projections of the superior colliculus in the cat. *J. comp. Neurol.*, **116**, 157–178.
CAJAL, S. RAMON Y (1909–11) *Histologie du Système Nerveux de l'Homme et des Vertébrés*. Maloine, Paris.
JOHNSEN, T. N. AND CLEMENTE, C. D. (1959) An experimental study of the fiber connections between the putamen, globus pallidus, ventral thalamus, and midbrain tegmentum in cat. *J. comp. Neurol.*, **113**, 83–101.
LORENTE DE NÓ, R. (1933) Vestibulo-ocular reflex arc. *Arch. Neurol. (Chicago)*, **30**, 245–291.
MABUCHI, M. AND KUSAMA, T. (1970) Mesodiencephalic projections to the inferior olive and the vestibular and perihypoglossal nuclei. *Brain Res.*, **17**, 133–136.
MATANO, S., ZYO, K. AND BAN, T. (1964) Experimental studies on the medial longitudinal fasciculus in the rabbit. II. The mesencephalic component of FLM and the central tegmental, medial tegmental and rubrospinal tracts. *Med. J. Osaka Univ.*, **15**, 169–191.
METTLER, F. A. (1935) Corticofugal fiber connections of the cortex of *Macaca mulatta*. The occipital region. *J. comp. Neurol.*, **61**, 221–256.
POMPEIANO, O. AND WALBERG, F. (1957) Descending connections to the vestibular nuclei. An experimental study in the cat. *J. comp. Neurol.*, **108**, 465–504.
SCHEIBEL, M. E. AND SCHEIBEL, A. B. (1958) Structural substrates for integrative patterns in the brain stem reticular core. In H. H. JASPER, L. D. PROCTOR, R. S. KNIGHTON, W. C. NOSHAY AND R. J. COSTELLO (Eds.), *Reticular Formation of the Brain*. Henry Ford Hospital Symposium. Little, Brown and Co., Boston, pp. 31–68.
SZENTÁGOTHAI, J. (1943) Die zentrale Innervation der Augenbewegungen. *Arch. Psychiat. Nervenkr.*, **116**, 721–760.
SZENTÁGOTHAI, J. UND RAJKOVITS, K. (1958) Der Hirnnervenanteil der Pyramidenbahn und der prämotorische Apparat motorischer Hirnnervenkerne. *Arch. Psychiat. Nervenkr.*, **197**, 335–354.
WOODBURNE, R. T., CROSBY, E. C. AND McCOTTER, R. E. (1946) The mammalian midbrain and isthmus regions. Part II. The fiber connections. A. The relations of the tegmentum of the midbrain with the basal ganglia in *Macaca mulatta*. *J. comp. Neurol.*, **85**, 67–92.

Descending Control of the Vestibular Nuclei: Physiology

C. H. MARKHAM

Department of Neurology, School of Medicine, University of California, Los Angeles, California, U.S.A.

This discussion of the descending influences acting on the vestibular system will move from higher functions and the least precise physiological information toward lower centers and more exact information.

Behavioral states clearly modify vestibular as well as other sensory input systems. 'Alertness' is a state which immediately follows 'arousal'; and in arousal, both cortical and brain stem mechanisms participate. Alertness, often well maintained by doing mental arithmetic or other mental tasks, enhances the amplitude and duration of caloric nystagmus (Collins, 1963). Conversely, 'reverie' or 'day dreaming' lessens the amplitude and duration of vestibular nystagmus. The way in which these states act on the vestibular system is unknown. 'Habituation', the decline of response following repeated stimuli, appears to have a main locus in the midbrain reticular formation. For example, the habituation of post-rotational nystagmus in cats is suppressed by lesions of the midbrain reticular formation (Hernández–Péon and Brust–Carmona, 1961) or by bilateral lesions of the superior and lateral vestibular nuclei (McCabe and Gillingham, 1964). Yet in man, mental tasks prevent a response decline on repeated trials of vestibular stimulation (Collins, 1963). Part of the problem is that arousal and habituation interact in a poorly understood way (Crampton and Schwam, 1961). Again, the way in which these higher functions, in conjunction with brain stem reticular elements, act on the vestibular system is unknown. Lastly, 'sleep', (a complex series of states in which brain stem adrenergic and serotonergic neurons, plus the reticular activating system, plus the cerebral cortex participate) modulates vestibular function. In sleep, caloric vestibular stimulus causes the eyes to deviate to the side of the slow phase of nystagmus, the quick phase being abolished. While this effect is probably mediated mostly at a brain stem level, a cortical role is not ruled out.

Childhood schizophrenia or infantile autism is one disorder of the higher central nervous system in which there is a significant disturbance in vestibular responsivity. The illness is characterized by (*i*) inability to relate to people, (*ii*) failure to use language for communication, (*iii*) apparent desire to be alone and to preserve sameness in the environment, and (*iv*) preoccupation with certain objects (Ritvo *et al.*, 1969). It is increasingly considered to have an organic basis (Ornitz and Ritvo, 1968), but there are no clear pathological findings. In view of the type of intellectual and behavioral disorder, we can conclude that the deficit mainly involves cortical and subcortical structures. There is no overt deficit in vestibular function: the children have normal balance,

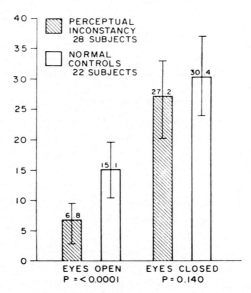

Fig. 1. Shows duration of post-rotatory nystagmus in normal and schizophrenic (perceptually inconstant) children. Significant differences occurred between the two groups when the test was done with eyes open in the light; but not with eyes held closed in the dark. From Ritvo *et al.* (1969).

posture, running, and eye movements. However, many of the afflicted children are preoccupied with whirling themselves and with rotating objects.

In childhood schizophrenia, post-rotational nystagmus performed in the light was much reduced as compared to controls (Colbert *et al.*, 1959; Ritvo *et al.*, 1969). However, when the test was performed in the dark, the duration of postrotational nystagmus was not significantly different from controls (Fig. 1) (Ritvo *et al.*, 1969). Caloric tests performed according to the Hallpike technique (Fitzgerald and Hallpike, 1942) gave markedly depressed values in the majority of children tested (Fig. 2). Further, the results of caloric testing showed more variation from one examination to another than did the control children (Fig. 3) (Colbert *et al.*, 1959). Vision was not evaluated in these caloric experiments, but the same children showed normal optokinetic eye nystagmus. Hyporeactivity and paradoxical vestibular reactions also have been seen in adult schizophrenics (Angyal and Blackman, 1941), suggesting a continuum with the childhood form.

These results fit with other data suggesting that in childhood schizophrenia there is a 'perceptual inconstancy', in which there is a dissociation between facilitatory and inhibitory systems which regulate sensory input. The major depression of evoked vestibular activity could be via the nucleus of Darkschewitsch inhibiting the vestibulo-oculomotor arc at a midbrain level (Szentágothai and Scháb, 1956; Scheibel *et al.*, 1961), via the interstitial nucleus of Cajal acting on inhibitory interneurons in the vestibular nuclei (Markham *et al.*, 1966; Markham, 1968), or via vestibular efferents (Gacek, 1960; Sala, 1965).

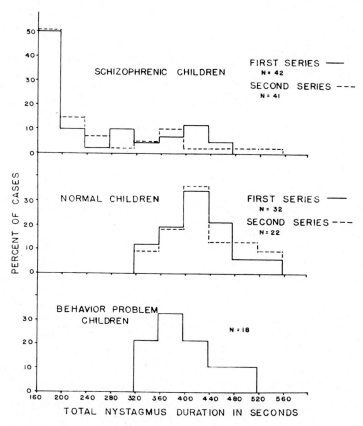

Fig. 2. Shows total durations of caloric nystagmus, made up of the sums of nystagmus durations following bilateral testing with water at 30°C, and at 44°C, in schizophrenic, normal and behavior problem children. From Colbert, Koegler and Markham (1959).

A variety of ablation studies confirm that cortical structures may influence vestibular-induced eye movements. Bauer and Leidler (1911) showed that post-rotational nystagmus was facilitated to the side of a resected cerebral hemisphere in the rabbit. Dusser de Barenne and deKleijn (1923) showed a similar response to caloric-induced nystagmus. Fitzgerald and Hallpike (1942) reported that caloric testing on patients with tumors of the temporal region showed a 'directional preponderance' toward the affected side. Four of the 10 patients had visual field defects implicating the optic radiation. Wycis and Spiegel (1953) showed in dogs and cats that post-rotatory nystagmus to the side of the lesion was enhanced by ablations of either the occipital lobe or of frontal lobe areas 4 and 6 (but not 8). They also showed that removal of the entire cortex had a greater effect than did the more limited frontal or occipital resections.

In addition to the occipital lesions noted above, other parts of the visual system influence the vestibulo-ocular reflex arc. Lesions of the lateral geniculate body or the optic tract enhance post-rotational nystagmus toward the operated side (Spiegel and Scala, 1945). And bilateral interruption of the optic nerves or optic tracts increased

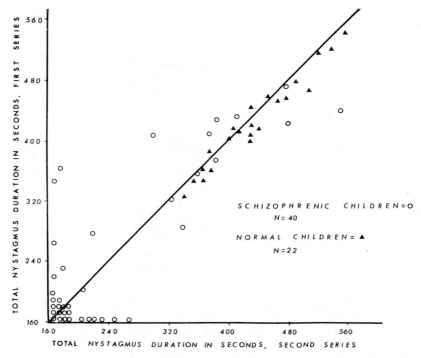

Fig. 3. Comparison of total nystagmus durations, the tests being done twice. They were done at 4–6 month intervals on the schizophrenic children, and a few days to 3 months on the normal children. The values of the normal children cluster about the 45° angle, indicating similar results. The schizophrenic children show much scatter, indicating much variation between the first and second tests. From Colbert, Koegler and Markham (1959).

the duration and number of beats of post-rotatory nystagmus (Spiegel and Scala, 1945). Post-rotatory nystagmus in man is also enhanced by doing the test in darkness (Mowrer, 1937). Lesions to the superior corpus quadrigeminum were followed by ipsilaterally directed post-rotational nystagmus which was more prolonged than that following complete ablation of one area striata (Spiegel and Scala, 1946). These results support the view that retinal influences exert a tonic inhibitory influence on the vestibulo-ocular reflex arc. Yet, vision or the visual apparatus are not the sole supratentorial modifiers of the vestibulo-ocular reflex arc. Frontal lobe ablations sparing area 8 also lead to directional preponderance (Wycis and Spiegel, 1953).

Most of these studies indicate that cortical lesions actually enhance or prolong vestibular nystagmus. This may suggest that the vestibulo-ocular arc is released from higher centers and supports the general concept of the cerebral cortex exerting an inhibitory type of modulation on lower centers. This receives some support from the observation of Scheibel *et al.* (1961) that stimulation of the internal capsule and cerebral peduncles, which contain a considerable proportion of corticifugal components, almost always inhibited vestibular nystagmus.

Stimulation of the temporo-occipital cortex of the rabbit induces a contra-adversive horizontal nystagmus (Manni, Azzena and Desole, 1964). Cortical nystagmus can still be induced after ablation of the vestibular nuclei, but it takes a more vertical vector (Spiegel, 1933; Manni and Giretti, 1969). Vestibular units, particularly in the lateral nucleus, have been shown to be responsive to both caloric labyrinthine stimulus and electrical stimulus of the temporal-parietal region of the guinea pig cortex (Manni and Giretti, 1968). The cortical nystagmogenic response could be abolished by an ipsilateral lesion of the diencephalic nystagmogenic area medial to the lateral geniculate, but the inverse was not true: nystagmus could still be elicited from stimulating the diencephalic area when the cortical area had been ablated (Manni, Azzena and Atzori, 1965). This suggests this variety of cortical modulation of vestibular function passes through the diencephalic eye movement center rather than directly to midbrain levels. These interlocking studies seem to indicate that there is an optokinetic type of nystagmus which is independent of the vestibular nuclei; a type of laterally directed cortical eye movement in which the vestibular neurons also participate; and one or both of these depend on the integrity of the lateral diencephalic nystagmogenic center.

Of several subcortical structures linked with the vestibular system, the caudate nucleus should be considered. Unilateral caudate lesions produced a circus movement to the same side which was then accentuated by ipsilateral rotation (Bergouignan and Verger, 1935); and this effect was enhanced by destruction of the lentiform nucleus (Delmas–Marsalet, Bergouigan and Verger, 1935). Scheibel *et al.* (1961) found that stimulating the caudate nucleus at low voltage and at frequencies of 100/sec caused increased amplitude and duration of vestibular nystagmus (Fig. 5).

Manipulation of the caudate produces two general kinds of behavioral responses: (*i*) inhibiting aspects such as the slow, sleepy or catatonic behavior produced by slow 5–12/sec stimuli in the hands of Akert and Andersson (1951), Heath and Hodes (1952), and Buchwald and Ervin (1957); deficits in conditioned responses produced by bilateral caudate lesions as seen by Gomez *et al.* (1958) and Knott *et al.* (1960); (*ii*) generally active or facilitatory responses such as contra-adversive turning by unilateral caudate stimulation at 30–60/sec (Forman and Ward, 1957; Akert and Andersson, 1951; Buchwald and Ervin, 1957). Such stimuli did not interfere with previously learned behavioral responses (Stevens *et al.*, 1961). It appears that the above described vestibular influences are more closely related to the facilitatory effects of the caudate. And it seems likely that the caudate facilitatory effects, quite different from the internal capsule inhibitory effects, pass via the globus pallidus to the interstitial nucleus of Cajal, nucleus of Darkschewitsch or other medial tegmental reticular sites (Johnson and Clemente, 1959; Woodburne *et al.*, 1946).

Stimulation in cats of a central core of the diencephalon extending from the centrum medianum–parafascicular complex caudally to the nucleus reticularis thalami rostrally also facilitated vestibular nystagmus (Scheibel *et al.*, 1961). So did stimulation of a limited area medial to the lateral geniculate body and including portions of the pulvinar, lateral posterior and lateral dorsal thalamic nuclei. This last region corresponds to a nystagmogenic area in rabbits described by Lachman *et al.* (1958) which when stimulated facilitates nystagmus induced from the contralateral vestibular nucleus or labyrinth; and inhibits nystagmus from the ipsilateral vestibular system (Fig. 4)

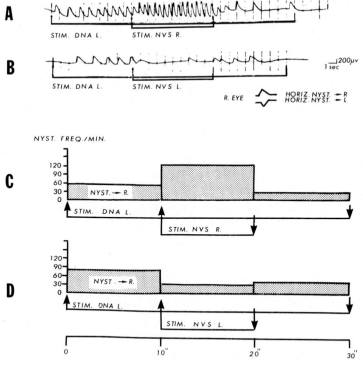

Fig. 4. Shows changes in nystagmus on combined stimulation of the left diencephalic area (DNA) with left and right superior vestibular nucleus (NVS). A and C show increase in nystagmus frequency and amplitude when the right superior vestibular nucleus stimulation is added to diencephalic stimulation. B and D show the effect of superimposed ipsilateral stimulation. Stimulations performed at 50/sec, 0.5–1.0 V. From Montandon and Monnier (1964).

(Montandon and Monnier, 1964). Further, nystagmus induced by stimulation of this lateral diencephalic area is enhanced by separating the frontal cortex and white matter rostral to the optic chiasm from the rest of the brain (Bergmann *et al.*, 1959).

It is not clear how the higher centers act on the vestibulo-ocular reflec arc. It may be action on the vestibular system itself via a midbrain way-station in the interstitial nucleus of Cajal (Pompeiano and Walberg, 1957). Szentágothai and Rajkovits (1958) also discuss and illustrate a direct pathway from frontal cortex to vestibular nuclei. Or it may be a more direct action on midbrain oculomotor mechanisms. Pathways do project to the interstitial nucleus of Cajal, the nucleus of Darkschewitch and possibly other midbrain tegmental sites from the pallidum (Johnson and Clemente, 1959; Woodburne *et al.*, 1946), from the striate cortex (Mettler, 1935), and from the frontal cortex (Szentágothai and Rajkovits, 1958; Kuypers and Lawrence, 1966). Further, one has to consider the path from cortex to midbrain reticular formation to Darksche-witch or interstitial nucleus of Cajal. These and other descending pathways will be discussed and evaluated by Walberg in this volume (see pp. 585–588). However, the likelihood is that there are several routes by which higher centers modulate the vestibular system, and several functions served.

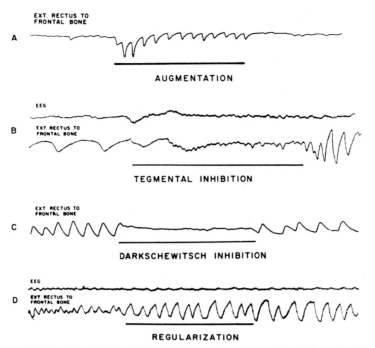

Fig. 5. Shows effect on laterally directed vestibular nystagmus on stimulating other brain sites at 100/sec, 1–4 V, 1 msec pulse duration. From Scheibel, Markham and Koegler (1961).

The descending influences the midbrain exerts on the vestibular system or the vestibulo-ocular reflex may be most important for head and eye coordination. Two midbrain nuclei are of particular interest: the nucleus of Darkschewitsch and the interstitial nucleus of Cajal. The former has an inhibitory effect on eye movements of vestibular or (?) spontaneous origin (Szentágothai and Scháb, 1956; Scheibel et al., 1961). On stimulation, eye movements stopped, and the eyes protruded slightly, presumably from the relaxation of extraocular muscles (Fig. 5). Stimulation of more lateral and inferior midbrain sites markedly modified the vestibular nystagmus, changing it to a fast, low amplitude shimmering nystagmus (Scheibel et al., 1961) closely resembling the tegmental stimulation effect on spinal motor activity (Fig. 5) (Magoun and Rhines, 1946). The nucleus of Darkschewitsch also may have an inhibitory effect on midbrain-induced head rotation: Mabuchi (1970) made lesions which included Darkschewitsch which had this effect (see his Fig. 8). The mechanism by which the nucleus of Darkschewitsch inhibits vestibular-induced eye movements and possibly eye and head movements induced from other sites is unknown. The nucleus of Darkschewitsch does not project caudally in the medial longitudinal fasciculus (Pompeiano and Walberg, 1957), nor does it seem to project the less-than-a millimeter distance to the oculomotor nucleus (Szentágothai and Scháb, 1956). The possibility exists that the nucleus of Darkschewitsch projects to short axoned inhibitory elements in the nearby reticular formation and these project back on the eye motor nuclei. Still another possible sub-

Another functional possibility: vestibular neurons responsive to labyrinthine stimulation may be facilitated or inhibited by pulling on a lateral rectus muscle (Weber and Steiner, 1965). Perhaps the interstitial nucleus participates in a feedback circuit from eye muscle to vestibular nuclei.

The interstitial nucleus of Cajal's strong inhibition of the vestibular substrate for horizontal eye movement may have another significance. It receives projections from the frontal (Szentágothai and Rajkovits, 1958) and striate cortex (Mettler, 1935) and globus pallidus (Johnson and Clemente, 1959; Woodburne et al., 1946). Influences from these higher centers could override, or modulate the vestibulo-ocular pathway concerned with laterally directed eye movements. For example, when the head is turned to the left, the eyes, under vestibular control, turn to the right. Yet it is often useful, particularly in decision-making situations, that the head and eyes turn in the same direction. The interstitial nucleus of Cajal-vestibular nuclei path might serve this purpose by acting to inhibit the vestibular substrate for horizontal eye movements.

SUMMARY

The vestibular system and the vestibulo-ocular reflex arc are influenced by a number of higher functions and centers. The phenomenon of 'alertness' has a cortical aspect; and it clearly facilitates vestibular activity. The role of the cortex in other behavioral states such as 'habituation' or sleep is less clear. Childhood schizophrenia, a severe thought and behavioral disorder, is accompanied by hypoactive and variable responses to caloric and post-rotatory nystagmus. The latter is strongly influenced by vision. Ablation of the occipital and frontal cortex tends to release vestibulo-ocular activity while stimulation studies of the same areas are not amenable to such generalizations. The ablation evidence, however, suggests that the cortex has a generally inhibitory effect in vestibular activity.

Both the caudate nucleus and an area medial to the lateral geniculate body act to augment, while the nucleus of Darkschewitsch inhibits vestibular nystagmus. The mechanisms of these actions are not clear.

The interstitial nucleus of Cajal, a center for head rotation and eye rotation and vertical movement, when stimulated, inhibits type-I vestibular neurons of the horizontal canal. The inhibitory action on type-I neurons of the anterior vertical canal is infrequent and weaker. This function may enhance rotatory head and eye movements; or may serve as a means by which cortical or subcortical stations could modulate vestibular-induced horizontal eye movement.

ACKNOWLEDGEMENTS

Various parts of the work reported were done in collaboration with Arnold Scheibel, Wolfgang Precht, Hiroshi Shimazu, Edward Ornitz, Edward Ritvo and Edward Colbert.

Partial support for the investigations reported has been from U.S. Public Health Service Grant NB 06658.

REFERENCES

AKERT, K. UND ANDERSSON, B. (1951) Experimenteller Beitrag zur Physiologie des Nucleus caudatus. *Acta physiol. scand.*, **22**, 281–298.

ANGYAL, A. AND BLACKMAN, N. (1941) Paradoxical vestibular reactions in schizophrenia under the influence of alcohol, of hyperpnea and CO_2 inhalation. *Amer. J. Psychiat.*, **97**, 894–903.

BAUER, J. UND LEIDLER, R. (1911) Über den Einfluss der Ausschaltung verschiedener Hirnabschnitte auf die vestibulären Augenreflexe. *Arb. Neurol. Inst. Univ. Wien*, **29**, 155–225.

BERGMANN, F., LACHMANN, J., MONNIER, M. AND KRUPP, P. (1959) Central nystagmus. III. Functional correlations in mesodiencephalic nystagmogenic center. *Amer. J. Physiol.*, **197**, 454–460.

BERGOUIGNAN, M. ET VERGER, P. (1935) Les réactions labyrinthiques chez le chien après lésion d'un noyau caudé. *C. R. Soc. Biol. (Paris)*, **118**, 1539–1541.

BUCHANAN, A. R. (1937) The course of secondary vestibular fibers in the cat. *J. comp. Neurol.*, **67**, 183–204.

BUCHWALD, N. A. AND ERVIN, F. R. (1957) Evoked potentials and behavior. A study of responses to subcortical stimulation in the awake, unrestrained animal. *Electroenceph. clin. Neurophysiol.*, **9**, 477–496.

CAMIS, M. (1930) *The Physiology of the Vestibular Apparatus*. Translated by R. S. Creed, Clarendon Press, Oxford, pp. XIV–310.

COHEN, B., SUZUKI, J.-I. AND BENDER, M. B. (1964) Eye movements from semicircular canal nerve stimulation in the cat. *Ann. Otol. (St. Louis)*, **73**, 153–169.

COLBERT, E. G., KOEGLER, R. R. AND MARKHAM, C. H. (1959) Vestibular dysfunction in childhood schizophrenia. *Arch. gen. Psychiat. (Chicago)*, **1**, 600–617.

COLLINS, W. E. (1963) Manipulation of arousal and its effects on human vestibular nystagmus induced by caloric irrigation and angular accelerations. *Aerospace Med.*, **54**, 124–129.

CRAMPTON, G. H. AND SCHWAM, W. J. (1961) Effects of arousal reaction on nystagmus habituation in the cat. *Amer. J. Physiol.*, **200**, 29–33.

DELMAS–MARSALET, P., BERGOUIGNAN, M. ET VERGER, P. (1935) Réactions vestibulaires chez le chien dont un noyau lenticulaire est détruit. *C. R. Soc. Biol. (Paris)*, **119**, 1219–1222.

DUSSER DE BARENNE, J. G. UND deKLEIJN, A. (1923) Über vestibuläre Augenreflexe. V. Vestibular-Untersuchungen nach Ausschaltung einer Grosshirnhemisphäre beim Kaninchen. *von Graefes Arch. Ophthal.*, **111**, 374–392.

FITZGERALD, G. AND HALLPIKE, C. S. (1942) Studies in human vestibular function. 1. Observation on the directional preponderance ('Nystagmusbereitschaft') of caloric nystagmus resulting from cerebral lesions. *Brain*, **66**, 115–137.

FORMAN, D. AND WARD, J. W. (1957) Responses to electrical stimulation of caudate nucleus in cats in chronic experiments. *J. Neurophysiol.*, **20**, 230–244.

GACEK, R. R. (1960) Efferent component of vestibular nerve. In G. L. RASMUSSEN AND W. F. WINDLE (Eds.), *Neural Mechanisms of Auditory and Vestibular Systems*. Thomas, Springfield, Ill., pp. 270–284.

GOMEZ, J. A., THOMPSON, R. L. AND METTLER, F. A. (1958) Effect of striatal damage on conditioned and unlearned behavior. *Trans. Amer. neurol. Ass.*, **83**, 88–91.

GREY, L. P. (1926) Some experimental evidence on the connections of the vestibular mechanisms in the cat. *J. comp. Neurol.*, **41**, 319–364.

HASSLER, R. UND HESS, W. R. (1954) Experimentelle und anatomische Befunde über die Drehbewegungen und ihre nervösen Apparate. *Arch. Psychiat. Nervenkr.*, **192**, 488–526.

HEATH, R. G. AND HODES, R. (1952) Induction of sleep by stimulation of the caudate nucleus in macaqus. Rhesus and man. *Trans. Amer. neurol. Ass.*, **77**, 204–210.

HYDE, J. E. AND ELIASSON, S. G. (1957) Brainstem induced eye movements in cats. *J. comp. Neurol.*, **108**, 139–172.

HYDE, J. E. AND TOCZEK, S. (1962) Functional relation of interstitial nucleus to rotatory movements evoked from zona incerta stimulation. *J. Neurophysiol.*, **25**, 455–466.

JOHNSON, T. N. AND CLEMENTE, C. D. (1959) An experimental study of the fiber connections between the putamen, globus pallidus, ventral thalamus, and midbrain tegmentum in cat. *J. comp. Neurol.*, **113**, 83–101.

KNOTT, J. R., INGRAM, W. R. AND CORRELL, R. E. (1960) Effects of certain subcortical lesions on learning and performance in the cat. *Arch. Neurol. (Chicago)*, **2**, 247–259.

KUYPERS, H. G. J. M. AND LAWRENCE, D. G. (1966) Organization of the cortical projections to the mesencephalon in the Rhesus monkey. *Anat. Rec.*, **154**, 469.

LACHMAN, J., BERGMANN, F. AND MONNIER, M. (1958) Central nystagmus elicited by stimulation of the mesodiencephalon in the rabbit. *Amer. J. Physiol.*, **193**, 328–334.

MABUCHI, M. (1970) Rotatory head response evoked by stimulating and destroying the interstitial nucleus and surrounding region. *Exp. Neurol.*, **27**, 175–193.

MAGOUN, H. W. AND RHINES, R. (1946) An inhibitory mechanism in the bulbar reticular formation. *J. Neurophysiol.*, **9**, 165–171.

MANNI, E., AZZENA, G. B. AND ATZORI, M. L. (1965) Relationships between cerebral and mesodiencephalic nystagmogenic centers in the rabbit. *Arch. ital. Biol.*, **103**, 136–145.

MANNI, E., AZZENA, G. B. AND DESOLE, C. (1964) Eye nystagmus elicited by stimulation of the cerebral cortex in the rabbit. *Arch. ital. Biol.*, **102**, 645–656.

MANNI, E. AND GIRETTI, M. L. (1969) Role of the vestibular nuclei in the cerebral eye nystagmus. *Europ. Neurol.*, **2**, 65–75.

MARKHAM, C. H. (1968) Midbrain and contralateral labyrinth influences on brain stem vestibular neurons in the cat. *Brain Res.*, **9**, 312–333.

MARKHAM, C. H., PRECHT, W. AND SHIMAZU, H., (1966) Effect of stimulation of interstitial nucleus of Cajal on vestibular unit activity in the cat. *J. Neurophysiol.*, **29**, 493–507.

McCABE, B. F. AND GILLINGHAM, K. (1964) The mechanism of vestibular suppression. *Ann. Otol. (St. Louis)*, **73**, 816–828.

METTLER, F. A. (1935) Corticofugal fiber connections of the cortex of the *Macaca mulatta*. The occipital region. *J. comp. Neurol.*, **61**, 221–256.

MONTANDON, P. AND MONNIER, M. (1964) Correlations of the diencephalic nystagmogenic area with the bulbovestibular nystagmogenic area. *Brain*, **87**, 673–690.

MOWRER, O. H. (1937) The influence of vision during bodily rotation upon the duration of postrotational vestibular nystagmus. *Acta oto-laryng. (Stockh.)*, **25**, 351–364.

MUSKINS, L. J. J. (1913–14) An anatomico-physiological study of the posterior longitudinal bundle in its relation to forced movements. *Brain*, **36**, 352–426.

ORNITZ, E. M. AND RITVO, E. R. (1968) Perceptual inconstancy in early infantile autism. *Arch. gen. Psychiat. (Chicago)*, **18**, 76–98.

POMPEIANO, O. AND WALBERG, F. (1957) Descending connections to the vestibular nuclei. An experimental study in the cat. *J. comp. Neurol.*, **108**, 465–503.

RITVO, E. R., ORNITZ, E. M., EVIATAR, A., MARKHAM, C. H., BROWN, M. B. AND MASON, A. (1969) Decreased postrotatory nystagmus in early infantile autism. *Neurology (Minneap.)*, **19**, 653–658.

SALA, O. (1965) The efferent vestibular system. Electrophysiological approach. *Acta oto-laryng. (Stockh.)*, Suppl. 197, 5–34.

SCHEIBEL, A., MARKHAM, C. AND KOEGLER, R. (1961) Neural correlates of the vestibulo-ocular reflex. *Neurology (Minneap.)* **11**, 1055–1065.

SHIMAZU, H. AND PRECHT, W. (1966) Inhibition of central vestibular neurons from the contralateral labyrinth and its mediating pathway. *J. Neurophysiol.*, **29**, 467–492.

SPIEGEL, E. A. (1933) Role of vestibular nuclei in the cortical innervation of the eye muscles. *Arch. Neurol. (Chicago)*, **29**, 1084–1097.

SPIEGEL, E. A. AND SCALA, N. P. (1945) Changes of labyrinthine excitability in lesions of optic tract or external geniculate body. *Arch. Ophthal.*, **34**, 408–410.

SPIEGEL, E. A. AND SCALA, N. P. (1946) Effects of quadrigeminal lesions upon labyrinthine nystagmus. *Confinia Neurol.*, **7**, 68–76.

STEVENS, J. R., KIM, C. AND MACLEAN, P. D. (1961) Stimulation of caudate nucleus. *Arch. Neurol. (Chicago)*, **4**, 47–54.

SZENTÁGOTHAI, J. (1943) Die zentrale Innervation der Augenbewegungen. *Arch. Psychiat. Nervenkr.*, **116**, 721–760.

SZENTÁGOTHAI, J. UND RAJKOVITS, K. (1958) Der Hirnnervenanteil der Pyramidenbahn und der prämotorische Apparat motorischer Hirnnervenkerne. *Arch. Psychiat. Nervenkr.*, **197**, 335–354.

SZENTÁGOTHAI, J. AND SCHAB, R. (1956) A midbrain inhibitory mechanism of the oculomotor activity. *Acta physiol. Acad. Sci. Hung.*, **9**, 89–98.

WEBER, G. UND STEINER, F. A. (1965) Labyrinthär erregbare Neurone im Hirnstamm und Kleinhirn der Katze. *Helv. physiol. pharmacol. Acta*, **23**, 61–81.

WOODBURNE, R. T., CROSBY, E. C. AND McCOTTER, R. E. (1946) The mammalian midbrain and the isthmus regions. Part II. The fiber connections. A. The relations of the tegmentum of the midbrain with the basal ganglia in *Macaca mulatta*. *J. comp. Neurol.*, **85**, 67–92.

WYCIS, H. T. AND SPIEGEL, E. A. (1953) Effect of cortical lesions and elimination of retinal impulses on labyrinthine nystagmus. *Arch. Otolaryng.*, **57**, 1–11.

Reticular Control of the Vestibular Nuclei: Physiology and Pharmacology

O. POMPEIANO

Institute of Physiology II, University of Pisa, Pisa, Italy

The anatomical observation that brain stem reticular neurons project axon collaterals to the vestibular nuclei (Cajal, 1909–11; Lorente de Nó, 1933; Scheibel and Scheibel, 1958; *cf.* Brodal *et al.*, 1962; Hauglie–Hanssen, 1968; Mehler, 1968) suggests that the reticular formation may influence vestibular functions. The demonstration that a spontaneous discharge of the vestibular neurons can still be observed after bilateral labyrinthectomy (Lorente de Nó, 1926; Spiegel and Sato, 1926) or bilateral section of the VIIIth nerves (Gernandt and Thulin, 1952; de Vito *et al.*, 1956), *i.e.*, in the absence of any specific afferents, indeed indicates the existence of an extralabyrinthine influence on second order vestibular neurons, which is probably reticular in origin.

The evidence of a reticular control on the vestibular reflex pathways to the oculo-motor nuclei and the spinal cord, however, is mainly based on experiments in which the reticular formation was either destroyed or stimulated (see for instance Yules *et al.*, 1966b). Unfortunately the intricate anatomic organization of the brain stem makes the interpretation of these studies rather problematic. Moreover, since some of the neurons intercalated in the vestibular efferent pathways to the oculomotor neurons and the spinal cord are located in the reticular formation, any change in the vestibular reflexes induced by stimulation or lesion of the reticular formation can be due in part at least to some interference with the relay stations interposed in these efferent vestibular projections.

Similar complexities emerge also from the study of the mechanisms responsible for the modulation of the labyrinthine nystagmus during the sleep-waking cycle. It is well established that the nystagmus is rather vigorous during wakefulness or attention, while it becomes greatly depressed during synchronized sleep (*cf.* Lenzi and Pompeiano, 1970, for references). The facilitation of the nystagmus during wakefulness can in part at least be referred to a direct influence of the reticular formation on the vestibular nuclei. This is shown by the fact that the activity of the vestibular neurons is greatly modified during the arousal reaction elicited by natural stimuli applied in the free-moving unanesthetized preparation (Bizzi *et al.*, 1964 a, b), as well as by electrical stimuli applied to the reticular formation (Dumont, 1960, 1964, 1966; Dumont–Tyč and Dell 1961) or to their efferent axons (Ito *et al.*, 1964, 1965, 1970). On the other hand the observation that no change in the spontaneous frequency and pattern of discharge of the vestibular neurons occurs during synchronized sleep with respect to quiet wakefulness (Bizzi *et al.*, 1964a, b) indicates that the depression of the nystagmus during this phase of sleep is due to some influence exerted by the sleep mechanisms on the brain stem reticular structures intercalated in the vestibulo-ocular pathway (*cf.* Lenzi and Pompeiano, 1970).

When considering the problem of the reticular control of the vestibular function we will restrict ourselves to the analysis of a remarkable phenomenon described during desynchronized sleep. It is well known that synchronized sleep in mammals is followed by a desynchronized phase of sleep, which is characterized by low voltage, fast cortical waves (Dement, 1958) and by a great depression of both the tonic activity of the postural muscles (Jouvet, 1962, 1967) and the spinal reflexes (Pompeiano, 1966, 1967). In addition to these tonic events, however, one observes also at irregular intervals phasic events, characterized by bursts of binocularly synchronous rapid eye movements, REM (Aserinsky and Kleitman, 1953, 1955; Dement, 1958, 1964). This state of REM sleep has also been described in man (Aserinsky and Kleitman, 1953, 1955; Dement and Kleitman, 1957a, b; Dement, 1964), where a striking relationship has been found between eye movements and dream activity. It will be shown in the following sections that the bursts of REM depend upon the extralabyrinthine activation of vestibulo-oculomotor mechanisms due to autochthonous excitation of a cholinergic reticular mechanism.

VESTIBULAR ORIGIN OF RAPID EYE MOVEMENTS DURING DESYNCHRONIZED SLEEP

Lesion experiments

A first attempt to localize the structures responsible for the bursts of REM indicates that these ocular phenomena still occur in the neodecorticate cat (Jouvet, 1962). They are actually present even after precollicular decerebration during the periods of transient collapse of the decerebrate rigidity (Rioch, 1952, 1954; Bard and Macht, 1958), which are thought to be homologous to the postural atonia during desynchronized sleep (Jouvet, 1962, 1967). The eye movements, on the other hand, disappear following a complete transection of the brain stem at the prepontine level, thus suggesting that the caudal part of the brain stem may be sufficient for the appearance of the REM during desynchronized sleep (*cf.* also Mouret, 1964; Jeannerod *et al.*, 1965). Experiments made by Pompeiano and Morrison (1965, 1966a) have recently shown that after bilateral lesion of all the vestibular nuclei or after lesions limited to the medial and descending vestibular nuclei the episodes of desynchronized sleep were still characterized by typical low voltage fast activity in the electroencephalogram and by atonia in the cervical antigravity muscles. However the bursts of REM were completely abolished. Fig. 1 illustrates the remarkable effect of the vestibular lesion on the ocular movements. Sporadic and isolated ocular movements make their appearance only rarely. The abolition of the typical bursts of REM lasted throughout the survival of the animal, *i.e.*, up to 36 days after the lesion. It is of interest, however, that REM could still be observed during desynchronized sleep after bilateral chronic section of

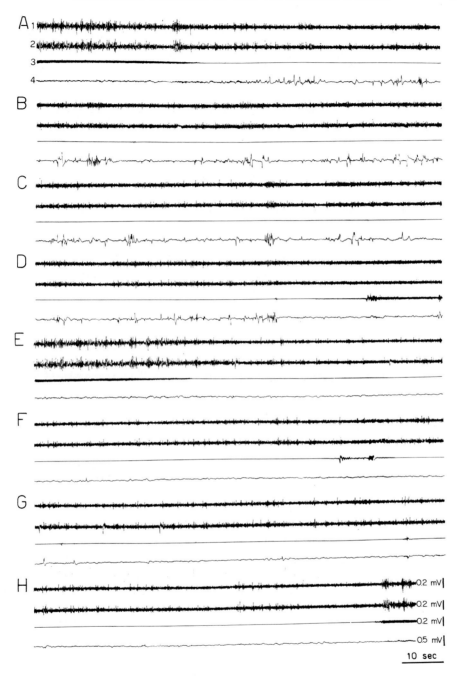

Fig. 1. Abolition of the bursts of rapid eye movements (REMs) during desynchronized sleep following total bilateral destruction of the medial and descending vestibular nuclei. The cat was unrestrained and unanesthetized. Bipolar records: 1, left parietooccipital; 2, right parietooccipital; 3, posterior cervical muscles; 4, ocular movements (electrooculogram). A–D, Episode of desynchronized sleep, recorded in the intact animal, 4 days after chronic implantation of the electrodes. Note the irregular occurrence of large bursts of REM and isolated ocular movements throughout the episode. E–H, Episode of desynchronized sleep recorded in the same animal 2 days following bilateral lesion of the medial and descending vestibular nuclei. From Pompeiano and Morrison (1965).

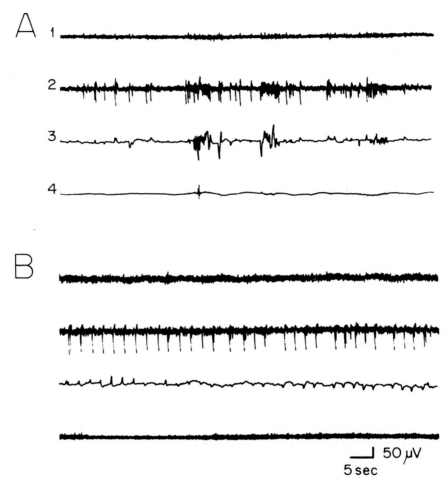

Fig. 3. Rhythmic ponto-geniculo-occipital activity occurring during desynchronized sleep or during the syndrome produced by reserpine. Unrestrained, unanesthetized cat. Bipolar records: 1, visual cortex; 2, lateral geniculate nucleus; 3, ocular movements; 4, posterior cervical muscles. A, Episode of desynchronized sleep, characterized by atonia of the posterior cervical muscles. Note the occurrence of rhythmic geniculate potentials which appear sometimes but not always related with the ocular movements. B, Syndrome induced by i.v. injection of 0.5 mg/kg of reserpine, characterized by cortical desynchronization, persistence of the tonic muscular activity and rhythmic geniculate potentials. Note the regular occurrence of the rhythmic geniculate potentials which appear to be related to ocular jerks. From Jeannerod (1965).

dealing, however, with two separate although mutually related phenomena is shown by the fact that (i) REMs occur only during the well developed episodes of desynchronized sleep, while monophasic potentials may occur also during synchronized sleep (cf. Morrison and Pompeiano (1966) for references) as well as during wakefulness at the time of the quick phases of nystagmus or during saccades (Brooks, 1968a, b; Cohen and Feldman, 1968; Feldman and Cohen, 1968); (ii) the REMs are generally grouped in bursts which occur at irregular intervals during desynchronized sleep,

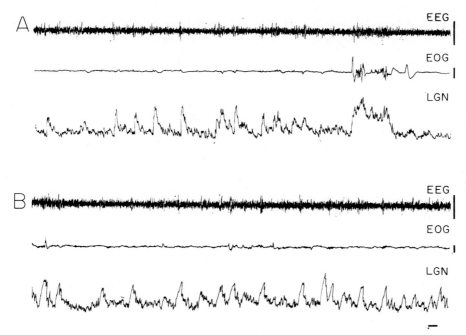

Fig. 4. Phasic increase in the lateral geniculate activity during REM and its abolition following vestibular lesion in the unrestrained unanesthetized cat. Bipolar records: EEG, electroencephalogram (left parietooccipital); EOG, electrooculogram; LGN, integrated geniculate activity. Time calibration, 1 sec. Voltage calibration, 0.2 mV. A, Experiment made 4 days after chronic implantation of the electrodes. Two kinds of activity are recorded from the lateral geniculate nucleus during desynchronized sleep. The first consists of regular, rhythmic enhancements, which are sometimes associated with small isolated ocular movements. The second type of activity is characterized by a phasic increase in the integrated geniculate discharge, larger in amplitude and longer in duration than those described above, which is strikingly related in time with a large burst of REM. B, Same animal as in A. Experiment made 6 days after chronic implantation of the electrodes and 2 days after complete bilateral lesion of the medial and descending vestibular nuclei. There is persistence during desynchronized sleep of the first type of rhythmic activity and abolition of the large bursts of REM and related enhancements of geniculate discharge. From Pompeiano and Morrison (1966).

while the deep sleep waves appear at a regular rate even during the intervals between the bursts of REM; (*iii*) a bilateral lesion of the vestibular nuclei abolishes selectively the REMs, while the rhythmic ponto-geniculate-occipital activity still persists after this lesion (Fig. 4) (Pompeiano and Morrison, 1966b; Morrison and Pompeiano, 1966).

Recent histochemical investigations have led to the discovery of two major systems, both located in the brain stem reticular formation. Neurons of one system, described by Dahlström and Fuxe (1964, 1965) and Fuxe (1965 a, b) contain monoamines, either a catecholamine (noradrenaline or dopamine) or 5-hydroxytryptamine, and are believed to be monoaminergic. Those of the other system, described by Shute and Lewis (1963, 1965), Holmes and Wolstencroft (1964), and Pavlin (1965), contain acetylcholinesterase and are believed to be cholinergic, releasing acetylcholine as a transmitter substance from their terminals.

According to Jeannerod (1965) and Jouvet (1967, 1969) a monoaminergic mechanism is responsible for the appearance of the phasic components of desynchronized sleep, including the REM. In fact the release of monoamines at monoaminergic terminals induced by reserpine is able to produce eye movements as well as ponto-geniculate-occipital activity without affecting the tonic components of desynchronized sleep (Fig. 3B). On the contrary, a cholinergic mechanism could play a role in the tonic phenomena of desynchronized sleep including postural atonia, but it would be unable to trigger the phasic phenomena of desynchronized sleep. The conclusion by Jouvet (1967, 1969) that all the phasic events depend upon release of monoamines is contradicted by the fact that reserpine produces only very discrete and isolated ocular jerks, which are related in time to the pontine waves (Fig. 3B), but they never appear to be grouped in bursts typical of the REM phase of sleep (Fig. 3A). On the other hand there is some evidence indicating that in cats decerebrated at precollicular or pre-pontine level (Matsuzaki and Kasahara, 1966; Matsuzaki *et al.*, 1967, 1968), or at midpontine level (Matsuzaki, 1968, 1969) intravenous injection of eserine sulphate, an anticholinesterase, elicits not only the tonic events of desynchronized sleep such as the abolition of the neck muscular activity, but also the phasic events such as pontine waves and rapid eye movements.

Since it is unlikely that the same event, for example, the pontine waves, are produced by two entirely different neuropharmacological mechanisms (the monoaminergic and the cholinergic one), we have postulated that there are two entirely different types of waves: (*i*) a *first* type of wave, triggered by a monoaminergic mechanism in the pons, which produces isolated ocular jerks independent of the vestibular system and (*ii*) a *second* type of wave, triggered by a cholinergic mechanism, which originates within the vestibulo-oculomotor system and leads to the occurrence of the typical bursts of REM.

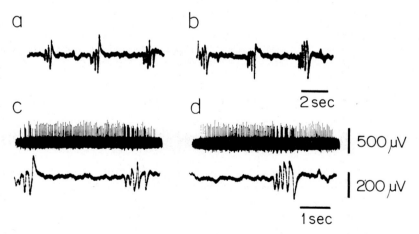

Fig. 5. Typical bursts of rapid eye movements induced by intravenous injection of eserine. Precollicular decerebrate cat. a, b, Typical bursts of rapid eye movements induced by i.v. injection of eserine sulphate (0.1 mg/kg). c, d, Changes in the pattern of discharge of a single neuron recorded from the medial vestibular nucleus (upper records) during the bursts of rapid eye movements (lower records) induced by the drug. From Magherini, Pompeiano and Thoden (1971b).

Magherini *et al.* (1971a, b, 1972) have recently shown that intravenous injection of eserine sulphate (0.1 mg/kg) in precollicular decerebrate cats abolishes not only the decerebrate rigidity as well as the tonic stretch reflex of the extensor muscles, but also produces bursts of conjugate rapid eye movements which generally occur in the horizontal plane at a regular frequency of one every 3.5–4 sec and continue for 15–25 min. Each burst consists of 2–6 nystagmus-like ocular movements which occur at the repetition rate of 4–5/sec and are generally directed either in one direction or in the other, although an alternation to both directions could also be observed (Fig. 5a, b). Monophasic potentials synchronous with the ocular movements were also recorded from the vestibular nuclei, the ascending medial longitudinal fasciculi, the oculomotor nuclei and the surrounding reticular formation. In no instance, however, were the potentials observed during the interval between the ocular bursts.

These potentials did not depend upon proprioceptive impulses from eye muscles since: (a) they preceded the ocular movements by 30 msec, and (b) they could still be induced by the anticholinesterase in spite of the absence of the ocular movements in low decerebrate preparations.

The rapid eye movements and the related monophasic potentials could still be elicited after bilateral section of the VIII cranial nerve and cerebellectomy but they were abolished after bilateral lesion of all the vestibular nuclei. This finding indicates that the monophasic potentials induced by eserine depend upon the rhythmic activity of the vestibular nuclei which is picked up at the level of the vestibular nuclei and their efferent projections (*cf.* Cook *et al.*, 1969). The effects elicited by eserine sulphate could be abolished within seconds by a 0.1–0.5 mg/kg dose of atropine sulphate, an anticholinergic drug. To control against the effects being of peripheral origin some animals were treated with neostigmine methylsulphate and atropine methylnitrate, agents which only poorly cross the blood-brain barrier. The effect was not produced by neostigmine (0.1 mg/kg, i.v.) and the eserine induced REMs were not abolished by atropine methylnitrate (1 mg/kg, i.v.).

Magherini *et al.* (1971a, b) and Thoden *et al.* (1972) have also performed experiments to study the effects of eserine sulphate on the spontaneous discharge of vestibular neurons in precollicular decerebrate preparations: 55 out of 125 vestibular neurons recorded before and after intravenous injection of eserine were investigated during the rapid eye movements induced by the drug. Among the 55 neurons tested, 27 showed typical changes in their pattern of discharge after eserine (Fig. 5c, d). These changes were generally characterized by bursts of unit activity during ocular movements in one direction and inhibition of the discharge during ocular jerks in the opposite direction (Fig. 6). In addition to these types of directional dependent units, a few units were encountered which were either excited or inhibited during ocular movements in both directions. The types of vestibular unit responses elicited by eserine resemble the four types of vestibular unit responses elicited by horizontal angular acceleration (Duensing and Schaefer, 1958). It is of interest that the responsive units were located particularly in the medial and occasionally in the superior, but never in the lateral vestibular nucleus. Systematic recordings from the descending vestibular nuclei were not performed.

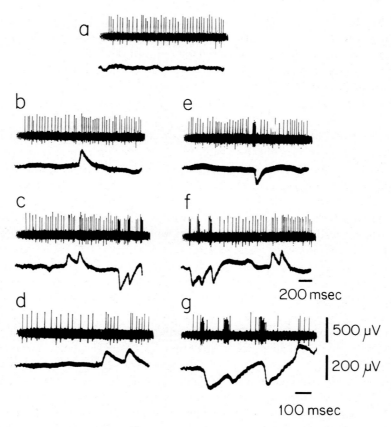

Fig. 6. Single unit activity recorded from the medial vestibular nucleus during rapid eye movements induced by eserine. Precollicular decerebrate cat. In all the traces the upper record corresponds to unit activity recorded from the right medial vestibular nucleus, the lower record to the eye movements. a, Regular unit discharge and absence of eye movements before injection of the drug. b–g, Changes in the pattern of unit discharge during the episodes of rapid eye movements induced by i.v. injection of eserine sulfate (0.1 mg/kg). Upward deflections of the electrooculogram, corresponding to eye movements towards the right side, are associated with inhibition of the unit discharge followed by rebound (b–d), while downward deflections, corresponding to eye movements towards the left side, are associated with bursts of high frequency discharge (e–g). Both changes in vestibular unit activity precede the occurrence of the rapid eye movements. From Magherini, Pompeiano and Thoden (1971 b).

The results of these experiments can be correlated with the finding that specific cholinesterase can be found in cells and fibers of different vestibular nuclei (Koelle, 1954; Shute and Lewis, 1963; Holmes and Wolstencroft, 1964) as well as in brain stem reticular structures (cf. Koelle, 1952, 1954; Gerebtzoff, 1959; Palmer and Ellerker, 1961; Pavlin, 1965), including the nucleus reticularis pontis oralis and caudalis (Shute and Lewis, 1963, 1965) and the nucleus reticularis gigantocellularis (Holmes and Wolstencroft, 1964). There is also physiological evidence indicating that many vestibular (Steiner and Weber, 1965; Yamamoto, 1967) and reticular neurons in the medulla and pons of the cat are cholinoceptive (Bradley and Wolstencroft, 1962,

1964, 1965, 1967; Salmoiraghi and Steiner, 1963; Krug *et al.*, 1970; Bradley *et al.*, 1964, 1966; Bradley and Mollica, 1958), and that eserine has marked and prolonged excitatory effects on most of the reticular neurons tested. These findings, together with our own observations, indicate the existence of a cholinergic mechanism, probably reticular in origin, which is responsible for the activation of the vestibulo-oculomotor system.

It should be pointed out here, that the *tonic* increase in the reticular unit discharge induced by eserine actually leads to *rhythmic* excitation and/or inhibition of the second order vestibular neurons which is ultimately responsible for the occurrence of the REM bursts. Future experiments are required to find out the neuronal mechanisms responsible for this rhythmic pattern of vestibular unit discharge. At present we may postulate that these rhythmic changes in firing discharge of the vestibular neurons are due to tonic activation of cholinergic neurons in the brain stem, whose discharge probably acts on the vestibular neurons through both excitatory and inhibitory pathways. In particular while the activation of the excitatory pathway leads to an increased activity of the vestibulo-oculomotor neurons, the rhythmicity of this discharge can be referred to periodic activity of inhibitory circuits, which leads to interruption of the vestibular unit discharge. These inhibitory circuits are probably located in part at least within and/or between the vestibular nuclei (Lorente de Nó, 1938; Horcholle and Dumont-Tyč, 1968; Shimazu, 1972). On the other hand the regular occurrence of the bursts of REM can be attributed to waxing and waning in the excitability of these neuronal mechanisms which lead to rhythmic excitation and inhibition of the vestibulo-oculomotor neurons.

It has already been mentioned that contrary to the eserine-induced bursts of REM, which occur at very regular intervals, the bursts of REM typical of desynchronized sleep appear at irregular intervals. The occurrence during this phase of sleep of monophasic potentials in the pontine reticular formation due to a monoaminergic mechanism is likely to be responsible for the disruption of the regular rhythm at which the cholinergic-induced bursts of REM appear.

NEUROCHEMICAL MECHANISM RESPONSIBLE FOR THE APPEARANCE OF ROTATORY NYSTAGMUS IN PRECOLLICULAR DECEREBRATE ANIMALS

Several investigators have studied the response characteristics of the second order vestibular neurons (Gernandt, 1959; Eckel, 1964; Duensing and Schaefer, 1958; Precht and Shimazu, 1965; Shimazu and Precht, 1965; Ryu *et al.*, 1969; *cf.* Precht 1972) as well as of the abducens neurons (Precht *et al.*, 1967, 1969) during horizontal angular acceleration. It is of interest that when this stimulus is applied in precollicular or intercollicular decerebrate cats it produces only steady changes in frequency of these unit discharges. On the contrary rhythmic changes of the discharge frequency occur only in non-decerebrate, unanesthetized animals, where they are closely related in time to the rhythmic eye movements characteristic of vestibular nystagmus (Schaefer, 1965). In order to explain why most of the vestibular and ocular motoneurons are devoid of rhythmic changes in response to angular acceleration following

References pp. 614-618

removal of the forebrain, it has been assumed that the triggering mechanism for the nystagmic rhythm had been severed by the decerebration. This assumption is in part at least supported by the fact that nystagmogenic structures are apparently located at cortical and subcortical levels (Dohlman, 1938; Crosby, 1953; Lachman *et al.*, 1958; Bergmann *et al.*, 1959; Di Giorgio and Manni, 1963; Manni *et al.*, 1964, 1965; Carmichael *et al.*, 1965; Monnier *et al.*, 1970).

It should be mentioned, however, that the rhythmicity of the nystagmic discharge is probably elaborated within the short circuits situated in the reticular formation (Lorente de Nó, 1928, 1933, 1938; Duensing and Schaefer, 1957a, b, 1960; Szentágo-thai, 1964) including the medullary reticular structures (Dumont–Tyč, 1964, 1966; Dumont–Tyč and Dell, 1962), and there are also recent experimental observations suggesting that the rhythmic firing of the vestibular nuclei is in part at least due to interneuronal activity located within (Horcholle and Dumont–Tyč, 1968) or between the vestibular nuclei (Shimazu, 1972). One may postulate, therefore, that the excita-bility of these interneurons is greatly depressed in the acute decerebrate cat.

Barale *et al.* (1971) have recently performed experiments to find out whether eserine is able to bring to the light a rotatory nystagmus in this type of preparation. Indeed it was shown (Fig. 7) that horizontal angular acceleration performed in precollicular decerebrate cats was unable to produce either a rotatory or a postrotatory nystagmus even when the turntable was rotated at the angular acceleration of $30°/sec^2$ as to reach the constant velocity of $250°/sec$. However, intravenous injection of eserine sulphate at a dose of 0.025–0.50 mg/kg (*i.e.*, lower than that responsible for the occurrence of

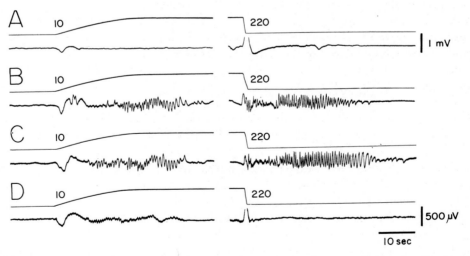

Fig. 7. Rotatory and postrotatory nystagmus induced by eserine in a precollicular decerebrate cat. In each record the upper traces indicate the movement of the turntable, the lower traces the electro-oculogram. The numbers on the left of each diagram give the acceleration rate (arc degree/sec²) and the number on the right indicates the constant speed of rotation (arc degree/sec). A, Absence of nystagmus in precollicular decerebrate cat. B, C, Rotatory and postrotatory nystagmus 5 and 35 min after intravenous injection of 0.5 mg/kg of eserine sulphate. D, 90 min after the injection. From Barale, Ghelarducci and Pompeiano (unpublished).

LORENTE DE NÓ, R. (1928) *Die Labyrinthreflexe auf die Augenmuskeln nach einseitiger Labyrinthexstirpation nebst einer kurzen Angabe über den Nervenmechanismus der vestibulären Augenbewegungen.* Urban und Schwarzenberg, Wien.

LORENTE DE NÓ, R. (1933) Vestibulo-ocular reflex arc. *Arch. Neurol. Psychiat. (Chicago)*, **30**, 245–291.

LORENTE DE NÓ, R. (1938) Analysis of the activity of the chains of internuncial neurons. *J. Neurophysiol.*, **1**, 207–244.

MAGHERINI, P. C., POMPEIANO, O. AND THODEN, U. (1971a) Cholinergic mechanism responsible for activation of vestibular neurones and rapid eye movements in decerebrate cat. *Proc. XXV int. Congr. physiol. Sci.*, Munich, IX, n. 1067, 360.

MAGHERINI, P. C., POMPEIANO, O. AND THODEN, U. (1971b) The neurochemical basis of REM sleep: a cholinergic mechanism responsible for rhythmic activation of the vestibulo-oculomotor system. *Brain Res.*, **35**, 565–569.

MAGHERINI, P. C., POMPEIANO, O. AND THODEN, U. (1972) Cholinergic mechanisms related to REM sleep. I. Rhythmic activity of the vestibulo-oculomotor system induced by an anticholinesterase in the decerebrate cat. *Arch. ital. Biol.*, **110**, 234–259.

MANNI, E., AZZENA, G. B. AND ATZORI, M. L. (1965) Relationship between cerebral and mesodiencephalic nystagmogenic centers in the rabbit. *Arch. ital. Biol.*, **103**, 136–145.

MANNI, E., AZZENA, G. B. AND DESOLE, C. (1964) Eye nystagmus elicited by stimulation of the cerebral cortex in the rabbit. *Arch. ital. Biol.*, **102**, 645–656.

MATSUZAKI, M. (1968) Differential effects of Na-butyrate and physostigmine on brain stem activities of para-sleep. *Brain Res.*, **11**, 251–255.

MATSUZAKI, M. (1969) Differential effects of sodium butyrate and physostigmine upon the activities of para-sleep in acute brain stem preparations. *Brain Res.*, **13**, 247–265.

MATSUZAKI, M. AND KASAHARA, M. (1966) Induction of para-sleep by cholinesterase inhibitors in the mesencephalic cat. *Proc. Jap. Acad.*, **42**, 989–993.

MATSUZAKI, M., OKADA, Y. AND SHUTO, S. (1967) Cholinergic actions related to paradoxical sleep induction in the mesencephalic cat. *Experientia (Basel)*, **23**, 1029–1030.

MATSUZAKI, M., OKADA, Y. AND SHUTO, S. (1968) Cholinergic agents related to para-sleep state in acute brain stem preparations. *Brain Res.*, **9**, 253–267.

MEHLER, W. R. (1968) Reticulovestibular connections compared with spinovestibular connections in the rat. *Anat. Rec.*, **160**, 485.

MONNIER, M., BELIN, I. AND POLC, P. (1970) Facilitation, inhibition, and habituation of the vestibular responses. *Adv. Oto-rhino-laryng.*, **17**, 28–55.

MORRISON, A. R. AND POMPEIANO, O. (1966) Vestibular influences during sleep. IV. Functional relations between vestibular nuclei and lateral geniculate nucleus during desynchronized sleep. *Arch. ital. Biol.*, **104**, 425–458.

MOURET, J. (1964) *Les Mouvements Oculaires au Cours du Sommeil Paradoxal. Recherches sur leur Nature et leurs Mécanismes chez le Chat et chez l'Homme.* Imprimerie des Beaux-Arts, Lyon, pp. 125.

MOURET, J., JEANNEROD, M. ET JOUVET, M. (1963) L'activité électrique du système visuel au cours de la phase paradoxale du sommeil chez le chat. *J. Physiol. (Paris)*, **55**, 305–306.

PALMER, A. C. AND ELLERKER, A. R. (1961) Histochemical localization of cholinesterases in the brainstem of sheep. *Quart. J. exp. Physiol.*, **43**, 344–352.

PAVLIN, R. (1965) Cholinesterases in reticular nerve cells. *J. Neurochem.*, **12**, 515–518.

POMPEIANO, O. (1966) Muscular afferents and motor control during sleep. In R. GRANIT (Ed.), *Nobel Symposium I. Muscular Afferents and Motor Control.* Almqvist and Wiksell, Stockholm, pp. 415–436.

POMPEIANO, O. (1967) The neurophysiological mechanisms of the postural and motor events during desynchronized sleep. *Res. Publ. Ass. nerv. ment. Dis.*, **45**, 351–423.

POMPEIANO, O. AND MORRISON, A. R. (1965) Vestibular influences during sleep. I. Abolition of the rapid eye movements during desynchronized sleep following vestibular lesions. *Arch. ital. Biol.*, **103**, 569–595.

POMPEIANO, O. AND MORRISON, A. R. (1966a) Vestibular origin of the rapid eye movements during desynchronized sleep. *Experientia (Basel)*, **22**, 60–61.

POMPEIANO, O. AND MORRISON, A. R. (1966b) Vestibular input to the lateral geniculate nucleus during desynchronized sleep. *Pflügers Arch. ges. Physiol.*, **290**, 272–274.

PRECHT, W. (1972) The physiology of the vestibular nuclei. In H. H. KORNHUBER (Ed.), *Handbook of Sensory Physiology. Vol. VI. The Vestibular Nuclei*, Springer, Berlin, in press.

PRECHT, W., GRIPPO, J. AND RICHTER, A. (1967) Effect of horizontal angular acceleration on neurons in the abducens nucleus. *Brain Res.*, **5**, 527–531.

Fig. 1 is a detailed summary of those areas on the dorsal lateral surface of the brain of the alert cervically transected *M. mulatta* which upon stimulation yielded contralateral conjugate eye movements. It can be readily seen that unilateral stimulation of almost the entire brain surface produced conjugate eye deviations toward the opposite side. One exception is the area caudal and rostral to the *rolandic sulcus*. The temporal lobe cortex was not explored thoroughly and is, therefore, surrounded by a broken line in Fig. 1. Upon stimulation of the subcortical temporal depths, however, eye movements were elicited.

Eye movements elicited from the posterior eye fields agree fairly well with the results obtained by previous investigators (Schäfer, 1888; Walker and Weaver, 1940). From the occipital pole to the superior temporal sulcus, stimulation of the dorsal and dorsal lateral surfaces produces a downward contralateral deviation. Stimulation of the infero lateral surface produces an upward contralateral deviation. Rostral to the superior temporal sulcus, on the other hand, only horizontal conjugate deviations are obtained by stimulation. Thorough exploration of the depths of the posterior portion of the brain yield complimentary results to those elicited by surface stimulation. Above the calcarine fissure, stimulation causes contralateral downward eye movements and stimulation below the fissure yields contralateral upward movements. Whether stimulating the surface or the depths, pure vertical movements, as well as pure horizontal movements, were much less frequent in occurrence than the oblique movements.

The frontal eye fields in the alert cervically transected monkey extends from the somatic motor area almost to the frontal pole. Laterally, it extends to the lower limb of the arcuate sulcus and, medially, it reaches to the level of the dorsal border of the genu of the corpus callosum. In the frontal fields, the threshold is lowest in the caudal portion, especially within the arms of the arcuate sulcus. However, threshold differences as one goes caudally are slight. Characteristics of eye movements are very similar throughout the whole frontal area; almost all movements are saccadic in nature.

There is a suggestion of a topographic distribution of upward and downward as well as horizontal movements (Fig. 1). The caudal limit of this frontal ocular motor area is difficult to determine since it overlaps the somatic motor area. In the lower part of this region, the threshold for facial movement was low and slightly suprathreshold stimuli often produced convulsions. On rare occasions, nystagmus and pupillary dilatation were obtained. These showed no consistency in their distribution. Stimulation of the depths of the frontal part of the brain also produced conjugate contralateral eye movements, but no particular pattern was observed. There was a greater frequency of loci both on the surface and in the depths which produced no response as compared to the occipital lobe and the middle portion of the brain. Of interest, in this regard, was the fact that stimulation of the caudate nucleus, putamen, and globus pallidus consistently produced contralateral conjugate eye movements upon stimulation. In contrast, Nashold (1971) did not see similar movements upon stimulation of basal ganglia of man.

Two recent studies of the frontal eye field on the unanesthetized monkey, by means of implanted electrodes, have yielded somewhat different results from those illustrated in Fig. 1 and different from each other (Brucher, 1966; Robinson and Fuchs, 1969). Both show the field to be more limited in extent. Brucher, essentially, duplicated the topographic map previously described by Crosby et al. (1952). The eye field delimited by the latter authors follows the contour of the arcuate sulcus and is limited to its anterior portion in this study and there is a distinct separation between horizontal contralateral eye movements, upward contralateral, and downward contralateral. The eye field described by Robinson and Fuchs was even smaller and limited to the upper portion of the arcuate. The inferior limb when stimulated in the latter study did not produce eye movements. These investigators limited the strength of stimulation used, and probably did not go much above the threshold strength. Furthermore, the parameters of stimulation such as frequency, pulse duration, and train duration were different in the various studies. Robinson and Fuchs, for example, used a train 30 msec long of one msec pulses delivered at 200/sec. They do state, however, that longer pulse trains did not change the results. Brucher used several combinations of parameters, each of which gave similar results.

In our own studies, summarized in Fig. 1, a train duration was often as long as 3 or 4 sec. As mentioned above, the threshold in the rostral portion of the frontal eye field was somewhat higher than in the caudal. Nevertheless, we convinced ourselves that submaximal stimuli did not evoke a response by means of spread through more excitable areas. Two important reasons are as follows. In the first place, increased depth of anesthesia reduces the extent of the excitable area quite markedly and increases the threshold for the response. Thus, under these conditions, even with higher strengths of stimulation outside the excitable area, no response is obtained. Secondly, in the occipital lobe at the margin between the upward contralateral locus and the downward contralateral locus, a movement of the electrode of 1 mm and often less, results in a change of the response to the appropriate direction. Thus, it seems clear that in order to consider the cortical control of eye movements, we must take into account the area as depicted in Fig. 1.

Our results are in agreement with those obtained by Lilly (1958) on alert rhesus monkeys with an implanted head piece enabling the stimulation of as many as 600 points in a single animal. The excitable area that he found in these monkeys was quite similar in extent to the one we have described. Lilly, furthermore, considered the various parameters of stimulation in great detail. He pointed out that the threshold is a function of pulse or pulse pair duration, the frequency of the train, and the duration of the train. He said, as we have also concluded, that trains were necessary for the buildup of most motor responses. A motor map either for eye movements or for the body and limb movements is dependent upon the parameters of stimulation used. Thus, we must accept the fact that the large area of the excitable cortex is indeed functionally significant.

This fact is important in considering the details of the projection from the cortex to the brain stem. Details of the projection must also be considered because of the different types of movements whether horizontal, obliquely up or down. With even finer methods of stimulation, and the consequent stimulation of smaller cell groups, we may expect, perhaps, that the types of movements seen would vary

References pp. 632–635

to a greater extent. This is borne out by the recent results of Robinson and Fuchs (1969), summarized above. These considerations lead to the conclusion that the anatomical pathways must be incredibly intricate and the integrating structures in the brain stem equally complex. Certainly in future anatomic studies, cortical areas outside of areas 8 and 17 must be taken into consideration regarding their roles in eye movements.

The problem is further compounded by the fact that stimulation of the same excitable cortical areas illustrated in Fig. 1 of the brain of an alert unrestrained animal via implanted electrodes invariably produces a head movement along with the eye movement. Furthermore, patterned body and limb movements appropriate to the movement of head and eyes are also obtained (Wagman, 1964). Isolated conjugate eye deviations are rarely seen under these conditions, although it is our impression that they may occur more often upon stimulation of the occipital lobe. Often, the eye deviation preceded the head movement, but this was an inconstant finding. It was usually impossible to determine whether the adversive movements were simultaneous or whether eye deviation preceded head movement or vice versa. The limb and body movements invariably followed eye and head movements. In man, Nashold (1971) found that eye movements frequently were not accompanied by head movements and that when they did occur the eyes moved first. Such apparent species differences need experimental clarification.

The head movement, of course, will give rise to vestibular stimulation and compensatory eye movement to maintain fixation. Thus, any relationship between cortical influence on eye movements and vestibular mechanisms may lie primarily in the motor behavioral effect due initially to cortical control. Patterned body and limb movements indicate, of course, that the vestibular descending systems as well as others, undoubtedly, are brought into play. Since cortical stimulation can initiate a sequence of events which may involve various motor mechanisms which are at the basis of postural adjustments of the animal, one important question for our present consideration is whether separate corticofugal systems bring about the eye and head movements which, in turn, initiate the complex postural adjustments.

The question has been at least partially answered by means of physiological experiments using the techniques of stimulation and lesioning of appropriate loci of the brain beginning in cerebral cortex and extending to midbrain and pons (Bender and Shanzer, 1964; Bender, Shanzer and Wagman, 1964). Contralateral deviation of the eyes is obtained upon stimulation above the third nerve nucleus; below this level the direction of eye movements becomes ipsilateral. Thus, there should be a decussation of the oculomotor pathway which mediates eye movements in the area of the third and fourth nerve nuclei. The change in direction of head turning does not occur at the same place. The decussation seems to be at more caudal and ventral levels. The crossing for the head movements is less sharply demarcated than that for eye movements (Bender *et al.*, 1964).

The oculomotor pathway delimited by means of stimulation and the effects of lesions is shown to descend from the cerebral areas and converge towards the pretectum and midbrain, passing via the fields of Forel and zona incerta. In the midbrain, the pathway is concentrated in the paramedian zone and, as mentioned above, crosses over at the level between the third and fourth nuclei. From here it continues to the paramedian zone of tegmentum of the pons (Bender and Shanzer, 1964). From this point on, the oculomotor pathway is unclear. Anatomically and physiologically it is known that the medial longitudinal fasciculus mediates impulses ascending to the oculomotor nuclei. In regard to the functional descending pathway outlined in the midbrain and pons for eye and head movements, we have little or no anatomical information. The fact that there may be two separate 'pathways' for eye and head movements is also suggested by the recent finding by Bizzi and Schiller (1970) that there are single units in the frontal eye fields of the monkey which respond only to head movements and other neurons responding only to saccadic eye movements.

The extensive representation of eye and head movements on the cortical surface and in the depths of the cortex suggests that these phenomena are important to a wide variety of normal behavioral functions. To begin with, it is more or less evident that these movements are integral parts of sensory functions such as visual and auditory. This is clearly seen in the occipital lobe on the basis of the movements elicited by cortical stimulation as well as from clinical, pathological material. When light hits the lower portion of the retina and comes therefore from the upper portion of the visual field, the projection is to the lower portion of the occipital lobe. Schäfer (1888) first noticed that stimulation of this part of the brain drove the eyes upward and contralateral. We agree with his interpretation just as other investigators have. Pathways from the occipital lobe have been shown to project to the tectum (Mettler, 1935; Crosby and Henderson, 1948), to the pons (Mettler, 1935; Sunderland, 1940) and lateral geniculate (Polyak, 1932). Recently, however, evidence has been presented that the pathways underlying opticokinetic nystagmus project to the medial reticular formation (Cohen and Feldman, 1968, 1971).

If we assume that the frontal eye fields play a role in the production and controls of saccades (Wagman et al., 1961; Robinson, 1968; Robinson and Fuchs, 1970; Westheimer, 1971), and since we know that a saccade results from a change in the location of the visual stimulus in the visual field, then it is clear that the role of eye movements elicited by frontal lobe activity may also be related to visual input. This can happen in one of two ways. In the first place, the occipital lobe may transmit an impulse to the frontal lobe which then triggers the appropriate response. The other alternative is that the visual stimulus which results in the saccadic eye movement is transmitted directly to the frontal lobe in parallel with its transmission to the occipital lobe. Bizzi (1968) found that the firing characteristics of frontal eye field neurons associated with saccades were not changed in darkness. Nevertheless, this does not negate the fact that the most frequent stimulus for a saccadic response is visual. It has been shown that a visual stimulus can project to the motor and premotor areas (Buser and Bignall, 1967). Of further interest is the fact that during the saccade vision may be inhibited; a fact which implies that they also involve the occipital lobe.

Eye and head movements are integral portions of other behavioral functions including arousal (Segundo et al., 1955), orientation reactions (Grastyán et al., 1959; Sokolov, 1960; Voronin and Sokolov, 1960) and defensive reactions (Hess, 1957). Eye movements are, of course, characteristic of REM sleep. These mechanisms implicate the reticular formation, the hippocampus, amygdala, and perhaps, other subcortical structures as well. If attention is included, it may also involve the nonspecific thalamic system. And finally, of course, the role of eye and head movements and associated body and limb movements are of unusual importance in the postural mechanisms which are essential in motor behavior associated with defense, arousal, orientation, as well as normal walking and standing. The functions of both the cerebellum and basal ganglia in the maintenance of equilibrium have, of course, been well documented. Eye and head movements are readily produced by stimulation of both structures (Wagman *et al.*, 1961; Wagman, 1964; Cohen *et al.*, 1965). Starr (1964) reported results which implicate the caudate nucleus of man in saccadic eye movements. Nashold (1971), however, as mentioned above, found that stimulation of the basal ganglia in man did not produce eye movements.

We can say, therefore, with some confidence that eye movements initiated at the cortical level are dependent upon sensory input and are associated with a variety of locomotor and behavioral patterns necessary for the adaptation of the animal. The elicited eye movements and the associated head and body postural reactions are appropriate to the input and are varied, complex, and exquisitely coordinated. One might assume that there is a corollary discharge from the cortex and perhaps, from the basal ganglia which act from motor systems on sensory ones to reset the latter (Teuber, 1970; Festinger, 1971). We may suggest that such pathways may be eventually discovered.

Since the final common pathways to the extraocular muscles are fixed, and since the coordinating mechanisms for eye and head movements and the structures underlying them provide for a remarkable flexibility of eye and associated movements which are dependent upon triggering signals from the cortex, consideration of the location of the areas upon which convergence must occur and where the final integration is achieved is of prime interest. It seems likely that these areas are located in the pontine reticular formation and/or the midbrain reticular formation (Bender and Shanzer, 1964; Cohen *et al.*, 1968; Cohen, 1971; Westheimer, 1971). Sites of convergence of various impulses both ascending from the labyrinth via the vestibular nuclei, as well as from other medullary and spinal structures, and descending from the cerebral cortex appear to be located in the lower midbrain and pontine tegmentum (Bender and Shanzer, 1964).

These conclusions have been revealed more clearly from physiological data than from extant anatomical information including new Nauta method studies. Nevertheless, detailed anatomical studies are absolutely essential to arrive at a clear understanding of the pathways. The present attempt to review the anatomical studies points out that even at present and after a great deal of consideration, only a beginning is at hand for the complete understanding of cerebral oculomotor pathways.

ANATOMICAL STUDIES

Since areas 8 and 19 of Brodmann have been, until recently, recognized as the frontal and occipital eye fields respectively, the anatomical projection studies have been almost entirely limited to considerations of those areas. In regard to the frontal cortex, even today as discussed above, some investigators located the frontal eye fields of the monkey only within the arcuate sulcus. In the chimpanzee and in man, only the low threshold frontal eye fields have been studied and are found to be located in the posterior part of the middle frontal convolution, an area also usually designated as area 8 (Penfield and Boldrey, 1937; Bucy, 1949). However, discrepancies with regard to the exact cortical location of the frontal eye field in the human are still not fully resolved (Smith, 1949; Lemmen et al., 1959). Stimulation of area 19 in man (Foerster, 1936) produces eye movements just as it does in the monkey. Whether or not such movements can be produced from wider areas in man as well is not determined. Let us now examine the more recent anatomical data on areas 8 and 19, and adjacent frontal and occipital projections, respectively.

The frontal lobe

Cytoarchitecturally, in those species that have been studied, area 8 is classified as a transitional type dysgranular cortex. It has been characterized by Krieg (1949) as having a thin internal granular layer IV, and by Scollo-Lavizzari and Akert (1963), as having a well-developed layer IV. Even these studies, therefore, are not in agreement.

Cortico-mesencephalic fibers originating from the region of the arcuate sulcus containing area 8 were observed by Levin (1936) and others in Marchi method anterograde fiber degeneration studies. Levin (1936), and later Brucher (1966), concluded that these fibers terminated only in the mesencephalic tegmentum, since they could not trace fibers directly to either the eye muscle nuclei nor to the tectum of the superior colliculus. Crosby et al. (1952), however, in comparable Marchi method studies reportedly traced corticobulbar fibers originating from the arcuate sulcus region into the pontine reticular formation where the fibers ". . . reach the lateral and ventrolateral side of the abducens nucleus, from which position degenerated fibers pass to this nucleus."

Studies with the more sensitive Nauta method, however, have failed repeatedly to confirm direct corticofugal fiber connections from the frontal or occipital cortex with cells of the abducens, trochlear or oculomotor nuclei (Myers, 1963a, b; Astruc, 1964, 1971; Kuypers, 1964; Kuypers and Lawrence, 1967). Experiments in subprimate species are no longer appropriate because, with only a few exceptions (Petras and Lehman, 1966), direct corticomotor neuron connections do not exist in these forms. Astruc (1971), therefore, has thoroughly restudied area 8 projections in the Macaque. Astruc's report confirms and extends the basic topology of area 8 fibers in the internal capsule reported by Levin (1936). He reiterates the relationship of a contingent of these projections at midbrain levels to the so-called 'pes lemniscus superficialis' of Dejerine as described by Crosby et al. (1952). Astruc found that these fibers terminate in the processus griseum pontis supralemniscalis, but he could confirm no connections or even degenerating fibers caudal to the pons as reported by the latter authors. Astruc's Nauta method investigation does confirm the existence of a fine-fibered cortico-mesencephalic system that traverses the subthalamic region and terminates chiefly in

References pp. 632–635

certain pretectal nuclei and in the intermediate layers or stratum lemnisci of the superior colliculus. Kuypers and Lawrence (1967) have noted that degenerating fibers to the upper midbrain which originate from any cortical area in front of the central sulcus share a common internal capsular and subthalamic course. De Vito and Smith (1964) also have described a similar subthalamic course via the H-fields for the prefrontal lobe projections to the midbrain tectum and central grey. While the latter authors also denied direct oculomotor connections, they did describe the possibility of bilateral terminations in the nucleus of Edinger-Westphal that have not been confirmed. Kuypers and Lawrence (1967) found, as we also have observed, that fronto-mesencephalic projections go chiefly to the dorsal central grey, a fact that in itself seems to preclude the Edinger–Westphal connections.

Before further detailed discussion is undertaken of the important question regarding the cortical connections with the nuclei of the posterior commissure of Darkschewitsch and the interstitial nucleus of Cajal, it is important to consider the role, if any, that these nuclei play in the control of eye movements. Recently, Carpenter *et al.* (1970) have addressed themselves to this question. Based upon Nauta studies of small differential lesions, they concluded that it is chiefly the interstitial nucleus in this triumvirate of upper midbrain nuclei that exhibits direct connections with the oculomotor and trochlear nuclei but not with the abducens. These interstitio-oculomotor fibers which, according to Carpenter *et al.* (1970) decussate in the ventral part of the posterior commissure, undoubtedly constitute some of the fibers noted by Pasik *et al.* (1969) and earlier investigators. The *lack* of discernible symptoms in Carpenter *et al.* (1970) interstitial nucleus lesion cases, however, leaves the question of the function of these oculomotor connections unanswered. The latter authors and Tarlov in the present volume discuss this question.

Pompeiano and Walberg (1957) found no interstitial or other upper midbrain nuclear connections with eye muscle nuclei in the cat. We also have never observed any terminal degeneration in these nuclei in cats with upper midbrain tectal or tegmental lesions. One case (CT 160)[1] of a lesion of the MLF at the trochlear nucleus level, however, reveals some preterminals in the ipsilateral abducens nucleus. While this case is not too significant in itself, it indicates that eye muscle nuclei preterminal afferent fibers, besides those of vestibular origin, can be demonstrated with the Nauta method.

Projections from area 8 to these nuclei have been recently reinvestigated by Astruc (1971). He found that area 8 connections with the interstitial nucleus of Cajal and Darkschewitsch's nucleus, both of which receive ascending vestibular connections, and with the nucleus of the posterior commissure are negligible compared to the density of terminations in the former two nuclei that arise from area 6 or the precentral gyrus. He found only some diffuse fiber projections to the neighboring ventrolateral central grey and to adjacent parts of the dorsal tegmentum often labelled as the 'mesencephalic reticular formation.' These scant latter projections most closely

---

[1] Nauta's Walter Reed collection.

approach the oculomotor complex, but based on what is known of the dendritic fields of these neurons, even these projections fail to suggest that less apparent axodendritic cell connections might exist.

Astruc's findings are consistent with the cases previously reported by Kuypers and Lawrence (1967), Petras (1969), and with the observations of one of us (Mehler) (see below). The interstitial connections reported by Astruc also were found by Kuypers and Lawrence to originate only from area 8. The interstitial nucleus of Cajal, there-fore, seems to be uniquely related to the area 8 frontal eye field. Direct occipital corticofugal connections with the interstitial nucleus, however, have not been reported but the nucleus' position as a major terminus of vestibular fibers ascending in the MLF is well documented. Astruc (1971) found no connections with the red nucleus in his cases but, like Kuypers and Lawrence (1967), we have found terminations in the dorso-medial subnucleus in both area 6 and 8 lesions as well as from ablations of the 'face' region of the precentral cortex. Owing to the intimate relationship of these rubral sub-divisions to the interstitial nucleus, the function and connections of this dorso-medial subnucleus buried in the rootlets of the oculomotor nerve should be re-examined. Some 'interstitio-oculomotor' fibers (Carpenter et al., 1970) might originate from this part of the red nucleus but it is more interesting to speculate that these rubral projec-tions, if they play any role in ocular function, probably go to facial nuclear cells con-trolling the orbicularis oculi. Smith (1949) got eye closure from stimulation of the posterior bank of the arcuate sulcus, and Wagman et al. (1961) got lid movements from both areas 6 and 8. Rubrofacial connections have been confirmed in several species (Kuypers, 1964; Courville, 1966; Martin and Dom, 1970), but the exact facial subdivision related to the orbicularis oculi in primates is still a disputed question (Hoyt and Loeffler, 1965).

To Astruc's 8 experiments we can add confirmatory data from another experiment on a *Macaca mulatta* and two cases involving extensive arcuate sulcus lesions in the New World Cebus monkey (*Cebus fatuellus*). These experiments were prepared as part of an ongoing study of the intra-cortical relationships of the so-called vestibular cortex in the monkey (Mehler and Fredrickson, 1970). In addition to the application of stan-dard variations of the Nauta method to the study of these cases, observations based upon series prepared by the Fink and Heimer (1967) method merit special comment. Astruc's (1971) more selective subpial ablations of the banks of the arcuate sulcus appear to have produced only limited fiber degeneration projecting into the dorso-lateral central grey around the aqueduct. Our observations, however, are based upon deeper lesions of the arcuate sulcus that impinged in some cases on subcortical white matter originating from the frontal cortex. Our material shows a considerable dense fine-fibered system which enters the central grey dorsolateral to the aqueduct immedi-ately under the posterior commissure dorsal to the oculomotor complex. Kuypers and Lawrence's (1967) arcuate sulcus case *1c* also suggests such dorsal central grey con-nections in addition to the cortico-tectal terminations in the intermediate layers of the tectum.

Little is known about the subcortical fiber projections of the pretectal nuclei in the monkey, or other species, in spite of considerable speculation in the older literature which is reflected in many textbooks. In the search for central eye muscle mechanisms, and in the absence of adequate evidence for direct cortico-oculomotor connections, 'tecto-oculomotor' connections were postulated (Crosby and Henderson, 1948). Tectofugal projections, however, have been recently re-evaluated with the Nauta method in the monkey (Myers, 1963b), cat (Altman and Carpenter, 1961), and rabbit (Tarlov and Moore, 1966). No 'tecto-oculomotor' connections were found in any of these studies in lesions restricted to the layers of the superior colliculus. Tecto-bulbar connections to the cuneiformis and subcuneiformis nuclear subdivisions of the so-called mesencephalic reticular formation, a region which also receives premotor (area 6) cortical projections, offer a potential link in a more probable reticulo-oculomotor circuit.

Frontal lobe cortico-tegmental projections reportedly distribute to medial and paramedially located nuclei in the limbic midbrain area of Nauta (1958) and to the medial part of the pontis oralis reticular nucleus according to initial, unconfirmed observations in a case with an ablation of the frontal cortex dorsal to the principal sulcus (Kuypers and Lawrence, 1967). Anatomically, therefore, confirmable frontal lobe projection patterns comparable to those envisioned by Cohen (1971) have been suggested but they still have not been adequately studied, especially with regard to eye movements. Only precentral 'face' area projections approximate to the functional pathways described.

The occipital lobe

Occipital ablations (Kuypers and Lawrence, 1967) or lobectomies (Myers, 1963a) have confirmed occipito-tectal connections which distribute extensively to the strata zonale, cinereum, and opticum and overlap to some degree with the fronto-tectal projections in the stratum intermedium. Occipitopontine connections with the lateral pontine nuclei are the caudalmost projections found, and a significant system of cortico-tegmental fibers cannot be demonstrated. There is no apparent mesencephalic tegmental or 'reticular' region where occipitofugal fibers might overlap frontal eye field projections as one would logically expect. The two functional eye field cortical regions, therefore, only appear to converge in the tectum and pretectum as Astruc (1971) has concluded. However, Spiegel and Scala (1937), and more recently, Pasik et al. (1969), found that the tectum per se is not indispensable to either vertical or horizontal ocular movements, respectively, in either the cat or dog. Although clinical evaluations continue to support the notion of tectal 'centers' in man (Cogan, 1964), clinical stereotaxic interventions allowing stimulation at upper mesencephalic levels (Nashold and Gills, 1967) appear to support the conclusions based upon stimulation experiments in animals.

Basal ganglia and thalamus

Physiological investigation (Wagman et al., 1961) indicate that the basal ganglia play an active role in conjugate eye movements. Projections from the globus pallidus to the vestibular nuclei or to the interstitial nucleus or Darkschewitsch nucleus have been considered to be the main pathways (Muskens, 1922). Neither projection actually appears to exist (Nauta and Mehler, 1966). The only pallido-mesencephalic connection that can be demonstrated with certainty is one to a tegmental nucleus called the pedunculo pontinus, pars compacta.

This cell group, lying on top of or partially intercalated in the brachium conjunctivum at the trochlear nucleus level, also receives precentral as well as premotor (areas 6 and 8) corticobulbar projections. The efferent connections of this 'reticular' nucleus, however, are still unknown, but initial studies of its projections in the monkey do not suggest that it has any direct eye muscle nuclei connections or that it feeds back to the vestibular nuclear complex.

Anatomically, cortical ablation studies in macaques reveal that only the pars multiformis, nucleus medialis dorsalis (Olszewski, 1952) is cortically dependent on area 8 (Scollo–Lavizzari and Akert, 1963). Reciprocal cortico-thalamic connections to this intralaminar nucleus also are described in Astruc's (1971) anterograde fiber degeneration study in addition to thalamic connections with the magnocellular part of the nucleus ventralis anterior and to nucleus parafascicularis. This paralamellar MDmf nucleus we consider part of the larger central lateral intralaminar region that receives spinal, trigeminal, and cerebellar afferent connections (Mehler, 1969). This central lateral nucleus, therefore, is well suited as a relay to convey various proprioceptive information, for example, into the striatum, area 8, and the frontal lobe relative to the coordination of eye, head, and body in contraversive movements (Hess, 1954; Montanelli and Hassler, 1964).

Intracortical connections

A detailed analysis of the intra- and intercortical connections are beyond the scope of this report, but it is of interest to consider briefly what is known about occipital and frontal lobe interconnections. Functionally, for example, movements produced by stimulation of the occipital cortex often can be superseded by frontal eye field stimulation. Similarly, ablation of the occipital cortex reportedly leads to malfunction of the ventral part of area 8 (Crosby, 1953). Occipital projections that terminate in the banks of the arcuate sulcus have been demonstrated, but monosynaptic reciprocal connections do not exist. Intimate neural relationships of the eye fields with the vestibular cortex are negligible.

A new era of analysis of cortical organization, especially pertinent to our discussion, is represented in the reports of Myers (1962, 1967), Kuypers et al. (1965), Pandya and Vignolo (1971), and Jones and Powell (1970), reports to which the reader interested in designing new visual field functional experiments is referred.

It appears, therefore, that in spite of considerable new functional and refined hodological data, there are still considerable discrepancies between known anatomical projections and (so-called) functional pathways delimited by electrical stimulation. A new approach is needed!

References pp. 632–635

SUMMARY

Under appropriate experimental conditions, especially using an encephale isolé rhesus monkey in the unanesthetized state, conjugate contralateral eye movements may be elicited by stimulation of wide areas of the cerebral cortex. Only the area caudal and rostral to the rolandic sulcus does not yield movements upon stimulation. The results are summarized in Fig. 1 which also indicates those areas which produce upward and downward components as well. Most eye movements obtained under the conditions noted are saccadic in nature. The state of consciousness, whether asleep or awake, whether anesthetized or not, is an important factor in the results obtained in mapping the eye fields. The maps described in the present paper show a wider distribution of sensitive points than do others.

Attempts to delimit the oculomotor pathways from cerebrum to brain stem by physiological means, that is, by studying the effects of lesions and stimulation, have been partially successful. The oculomotor pathway found by means of stimulation and effects of lesions is shown to descend from the cerebral areas and converge toward the pretectum and midbrain, passing via the fields of Forel and zona incerta. In the midbrain, the pathway is concentrated in the paramedian zone and crosses over at the level between the third and fourth nerve nuclei. From here, it continues to the paramedian zone of the tegmentum of the pons.

Details of projections from different areas of the cortex cannot easily be outlined by physiological methods. There is evidence to indicate that the pathways underlying opticokinetic nystagmus project to the medial reticular formation. Of further interest is the fact that in the monkey, stimulation of caudate nucleus, putamen and globus pallidus consistently produces contralateral conjugate eye movements.

If the excitable areas of the brain are stimulated via implanted electrodes in normal, unrestrained monkeys, the result is patterned head and eye movements along with appropriate body and limb movements. The results obtained during both acute and chronic experiments indicating widespread excitable brain areas and a variety of responses, show that conjugate eye movements are integral portions of many behavioral functions, including vision, audition, arousal, orientation, and defensive reactions, and, of course, postural and equilibrium motor behavior.

Thus, it seems that the pathways mediating eye movements and the integrating mechanisms in brain stem and the underlying anatomical structures, are varied and complex. To date, however, the anatomical projection studies have been almost entirely limited to considerations of Brodmann areas 8 and 19, because these have been, until recently, recognized as the frontal and occipital eye fields, respectively. The physiological results point the way to further anatomical studies since the newer and more sensitive methods may be expected to reveal many of the suggested projections from the forebrain which play a role in control of eye and body movements.

REFERENCES

ALTMAN, J. AND CARPENTER, M. B. (1961) Fiber projections of the superior colliculus in the cat. *J. comp. Neurol.*, **116**, 157–178.

ASTRUC, J. (1964) Corticofugal fiber degeneration following lesions of area 8 (frontal eye field) in *Macaca mulatta*. *Anat. Rec.*, **148**, 256.

ASTRUC, J. (1971) Corticofugal connections of area 8 (frontal eye field) in *Macaca mulatta*. *Brain Res.*, **33**, 241–256.

BENDER, M. B. AND SHANZER, S. (1964) Oculomotor pathways defined by electric stimulation and lesions in the brainstem of monkey. In M. B. BENDER (Ed.), *The Oculomotor System*, Harper and Row, New York, pp. 81–140.

BENDER, M. B., SHANZER, S. AND WAGMAN, I. H. (1964) On the physiologic decussation concerned with head turning. *J. comp. Neurol.*, **24**, 169–181.

BIZZI, E. (1968) Discharge of frontal eye field neurons during saccadic and following eye movements in unanesthetized monkeys. *Exp. Brain Res.*, **6**, 69–80.

BIZZI, E. AND SCHILLER, P. H. (1970) Single unit activity in the frontal eye fields of unanesthetized monkeys during eye and head movement. *Exp. Brain Res.*, **10**, 151–158.

BRUCHER, J. M. (1966) The frontal eye field of the monkey. *Int. J. Neurol.*, **5**, 262–281.

BUCY, P. C. (1949) *The Precentral Motor Cortex*. Univ. of Illinois Press, Urbana, Ill., pp.XIV-615.

BUSER, P. AND BIGNALL, K. E. (1967) Nonprimary sensory projections on the cat neocortex. *Int. Rev. Neurobiol.*, **10**, 111–165.

CARPENTER, M. B., HARBISON, J. W. AND PETER, P. (1970) Accessory oculomotor nuclei in the monkey: projections and effects of discrete lesions. *J. comp. Neurol.*, **140**, 131–154.

COGAN, D. G. (1964) Brain lesions and eye movements in man. In M. B. BENDER (Ed.), *The Oculomotor System*. Hoeber Medical Division, Harper and Row, New York, pp. 417–427.

COHEN, B. (1971) Vestibular ocular relations. In P. BACH-Y-RITA, C. C. COLLINS AND J. E. HYDE (Eds.), *The Control of Eye Movements*. Academic Press, New York, London, pp. 104–148.

COHEN, B. AND FELDMAN, M. (1968) Relationship of electrical activity in pontine reticular formation and lateral geniculate body to rapid eye movements. *J. Neurophysiol.*, **31**, 806–817.

COHEN, B. AND FELDMAN, M. (1971) Potential changes associated with rapid eye movement in the calcarine cortex. *Exp. Neurol.*, **31**, 100–113.

COHEN, B., GOTO, K., SHANZER, S. AND WEISS, A. (1965) Eye movements induced by electric stimulation of the cerebellum in the alert cat. *Exp. Neurol.*, **13**, 145–162.

COHEN, B., KOMATSUZKA, A. AND BENDER, M. B. (1968) Electrooculographic syndrome in monkeys after pontine reticular formation lesions. *Arch. Neurol.*, **18**, 78–92.

COURVILLE, J. (1966) Rubrobulbar fibres to the facial nucleus and the lateral reticular nucleus (nucleus of the lateral funiculus). An experimental study in the cat with silver impregnation methods. *Brain Res.*, **1**, 317–337.

CROSBY, E. C. (1953) Relation of brain centers to normal and abnormal eye movements in the horizontal plane. *J. comp. Neurol.*, **99**, 437–479.

CROSBY, E. C. AND HENDERSON, J. W. (1948) The mammalian midbrain and isthmus regions. Part II. Fiber connections of the superior colliculus. B. Pathways concerned in automatic eye movements. *J. comp. Neurol.*, **88**, 53–91.

CROSBY, E. C., YOSS, R. E. AND HENDERSON, J. W. (1952) The mammalian midbrain and isthmus region. Part II. The fiber connections. D. The pattern for eye movements on the frontal eye field and the discharge of specific portions of this field to and through midbrain levels. *J. comp. Neurol.*, **97**, 257–383.

DE VITO, J. L. AND SMITH, O. A., JR. (1964) Subcortical projections of the prefrontal lobe of the monkey. *J. comp. Neurol.*, **123**, 413–424.

EVARTS, E. V., BIZZI, E., DELONG, M. AND THACH, W. T., JR. (1971) Central control of movement. *Neurosci. Res. Progr. Bull.*, **9**, 1–170.

FESTINGER, L. (1971) Eye movements and perception. In P. BACH-Y-RITA, C. C. COLLINS AND J. E. HYDE (Eds.), *The Control of Eye Movements*. Academic Press, New York, London, pp. 259–273.

FINK, R. P. AND HEIMER, L. (1967) Two methods for selective silver impregnation of degenerating axons and their synaptic endings in the central nervous system. *Brain Res.*, **4**, 369–374.

FOERSTER, O. (1936) Symptomologie der Erkrankungen des Grosshirns. Motorische Felder und Bahnen. In O. BUMKE UND O. FOERSTER (Eds.), *Handbuch der Neurologie. Vol. 6*. Springer, Berlin, pp. 1–448.

GRASTYÁN, E., LISSÁK, K., MADARÁSZ, I. AND DONHOFFER, H. (1959) Hippocampal electrical activity during the development of conditioned reflexes. *Electroenceph. clin. Neurophysiol.*, **11**, 409–430.

HESS, W. R. (1954) *Das Zwischenhirn*. 2. Aufl. Schwabe, Basel, pp. 218.

HESS, W. R. (1957) *The Functional Organization of the Diencephalon*. In J. R. HUGHES (Ed.), Grune and Stratton, New York, pp. 121–125.

HOYT, W. F. AND LOEFFLER, J. D. (1965) Neurology of the orbicularis oculi. In J. L. SMITH (Ed.), *Neuro-ophthalmology. Vol. 2.* C. V. Mosby Co., St. Louis, pp. 167–205.

JONES, E. G. AND POWELL, T. P. S. (1970) An anatomical study of converging sensory pathways within the cerebral cortex of the monkey. *Brain, 93,* 793–820.

KRIEG, W. J. S. (1949) Connections of the cerebral cortex II. The macaque. C. Frontal areas and subareas. *J. comp. Neurol., 91,* 467–506.

KRIEGER, H. P., WAGMAN, I. H. AND BENDER, M. B. (1958) Changes in state of consciousness and patterns of eye movements. *J. Neurophysiol., 21,* 224–230.

KUYPERS, H. G. J. M. (1964) The descending pathways to the spinal cord, their anatomy and function. In J. C. ECCLES AND J. P. SCHADÉ (Eds.), *Progress in Brain Research. Vol. 11. Organization of the spinal cord.* Elsevier, Amsterdam, pp. 178–202.

KUYPERS, H. G. J. M. AND LAWRENCE, D. G. (1967) Cortical projections to the red nucleus and the brainstem in the rhesus monkey. *Brain Res., 4,* 151–188.

KUYPERS, H. G. J. M., SZWARCBART, M. K., MISHKIN, M. AND ROSVOLD, H. E. (1965) Occipito-temporal corticocortical connections in the rhesus monkey. *Exp. Neurol., 11,* 245–262.

LEMMEN, L. J., DAVIS, J. S. AND RADNOR, L. L. (1959) Observations on stimulation of the human frontal eye field. *J. comp. Neurol., 112,* 163–168.

LEVIN, P. M. (1936) The efferent fibers of the frontal lobe of the monkey (*Macaca mulatta*). *J. comp. Neurol., 63,* 369–419.

LILLY, J. C. (1958) Correlations between neurophysiological activity in the cortex and short-term behavior in the monkey. In H. F. HARLOW AND C. N. WOOLSEY (Eds.), *Biological and Biochemical Bases of Behavior.* University of Wisconsin Press, Madison, pp. 83–100.

MARTIN, G. F. AND DOM, R. (1970) Rubrobulbar projections of the opossum (Didelphis virginiana). *J. comp. Neurol., 139,* 199–214.

MEHLER, W. R. (1969) Some neurological species differences — a posteriori. *Ann. N. Y. Acad. Sci., 167,* 424–468.

MEHLER, W. R. AND FREDRICKSON, J. M. (1970) Interrelations of the vestibular, auditory and somatosensory cortices in the rhesus monkey. *Anat. Rec., 166,* 408.

METTLER, F. A. (1935) Corticofugal fiber connections of the cortex of *Macaca mulatta.* The occipital region. *J. comp. Neurol., 61,* 221–256.

MONTANELLI, R. P. AND HASSLER, R. (1964) Motor effects elicited by stimulation of the pallido-thalamic system in the cat. In W. BARGMANN AND J. P. SCHADÉ (Eds.), *Progress in Brain Research. Vol. 5. Lectures on the diencephalon.* Elsevier, Amsterdam, pp. 56–66.

MUSKENS, L. J. J. (1922) The central connections of the vestibular nuclei with the corpus striatum and their significance for ocular movements and for locomotion. *Brain, 45,* 454–478.

MYERS, R. E. (1962) Commissural connections between occipital lobes of the monkey. *J. comp. Neurol., 118,* 1–16.

MYERS, R. E. (1963a) Projections of superior colliculus in monkey. *Anat. Rec., 145,* 264.

MYERS, R. E. (1963b) Cortical projections to midbrain in monkey. *Anat. Rec., 145,* 337–338.

MYERS, R. E. (1967) Cerebral connectionism and brain function. In F. L. DARLEY (Ed.), *Brain Mechanisms Underlying Speech and Language.* Grune and Stratton, New York, pp. 61–72.

NASHOLD, B. S. (1971) Ocular reactions from brain stimulation in conscious man. In J. L. SMITH (Ed.), *Neuro-ophthalmology. Vol. 5.* Huffman Publishing Co., Hallandale, Fla., pp. 92–103.

NASHOLD, B. S. AND GILLS, J. P. JR. (1967) Ocular signs from brain stimulation and lesions. *Arch. Ophthal. (Chicago), 77,* 609–618.

NAUTA, W. J. H. (1958) Hippocampal projections and related neural pathways to the midbrain in the cat. *Brain, 81,* 319–340.

NAUTA, W. J. H. AND MEHLER, W. R. (1966) Projections of the lentiform nucleus in the monkey. *Brain Res., 1,* 3–42.

OLSZEWSKI, J. (1952) *The Thalamus of the Macaca mulatta.* S. Karger, Basel, pp. 93.

PANDYA, D. N. AND VIGNOLO, L. A. (1971) Intra- and interhemispheric projections of the precentral premotor, and arcuate areas in the rhesus monkey. *Brain Res., 26,* 217–233.

PASIK, P. AND PASIK, T. (1964) Oculomotor functions in monkeys with lesions of the cerebrum and the superior colliculi. In M. B. BENDER (Ed.), *The Oculomotor System.* Hoeber Medical Division, Harper and Row, New York, pp. 40–80.

PASIK, P., PASIK, T. AND BENDER, M. B. (1960) Oculomotor function following cerebral hemidecortication in the monkey. *Arch. Neurol., 3,* 298–305.

PASIK, P., PASIK, T. AND BENDER, M. B. (1969) The pretectal syndrome in monkeys. I. Disturbances of gaze and body posture. *Brain, 92,* 521–534.

PENFIELD, W. P. AND BOLDREY, E. (1937) Somatic motor and sensory representation in the cerebral cortex of man as studied by electrical stimulation. *Brain*, **60**, 389–443.

PENFIELD, W. AND JASPER, H. (1954) *Epilepsy and the Functional Anatomy of the Human Brain.* Little, Brown and Co., Boston, pp. XV–896.

PETRAS, J. M. (1969) Some efferent connections of the motor and somatosensory cortex of simian primates and felid, canid, and procyonid carnivores. *Ann. N. Y. Acad. Sci.*, **167**, 469–505.

PETRAS, J. M. AND LEHMAN, R. A. W. (1966) Corticospinal fibers in the raccoon. *Brain Res.*, **3**, 195–197.

POLYAK, S. (1932) The main afferent fiber systems of the cerebral cortex in primates. *Univ. Calif. Publ. Anat.*, **2**, 1–370.

POMPEIANO, O. AND WALBERG, F. (1957) Descending connections to the vestibular nuclei. An experimental study in the cat. *J. comp. Neurol.*, **108**, 465–503.

ROBINSON, D. A. (1968) Eye movement control in primates. *Science*, **161**, 1219–1224.

ROBINSON, D. A. AND FUCHS, A. F. (1969) Eye movements evoked by stimulation of frontal eye fields. *J. Neurophysiol.*, **32**, 637–648.

SCHÄFER, E. A. (1888) Experiments on the electrical excitation of the visual area of the cerebral cortex in the monkey. *Brain*, **11**, 1–6.

SCOLLO-LAVIZZARI, G. AND AKERT, K. (1963) Cortical area 8 and its thalamic projection in *Macaca mulatta. J. comp. Neurol.*, **121**, 259–270.

SEGUNDO, J. P., ARANA, R. AND FRENCH, J. D. (1955) Behavioral arousal by stimulation of the brain in monkey. *J. Neurosurg.*, **12**, 601–613.

SMITH, W. K. (1949) The frontal eye fields. In P. C. BUCY (Ed.), *The Precentral Motor Cortex.* Univ. of Illinois Press, Urbana, Ill., pp. 307–352.

SOKOLOV, E. N. (1960) Neuronal models and the orienting reflex. In M. A. B. BRAZIER (Ed.), *The Central Nervous System and Behavior.* Transactions of the IIId Conference, J. M. Macy, Jr. Foundation, New York, and National Science Foundation, Washington, D.C., pp. 187–276.

SPIEGEL, E. A. AND SCALA, N. P. (1937) Ocular disturbances associated with experimental lesions of the mesencephalic central gray matter. *Arch. Ophthal. (Chicago)*, **18**, 614–632.

STARR, A. (1964) A disorder of rapid eye movements in Huntington's Chorea. *Brain*, **90**, 545–564.

SUNDERLAND, S. (1940) The projections of the cerebral cortex on the pons and cerebellum in the Macaque monkey. *J. Anat. (Lond.)*, **74**, 201–226.

TARLOV, C. E. AND MOORE, R. Y. (1966) The tecto-thalamic connections in the brain of the rabbit. *J. comp. Neurol.*, **126**, 403–422.

TEUBER, H.-L. (1970) Subcortical vision: a prologue. *Brain Behav. Evol.*, **3**, 7–15.

VORONIN, L. G. AND SOKOLOV, E. N. (1960) Cortical mechanisms of the orienting reflex and its relation to the conditioned reflex. In H. H. JASPER AND G. D. SMIRNOV (Eds.), *Moscow Colloquium in Electroencephalography of Higher Nervous Activity. EEG clin. Neurophysiol.*, Suppl. 13, 335–346.

WAGMAN, I. H. (1964) Eye movements induced by electric stimulation of cerebrum in monkeys and their relationship to bodily movements. In M. B. BENDER (Ed.), *The Oculomotor System*, Harper and Row, New York, pp. 18–39.

WAGMAN, I. H., KRIEGER, H. P. AND BENDER M. B. (1958) Eye movements elicited by surface and depth stimulation of the occipital lobe of *Macaque mulatta. J. comp. Neurol.*, **109**, 169–194.

WAGMAN, I. H., KRIEGER, H. P., PAPATHEORODOU, C. A. AND BENDER, M. B. (1961) Eye movements elicited by surface and depth stimulation of the frontal lobe of *Macaque mulatta. J. comp. Neurol.*, **117**, 179–188.

WALKER, E. A. AND WEAVER, T. A., JR. (1940) Ocular movements from the occipital lobe in the monkey. *J. Neurophysiol.*, **3**, 353–357.

WESTHEIMER, G. (1971) Saccadic eye movements. In *Eye Movement and Brain Function.* Slovak Academy of Sciences, Bratislava, in press.

WURTZ, R. H. (1968) Visual cortex neurons: response to stimuli during rapid eye movements. *Science*, **162**, 1148–1150.

COMMENTS TO CHAPTER VIII

Some Reflexions on the Relations between the Reticular Formation and the Vestibular Nuclei

A. BRODAL

Anatomical Institute, University of Oslo, Oslo, Norway

From the preceding presentations it is obvious that there are intimate structural and functional relations between the vestibular nuclei and the reticular formation. It is equally clear, however, that we have little precise knowledge about these relations. No doubt, in the years to come much research will be devoted to this subject. It may be worthwhile, therefore, to consider briefly some general features which should be kept in mind in future studies.

Contrary to what was often said in the fifties, the reticular formation (RF) is no diffuse conglomerate of cells. Even if the borders between different subdivisions (nuclei) are not as distinct as in the vestibular nuclei, there can be no doubt that different parts of the RF differ anatomically, architectonically as well as with regard to fiber connections, and therefore, presumably, also functionally. This is especially evident with regard to those parts of the RF which send their fibers to the cerebellum: the lateral reticular nucleus, the nucleus reticularis tegmenti pontis and the paramedian reticular nucleus. They all form rather well delimited cell groups. Concerning the remaining parts of the RF (the 'main' RF) there are clear differences between the medial two thirds and the lateral third. Within the former there are again differences between various levels of the brain stem, for example, with regard to the sources of their afferents. (For some data on these aspects see, for example, Brodal, 1957; Rossi and Zanchetti, 1957; Pompeiano, 1972). Our study of the vestibuloreticular projection (Ladpli and Brodal, 1968) adds another piece of evidence in favour of the above view, since the projections of the various vestibular nuclei onto the RT differ, as I have discussed in my lecture. We hope now to be able to study experimentally the projections from the RF back to the vestibular nuclei. Even if this is technically difficult and final conclusions may not be possible concerning all relevant questions, I have little doubt that the various reticular nuclei will turn out to differ in their projections onto the vestibular nuclei.

The fact that the RF is no diffusely organized mass of cells makes it imperative to indicate precisely the region under consideration in any study of the RF. The sites of lesions, of cell changes or of terminations of fibers must be mapped as accurately as possible, and in physiological studies the sites recorded from or stimulated must be indicated exactly in drawings or maps of the RF. If this is not done, much work devoted to the study of, for example, the behaviour of units and the convergence of impulses on cells in the RF, will certainly have to be done over again in the future.

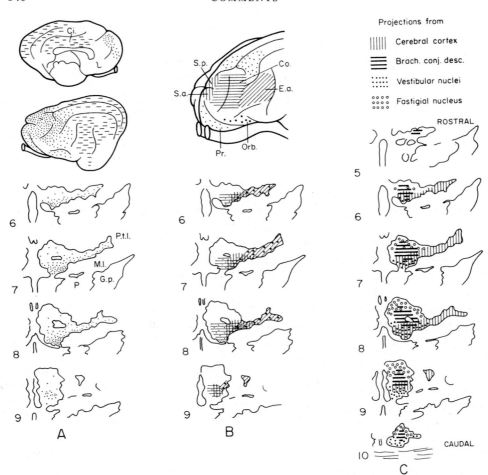

Fig. 1. Projections onto the nucleus reticularis tegmenti pontis (N.r.t.) in the cat as studied experimentally. A shows the cerebral cortical areas (dotted) which send fibers to the N.r.t. and their termination within this. The N.r.t. is shown in transverse sections from rostral to caudal (6–9). G.p.: pontine nuclei; M.l.: medial lemniscus. Note restricted distribution of cortical fibers chiefly to ventral regions of the N.r.t. B shows details in the projection from the cerebral cortex onto the N.r.t. C shows the areas of terminations within the N.r.t. of fibers from different sources (see key for symbols above). Note preferential distribution of different contingents of afferents. Overlapping is more extensive than shown in the diagram. From A. Brodal and P. Brodal (1971).

It is generally agreed that the anatomical organization of the RF is such that it provides possibilities for an extensive integration of impulses from many sources. This, however, does not invalidate the notion of the RF as being composed of a number of units (although not all sharply delimited). For example, the two large cerebellar projecting reticular nuclei, the lateral reticular nucleus and the nucleus reticularis tegmenti pontis, are both supplied by fibres from different, but not identical, sources. For example, they do not receive identical inputs from the vestibular nuclei, as I have discussed in my lecture. Furthermore, in both of them the various afferent contingents supply preferentially certain regions of the nuclei, although with considerable over-lapping. Fig. 1 shows a diagram of the distribution of the main afferents to the nucleus reticularis tegmenti pontis in the cat as inferred from experimental studies in our laboratory. It appears that this nucleus is organized so as to make possible an integra-tion of impulses from the cerebral cortex, the fastigial nucleus, the dentate and inter-positus anterior (via the brachium conjunctivum) and from the superior and lateral vestibular nuclei, before it exerts its action on the cerebellum (vermis as well as hemi-spheres). It seems a likely assumption that integration will be especially marked between impulses entering in fiber contingents which end in the same or adjoining regions of the nucleus (see Fig. 1).

The tegmental reticular pontine nucleus appears to be in the first place an important link in a cerebello-reticular feedback circuit. In addition it is a station in the cerebro-cerebellar and the vestibulocerebellar pathways and certainly deserves attention in physiological studies of the vestibulocerebellar relations. So far it has apparently been entirely neglected in physiological studies of cerebrocerebellar relationships.

In many respects, but not in all, the pontine reticular tegmental nucleus is similar in its organization to the lateral reticular nucleus (see Brodal *et al.*, 1967).

I have mentioned these features in our present knowledge of the two precerebellar reticular nuclei for two reasons. In the first place in order to invite neurophysiologists to study the role of these nuclei in vestibulo-cerebellar relations, in the second place, because there is reason to believe that the other reticular nuclei are organized accord-ing to similar principles. If this is so, it will be essential in future experimental studies to be very accurate as to the geography of sites of lesions, stimulations or recordings, when the role played by the RF for vestibular influences on the spinal cord as well as 'higher levels' of the brain is studied.

REFERENCES

BRODAL, A. (1957) *The Reticular Formation of the Brain Stem. Anatomical Aspects and Functional Correlations*. Oliver and Boyd, Edinburgh, pp. VII–87.
BRODAL, A. AND BRODAL, P. (1971) The organization of the nucleus reticularis tegmenti pontis in the light of experimental anatomical studies of its cerebral cortical afferents. *Exp. Brain Res.*, **13**, 90–110.
BRODAL, P., MARŠALA, J. AND BRODAL, A. (1967) The cerebral cortical projection to the lateral retic-ular nucleus in the cat, with special reference to the sensorimotor cortical areas. *Brain Res.*, **6**, 252–274.
LADPLI, R. AND BRODAL, A. (1968) Experimental studies of commissural and reticular formation projections from the vestibular nuclei in the cat. *Brain Res.*, **8**, 65–96.
POMPEIANO, O. (1972) Reticular formation. In A. IGGO (Ed.), *Handbook of Sensory Physiology*. *Vol. II. Somatosensory System*, Springer, Berlin, in press.
ROSSI, G. F. AND ZANCHETTI, A. (1957) The brain stem reticular formation: Anatomy and physio-logy. *Arch. ital. Biol.*, **95**, 199–435.

Labyrinthine Input to Reticular Neurons

B. W. PETERSON

The Rockefeller University, New York, N.Y., U.S.A.

We have recently been investigating labyrinthine input to neurons of the medial ponto-bulbar reticular formation. Experiments have been performed on cerebellectomized cats under chloralose-urethane anesthesia. We activate the labyrinth and VIII nerve by applying shocks to a pair of electrodes implanted in the scala vestibuli. Shock intensity is adjusted to produce large field potentials in the vestibular nuclei but no input to facial or cochlear nuclei. As illustrated in Fig. 1 such stimulation can produce excitatory and inhibitory postsynaptic potentials (EPSPs and IPSPs) with latencies as short

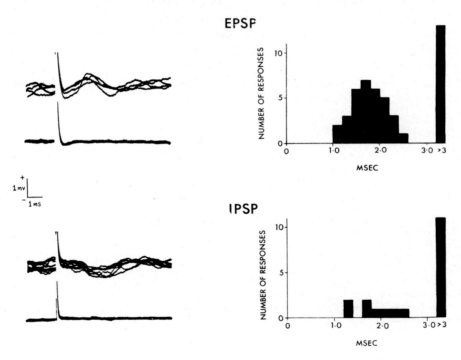

Fig. 1. Synaptic potentials evoked in reticular neurons by stimulation of labyrinth. Pairs of oscilloscope traces at left are examples of the short latency EPSPs and IPSPs recorded intracellularly in reticular neurons following labyrinthine stimulus. Upper trace in each pair contains several superimposed intracellular responses, lower trace shows extracellular potential recorded nearby. Histograms at right show number of EPSPs and IPSPs recorded at various latencies following stimulation of ipsilateral labyrinth.

as 1.0 msec. Since vestibular neurons fire as early as 0.7 msec after labyrinthine stimulation, the early reticular responses are probably disynaptic. Short latency (1.0 to 2.5 msec, see Fig. 1) EPSPs have been observed in 45% of the reticular neurons studied, short latency (1.3–2.5 msec) IPSPs in 12%. Another 21% exhibited EPSPs or IPSPs of longer latency and 22% did not respond.

In experiments in which we identified reticulospinal neurons by stimulating the spinal cord we have observed short latency EPSPs and IPSPs in neurons projecting to both cervico-thoracic and lumbo-sacral levels. With extracellular recording only 8% of these cells fired at latencies ranging from 1.8 to 3.0 msec while another 27% fired at longer latencies. By contrast we have found that 90% of reticulospinal neurons fire in response to stimulation of cerebral cortex, 72% in response to stimulation of optic tectum and 48% in response to cutaneous stimulation. Thus, although reticulospinal neurons receive both short and long latency labyrinthine input, this input is less likely to evoke firing than are inputs from other sources.

Vestibular Influences on the Lateral Geniculate Nucleus

O. POMPEIANO

Institute of Physiology II, University of Pisa, Pisa, Italy

The demonstration that vestibular and visual impulses converge on the cat's visual cortex is well established. The possibility, however, that some integration of vestibular and visual impulses occurs at the level of the lateral geniculate nucleus (LGN) should also be considered. The demonstration that vestibular volleys impinge upon the LGN has been given in unrestrained, unanaesthetized cats during the rapid eye movements (REM) phase of desynchronized sleep (Pompeiano and Morrison, 1966; Morrison and Pompeiano 1966; *cf.* also Ghelarducci and Pompeiano, 1971). In these experiments the integrated activity of the all-or-none events in the LGN has been recorded during desynchronized sleep, before and after bilateral electrolytic lesion of the medial and descending vestibular nuclei.

Two kinds of geniculate activity have been differentiated with this technique (Fig. 4 in Pompeiano, 1972). The first type of activity is represented by short-lasting rhythmic enhancements, referred to as type-I LGN waves, which may be related only with single ocular jerks. The second type of geniculate activity is characterized by phasic increases, 1.5 to 2.0 times larger in amplitude and 2 to 6 times longer in duration than those described above. Only these waves, designated as type-II LGN waves, are strictly related in time with the large bursts of REM.

Following a bilateral lesion of the vestibular nuclei the type II lateral geniculate waves disappear and the related bursts of REM are abolished. However, the rhythmic type-I activity, which is apparently unrelated with the large bursts of REM, persists throughout the episodes of desynchronized sleep.

The results of these experiments suggest that two extraretinal inputs influence the LGN during desynchronized sleep: (*i*) a vestibular input, originating from the medial vestibular nuclei, which impinges upon the LGN at the time of the large bursts of REM, and (*ii*) an extravestibular input, which affects rhythmically the geniculate activity throughout the episode of desynchronized sleep. Stimulation (Bizzi and Brooks, 1963) and lesion experiments (Hobson, 1965) indicate that this endogenous influence on the LGN originates from the pontine reticular formation.

It has been assumed for years that the vestibular nuclei represent a premotor center which control the oculomotor activity. The experiments performed during REM sleep clearly indicate that efferent discharges originating from the vestibular nuclei impinge upon the LGN simultaneously with the efferent discharges which give rise to contraction of the extrinsic eye muscles. Since a striking relation exists between rapid eye movements and dream activity in man (Dement, 1964) we have postulated that the medial vestibular nuclei represent the source for the "internal sensory input" which may explain the occurrence of the visual imagery during dreams (Pompeiano, 1970). As a further development of these observations one may also postulate that vestibular impulses reach the LGN not only during REM sleep, but also during natural labyrinthine stimulation in the awake animal. It is well known that impulses originating selectively from the maculae and the cristae lead to static and dynamic oculomotor responses. The interaction of vestibular and visual signals in the LGN may account for the perceptual constancy of the environment during these reflex-induced ocular movements. Systematic experiments, however, are required to verify this hypothesis. Experiments so far performed in acute preparations have clearly shown that electrical stimulation of the vestibular nuclei enhances the excitability of the intra-geniculate optic tract endings (Marchiafava and Pompeiano, 1966) and modulates the discharge of lateral geniculate neurons (Papaioannou, 1969, 1972a, b; Jeannerod and Putkonen, 1971).

REFERENCES

BIZZI, E. AND BROOKS, D. C. (1963) Functional connections between pontine reticular formation and lateral geniculate nucleus during deep sleep. *Arch. ital. Biol.*, **101**, 666–680.

DEMENT, W. C. (1964) Eye movements during sleep. In M. B. BENDER (Ed.), *The Oculomotor System*, Hoeber Medical Division, Harper and Row, New York, pp. 366–416.

GHELARDUCCI, B. AND POMPEIANO, O. (1971) Oscillatory potentials in the lateral geniculate nucleus during sleep and wakefulness. *Arch. ital. Biol.*. **109**, 37–58.

HOBSON, J. A. (1965) The effects of chronic brain-stem lesions on cortical and muscular activity during sleep and waking in the cat. *EEG clin. Neurophysiol.*, **19**, 41–62.

JEANNEROD, M. AND PUTKONEN, P. T. S. (1971) Lateral geniculate unit activity and eye movements: saccade-locked changes in dark and in light. *Exp. Brain Res.*, **13**, 533–546.

MARCHIAFAVA, P. L. AND POMPEIANO, O. (1966) Enhanced excitability of intra-geniculate optic tract endings produced by vestibular volleys. *Arch. ital. Biol.*, **104**, 459–479.

MORRISON, A. R. AND POMPEIANO, O. (1966) Vestibular influences during sleep. IV. Functional relations between vestibular nuclei and lateral geniculate nucleus during desynchronized sleep. *Arch. ital. Biol.*, **104**, 425–458.

PAPAIOANNOU, J., (1969) Vestibular influences on the spontaneous activity of neurones in the lateral geniculate nucleus of the cat. *J. Physiol. (Lond.)*, **202**, 87P.

PAPAIOANNOU, J. (1972a) Electrical stimulation of vestibular nuclei: effects on spontaneous activity of lateral geniculate nucleus neurones. *Arch. ital. Biol.*, **110**, 217–233.

PAPAIOANNOU, J. (1972b) Electrical stimulation of vestibular nuclei: effects on light-evoked activity of lateral geniculate nucleus neurones. *Pflügers Arch. ges. Physiol.*, **334**, 129–140.

POMPEIANO, O. (1970) Mechanisms of sensorimotor integration during sleep. In E. STELLAR AND J. M. SPRAGUE (Eds.), *Progress in Physiological Psychology*. Academic Press, New York, London, **3**, 1–179.

POMPEIANO, O. (1971) Vestibular influences on the visual system during the rapid eye movements of sleep. In *Visual Information Processing and Control of Motor Activity*, Proc. int. Symp., Bulgarian Academy of Sciences, Sofia, pp. 67–77.

POMPEIANO, O. (1972) Reticular control of the vestibular nuclei: physiology and pharmacology. In A. BRODAL AND O. POMPEIANO (Eds.), *Progress in Brain Research. Vol. 37. Basic aspects of central vestibular mechanisms*. Elsevier, Amsterdam, pp. 601–618.

POMPEIANO, O. AND MORRISON, A. R. (1966) Vestibular input to the lateral geniculate nucleus during desynchronized sleep. *Pflügers Arch. ges. Physiol.*, **290**, 272–274.

Author Index

Subject Index

Where a subject is treated on more than one page, an italicized page number indicates the place where it is most completely described. n. indicates reference to a footnote.